INTERVENTIONAL
MRI

INTERVENTIONAL MRI

Robert B. Lufkin, M.D.

Professor of Radiological Sciences
University of California, Los Angeles, School of Medicine
Chief of Head and Neck Radiology
UCLA Medical Center
Los Angeles, California

With 548 illustrations
including 21 color plates

Mosby

St. Louis Baltimore Boston Carlsbad
Chicago Minneapolis New York Philadelphia Portland
London Milan Sydney Tokyo Toronto

Mosby
Dedicated to Publishing Excellence

A Times Mirror Company

Editor: Elizabeth Corra
Associate Development Editor: Catherine Gray
Project Manager: David Orzechowski
Production Editor: Susie Coladonato
Designer: Carolyn O'Brien
Cover Designer: Carolyn O'Brien/Maria Bellano
Manager of Manufacturing and Production-Philadelphia: William A. Winneberger, Jr.
Publisher: Geoff Greenwood

Composition by Graphic World Inc.
Lithography by Trinity Graphics
Printing/binding by Maple Vail, York

Mosby, Inc.
11830 Westline Industrial Drive
St. Louis, Missouri 63146

Library of Congress Cataloging in Publication Data

Interventional MRI / [edited by] Robert B. Lufkin. — 1st ed.
p. cm.
Includes bibliographical references and index.
ISBN 0-8151-4545-4
1. Interventional magnetic resonance imaging. I. Lufkin, Robert B.
[DNLM: 1. Magnetic Resonance Imaging. 2. Radiography, Intervention—methods. WN 185I614 1999]
RD33.56.I59 1999
616.07'548—dc21
DNLM/DLC
for Library of Congress 98-39428
CIP

99 00 01 02 03 /9 8 7 6 5 4 3 2 1

CONTRIBUTORS

Elliot Abemayor, M.D., Ph.D.
Professor and Vice Chief
Division of Head and Neck Surgery
UCLA School of Medicine
Los Angeles, California

Eben Alexander, III, M.D.
Associate Professor of Neurosurgery
Harvard Medical School
Neurosurgeon
Brigham & Women's Hospital
Children's Hospital
Dana Farber Cancer Institute
Boston, Massachusetts

Chris J. G. Bakker, Ph.D.
University Hospital Utrecht
Utrecht, The Netherlands

Keith L. Black, M.D.
Professor and Chairman
Department of Neurosurgery
UCI Medical Center
Orange, California
Director
Cedars-Sinai Neurosurgical Institute
Cedars-Sinai Medical Center
Los Angeles, California

Peter M. Black, M.D., Ph.D.
Franc D. Ingraham Professor of Neurosurgery
Harvard Medical School
Neurosurgeon in Chief
Brigham & Women's Hospital
Chairman, Department of Surgery
Children's Hospital
Chief of Neurosurgical Oncology
Dana Farber Cancer Institute
Boston, Massachusetts

Travis L. Boaz, M.D.
University Hospitals of Cleveland
Case Western Reserve
Cleveland, Ohio

Alexandra R. Borges, M.D.
Clinical Instructor
Head and Neck Radiology
UCLA Medical Center
Los Angeles, California
Radiologist
Cancer Institute of Lisbon
Lisbon, Portugal

Stephen G. Bown, M.D.
Professor of Laser Medicine and Surgery
Director of National Medical Laser Centre
University College London Medical School
Consultant Physician
University College London Hospitals
London, United Kingdom

Angela M. Browne, M.D.
Resident in Anesthesiology
Department of Anesthesiology
Heidelberg University Hospital
Heidelberg, Germany

Martin Busch, M.D.
Managing Director
Systems and Instruments for Magnetic Resonance
Tomography Mediport Simag GmbH
Berlin, Germany

Alfonso F. Cardenas, B.S., M.S., Ph.D.
Professor
Department of Computer Science
UCLA
Los Angeles, California

Dan J. Castro, M.D.
Associate Professor
UCLA
Otolaryngologist
UCLA School of Medicine
Los Angeles, California

Simon Cherry, Ph.D.
Associate Professor
Department of Molecular and Medical Pharmacology
UCLA School of Medicine
Los Angeles, California

Yiu Cho Chung, M.Phil.
Research Assistant
Department of Biomedical Engineering
Case Western Reserve University
University Hospitals of Cleveland
Cleveland, Ohio

John G. Curran, M.D.
Assistant Professor, Radiological Sciences
UCLA School of Medicine
Pediatric Neuroradiologist
UCLA Medical Center
Los Angeles, California

Jevan Damadian, B.S.E.E.
Electrical Engineer
FONAR Corporation
Melville, New York

Raymond V. Damadian, M.D.
President and CEO
FONAR Corporation
Melville, New York

Gordon Danby, Ph.D.
Consultant
FONAR Corporation
Melville, New York

Jörg F. Debatin, M.D.
Associate Professor of Radiology
University Hospital Zürich
Zürich, Switzerland

Martin Deli, M.S.
EFMT
Institute for Microtherapy
Bochum, Germany

Antonio A. F. DeSalles, M.D., Ph.D.
Associate Professor
UCLA School of Medicine
Head, Stereotactic Surgery Section
Division of Neurosurgery
Los Angeles, California

Jeffrey L. Duerk, Ph.D.
Associate Professor
Department of Radiology and Biomedical Engineering
University Hospitals of Cleveland
Director, Physics Research, University Hospitals, Radiology
Case Western Reserve University
Radiology and Biomedical Engineering
Cleveland, Ohio

Charles L. Dumoulin, Ph.D.
Associate Professor of Radiology
Albany Medical College
Albany, New York
Research Scientist
General Electric Research and Development Center
Schenectady, New York

Jay Dworkin, Ph.D.
Product Marketing Manager
FONAR Corporation
Melville, New York

Keyvan Farahani, Ph.D.
Assistant Professor
Department of Radiological Sciences
UCLA School of Medicine
Los Angeles, California

Christian Frahm, M.D.
Medical University of Lübeck
Department of Radiology
Lübeck, Germany

Hans-Björn Gehl, M.D.
Medical University of Lübeck
Department of Radiology
Lübeck, Germany

John C. Gilbert, Ph.D.
Assistant Professor
Department of Radiology, UCSF
San Francisco, California

Susanne Charlotte Göhde, M.D.
Department of Medical Radiology
University Hospital
Zürich, Switzerland

Jonathan G. Goldin, M.D., Ph.D.
Assistant Professor of Radiology, Thoracic Imaging
UCLA Medical Center
Los Angeles, California

Dietrich Grönemeyer, M.D.
Professor and Chairman
University of Witten/Herdecke
Department of Radiology and Microtherapy
EFMT - Bochum
Bochum, Germany

Margaret A. Hall-Craggs, M.D.
Consultant Radiologist
The Middlesex Hospital
University College London Hospitals Trust
London, United Kingdom

Nobuhiko Hata, Ph.D.
Research Fellow
Harvard Medical School
Brigham & Women's Hospital
Boston, Massachusetts

Andreas Heuck, M.D.
Assistant Professor
Department of Diagnostic Radiology
Klinikum Großhadern
Ludwig-Maximilians-Universität
Munich, Germany

Paul R. Hilfiker, M.D.
MR Center
Research Fellow
Department of Medical Radiology
University Hospital Zürich
Zürich, Switzerland

Gregory C. Hurst, Ph.D.
Chief of Imaging Science
Field Effects
Division of Intermagnetics General Corporation
Tyngsboro, Massachusetts

Stephen G. Hushek, Ph.D.
General Electric Medical Systems
Milwaukee, Wisconsin

Kullervo Hynynen, Ph.D.
Associate Professor
Harvard Medical School
Director of Therapeutic Ultrasound Research
Brigham & Women's Hospital
Boston, Massachusetts

Ferenc A. Jolesz, M.D.
Professor of Radiology
Harvard Medical School
Director, Division of MRI and Image Guided Therapy
Brigham & Women's Hospital
Boston, Massachusetts

Thomas Kahn, M.D.
Professor of Radiology
Heinrich-Heine-Universität
Institute of Diagnostic Radiology
Düsseldorf, Germany

Joachim Kettenbach, M.D.
Instructor, Department of Radiology
University of Vienna
General Hospital of Vienna
Department of Radiology
Vienna, Austria

Ron Kikinis, M.D.
Associate Professor of Radiology
Harvard Medical School
Director, Surgical Planning Laboratory
Brigham & Women's Hospital
Boston, Massachusetts

Karl Kipfmüller, M.D.
Assistant Professor
University Witten/Herdecke
Head, Department of Surgery
St. Marien Hospital
Mülheim, Germany

Michael Knauth, M.D.
Department of Neuroradiology
University of Heidelberg
Oberarzt
University Clinic Heidelberg
Heidelberg, Germany

John Kurhanewicz, Ph.D.
Asssistant Professor of Radiology
Pharmaceutical Chemistry and Bioengineering
University of California, San Francisco
San Francisco, California

Lee Min Lai, F.R.C.S.
Research Fellow
University College, London
National Medical Laser Centre
University College London Hospitals Trust
London, United Kingdom

Gerald W. Lenz, Ph.D.
Medical Engineering
MR Applications
Siemens AG
Erlangen, Germany

Jonathan S. Lewin, M.D.
Associate Professor
Vice Chairman for Research and Academics, Radiology
Case Western Reserve University School of Medicine
Director, Magnetic Resonance Imaging
University Hospitals of Cleveland
Cleveland, Ohio

John Linardos, M.S.E.E.
Director of Digital Engineering
FONAR Corporation
Melville, New York

David S. K. Lu, M.D.
Associate Professor of Radiology
UCLA
Director, Abdominal Interventional Radiology
UCLA Medical Center
Los Angeles, California

Robert B. Lufkin, M.D.
Professor of Radiological Sciences
UCLA School of Medicine
Chief of Head and Neck Radiology
UCLA Medical Center
Los Angeles, California

Martin G. Mack, M.D.
Humboldt - Universität Berlin
Campus Virchow - Klinikum
Department of Radiology
Berlin, Germany

Alastair J. Martin, Ph.D.
Assistant Professor
University of Minnesota
Department of Radiology
Clinical Scientist
Philips Medical Systems
Minneapolis, Minnesota

Eike Martin, M.D.
Chairman, Department of Anesthesiology
Medical Director
University Hospitals Heidelberg
Heidelberg, Germany

Andreas Melzer, M.D., D.D.S.
Director of Research and Development and Interventional MRI
University Witten/Herdecke
Institute for Diagnostic and Interventional Radiology
Mülheim/Ruhr, Germany

Thomas M. Moriarty, M.D., Ph.D.
Assistant Professor of Neurological Surgery
University of Louisville
Louisville, Kentucky

Ullrich G. Müeller-Lisse, M.D., B.A.
Department of Diagnostic Radiology
Klinikum Großhadern
Ludwig-Maximilians-Universität
Munich, Germany

Jörg M. Neuerburg, M.D.
Assistant Professor of Diagnostic Radiology
Department of Diagnostic Radiology
University of Aachen
Aachen, Germany

Thomas Oshiro, M.S.
UCLA Department of Radiological Sciences
Los Angeles, California

Martyn Paley, Ph.D.
Senior Lecturer in M.R. Physics
University of Sheffield
Royal Hallamshire Hospital
Sheffield, United Kingdom

Jürgen Plaßmann, M.D.
University of Witten/Herdecke
Institute of Diagnostic and Interventional Radiology
Medical Computer Science
Mülheim, Germany

Heinrich Polarz, M.D.
Staff in Anesthesiology
Department of Anesthesiology
Heidelberg University Hospital
Heidelberg, Germany

Gregory J. Rubino, M.D.
Assistant Professor
Director, UCLA Brain Metastatic Tumor Program
UCLA Medical Center
Los Angeles, California

Armin Schmidt, M.D.
University of Witten/Herdecke
Institute of Diagnostic and Interventional Radiology
Mülheim, Germany

Mitchell D. Schnall, M.D., Ph.D.
Associate Professor of Radiology
University of Pennsylvania
Chief of MRI
University of Pennsylvania Health System
Philadelphia, Pennsylvania

Peter Schneede, M.D.
Department of Urology
Klinikum Großhadern
Ludwig-Maximilians-Universität
Munich, Germany

Martin Scholz, M.D.
Neurosurgeon
Department of Neurosurgery
Ruhr-University Bochum
Bochum, Germany

Richard Schwartz, M.D., Ph.D.
Associate Professor of Radiology
Harvard Medical School
Assistant Director of Neuroradiology
Brigham & Women's Hospital
Boston, Massachusetts

Hans-Joachim Schwarzmaier, M.D.
Heinrich-Heine University
Department of Laser Medicine
Düsseldorf, Germany

Cornelia Sehnert, M.D.
University of Witten/Herdecke
Institute of Diagnostic and Interventional Radiology
Mülheim, Germany

Rainer M. M. Seibel, M.D.
Professor
University of Witten/Herdecke
Institute of Diagnostic and Interventional Radiology
Mülheim, Germany

Joel Sercarz, M.D.
Assistant Professor
UCLA School of Medicine
Los Angeles, California
Attending Surgeon
Harbor-UCLA Medical Center
Torrance, California

Yiping Shao, Ph.D.
Assistant Researcher
Crump Institute
UCLA School of Medicine
Los Angeles, California

Frank G. Shellock, Ph.D.
Clinical Professor of Radiology
University of Southern California School of Medicine
Los Angeles, California

Stuart G. Silverman, M.D.
Associate Professor
Harvard Medical School
Director of Abdominal Imaging
Brigham & Women's Hospital
Boston, Massachusetts

Shantanu Sinha, Ph.D.
Associate Professor
Department of Radiological Sciences
UCLA School of Medicine
Los Angeles, California

Usha Sinha, Ph.D.
Assistant Professor
Department of Radiological Sciences
UCLA School of Medicine
Los Angeles, California

Randal B. Slates, B.S.
Graduate Student Researcher
Crump Institute for Biological Imaging
UCLA
Los Angeles, California

Henk F. M. Smits, M.D.
University Hospital Utrecht
Utrecht, The Netherlands

Andreas Staubert, Dipl. Phys.
Physicist
University of Heidelberg
Neurosurgical Department, Kopfklinik
Heidelberg, Germany

Philip E. Stieg, Ph.D., M.D.
Associate Professor
Harvard Medical School
Associate Chief of Neurosurgery
Brigham & Women's Hospital
Boston, Massachusetts

Dieter Stoeckel, Ph.D.
Professor
Nitinol Devices and Components, Inc.
Fremont, California

Masao Sugita, M.D.
Yamanashi Medical University
Department of Neurosurgery
Tamaho-machi, Yamanashi, Japan

Ricky K. Taira, Ph.D.
Associate Professor
University of Washington
Medical Physicist
Children's Hospital and Regional Medical Center
Seattle, Washington

Wolfram Triebe, M.D.
University Witten/Herdecke, MRI
Mülheim/Ruhr, Germany

Volker M. Tronnier, M.D., Ph.D.
Associate Professor
Heidelberg College of Medicine
Department of Neurological Surgery
University Hospital Heidelberg
Heidelberg, Germany

Frank Ulrich, M.D.
Neurosurgeon
Heinrich Heine University of Düsseldorf
Director, Department of Neurosurgery
Klinikum Krefeld
Krefeld, Germany

Joop J. van Vaals, Ph.D.
Senior Clinical Scientist
Philips Medical Systems
Clinical Science MR
Best, The Netherlands

J. Pablo Villablanca, M.D.
Assistant Professor
UCLA Medical Center
Division of Neuroradiology
Los Angeles, California

Thomas J. Vogl, M.D.
Professor of Radiology
Charitè-Berlin
Virchow-Klinikum
Humboldt-University of Berlin
Strahlenklinik und Poliklinik
Berlin, Germany

Gustav K. von Schulthess, M.D., Ph.D.
Professor of Nuclear Medicine
University of Zürich
Director, Division of Nuclear Medicine
University Hospital
Zürich, Switzerland

Christian R. Wirtz, M.D.
University of Heidelberg
Department of Neurosurgery, Kopfklinik
Heidelberg, Germany

Eric J. Woodard, M.D.
Instructor in Surgery
Harvard Medical School
Associate Surgeon
Brigham & Women's Hospital
Children's Hospital
Boston, Massachusetts

Ian R. Young, Ph.D.
Professor
Imperial College School of Medicine
Hammersmith Hospital
London, United Kingdom

Zong-Ping Zhao, Ph.D.
(Formerly) Manager of Magnet Engineering
Magna-Lab, Inc.
Hicksville, New York

To my family

PREFACE

The concept of using magnetic resonance (MR) imaging to guide biopsy or aspiration cytology was first reported in the mid 1980s. Today there are applications in the breast, brain, mediastinum, abdomen, musculoskeletal system, head and neck, and other areas. As interesting as the notion of MR-guided biopsy is, in many ways it is really only the first step in the field of interventional MRI, which now includes many other MR-guided interventions. In fact, if it were not for more advanced techniques like MR-guided therapy, the phrase *interventional MRI* would still be an oxymoron and MR-guided biopsy would be just one more derivative form of image-guided biopsy including fluoroscopic-, ultrasound-, and computed tomography-guided techniques.

MR has been described as the most powerful stereotactic soft-tissue imaging technique ever conceived and realized by humankind. To employ this technology for diagnosis only is shortsighted. Many experts believe that the unparalleled soft-tissue imaging capabilities of MRI also make it the most powerful imaging technique available to guide interventional procedures of an interstitial nature. *Interstitial* is meant to imply a direct percutaneous soft-tissue route and not necessarily endovascular or endoluminal routes, although MRI may play an increasing role there.

The use of MR to guide therapeutic procedures has been largely limited to small series in research centers and is only now beginning to receive mainstream clinical validation. For example, there is growing experience with MR-guided procedures in the spine, including discectomy and combined MR-endoscopic approaches. Benign breast disease is treated with MR-guided focused ultrasound, and the use of MR-guided laser ablation in the management of breast cancer is under investigation. Head and neck cancer management with MR-guided laser ablation is being studied. MR monitoring of liver and prostate therapy and endoluminal coil therapeutic approaches are being investigated by other groups. The treatment of primary and metastatic brain tumors using MR-guided radiofrequency and laser ablation is under study.

Despite the modest clinical accomplishments of the field and a lukewarm MR marketplace, there has recently been an unprecedented emphasis on technology developments from MR manufacturers. In the early 1990s, as healthcare reform and managed care became more significant issues in the United States, development in many areas of diagnostic MR as well as sales in this area slowed dramatically. An interesting thing happened in this stalled environment. New MR scanners were introduced from almost every major MR manufacturer. Although only two or three were referred to as *interventional*, they all had the common features of a more open design with improved patient access. Along with the main magnet design an industry of support workstations, monitors, trackers, needles, and other hardware and software has developed for MR-guided procedures.

One reason for this vendor reaction is economic (or maybe the reason for vendor reaction is always economic). Even in the current United States environment that results in an increasingly flat economy for diagnostic MR scanners, there is a strong growth potential for interventional MRI. In the case of diagnostic MR examinations, even the most exciting new wrinkle (e.g., kinematic dynamic fat-suppressed, diffusion-weighted magnetization transfer MR of the larynx) is in most cases still reimbursed at the overall rate for diagnostic MRI of the larynx. That is, it is a zero sum game for each diagnostic evaluation—the goal is to try to maintain quality with less money. This same concept also holds for newer, non-fee-for-service reimbursement schemes.

Using interventional MR as a therapeutic technique rather than a purely diagnostic technique, creates new fee schedules for new procedures (in many cases heretofore untapped by MR service providers). Often these fees are based on in-patient procedures with high rates for cost-shifted (i.e., inflated) hospital-based charges for operating rooms and other services that make lower-priced imaging-guided outpatient procedures particularly appealing. If the potential for interventional MR in this therapeutic arena can be realized, tremendous growth potential obviously exists.

What is needed for this growth to occur? Progress, such as that described in this text, and the various versions of "open" designed magnets that are being promoted by every major MR manufacturer help to make routine clinical interventional MRI a reality. Unfortunately high technology and instrumentation alone are no longer sufficient to drive development. Unlike the 1980s and 1990s when such descriptors as "high technology," "interesting concept," "great potential," and "fantastic research tool" were sufficient to drive clinical interest and sales, in the late 1990s and onward, this is no longer true. In fact, "high technology" has been branded as fiscally evil by many architects of the new healthcare system. These same critics may soon be forced to admit that the use of MR to guide therapeutic procedures that replace more costly invasive procedures may actually be a powerful means to lower the cost of medical care. Some experts speculate that interventional MRI could become the most cost-saving clinical application of MR ever developed.

As has been the case with other new techniques for lower-cost, minimally invasive therapy, the usual caveat exists. Although these new procedures should lower the cost of medical care overall given current rates, there is always the possibility of actually increasing overall costs because of increased use of the minimally invasive technique. This has been described in some studies of percutaneous cholecystectomy and other minimally invasive techniques. The issues involved in analyzing this situation are broad and complex.

"High technology" and powerful instrumentation alone are not sufficient to drive the field of interventional MRI forward. What is now necessary is development and clinical validation of

MR-guided procedures. We must move beyond the feasibility stage; questions that are more important must now be addressed in order to place the potential treatment option in a clinical perspective. What is the cost compared to other treatment options? What is the morbidity and outcome of the procedure compared to other treatments? Ideally these and other questions will soon be addressed in appropriate prospective randomized clinical studies.

Turf issues are a frequent concern in any discussion of interventional MRI. Each procedure will demand different technical expertise. In our laboratory, some procedures are performed entirely by radiologists and others are performed with joint staffing by radiology and surgery. With more experience this model will surely evolve and may someday resemble the neuroendovascular therapy teams that are so effective today.

For now, we put turf issues aside as much as possible in our center. Although it is difficult to overcome the barriers that are put up by God, Mother Nature, and the laws of physics, the barriers that we create for ourselves can be even more problematic.

Much of the basic instrumentation development and basic science animal studies are complete. The specification of clearcut clinical indications and large clinical trials to define the ultimate value of the techniques are essential now. As we look past the millennium it is possible to imagine interventional MR systems for novel, minimally invasive treatment approaches in what may become a major therapy paradigm for the twenty-first century.

Interventional MRI is in an exciting phase of development as evidenced by the brilliant work summarized in the following chapters by the world's experts in the field. The value of MR-guided procedures has been confirmed with human clinical studies, but the ultimate future of MR-guided therapy remains to be defined. With the new open design interventional MR scanners, supporting hardware, and even brighter new investigators in the field, this work will be rapidly forthcoming.

Robert B. Lufkin, M.D.
Los Angeles, 1998

CHAPTERS

I INSTRUMENTATION

II INTERVENTIONAL MR–GUIDANCE TECHNIQUES

III MR–GUIDED TREATMENT TECHNIQUES

IV CLINICAL APPLICATIONS

Part I

INSTRUMENTATION

Chapter 1

OVERVIEW OF INTERVENTIONAL MRI MAGNETS

Zong-Ping Zhao

Since the discovery of nuclear magnetic resonance (NMR) by Bloch at Stanford and Purcell at Harvard in 1945, for which they received the Nobel prize, its uses have continued to increase. For example, magnetic resonance imaging (MRI) was introduced in the middle 1970s. Today, MRI is an irreplaceable diagnostic tool. As MRI technology matures, there is an increasing demand to use MRI to guide interventional procedures.

The more open-magnet designs used for interventional MRI enable the patient to be accessible for clinical procedures during scanning, may make claustrophobic patients more comfortable, and may allow for new applications (e.g., kinematic musculoskeletal studies). In principle, other than the more open-type magnet geometry used in interventional MRIs, magnet design principles do not differ between traditional MRI and interventional MRI. Open MRI magnets have evolved to include low to high field systems using electromagnets, permanent magnets, superconducting magnets, or a combination of these magnets.

Of primary concern in MRI magnet design are (1) the magnetic field strength, uniformity, and stability, to which MRI resolution and sensitivity are directly related, and (2) the fringe field size, magnet weight, and cost. Interventional MRI magnets have additional concerns: increasing openness and patient accessibility versus maintaining a quality field for imaging.

MAGNETIC FIELD STRENGTH, RESONANCE FREQUENCY, AND MAGNETIC RESONANCE IMAGING RESOLUTION

MRI involves nuclear spins induced at a radiofrequency (RF) given by the Larmor relation $f = \gamma B_0$, where f is the resonance frequency, γ is the nuclear gyromagnetic ratio that characterizes a nuclear species, and B_0 is the magnetic field produced by the magnet.

Hydrogen comprises 80% of all atoms found in humans. The hydrogen nucleus (i.e., the proton) has a gyromagnetic ratio of 42.6 MHz/Tesla (T). If the magnet field is 1 T, the MRI precessional center frequency for protons is 42.6 MHz. Likewise, for a field of 0.5 T, precessional frequency is 21.3 MHz. In terms of resonance frequency, MRI systems are commonlyclassified according to magnetic strength: low field, approximately 0.2 T, midfield, 0.2 to 0.5 T; and high field, greater than 0.5 T.

The principal advantage of a high-field magnet is increased frequency resolution. Within a nuclear species, more than one resonance frequency exists in the spectrum because of the different chemical structures of the molecule in which a particular nucleus is bound. This pattern of resonance frequency displacement, resulting from the magnetic fields generated by the motion of the bonding electrons, is called a *chemical shift*. The number of resonant frequencies correlates with the number of chemically distinct groups in the molecule. As field strength increases, the frequency difference and chemical shift increase, therefore increasing the MRI frequency resolution. These factors are a key advantage in MR spectroscopy, in which the goal is to resolve separate chemical species based on frequency differences. Another major advantage of a high-field magnet is an increased signal-to-noise ratio (SNR) because, at a higher field, increased nuclear magnetization produces stronger MR signals. Thus, fewer averages are required to display the signals. As a result, an MRI obtained at a high field tends to have a shorter examination time than does a similar study at a low field.

Open magnets create more space for the patient's body but sacrifice magnetic energy efficiency when compared with traditional closed magnets. The magnet openings disrupt the natural flow of magnetic flux through the field, which increases the difficulties in homogenizing the field. As the magnetic field strength increases, this problem becomes more prominent, resulting in a larger magnet and therefore excessive weight and costs. It is for this reason that most open MRIs operate at low- and midfield strength, whereas closed MRIs operating at high-field strength are widely available.

FIELD UNIFORMITY, STABILITY, AND FRINGE FIELD

MRI requires a homogenous magnetic field (in combination with the magnetic fields of its gradient coils) to produce accurate spatial location information. Field uniformity is a measure of maximum field variations (in parts per million [ppm]) over a volume of interest at the magnet center. For a 1-T magnet, a 10-ppm 45-cm diameter-spherical-volume uniformity refers to a field variation of 10^{-5} T or a resonance frequency variation of 426 hertz (Hz) over 45-cm diameter-spherical volume. The same uniformity will represent a variation of 5×10^{-4} T or 213 Hz in a 0.5-T MRI magnet.

A highly homogenous magnet is obtained through careful magnet design, construction, and shimming. Adjusting the main magnet field by insertion of ferromagnetic pieces (e.g., soft iron) onto the magnet bore is called *passive shimming*, whereas adjusting the field by the means of shim coils is called *active shimming*. Passive shimming permanently alters the magnetic field and therefore requires no maintenance. Active shimming, however, requires an external power supply with frequent adjustment. In general, open magnets are more difficult to shim because the magnetic field distributions are more complex than those in closed magnets.

The field stability or drift is a measure of maximum field variations over a given time (e.g., an 8-hour working day). Magnet field stability varies according to the type of magnet; the best superconducting magnets are below 1% ppm/hr. Stability is not intrinsically different between open and closed magnets.

Fringe magnetic field is the main field component that extends outside the magnet and its housing. The fringe field is normally evaluated by using a 5-gauss (G) or 50-milliTesla (mT) isomagnetic line. Inside this line, public access should be restricted to avoid inadvertent magnetic field effects on pacemakers and other implanted medical devices (see Chapter 10). The 5-G line, which is about 10 times stronger than the earth's magnetic field, can extend beyond the RF-shielded room depending on the strength of the magnet and magnet shielding. In general, fringe fields correspond with magnet field strength. Open magnets exhibit larger fringe field than closed types for a given field strength.

RESISTIVE ELECTROMAGNETS

Electromagnets are based on the principle that a circular coil creates a uniform magnetic field at the coil center and a spherical coil produces a homogeneous field inside (Fig. 1-1).[1] Separating two sets of coils produces a useful field in between, which may allow an open design. The most common design of open resistive electromagnets is the classic C or H-shape with a frame of soft iron serving as a flux return path and as a structural support. Aluminum strips are normally chosen for winding the coils over copper strips, reducing weight and cost.

A resistive electromagnet can be built to field strength of about 0.3 T for an 18- to 20-inch magnet gap with less than 80-kW electricity. Beyond this measurement, extensive cooling systems become necessary, making the design more challenging. Removing the heat generated by the coils is often accomplished by constantly circulating cooling water.

The main advantages of resistive magnets are (1) they are relatively inexpensive to build in comparison with permanent or superconducting magnets; (2) they are easy to ramp up to the operating field and may be switched off during off-work hours; and (3) they weigh less. The major disadvantages are (1) field instability is caused by the dependence of a continuous electrical power supply and (2) they require cooling facilities. Unlike some permanent magnets, resistive magnets generally are not assembled on-site and thus have large accessibility requirements for installation.

PERMANENT MAGNETS

Permanent magnets are the oldest and most familiar type of magnets but are also the most promising. Open permanent magnets are built in C- or H-shapes with two parallel ferromagnetic poles facing each other. One or more iron posts support the poles while providing the flux return path. Beneath each pole is the housing for an array of permanent magnet bricks oriented in one direction, forming a transverse magnetic field from one pole to the other across the magnet gap.

The principle of permanent MRI magnets lies in the theory that two infinite-sized parallel magnet blocks of same magnetization form a perfect homogeneous field in between. Permanent MRI magnets can also be built based on the concept that an egg-type permanent magnet block with a spherical hollow center has a perfect uniform field inside the hollow center. In practice, applying such principles with a large magnet gap and limited pole size requires delicate designs to shape the field and achieve desirable field intensity (Fig. 1-2).[2] Permanent magnet shimming often involves magnet structural adjustments and passive shimming with iron pieces in permanent magnets. Iron pieces behave differently on ferromagnetic pole surfaces, unlike in superconducting magnets, in which no ferromagnetic material exists.

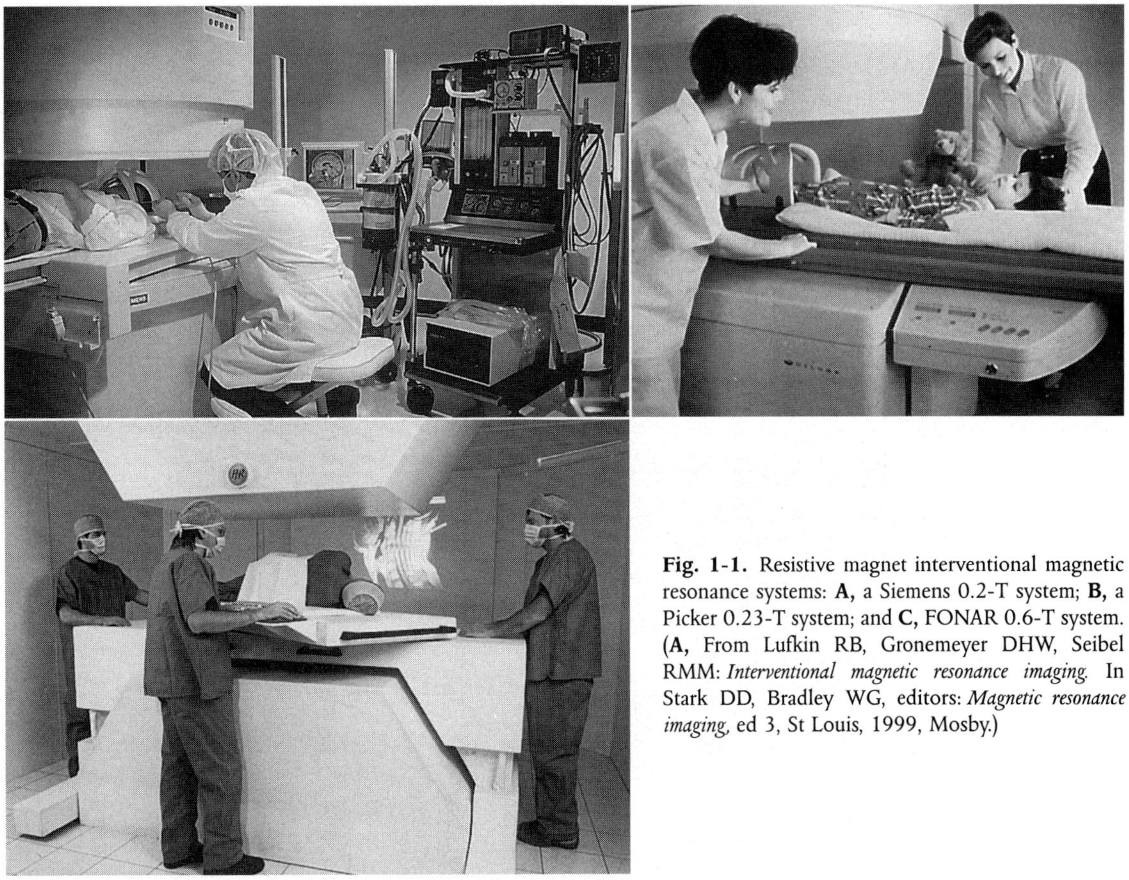

A

B

C

Fig. 1-1. Resistive magnet interventional magnetic resonance systems: **A,** a Siemens 0.2-T system; **B,** a Picker 0.23-T system; and **C,** FONAR 0.6-T system. (**A,** From Lufkin RB, Gronemeyer DHW, Seibel RMM: *Interventional magnetic resonance imaging.* In Stark DD, Bradley WG, editors: *Magnetic resonance imaging,* ed 3, St Louis, 1999, Mosby.)

Open permanent magnets have been built up to 0.35 T for a 16- to 18-inch magnet gap by using ferrite or rare earth magnetic materials. Exceeding 0.35 T is difficult because of weight and costs. Ferrite is very inexpensive compared with rare earthmaterials. The energy product is normally below 5×10^6 G-Oersted, (5 MGOe). The rare earth ceramic material, which is made of neodymium, boron, and iron, is the latest (about 15 years old) and highest energy permanent magnetic material.[3] Although the energy products for neodymium materials have reached 50 MGOe in laboratory studies, most MRI magnets use 35-MGOe materials because of the cost. Because of the material's magnetic field sensitivity to temperature variations (0.1%/° C), an advanced temperature control is often required for better field stability. Commonly, raising the magnet system temperature slightly above room temperature serves this purpose.

Permanent MRI magnets are best known for their insignificant fringe field, minimal maintenance requirement, and minimal electrical power consumption. The 5-G line for a typical 0.3-T open permanent magnet is only a few feet from the magnet isocenter. Small fringe fields eliminate the need for magnet shielding. Unless problems related to temperature stability arise, scan interruption is virtually nonexistent. The primary disadvantages of permanent magnets are the relatively poor field homogeneity (normally 30 to 50 ppm) and large weight (greater than 10 tons). Eddy currents contribute the most to poor homogeneity. Techniques such as slicing the poles and using eddy current–resistive ferromagnetic materials on the pole surfaces have been developed to improve the eddy current characteristics.

SUPERCONDUCTING MAGNETS

A superconducting magnet is a special type of electromagnet in which superconducting wires (rather than common conductors, such as aluminum) are used to wind the coils. A superconductor exhibits no resistance when a certain magnetic flux density (B), electrical current density (J), and temperature (T), the so-called B-J-T surface, are met. Therefore, it has the ability to carry enormous currents to create strong magnetic fields that are unobtainable by other means. Although large-bore superconducting MRI magnets have been built with a field intensity ranging from 0.5 to 8 T, the United States Food and Drug Administration limits routine clinical use up to only 2 T. Most superconducting magnets are in tunnel shapes built with solenoid coils.[4]

Niobium-tin or niobium-titanium superconductors are normally used in MRI magnets (Fig. 1-3). They require cooling in cryostats at a liquid helium temperature of −277° C. Cryogen is very expensive and hence increases the operation cost. Once ramped to a desirable field, the main magnet requires no external electrical supply. Only regular refilling for liquid helium or nitrogen is necessary. Charging or discharging a magnet is not simple because of the possibility of a magnet quench,[5] a process of boiling off cooling liquids and burning the magnet.

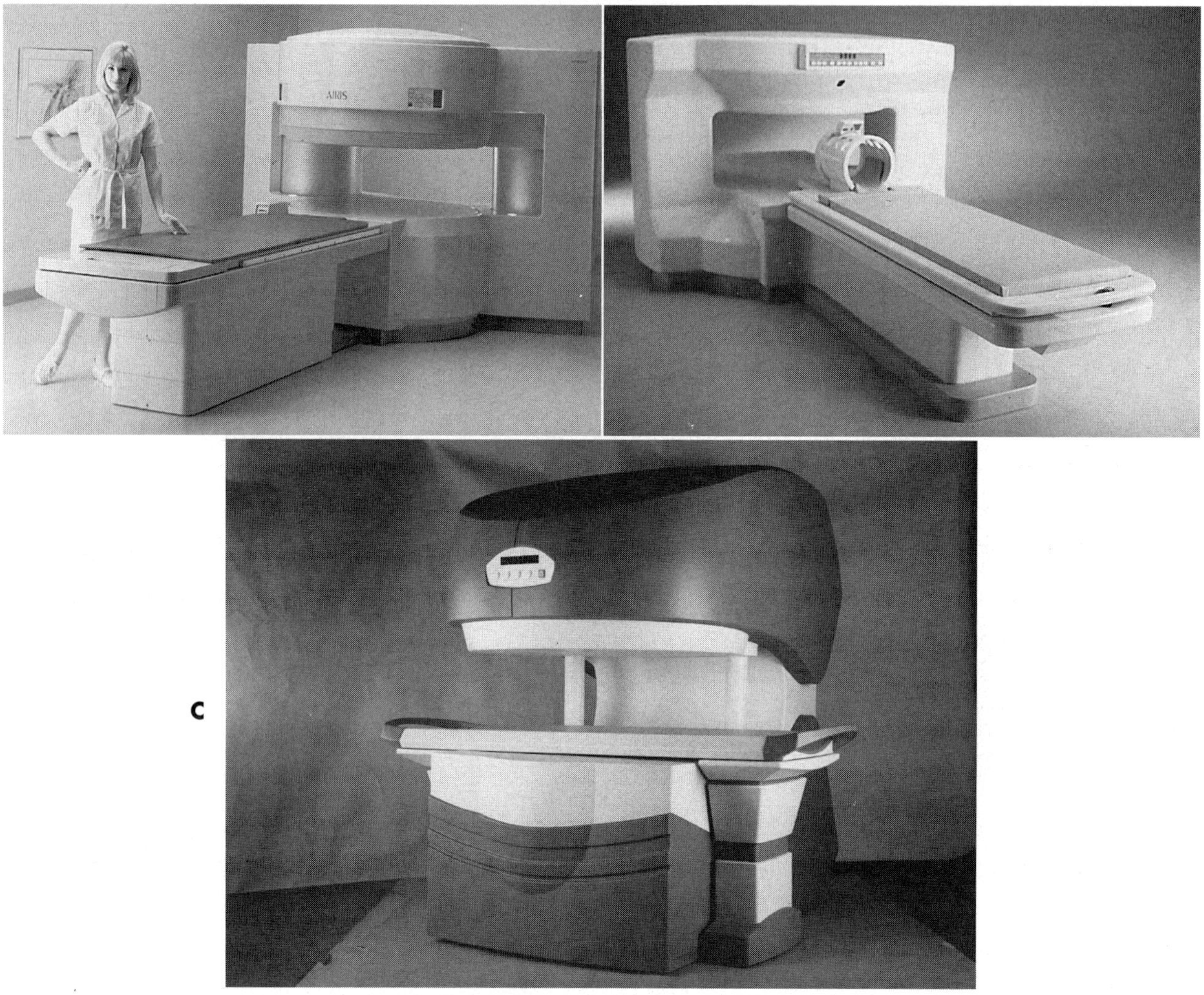

A B C

Fig. 1-2. Permanent magnet interventional magnetic resonance systems: **A,** a Hitachi 0.35-T system. **B,** A General Electric 0.2-T system. **C,** A Score Medical 0.35-T system.

Superconducting magnets can be shimmed to a field uniformity that is unachievable for electromagnets or permanent magnets. Also, they possess the highest field stability and least eddy current effect. Commercial superconducting MRI magnets usually have a field uniformity less than 10 ppm over a 45-cm diameter-spherical-volume and a field stability of 1 ppm/hr or less. High-field magnets inevitably create large fringe fields.

There is a trend toward increased patient access with shorter bore superconducting magnets, which are being used for interventional magnets. Magnet shielding techniques, (e.g., passive shielding with soft iron, active shielding with coils) are applied to counteract the main field, resulting in less magnetic energy efficiency and therefore high cost. The 5-G line for a good active shield superconducting magnet can be 3 to 5 m away from the magnet.

TRENDS IN INTERVENTIONAL MAGNETIC RESONANCE IMAGING MAGNET DEVELOPMENT

The most recent advance in intervention system design is a new system that allows 360° access (OR-360, Fonar Corporation, Melville, NY), which is also discussed in Chapter 4 (see Fig. 1-1). The new electromagnet design operates at 0.6 T. Other electromagnetic systems operating at approximately 0.2 T are available from Siemens and Picker (see Fig. 1-1). Another recent advance in interventional MRI has been the development of a T-split solenoid or double-donut magnet with radial access for physicians and horizontal access for patients.[6] It is a novel combination of permanent magnets and superconducting coils (see Chapter 3). The niobium-tin coils in the magnet are cooled by conduction from a mechanical cooler rather than from the conventional liquid helium in a cryostat (see Fig. 1-2). An open superconducting MRI fabricated at Toshiba,[7] resembles an open permanent magnet and is a cryogen-free 0.35-T system. Siemens built a 1.5-T specialty head imager in which the superconducting magnet is of the traditional solenoid type but is much thinner so it produces a more limited volume. Philips has a short-bore superconducting 1.5-T magnet that may be used for interventional work. All of these systems benefit from the flexibility of an open structure and the image quality of superconducting magnets.

A B C

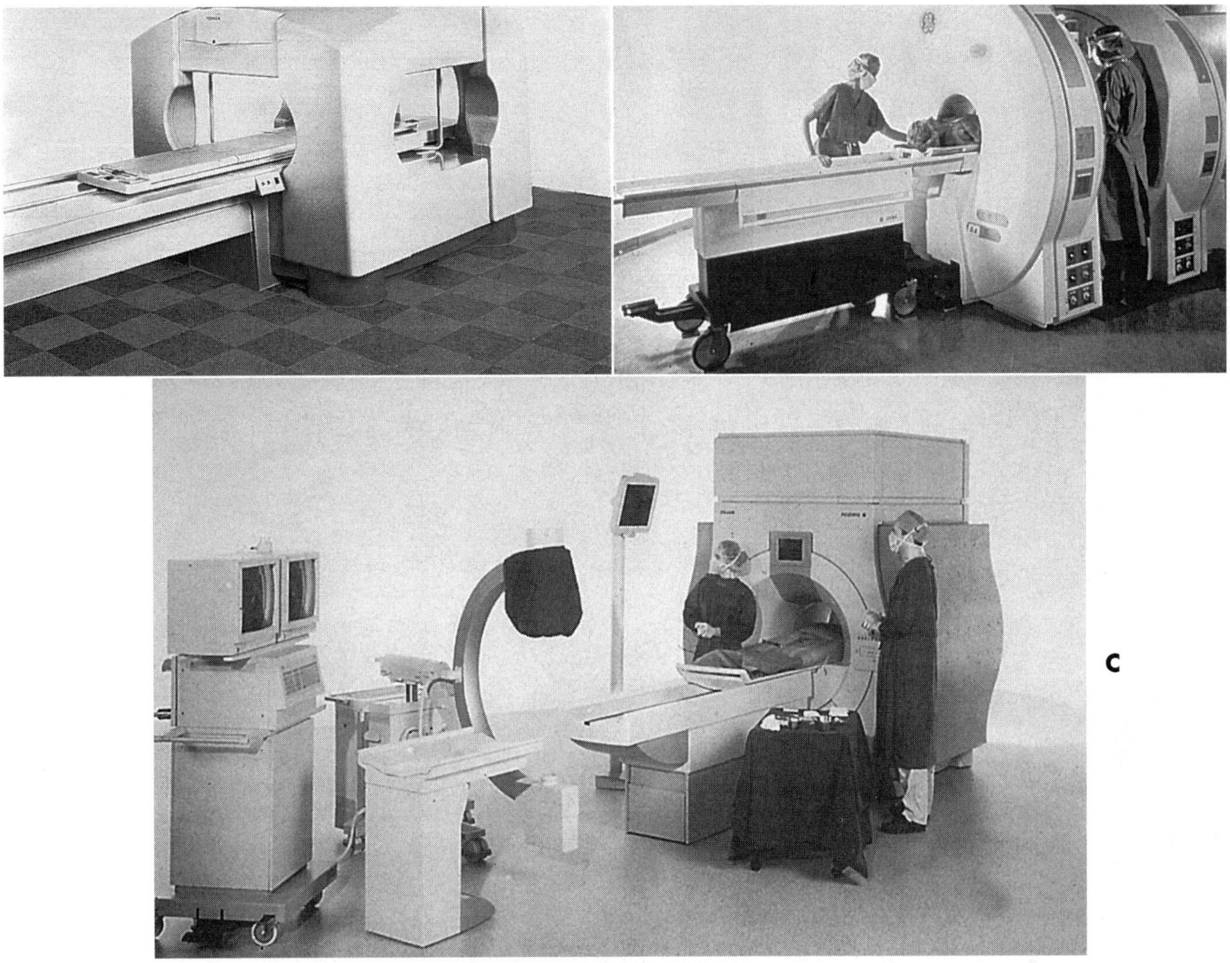

Fig. 1-3. Superconducting magnets for interventional magnetic resonance imaging: **A,** a Toshiba 0.35-T system; **B,** a General Electric 0.5-T system; and **C,** a Philips 1.5-T system. (**B,** From Lufkin RB, Gronemeyer DHW, Seibel RMM: *Interventional magnetic resonance imaging.* In Stark DD, Bradley WG, editors: *Magnetic resonance imaging,* ed 3, St Louis, 1999, Mosby.)

Low-field open designs using permanent magnets have been widely used in MRI. These designs include 0.2- to 0.3-T magnets from Hitachi and General Electric (see Fig. 1-3). These low-field MRI systems are less expensive than high-field systems. Other specialty imagers (e.g., head, shoulder, mammography, spine, extremity, prostate MRIs) can be built with open magnets.

Although most MRI systems use closed superconducting magnets, low- and midfield systems with open resistive and permanent magnets are the fastest growing types. Of the 10,000 or more systems worldwide, it is estimated that more than 10% are low-field systems that have only recently been installed. Future interventional MRIs will require wide magnet gap, high–image quality magnets; fast imaging for efficient use; and low-cost systems in design and operation.

Open resistive electromagnets seem to have an upper limit at which field strength is obtainable without excessive electrical power supply and cooling requirements. Open permanent magnets offer great flexibility in design and structure but are limited by available magnetic materials. New developments in materials (e.g., high-temperature superconductors, high-energy rare earth permanent magnetic materials), will inevitably lead to more MRI applications and will make interventional systems more economically feasible.

REFERENCES

1. Smythe WR: *Static and dynamic electricity,* ed 3, New York, 1989, Hemisphere.
2. Abele MG: *Structures of permanent magnet: generation of uniform fields,* New York, 1993, John Wiley & Sons.
3. Parker RJ: *Advances in permanent magnetism,* New York, 1990, John Wiley & Sons.
4. Wilson MN: *Superconducting magnets,* Oxford, 1983, Oxford Science.
5. Iwasa Y: *Case studies in superconducting magnets: design and operational issues,* New York, 1994, Plenum Press.
6. Dorri B, Laskaris ET: *Open MRI magnet with homogeneous imaging volume,* November 1996, US patent 5,574,417.
7. Breneman BC, Sarwinski RE, Hsu YH: *Open access superconducting MRI magnet,* May 1995, US patent 5,412,363.

Chapter 2

INTERVENTIONAL MAGNET AND SYSTEM DESIGN AT LOW FIELD

Gerald W. Lenz

Interventional magnetic resonance imaging (MRI) is a fairly new discipline, with origins in radiology and in surgery. In the past decade, the dramatic change in the healthcare environment toward managed care has converted many radiology departments from profit centers charging fees for scanning services into cost centers. Although the demand for diagnostic services is stagnating, radiologists extend their expertise in imaging into treatment as can be seen in the growing number of image-guided therapy techniques.

For many years, conventional x-ray fluoroscopy, computed tomography (CT), and ultrasound (US) have been used as interventional diagnostic and therapeutic procedures. With the advent of open magnet technology and the progress in fast imaging techniques, MR-guided interventional procedures are being developed.[1–3] Unique advantages of MRI, besides (ionizing) radiation-free imaging, are the excellent soft-tissue contrast, the ability to acquire images in any arbitrary slice orientation, three-dimensional (3D) imaging capabilities, and most importantly, the ability to image tissue response to thermal treatment.[4–7]

In surgery, there are two main reasons for the interest in intraoperative MRI. Although a variety of sophisticated diagnostic imaging systems can provide an incredible amount of information about each patient, this information is not usually transferred and available in the operating room (OR), where often simple view boxes for radiologic films are being used. Neurosurgeons were the first to use navigation systems to relate image information to the surgical field for each patient. As a natural extension of this development, intraoperative imaging systems guide the surgeon and control the surgical results immediately. However, cost containment in healthcare accelerates the development of minimally invasive procedures on an outpatient basis. Although interest in tissue-conserving methods with few complications was once dominant, the focus today is on improving the cost-effectiveness of medical services through shorter hospitalization and faster recuperation. The limited access to the region of treatment that makes these techniques possible mandates the use of image-assisted methods to control instruments or to monitor therapy.

Hence, interventional radiology and image-assisted surgery develop slowly together, creating an opportunity for interventional MRI because investment in expensive technology cannot be justified unless a baseline number of procedures is performed. With the current lack of reimbursement for many MR-guided procedures, dedicated interventional MRI is limited to a few research centers that can perform only a few patient studies. Therefore, a valid and ideal solution for many centers seems to be an open MR scanner that combines diagnostic and interventional imaging, minimizing financial risk.

TECHNICAL PREREQUISITES

The most important prerequisite for interventional MRI is an open magnet system that allows access to the patient during the procedure. Low-field systems with permanent or resistive magnets have always been more open than closed-bore superconducting magnets, but the MAGNETOM Open system (Siemens AG, Erlangen, Germany) was one of the first to combine openess with powerful imaging capabilities.[8] Its C-shaped magnet has a vertically oriented field of 0.2 T between horizontal poles (Fig. 2-1). This design allows lateral patient access of approximately 280° circumferentially for interventional and intraoperative procedures (Fig. 2-2). In particular, claustrophobic or obese patients benefit from the patient-friendly design, but advantages also exist for imaging patients in the emergency department who require ventilation or pediatric patients. With a maximum field of view (FOV) of more than 36 cm, this all-purpose imager is suitable for all head and body interventions. The use of a resistive instead of a permanent magnet enables the magnet to be switched off in less than 1 sec in case of an

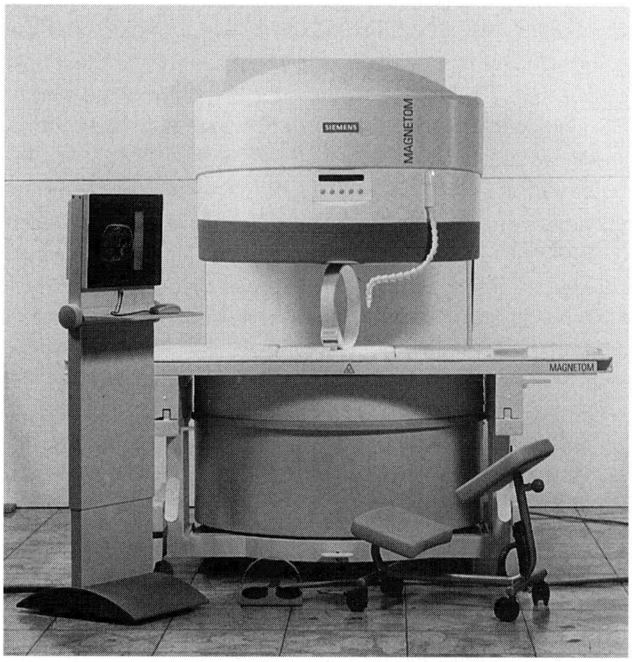

Fig. 2-1. MAGNETOM Open Viva unit (Siemens AG, Erlangen, Germany) with the in-room magnetic resonance console and components of the magnetic resonance–guided procedure package (e.g., inbore light, foot switch, open body coil, sterile drape, ergonomic knee chair).

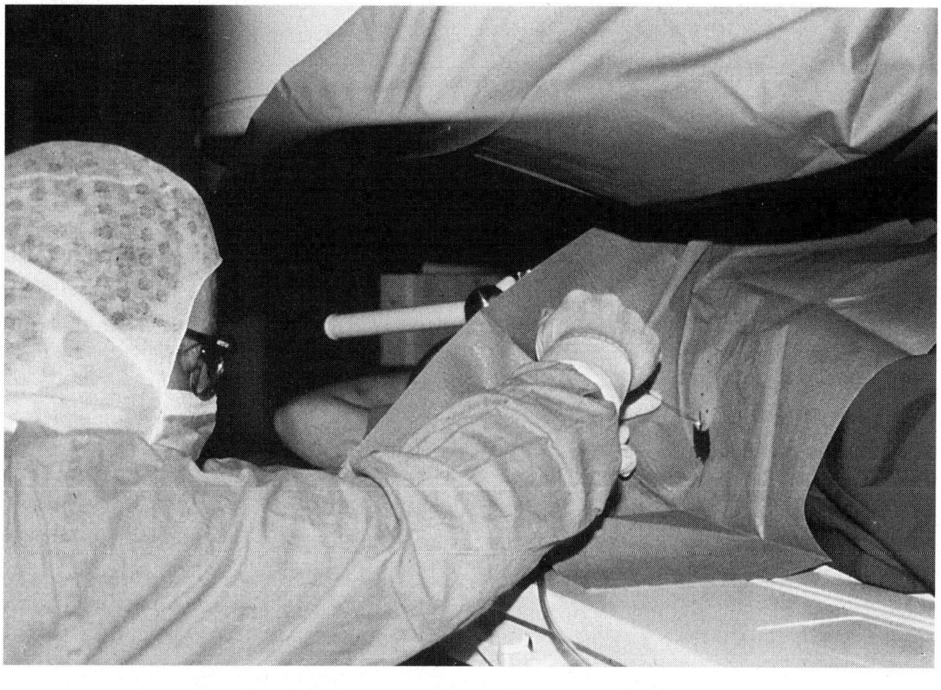

Fig. 2-2. Patient access during a magnetic resonance–guided procedure.

emergency or when not in use. The small magnetic fringe field at 0.2 T results in space requirements of less than 320 ft^2 (30 m^2) and enables convenient site planning in existing radiologic suites or operating rooms. More importantly, MR-guided procedures require that the physician and patient be exposed to a magnetic field for an extended time. Based on standards established by the American Conference of Governmental Industrial Hygenists, this low-field system allows for more than 8-hr exposures per day. This approach provides a safe environment for the patient and hospital staff and allows one person to perform several procedures per day, if necessary.

Very effective annular coils can be used as interventional receiver coils because of the vertical magnetic field orientation. These flexible coils are placed around the patient's body and provide an optimal filling factor. When the coils are covered with a sterile drape, the physician has an interventional field on either side of the coil, fulfilling all sterility requirements without the receiver coil being an obstruction. If the annular coil is slightly tilted relative to the long axis of the patient's body, the region of interest can be positioned in the center of the coil, providing the best signal-to-noise ratio (SNR) and the shortest possible access from the side. Of economic importance, these coils are reusable.

Interventional MRI guides instruments with near real-time measurement sequences into the target region and accurately controls the position of instruments, with sequences providing a good contrast-to-noise ratio and showing only small susceptibility artifacts. A prerequisite for fast imaging is a powerful gradient system with a high duty cycle. The MAGNETOM Open unit features a flat, actively shielded gradient system with 15 mT/m and an ultrashort rise time of 900 μsec for 15 mT/m. Because of water cooling, a maximum duty cycle of 100% becomes possible. The fastest MRI technique is in general echoplanar imaging (EPI). However, EPI is very sensitive to any local field distortion caused by interventional instruments and has not been successfully used for interventional MRI. At low-field strength, steady-state gradient-echo sequences provide maximum SNR per unit time. Combined with rectangular FOV for improved resolution, image frame rates of less than 1 sec are possible, which is sufficient for near real-time guidance of instruments. Autodisplay software ensures that all measured data sets are automatically reconstructed and displayed at the local monitor during the ongoing measurement. Thus, continuous acquisition, similar to that in fluoroscopy, can be implemented on the MAGNETOM Open system. Passive interventional tools are not directly visible in MR but are depicted by the local susceptibility artifact they create. The size of the artifact and the augmented width of the instrument depend on sequence parameters, field strength, and main field orientation.[9,10] At low field strength, the typical materials used for instruments (e.g., stainless steel, titanium alloys) create an acceptably small artifact, whereas at higher field strength the artificial augmentation of the tool size increases, thus decreasing the position accuracy.[11]

As in x-ray fluoroscopy a local monitor placed close to the magnet bore provides immediate image feedback. Because of the magnetic fringe field, only liquid crystal display technology is recommended. With the mobile and adjustable in-room MR console, a large liquid crystal display screen shielded from radiofrequencies (RF) can be operated inside the RF room without disturbing image acquisition. The resolution is sufficient to display up to four images simultaneously and all control and operating windows. Using a shielded mouse, the in-room MR console allows operation of the MR scanner next to the patient. A modified version of this monitor is color capable and can handle various input sources of data. In addition to the imager output signal, a video input allows the display of endoscopic or US video images or the display of dedicated software of a scientific workstation.

In addition to the in-room MR console, fluoroscopic sequences, and accessible receiver coils, a few other components complete a commercially available MR-guided procedures package: a fiberoptic lamp with a goose-neck extension provides a cold light source for the interventional working area. A customized drape covers the upper pole shoe of the magnet to guarantee sterility. Patient positioning using the light localizer is still possible through a transparent plastic cover. A specially adapted knee chair ensures an ergonomic sitting position for the physician during the interventional procedure. The knee chair has a foot switch to start or stop the fluoroscopic imaging mode. The physician can concentrate on the patient and still operate the system interactively.

Proper localization of needle insertion is often a problem when performing interventional MRI. The most straightforward approach uses the physician's finger to match the location of the current image plane with the patient's body. Alternatively, an MR-visible grid positioned on the patient during the acquisition of the localizer images is available for procedure planning. Likewise, a small tube filled with contrast agent can be used. A more sophisticated solution is integration of a 3D tracking system to control the scan plane.[12] Although active optical systems require a free line of sight, they are most accurate and versatile. With a digitizer probe, procedure planning is easy, and the optimal insertion point and slice angulation can be determined quickly. During the interventional procedure, interactively changing the position or orientation of the imaging plane is often necessary because the biopsy needle does not always follow a straight line. With the MAGNETOM Open system, this is accomplished with an MR-compatible version of the optical tracking system POLARIS (Northern Digital, Waterloo, Ontario, Canada), in which the digitizer probe serves as instrument holder. The position information of the instrument holder is communicated to the measurement control system of the MAGNETOM Open system and used for the next measurement (Fig. 2-3). Because markers are attached to the cover of the MR scanner at a fixed distance from the isocenter of the magnet, the camera system can be easily repositioned between interventional procedures without the need for time-consuming calibration procedures to match the

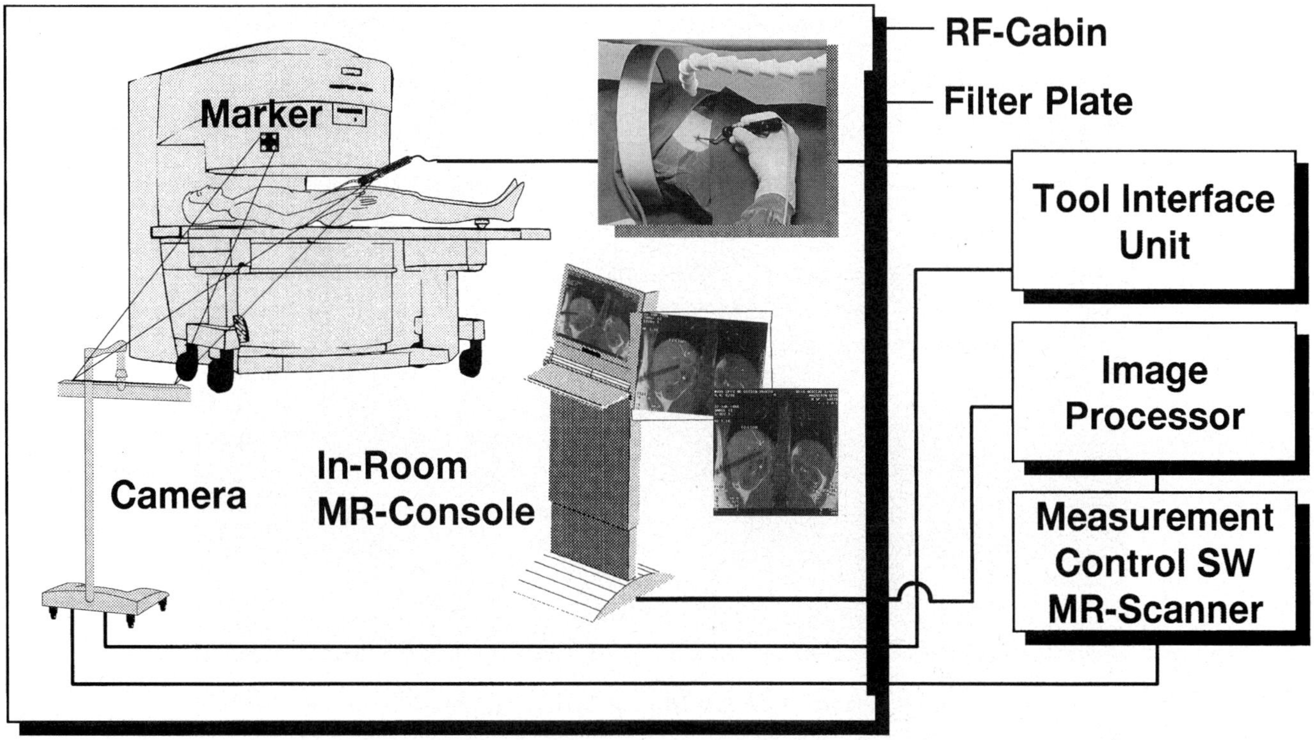

Fig. 2-3. Interactive scan plane control is integrated into the MAGNETOM Open Viva unit (Siemens AG, Erlangen, Germany) using the magnetic resonance–compatible optical tracking system POLARIS (Northern Digital, Waterloo, Ontario, Canada).

coordinate system of the imager and the tracking system. Calibration of the markers at the magnet cover is done once during installation using an automated calibration procedure. When additional markers are placed directly on the patient or on the patient table, the optical tracking system can be used even when the patient table is pulled out of the magnet.

Because interventional MRI is fairly new, various questions are still being considered: what indications for MR-guided procedures versus other imaging modalities can be developed? Which interventional procedures controlled by other imaging methods can be replaced by interventional MRI using its specific advantages (e.g., superior soft-tissue contrast, arbitrary slice orientation, 3D imaging, low complication risk, safe contrast media)? Radiation-free imaging will be an issue for longer procedures and pediatric management. Multiple studies are being performed to show the benefits of interventional MRI, including its cost advantages.

Potential applications of interventional MRI include:

- Diagnostic biopsy of primary tumors, metastases, and lymph nodes in the head and neck, liver, and lower pelvis[12–14] whenever better soft-tissue contrast is advantageous or other imaging modalities are too difficult
- Drainage of cysts, abscesses, and hematomas[15]
- Degenerative spinal diseases with pain syndrome requiring nerve root management[16,17] and MR-guided sympathectomies
- Interstitial laser therapy[18–20]
- Local tumor therapy with RF ablation[21, 22]
- MR-guided focused US[23,24]
- MR-guided cryosurgery[25]
- Local drug therapy and chemoablation[26,27]
- Vascular intervention[28]

DEVELOPMENTS FOR INTRAOPERATIVE USE

In neurosurgery, complex surgical planning and intraoperative neuronavigation techniques based on 3D imaging data are being applied more often. Neurosurgeons are among the first to use MRI in the OR[29–31] because it offers outstanding demarcation of pathologic structures in the brain and spinal cord. Use of the same MR scanner for surgical planning, intraoperative surgical monitoring, postoperative control, and, in exceptional cases, preoperative diagnosis ensures greater imaging system use. In neuronavigation, certain position points in the operating area are projected into the preoperative MR data, thus allowing the surgeon to determine the position of deeper structures or lesions. Also, certain invasive tumors often cannot be clearly demarcated even by microsurgery. The goals of neuronavigation systems are to improve microsurgical precision and to minimize the amount of residual tumor tissue. However, the main disadvantage of all systems of this type, regardless of whether they are mechanical, optical, acoustic, or electromagnetic, is that they are all based solely on preoperative image data. Discharge of

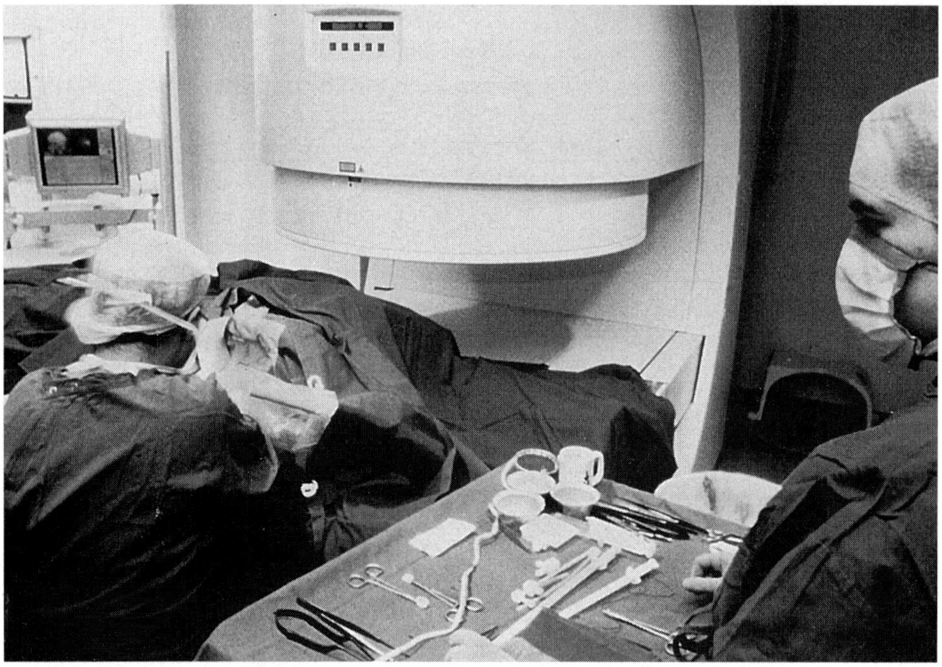

Fig. 2-4. Intraoperative installation of the MAGNETOM Open unit (Siemens AG, Erlangen, Germany) at the University of Heidelberg, Germany, showing the adjacent operating room in the background. The neurosurgical procedure is performed at the patient table of the magnetic resonance scanner. Intraoperative control images can be acquired when necessary during the procedure.

cerebrospinal fluid after the cranial cap and dura have been opened and use of brain retractors during tumor resection will alter anatomy. With intraoperative MRI, these alterations of brain structures can be detected, resulting in increased spatial accuracy of neuronavigation, which should reduce morbidity and further improve surgical precision.

At the University of Heidelberg, Germany, and the University of Erlangen, Germany, the MAGNETOM Open system has been installed inside the OR (Fig. 2-4). An important criterion in planning these installations was availability of intraoperative MRI when needed, while minimizing the need for change of the surgical routine. Both institutions also use sophisticated surgical microscopes with built-in neuronavigation systems for stereotactic guidance; these microscopes are not MR-compatible. Therefore, the RF cabin for the MR scanner occupies only part of the OR, and the surgeons work outside of the cabin. By having a second entrance to the RF cabin, the MR scanner can be used independently of the adjacent OR for preoperative scanning. During surgery, time-consuming preparation of the tumor is best done in the OR. After craniotomy, the patient undergoes MRI to obtain an updated, intraoperative 3D data set for neuronavigation systems. This technique guarantees the greatest precision for the remaining stage of surgery outside of the RF cabin. If required, intraoperative control images can be repeated before tumor resection. Contrast-enhanced MRI after tumor resection reduces the risk of residual tumor.[30] A specially designed transport system ensures shock-free transportation using an air pillow, and it avoids the need for patient repositioning during surgery. Mounted on the patient table is an MR-compatible ceramic head holder with plastic screws and ceramic tips that provides metal-free support and avoids additional susceptibility artifacts. A specially designed receive head coil beside the head holder allows unobstructed patient access. The upper part of the coil can be easily removed and is only present during imaging, not during surgery. Anesthesia and life-support systems were carefully chosen for MR compatibility and for lack of interference with the RF system of the MR scanner.

For frameless stereotactic procedures and less demanding surgeries, patient transport is unnecessary. Having gained more experience with intraoperative MRI, physicians are more frequently performing procedures under MR guidance inside the scanner (e.g., free hand brain biopsy, drainage of cysts and abscesses, catheter placement for brachytherapy). This principle can be extended by placing an MR-compatible surgical microscope at the far end of the table position range, allowing certain procedures to be performed next to the magnet. Transsphenoidal pituitary surgeries, for example, can benefit from immediate control of MRI after surgery to guarantee no residual tumor is present. If necessary, surgery can be continued until completion. As MR-compatible neuroendoscopes become commercially available, the range of intraoperative procedures is likely to increase.

A logical consequence of this development from a manufacturer's point-of-view is to integrate the surgical working place next to the magnet. This principle is depicted in Figure 2-5, in which an MR-compatible table top is mounted on a revolving

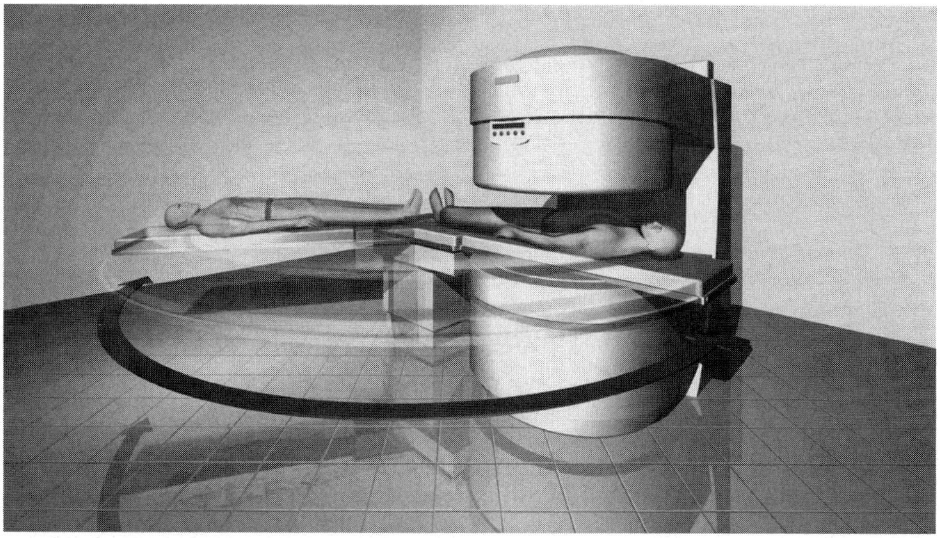

Fig. 2-5. Intraoperative installation of the MAGNETOM Open Viva unit (Siemens AG, Erlangen, Germany) with a revolving operating table. Surgery is done in a low magnetic fringe field with limited need for magnetic resonance–compatible surgical instruments.

operating table base. As in conventional surgery, the OR table can be height-adjusted and tilted according to the surgeon's need. Surgery is performed in a very low magnetic fringe field without time restrictions. At this distance to the low-field magnet, the need for MR-compatible instrumentation is limited. Connections from the anesthesia equipment to the patient are positioned at the foot of the table. Hence, anesthesia need not be moved when the patient is rotated into the scanner. Patient relocation can be done fairly quickly, and MRI is readily available when needed during surgery.

CONCLUSIONS

Use of interventional radiology and image-guided surgery is increasing. Radiologists extend their expertise in interventional radiology toward local tumor therapy and more invasive procedures, whereas neurosurgeons, ear, nose, and throat surgeons, and implant surgeons use navigation systems and intraoperative imaging to improve the procedure quality. State-of-the-art open low-field scanners are valid for interventional and intraoperative research and development. Although many interventional procedures (e.g., MR-guided biopsy) are done routinely in several institutions, new approaches to local tumor management (e.g., interstitial laser therapy, RF ablation, high-intensity focused US) require more time to become accepted alternatives to conventional surgery. Clinical research must continue over the next years. As clinical procedures are further developed, their technical requirements will become obvious. Thus, clinical validation, outcome analysis, and prospective randomized clinical trials are needed. Dedicated MR scanners will be developed to support those procedures, but a single design will unlikely satisfy all needs. Therefore, dedicated scanners with different magnet design are soon likely to be developed for various procedures.

REFERENCES

1. Jolesz FA, Kikinis R: Intraoperative imaging revolutionizes therapy, *Diagn Imaging* 9:62, 1995.
2. Lufkin RB: Interventional MR imaging, *Radiology* 197:16, 1995.
3. Schenck JF, and others: Superconducting open-configuration MR imaging system for image-guided therapy, *Radiology* 195:805, 1995.
4. De Poorter J, and others: Noninvasive MRI thermometry with the proton resonance frequency (PRF) method: in vivo results in human muscle, *Magn Reson Med* 33:74, 1995.
5. Le Bihan D, Delannoy J, Levin RL: Temperature mapping with MR imaging of molecular diffusion: application to hyperthermia, *Radiology* 171: 853, 1989.
6. Matsumoto R, and others: Tissue temperature monitoring for thermal interventional therapy: comparison of T1-weighted MR-sequences, *J Magn Reson Imaging* 4:65, 1994.
7. Sinha S, and others: Temperature measurements using phase-shift imaging on an open 0.2 T interventional MR scanner, *Radiology* 197:423, 1995.
8. Lenz GW, Dewey C: *An open MRI system used for interventional procedures: current research and initial clinical results.* In Lemke HU, and others, editors: *Computer assisted radiology,* Berlin, 1995, Springer.
9. Luedecke KM, Roeschmann P, Tischler R: Susceptibility artifacts in NMR imaging, *Magn Reson Imaging* 3:329, 1985.
10. Shellock FG, Morisoli S, Kanal E: MR procedures and biomedical implants, materials, and devices, *Radiology* 189:587, 1993.
11. Lewin JS, and others: Needle localization in MR-guided biopsy and aspiration: effects of field strength, sequence design, and magnetic field orientation, *Am J Roentgenol* 166:1337, 1996.
12. Silverman SG, and others: Interactive MR-guided biopsy in an open-configuration MR imaging system, *Radiology* 197:175, 1995.
13. Duckwiler G, and others: Head and neck lesions: MR-guided aspiration biopsy, *Radiology* 170:519, 1989.
14. Frahm C, and others: Technik der MRT-gesteuerten Stanzbiopsie im Abdomen an einem offenen Niederfeldgerät: Durchführbarkeit und erste klinische Ergebnisse, *Rofo Fortschrgeb Rontgenstr Neuen Bildgeb Verfahr* 164:64, 1996.
15. Gehl HB, and others: Technik der MRT-gesteuerten abdominellen Drainage an einem offenen Niederfeldmagneten, *Rofo Fortschrgeb Rontgenstr Neuen Bildgeb Verfahr* 165:70, 1996.

16. Groenemeyer DHW, and others: Image-guided access techniques, *Endoscopic Surgery* 3:69, 1995.
17. Seibel RM, and others: Computed tomography- and magnetic resonance imaging-guided microtherapy, *Seminars in Laparoscopic Surgery* 4:61, 1997.
18. Kahn T, and others: MRI-guided laser-induced interstitial thermotherapy of cerebral neoplasms, *J Comput Assist Tomogr* 18:519, 1994.
19. Pushek T, and others: Dynamic MRI-guided interstitial laser therapy: a new technique for minimally invasive surgery, *Laryngoscope* 105:1245, 1995.
20. Vogl TJ, and others: Recurrent nasopharyngeal tumors: preliminary clinical results with interventional MR imaging-controlled laser-induced thermotherapy, *Radiology* 196:725, 1995.
21. Anzai Y, and others: Preliminary experience with MR-guided thermal ablation of brain tumors, *Am J Neuroradiol* 16:39, 1995.
22. Farahani K, and others: Hyperacute thermal lesions: MR imaging evaluation of development in the brain, *Radiology* 196:517, 1995.
23. Cline HE, and others: Focused US system for MR imaging-guided tumor ablation, *Radiology* 194:731, 1995.
24. Hynynen K, and others: Clinical, noninvasive, MR imaging-monitored ultrasound surgery method, *Radiographics* 16:185, 1996.
25. Pease GR, and others: MR image-guided control of cryosurgery, *J Magn Reson Imaging* 5:753, 1995.
26. Bartolozzi C, and others: Hepatocellular carcinoma: CT and MR features after transcatheter arterial embolization and percutaneous ethanol injection, *Radiology* 191:123, 1994.
27. Sironi S, and others: Small hepatocellular carcinoma treated with percutaneous ethanol injection: unenhanced and gadolinium-enhanced MR imaging follow-up, *Radiology* 192:407, 1994.
28. Wildermuth S, and others: MR imaging-guided intravascular procedure: initial demonstration in a pig model, *Radiology* 202:578, 1997.
29. Tronnier VM, and others: Intraoperative diagnostic and interventional magnetic resonance imaging in neurosurgery, *Neurosurgery* 40:891, 1997.
30. Huang AY, and others: Interventional MRI for neurosurgery, *Perspectives in Neurological Surgery* 6:44, 1995.
31. Jolesz FA, Shtern F: The operating room of the future, *Invest Radiology* 27:326, 1992.

Chapter 3

DESIGN OF A MID-FIELD INTRAOPERATIVE MR SYSTEM AT 0.5 TESLA

Stephen G. Hushek

BACKGROUND

The 0.5-T Signa SP (GE Medical Systems, Milwaukee, Wis.) intraoperative magnetic resonance (MR) system was designed for MR guidance of minimally invasive surgery. The project team created a system that allowed physicians to walk up to a patient lying on a surgical table and perform an operation as usual. The search for a magnet that would form the basis of the system began with the open magnet concepts that already existed in the late 1980s. An early example of such a magnet was designed by the Aberdeen Group in the late 1970s and early 1980s.[1] The Aberdeen design incorporated "pole pieces" that created a horizontal gap. These horizontal gap magnets, although potentially adequate for several minimally invasive procedures, did not allow the type of access physicians required and thus were rejected. A new magnet configuration was required for what appeared to be the initiation of a new modality.

Several magnet design concepts were discussed, including a magnet so large that the entire operating room was in the imaging field of the magnet (see Chapter 4). A magnet of this size would have required a large amount of power, but the B_0 homogeneity would have been excellent; with the use of flat gradient coils built into the surgical table top, the system would have been largely transparent to the physician. However, this design had significant problems with the cost, siting, stray field, and field strength requirements. Ultimately, a vertical gap design with dual air core superconducting solenoidal (DACSS) magnets provided the preferred surgical access to the patient and the potential for many patient positions for orthopedic or other types of studies (Fig. 3-1).

MAGNET

The DACSS magnet achieves the goals of a surgical MR system by constructively combining what are effectively the stray fields of each magnet half; the two halves of the system combine to form a field of 0.5 T in a 30-cm diameter spherical volume (DSV). The 30-cm DSV is located coaxially with the two

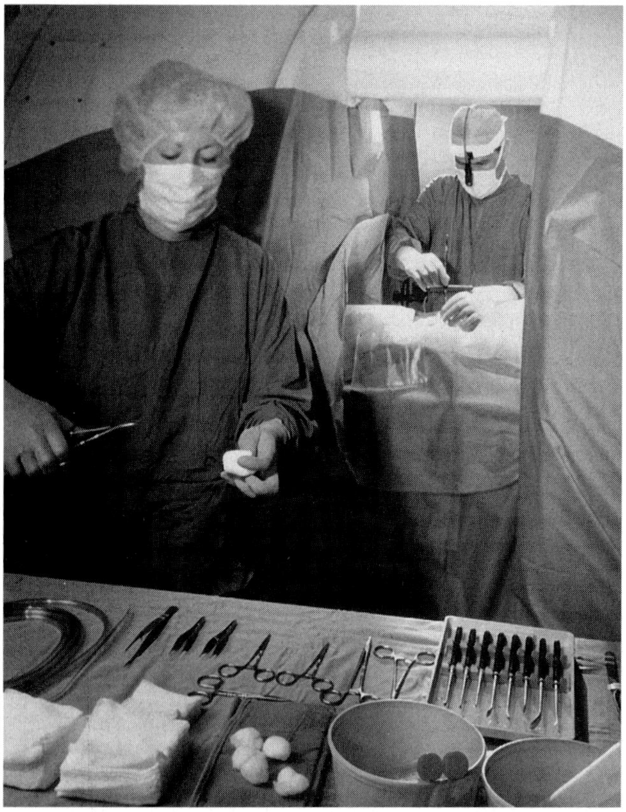

Fig. 3-1. View from the side of a draped magnet, showing a physician in the gap inserting a trocar through a Flashpoint™ handpiece and an assistant handling an array of magnetic resonance–compatible surgical instruments.

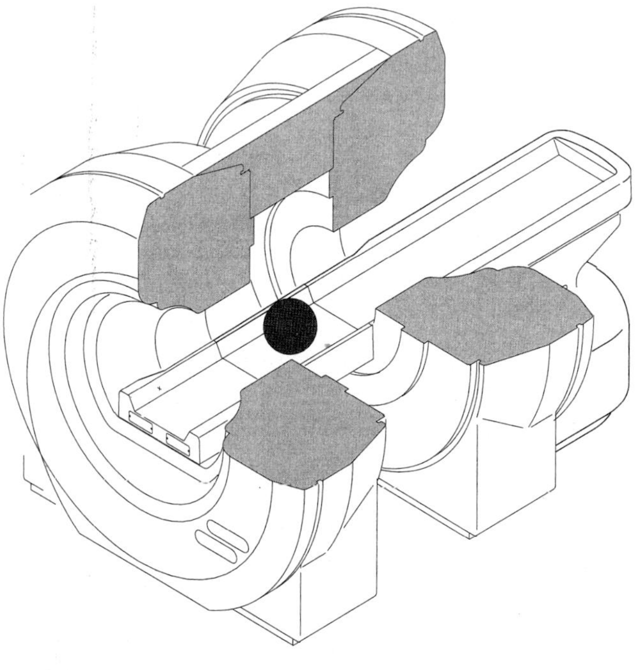

Fig. 3-2. View of the magnet with the upper quarter removed, showing location of a 30-cm diameter spherical imaging volume represented by a grey sphere.

magnets and halfway between them, so that no magnet structure is located in the immediate vicinity of the imaging volume (Fig. 3-2). The gap between the magnet halves is 58 cm, allowing the physician to walk between the magnet halves and have customary contact with a patient entering the system on a support bed that is coaxial with the magnet. Thus, the physician can easily and directly interact with the patient anatomy during imaging. No delay occurs while the patient is transferred from an imaging to an operating location; the working and the imaging volumes are the same.

Horizontal gap systems do not provide access to the imaging volume from above, but the physician can reach into the imaging volume from the lateral extent of the magnet. Although this approach may be adequate for several percutaneous procedures, it does not meet the requirements for most surgeries.[2] However, a vertical gap alone is not sufficient to provide true surgical access for most procedures. Some conventional horizontal gap systems may be turned on their side to create a vertical gap system (Fig. 3-3), but this position allows normal surgical access for only a few cranial procedures. The solid pole faces of these magnets prevent a patient from entering the gap along the axis. The air core solenoidal design allows the patient to be inserted through the hole along the axis of the solenoid and between the two solenoids, permitting surgical access to any portion of the body.

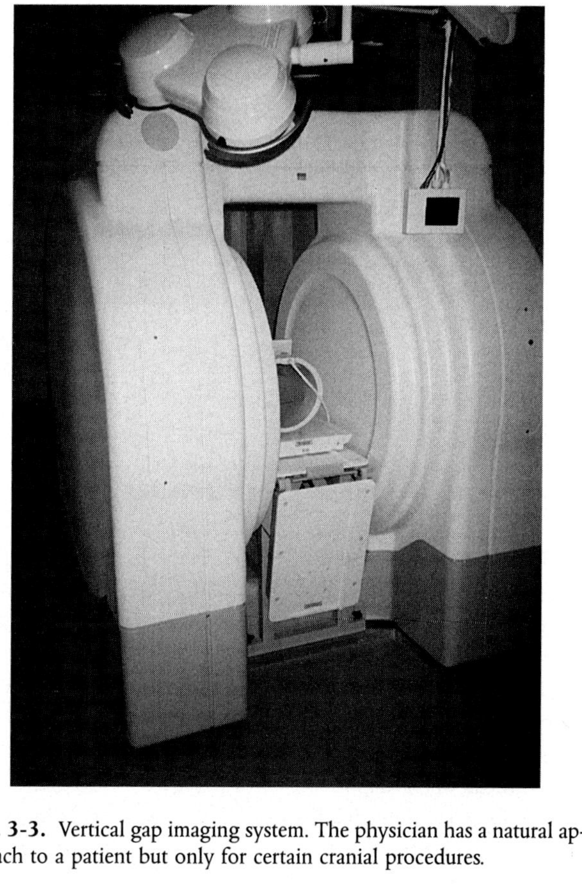

Fig. 3-3. Vertical gap imaging system. The physician has a natural approach to a patient but only for certain cranial procedures.

The magnet designers were challenged to achieve as high a magnetic field as possible, while maintaining a useful gap between the magnet halves. The field decreases as distance from the magnet increases ($B \propto \frac{1}{d^3}$), with a rate proportional to the distance from the magnet to the third power, so increases in gap width significantly decrease the field strength. The system design can generate a 0.5-T field while maintaining a 58-cm gap. Human-factors studies and tests with full-size mock-ups determined that this gap distance allowed many procedures to be performed in the new system, including most, if not all, of the targeted procedures.

The magnet designers were next faced with the challenge of generating a homogeneous field from two inherently inhomogeneous fields. The current in the magnet windings is distributed among various locations within the magnet cryostat to maximize the uniformity of the field in the imaging volume. In addition, ferromagnetic material is built into the magnet structure to "focus" the flux generated by this current, further improving the field uniformity in the imaging volume.[3] A map of the static magnetic field shows the homogeneity achievable with the magnet design (Fig. 3-4).

The homogeneity of the main magnetic field can be further improved through the use of passive shimming. A cylindrical structure known as a shim drum is placed against the inner cylindrical wall of each magnet half; precise amounts of iron are positioned at strategic locations on the shim drum. An iterative process is used to determine the location and amount of the shims required to optimize the field homogeneity. The shimming procedure is performed only once as part of the system installation procedure, and no adjustments are necessary unless major changes occur in the magnet environment (e.g., the addition of a new magnet in an adjoining room would require another shim iteration). The shimming procedure can produce homogeneity better than 15 ppm in the 30-cm DSV.

The magnets are constructed of a superconductor composed of Nb_3Sn, which can maintain superconductive properties at temperatures as high as 14° to 16° K. Superconductors in more typical magnets maintain their superconductive properties only

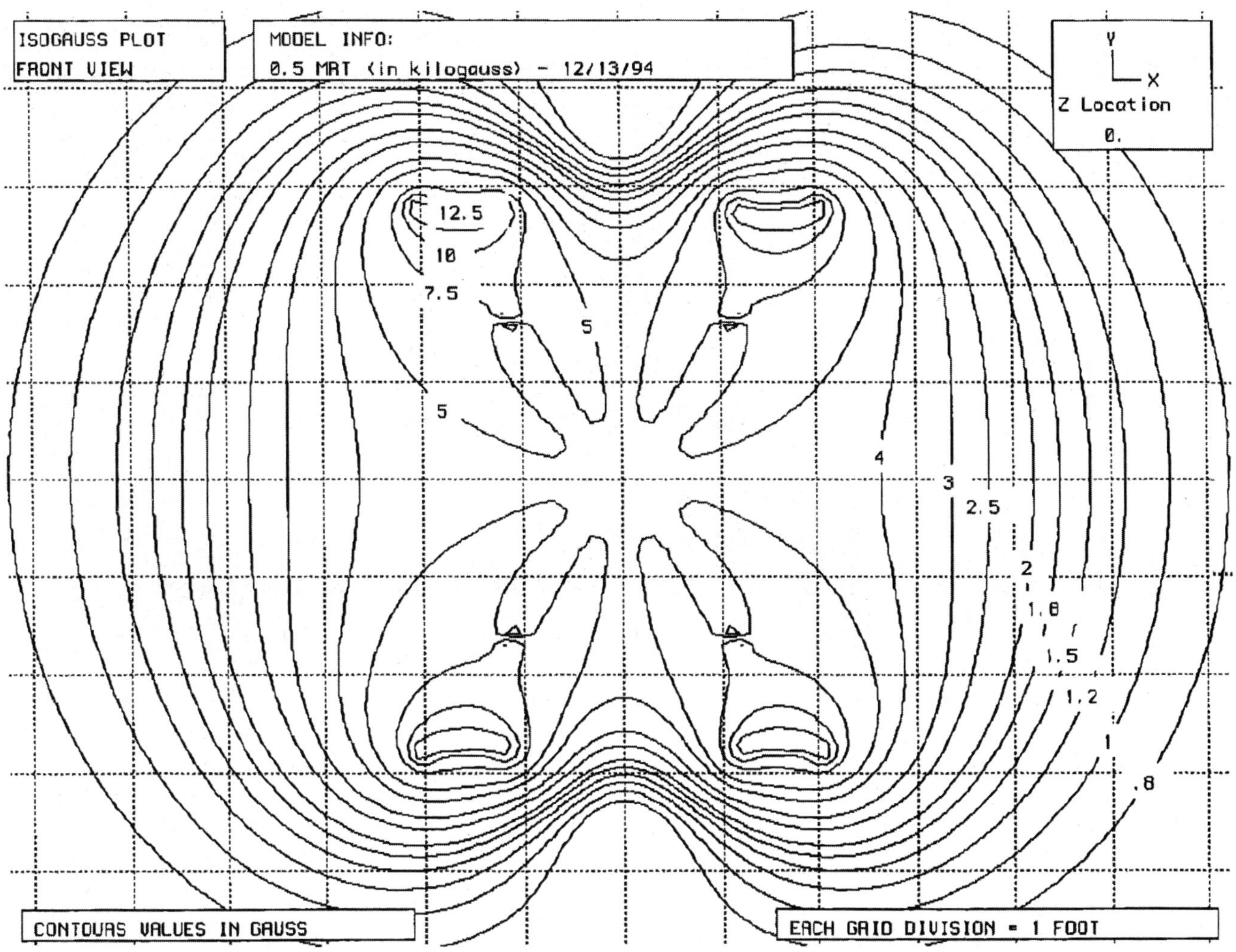

Fig. 3-4. Map of the main magnetic field in the axial plane through the isocenter. The field is very homogeneous in the imaging volume but has significant variations outside the 30-cm diameter sphere.

up to 4° to 5° K. The relatively high temperature at which these superconductors operate allows the magnet to be cooled exclusively by a thermal conduction system rather than by liquid cryogens. Elimination of the liquid cryogens decreased the size of the magnet structure, thereby increasing the room available for the physician in the magnet gap.

Conduction cooling is accomplished by cooling the entire mass of superconducting material from one point. Heat generated anywhere in the superconducting material flows through the material itself and through a copper overwrap until it reaches a structure known as the *thermal busbar,* where the superconductor material is connected to a cryocooling refrigeration system. The cryocooling refrigeration system can maintain the entire mass of superconductor at superconductive temperatures with one cryocooler, the active cooling device. In the system design, a second cryocooler was added to improve the system reliability.

The most significant magnet design criterion is the relationship between the magnet coil windings and the imaging volume, but other design requirements also play major roles. The magnet structural supports are critical to the function of the magnet, but they should be positioned to preserve access to the imaging volume from as many directions as possible. The supports provide electrical, mechanical, thermal, and vacuum continuity between the magnet halves. The magnet coil windings are aligned; the south pole of one coil winding faces the north pole of the other, so the force between them is attractive. The strength of the magnetic field produces a mechanical force on the windings of approximately 20 tons. However, the coil windings must be suspended in vacuum and thermally insulated from the cryostat to maintain their low temperature and thus their superconductivity. To provide a strong mechanical structure with excellent thermal and electrical insulation, careful material selection and mechanical design are important. The de-

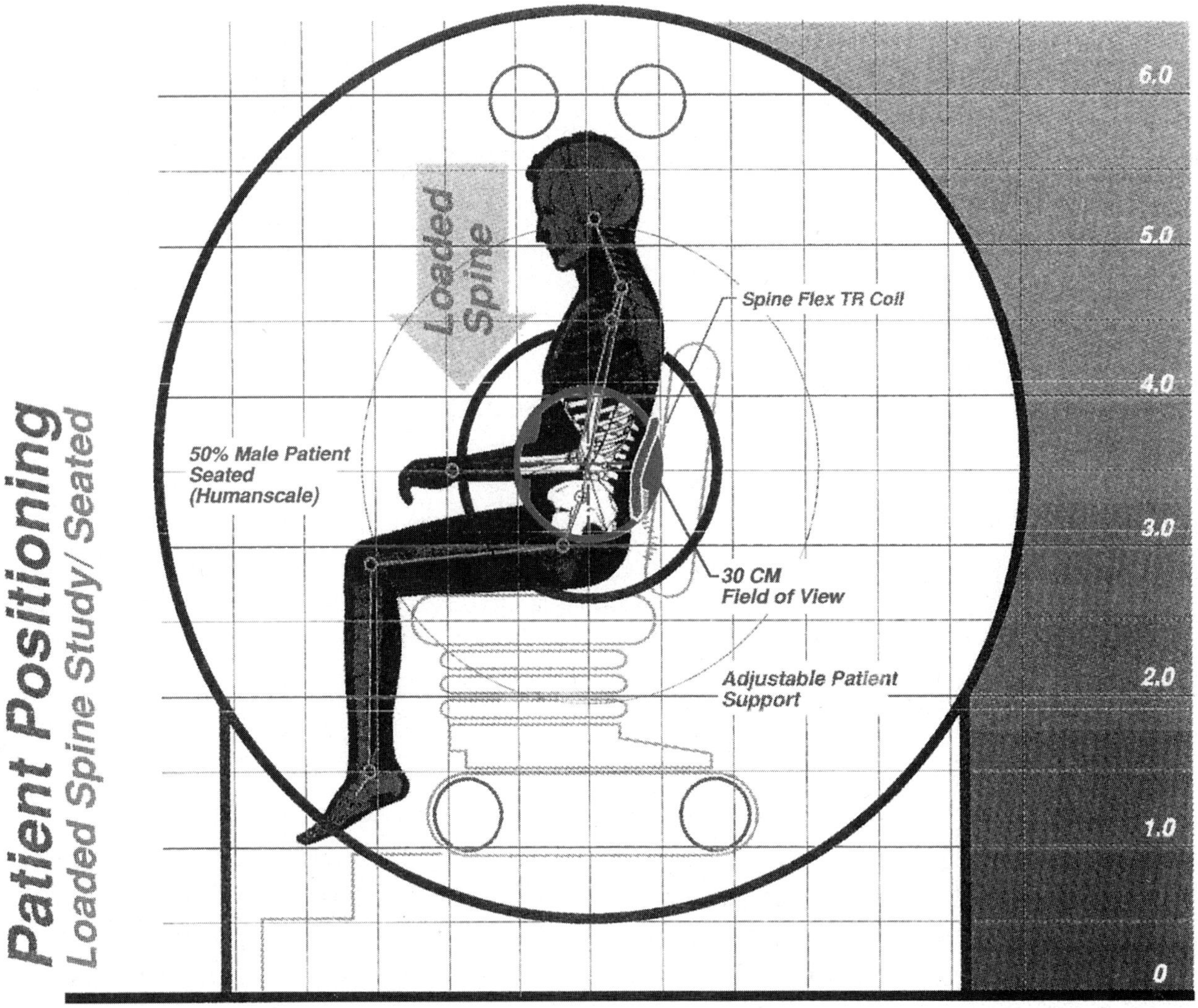

Fig. 3-5. Diagram of a patient positioned for a seated, loaded lumbar spinal examination. The circles near the patient's head represent the upper magnet structural supports.

sign minimizes mechanical contact with the superconducting coil structure while providing high strength.

The solution accommodates the mechanical forces while allowing most of the gap to be open. The structural supports are positioned at the top and bottom of the magnet and at the maximum radial extent of the cryostat. In this configuration, they are over and under the patient for axial and side entry surgical applications, and they produce minimal inconvenience for the physician. They are also positioned sufficiently far from isocenter so the upper support only slightly interferes with a patient's head during a "loaded" or weight-bearing lumbar spine study (Fig. 3-5). The lower structural support is sufficiently low to allow the patient to sit in the gap for a vertical cervical spine imaging study (Fig. 3-6). In addition, the upper structural supports bracket the upper enclosure, which houses various cameras and lights used during the procedures.

Another important aspect of the magnet design was the overall dimension of the entire structure. It is desirable to keep the magnet profile as small as possible. Although imaging volume access is acceptable for two physicians standing adjacent to the patient, access to those two physicians needs to be as great as possible. The passage of surgical instruments in and out of the gap, space for in-bore displays, general anesthesia tubing passage, and various other requirements mandate that the system be as open as possible. Thus, the radius and length of the system have been reduced to the absolute minimum. The entire length of the magnet can be draped so the surgical trays can be positioned outside the magnet. However, when one physician is working in the bore, the trays can be positioned across the patient so the surgical instruments are readily available.

Performance of surgical and interventional procedures in these systems is a team effort, so the needs of each member of

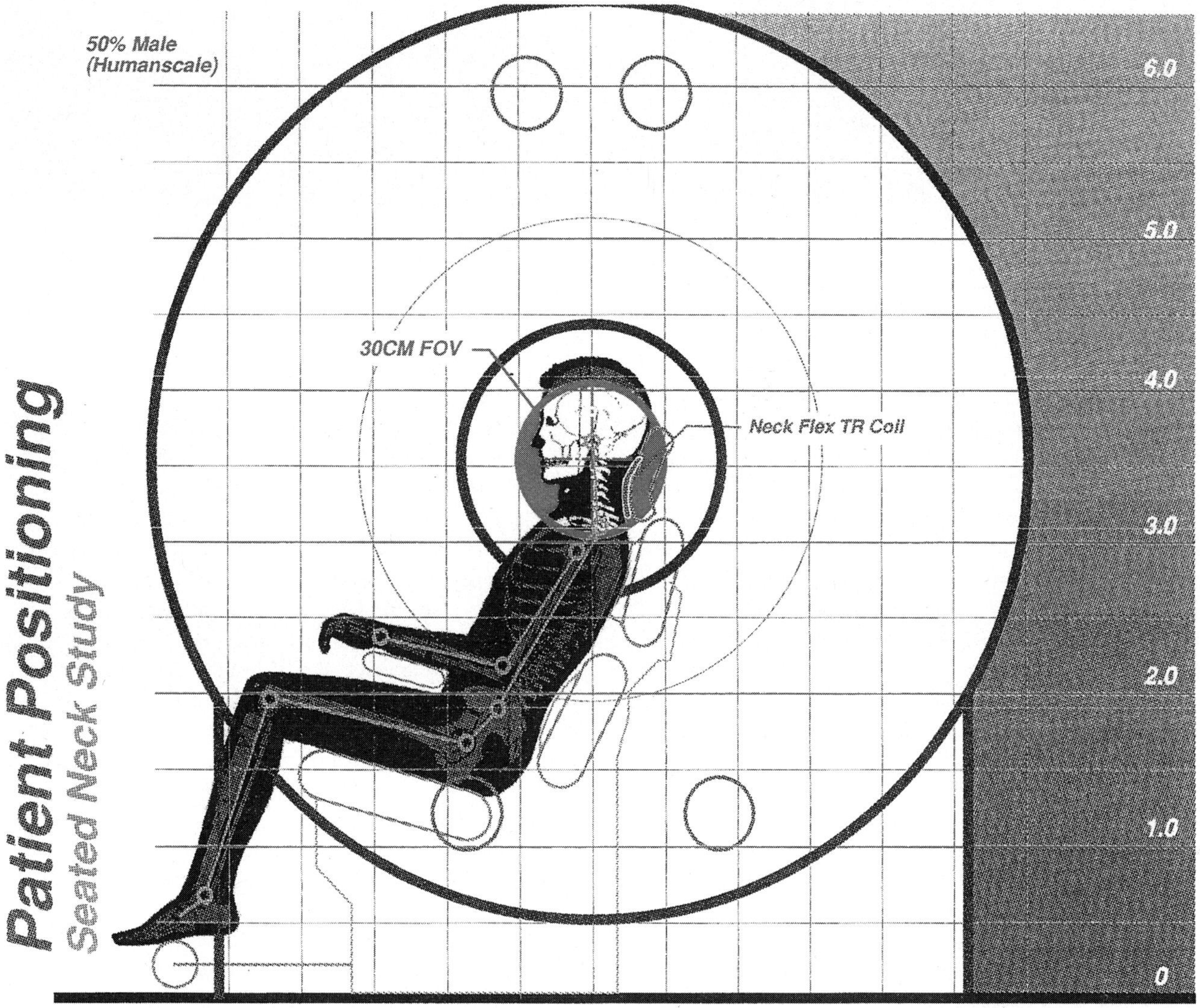

Fig. 3-6. Diagram of a patient positioned for a seated, loaded, cervical spinal examination. The circles near the patient's pelvis represent the lower magnet structural supports.

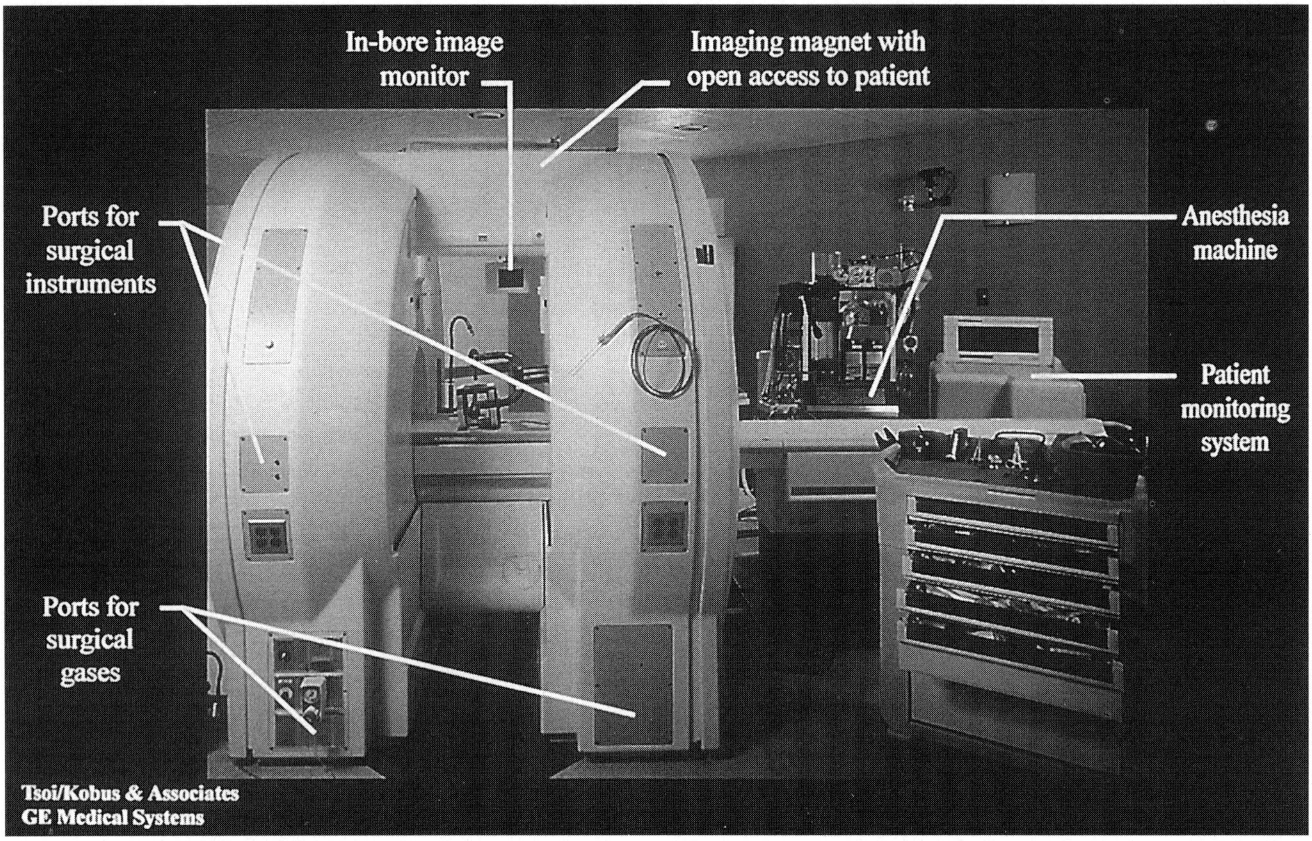

Fig. 3-7. Tool panels, surgical instrument port panels, and ancillary equipment.

the team are considered. The anesthesiologist requires surgical gas ports built into the enclosures. Tool panels for connecting intercom headsets, microphones, 3D locator handpieces, laser fibers, radiofrequency (RF) handpieces, and cryosurgical probes are also provided (Fig. 3-7). The connections for these interventional tools and other ancillary systems are located under the floor of the room in three 4-inch diameter pipes that run from the penetration panels to the magnet footing. The cables or gas lines run from the magnet footing up behind the enclosures to the tool panels. The enclosures cover only the peripheral surfaces of the magnet. The surfaces of the gap and the bore are the surfaces of the gradient coils and the cryostat to avoid unnecessary encroachment into the space in the gap between the magnets or the patient bore.

GRADIENT DESIGN

The magnet design provides the access to the patient, which is the first step in a series of advances that allow new procedures to be performed under MR guidance. The gradient design should maintain the patient access made possible by the magnet design, which is accomplished by adding a flange to the gradients to give them a top-hat shape (Fig. 3-8).[4] The current paths are continuous from the cylindrical portion of the coil onto the flange portion. This concept increases the gradient strength and provides the same linearity as a standard 0.5-T system within the 30-cm DSV, but with reduced efficiency because the gradient windings are farther from the imaging volume. In addition, the gradients are actively shielded, which reduces eddy currents in the magnet cryostat but also reduces their efficiency. The trade-off is acceptable because gradient inefficiencies can be overcome at relatively little cost, but eddy currents can significantly degrade the performance of an MRI system.

Stronger gradient amplifiers are required in this system to maintain gradient performance equivalent to that in conventional designs. However, the additional current through the coils produces more heat than desired. The gradient coils are cooled by controlled chilled water and have integrated thermocouples for monitoring internal temperature at various points on the coil. The temperature monitoring system is controlled by the workstation, which adjusts the scanning modes depending on the temperature measured in the gradient coils. The system notifies the operator if the first temperature limit is exceeded. If the second limit is exceeded, the scan in interrupted until the temperature decreases, and if the third limit is exceeded, the power to the gradient amplifiers is interrupted. This feature protects the hardware from dangerous temperatures and allows the operator to intervene and modify the scanning procedures to prevent high temperatures.

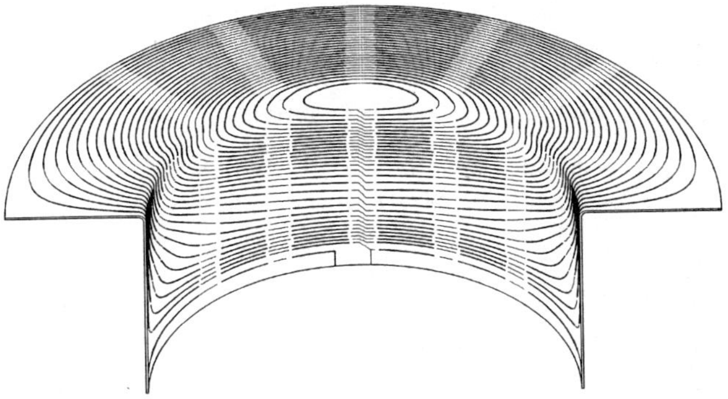

Fig. 3-8. Diagram of the open gradient coil, showing the winding pattern on one half of the top-hat–shaped structure, with continuity of the windings from the cylindrical to the flange portion.

DB/DT

The unique shape of the gradient coil and the proximity of the physician to the gradient coil in this system make it more possible for personnel to be exposed to rapidly changing magnetic fields than in a conventional MR system. Rapidly changing magnetic fields can induce nerve firings, which typically manifest as tingles or twitches in peripheral nerves or light flashes, buzzes, or random tastes in the associated sensory nerves. A computer analysis of the rate of change of the magnetic fields in the system (dB/dt) was conducted, based on the gradient coil design, and experiments were conducted to verify the accuracy of the computer model. The maximum dB/dt occurred when all three gradient axes were changing simultaneously, at a location 45° between the axial and sagittal planes and elevated approximately 45° from the coronal plane. The dB/dt cannot be limited by computing the gradient waveforms during scan plane prescription because all scan planes are possible with the interactive scan plane guidance used on the system (see below). Instead, the minimum ramp times are set to maintain dB/dt within the limits mandated by various national and international regulatory agencies (see Chapter 10).

GRADIENT PERFORMANCE SUMMARY

The gradient design provides linearity equivalent to a standard 0.5-T imager over the 30-cm DSV imaging volume, but a more powerful gradient amplifier subsystem is required to compensate for the reduced efficiency of the open gradient coils. The more powerful gradient amplifiers drive more current through the coils, necessitating gradient cooling and temperature monitoring. The gradient temperature monitoring system allows the operator to scan as desired, while protecting the gradient coil hardware from dangerous high temperatures. The dB/dt of the system was analyzed and a solution implemented to prevent dB/dt levels from exceeding regulatory guidelines in the patient- or physician-accessible volume. These factors combined provide a gradient performance equivalent to that of a standard 0.5-T scanner. Equivalent gradient performance, combined with equivalent magnet homogeneity, enabled the team to achieve the goal of providing image quality equivalent to that of a standard 0.5-T imager over the slightly reduced imaging volume of 30 cm.

GRADIENT MANUFACTURABILITY

The gradient design delivered the intended performance. However, the top-hat–shaped structure, combined with the significant currents that would be driven through the coil, required a method significantly different from the photo etching of flat copper sheets used for standard closed bore cylindrical systems. The top-hat–shaped coil can be formed by welding the flat, annular flange onto the cylindrical portion of the coil; spinning an annular flange at high speed and flaring its inside edge into a cylinder; or spinning a cylinder and flaring one end into a flange. Whichever method is used to form the structure, the current distributions are achieved by cutting the copper along specific patterns. Cutting a spiral groove in the irregularly shaped structure is difficult but can be accomplished via a computer numerically controlled water jet cutting tool.

The patented cutting process mounts the coil on a support structure, then directs the cutting tool in a direction perpendicular to the gradient coil surface.[5] The cutting process is completed in a minimum of two steps. In the first step, several sections of each groove are cut, with some distance between each section. Next, the cut portions are filled with epoxy, or holding strips are applied to maintain the spatial relationship between the runs. Additional sections of the groove are cut and subsequently fixed in place, and the process is repeated until the entire groove has been cut. If the cut length is the same as the distance between the cuts, the cutting process can be completed in two steps. More typically, the distance between the cuts is two to three times the cut length, so the process is usually complete in three to four steps. In this way, the coil does not deform during the cutting process and maintains its structural integrity. The water jet can cut through 12-inch–thick steel, which makes cutting of the 0.125-inch–thick copper sheet fairly quick. The cutting tool is very precise and can cut a groove of 0.04 inches, which allows wider runs for lower resistance or higher density of runs for a given coil area. After the cutting process, the gradient coils are filled with an epoxy composite. The epoxy composite filler suppresses noise, provides electrical isolation between the gradient runs, helps distribute the thermal load generated by the coil, and enhances the structural integrity of the entire assembly.

RADIOFREQUENCY SYSTEM

The magnet and gradient designers provided openness that would allow contact between the physician and the patient, which is unique among MR systems. The RF subsystem also had to maintain this openness, so a standard birdcage-style body coil was not an option. Furthermore, the gradient and magnet designs can achieve excellent uniformity and linearity, respectively, within the 30-cm DSV imaging volume. However, outside that volume, the homogeneity and linearity degrade more quickly than is typical of standard imaging systems.

Superposition of the gradient fields on the inhomogeneous B_0 field produces aliased fields, in which the field strength is the same in different portions of the patient space. If a large body coil is used for imaging in the system, uncontrolled wrap-around artifacts could occur.

The disadvantages of a body coil are overcome by developing a series of transmit/receive (T/R) flexible surface coils. The coil set includes simple loop, rectangular, and Helmholtz pair (a figure 8 shape)–type coils in various sizes. The various coils included in the system allow many imaging applications to be conducted on every anatomic region. The coils are constructed with minimal mechanical cross section, so surgical procedures can be performed through the coils.

The RF monitoring and control system is modified to accommodate the use of the T/R surface coils. MRI systems generally control the amount of RF energy that can be deposited in the patient's body. Regulatory agencies provide guidelines for whole-body average and peak specific absorption ratios (SAR). In this system, the lack of a body coil and the relatively low power levels required at 0.5 T combine to virtually eliminate whole-body SAR as a relevant limit. However, the proximity of the transmit coil to the patient can produce higher levels of peak SAR delivered into the worst-case gram of tissue than found with a whole-body birdcage coil. Thus, each coil was tested independently, and the power level that produced a peak SAR of 7.5 W/kg for the coil under worst case conditions, was determined. This precaution ensures that the system always operates with an appropriate safety buffer.

Magnets, gradient coils and amplifiers, and RF coils and amplifiers are parts of every MR imaging system; they needed to be radically redesigned for the new intraoperative imaging applications. Although the applications were new, the function of these systems remained essentially the same: acquire the best possible images. However, hardware and software not previously used on MR systems were required to enable the new and unique procedures as envisioned by the program team.

REAL-TIME SOFTWARE CONTROL

First, real-time scanning software that allowed an infinite number of single slice images to be acquired was developed. Scan plane orientation needed to be changed with one button click, and arbitrary offsets from the isocenter were required. These adjustments were implemented via sliders or text fields (Fig. 3-9). The ability to change the slice thickness in real-time was provided to facilitate rapid target localization. Dynamic slice-thickness changes were limited to the original slice thickness or to larger values to simplify gradient waveform calculations. Dynamic control of receiver gain was also provided, for the situations in which the signal level varied significantly between various dynamically prescribed slices. Finally, an automatic averaging mode was implemented, so if multiple images are acquired from the same location, the operator can automatically average these images. In this way, if the operator finds an optimum slice, the displayed image quality improves the longer that slice is imaged. The operator can choose to average up to eight images from one location. If the location remains constant beyond the value selected by the user, the most recent images are averaged using a rolling average approach.

INTERACTIVE SCAN GUIDANCE

Another key component for surgical guidance is the Flashpoint™ (Image-Guided Technologies, Boulder, Colo) optical tracking subsystem, which serves as a major interface between the operator and the system. The tracking subsystem allows a point-and-shoot approach to MR and is based on the concept of a handpiece together with a "needle." A handpiece is an arbitrarily shaped device with two or more light-emitting diodes (LEDs) (Fig. 3-10). A computer profile of the handpiece, to-

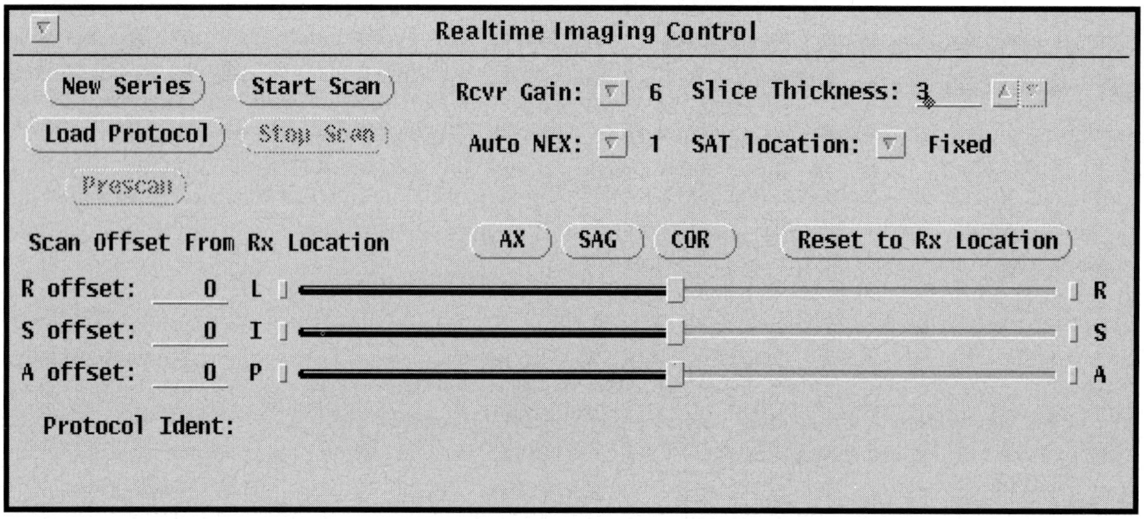

Fig. 3-9. Real-time Scan Guidance interface, showing variables such as position, orientation, and slice thickness, which can be controlled in real-time. (Courtesy of GE Medical Systems, Milwaukee, Wis.)

gether with the needle length, relates the LED positions to the trajectory and tip of a needle. The handpiece is selected from a list, and the needle length associated with the handpiece is also entered. The subsystem operates by optically locating the infrared LEDs that are built into the handpiece. The optical system first compares the LED positions to the handpiece computer profile to determine if the handpiece matches that selected by the user. If so, the needle tip position, the needle trajectory vector, and a transverse normal vector are calculated. The optical system communicates the tip position and the vectors to the computer workstation via a serial line.

Interactive scan guidance software was designed to exploit optical tracking and real-time imaging capabilities. The interactive scan guidance software allows handpiece-guided MR scanning to resemble hand-held ultrasound scanning. The workstation uses the needle tip position, the needle trajectory vector, and the transverse normal vector provided by the optical system to determine the magnet coordinates of the needle tip. A calibration procedure is executed during system installation, which relates the optical coordinates to the magnet coordinates. This calibration procedure only needs to be done once and remains constant regardless of the patient position or orientation. The interactive scan guidance capability can be used any time the handpiece is in the field of view (FOV) of the Flashpoint™ cameras (Fig. 3-11). Intraprocedural verification processes allow the physician to rapidly and graphically verify the validity of the calibration.

This capability was further exploited to enable automatic scan-plane prescriptions to be determined by the position of the handpiece. In the most straightforward mode, axial, sagittal,

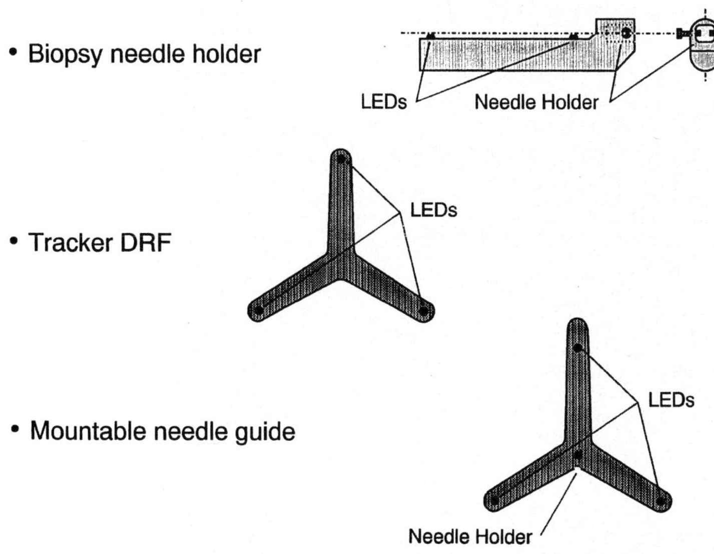

Fig. 3-10. Two handpieces used for interactive scan guidance.

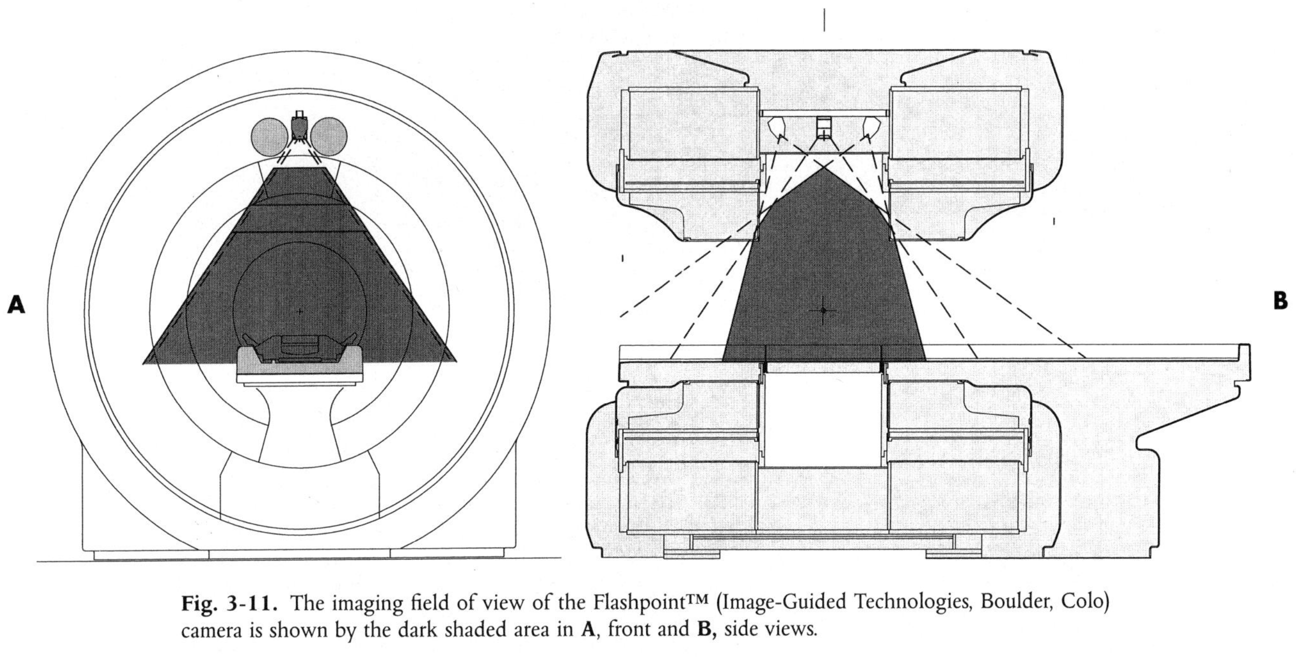

Fig. 3-11. The imaging field of view of the Flashpoint™ (Image-Guided Technologies, Boulder, Colo) camera is shown by the dark shaded area in **A**, front and **B**, side views.

and coronal scans can automatically be obtained, with the center of the image at the needle tip. In a different mode, images referenced to the needle trajectory are possible with in-plane modes that scan along the axis of the needle. Image planes that are predominantly vertical (in-plane 90° or − 90°) or horizontal (in-plane 0°) are possible, with arbitrary rotation angles possible via text field entry (Fig. 3-12). Annotation is added to the image to represent the calculated needle position and the needle trajectory. In addition, a perpendicular or "archer's view" for scanning is possible. The slice can be "slid up and down the needle" by entering a value in the Offset field on the Interactive Scan Guidance graphical user interface. This approach enables the physician to scan ahead of the needle to verify what tissue will be intersected as the needle is advanced. In this mode, the needle annotation is a cursor with a variable shape, depending on the tip's position relative to the slice. If the needle tip is in the slice, the cursor appears as an X. If the tip is proximal to the slice, the cursor appears as an □ and if the tip is distal to the slice, the cursor appears as an ⊠ (Fig. 3-13).

A modified version of the in-plane modes are the single-angle oblique modes. In these modes, the image plane is rotated around an axis until the needle trajectory is captured in the image plane, but the image plane is not rotated to make the needle trajectory parallel to the image axis. In this mode, the needle will usually appear to enter the image at an angle. The in-plane modes always have the needle entering the image from

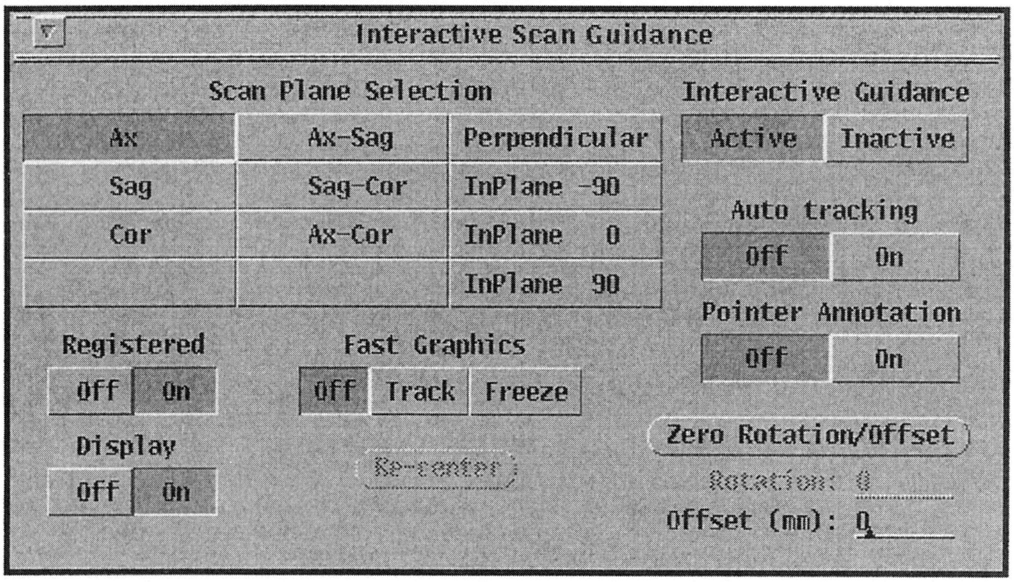

Fig. 3-12. Interactive Scan Guidance graphical user interface, showing the buttons that allow rapid transitions between scan-plane orientations; rotation and offset values are input via text fields in the lower right corner. (Courtesy of GE Medical Systems, Milwaukee, Wis.)

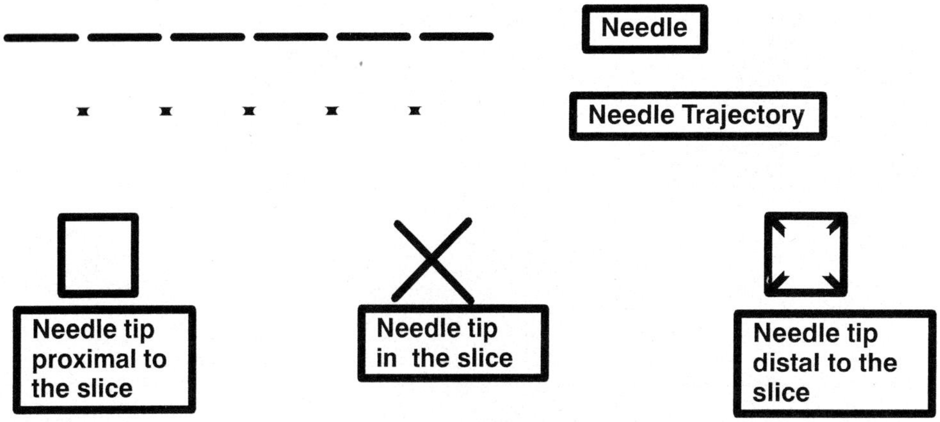

Fig. 3-13. Annotation representing the position of the needle tip and needle trajectory relative to the displayed slice.

the top of the FOV. The operator can switch from the various in-plane modes to the single-angle oblique modes to the orthogonal planes with one button click. This allows 10 scan-plane orientations to be selected from one handpiece position, a significant improvement from the single scan plane selected with one ultrasound transducer position.

All interactive modes function by reading the needle vectors and tip position, adding any offsets entered by the user and imaging at that location. New position data are continually acquired during initial image data acquisition; and when all data are acquired, the system uses the most recent position data to determine where the second image should be acquired. Reconstruction and display of the initial image occur while acquisition of the second image starts. Annotation of the needle location at the start of the initial image is superimposed on the image after reconstruction. This annotation can be "burned into the image," replacing the image pixels if desired. In this mode, a delay occurs between the actual needle position and the displayed needle position. If the image is a fast gradient echo scan, the delay can be as little as 1 sec. However, if longer imaging times are used for improved image quality, the delay can be significant. This delay was deemed acceptable because the annotation represented the reason for the location of the image, and the needle position at the initiation of the scan was the only needle position guaranteed to have a reliable relationship with the image.

However, the delay was inappropriate for some modes of operation, so an alternative mode was added to accelerate the needle annotation update rate. In this fast graphics mode, the needle annotation superimposed on the image is updated at the needle position update rate of four times per sec. This advantage allows the physician to immediately see the relationship between the handpiece position and the displayed slice and to relocate the handpiece position accordingly.

VIDEO SYSTEM

The need to display images inside the magnet is implicit. The system is equipped with two in-bore displays mounted on articulating arms, so they can be positioned on either side of the patient space or put on one side. The displays are 6.4-inch (diagonal) liquid crystal displays with a resolution of 640 × 480, driven by NTSC or PAL video. The system is also equipped with three video monitors mounted in the control area. The video sources for all of these displays include a camera immediately above the imaging volume; two magnet room, wall-mounted cameras; a video cassette recorder; the scanner console monitor; and the output of a screen capture system that allows a segment of the workstation screen to be seen as video. The workstation screen capture is usually used to view the real-time images that are displayed on the workstation but not on the scanner console. Additional video sources can be added to the system, so outside video sources (e.g., endoscopic video, patient monitor video) can be displayed on the screens.

The entire video system is controlled by a video router that allows any of 16 inputs to be piped to any of 16 outputs. The video router is controlled from the workstation (Fig. 3-14). The

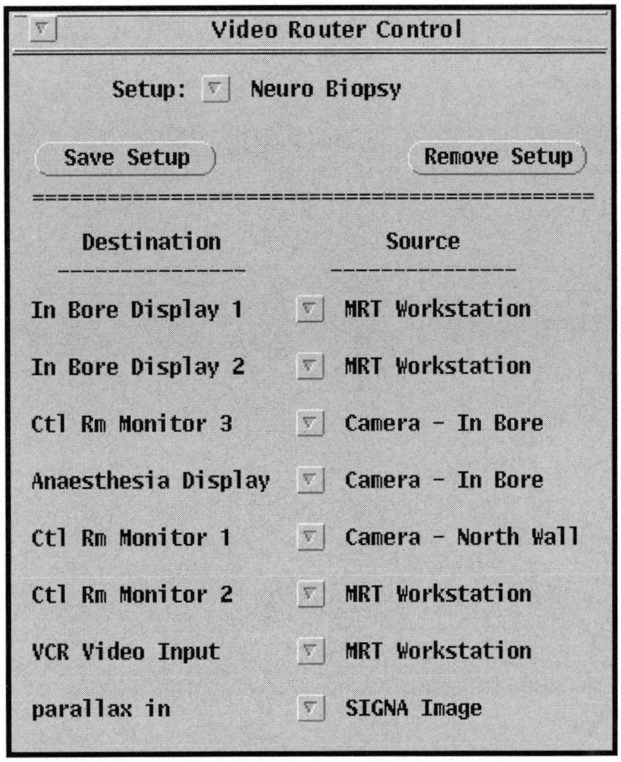

Fig. 3-14. The video router user interface, showing possible inputs and outputs. Any input can be connected to any output. (Courtesy of GE Medical Systems, Milwaukee, Wis.)

software allows preset combinations to be labeled and loaded with one button click, so transitions from neurosurgery cases to endoscopic cases to orthopedic cases do not require extensive setting changes. The video system also can control and drive additional displays at remote locations. One institution has exploited this capability to create a remote video-equipped conference room for visitors to view procedures. The conference room has several monitors and a computer, which is connected to the workstation and controls the monitors in the conference room only, preventing observers from accidentally changing the physician's display. The visitors use the computer to select which video source is displayed on their monitors, often selecting a wall camera to observe the dynamics of the surgical personnel, the in-bore camera to observe the surgical field, and the workstation monitor to review the real-time images as they are acquired. This set-up reduces crowding in the magnet room while allowing many persons to view the new and unique procedures performed in these systems.

SAMPLE CLINICAL CASES

The types of cases performed with this system are constantly increasing, but several examples can show the advantages of the system for the physician. One case shows how intraoperative images without the real-time or interactive guidance capabilities of the system can improve a procedure. A 21-year-old woman with no significant medical history presented with a new onset of generalized seizures. A small lesion, which enhanced with gadolinium, and an associated cyst were found in the mesial left temporal lobe (Fig. 3-15, *A*). Image-guided resection with intraoperative MRI was performed (Fig. 3-15, *B*). These images were valuable because the tumor was clearly discrete on MR but was barely discernible from normal brain by visual or tactile discrimination.

The configuration of the magnet makes certain procedures possible, such as weight-bearing spine studies (Fig. 3-16). In a 30-year-old man with a several-month history of severe back and right L_5-S_1 pain after a fall, conventional MRI in a supine position with knees bent showed a small disk bulge at L_5-S_1 without evidence of thecal sac or nerve root compression. Conservative management did not relieve the patient's pain. Images acquired in the vertical gap system with the patient seated under normal physiologic axial load and with extension of the spine showed disk herniation, with repeatable pain. Conventional microdiscectomy showed a markedly boggy and bulging disk, and several prominent free fragments were removed. The patient is currently pain-free with no medications and is back at work.

These novel patient positioning possibilities are creating many unique diagnostic applications beyond loaded spine. Orthopedic surgeons and radiologists are doing range-of-motion studies on various joints; software was added to the system to automatically annotate an image with a joint angle to facilitate these studies. The ability to manipulate a joint while imaging represents a new, potentially valuable weapon in an orthopedic surgeon's arsenal. Stress studies with the patient exercising in the magnet are also possible with the system. Many studies in which gravity is a factor (e.g., female incontinence studies), can benefit from the unique patient positioning possibilities. Interactive scan guidance capabilities have been used in some applications to maintain the image plane through the anatomy of interest despite patient motion. The continuous imaging capabilities have also been invaluable in certain applications. The openness of the system has allowed imaging of severe claustro-

A

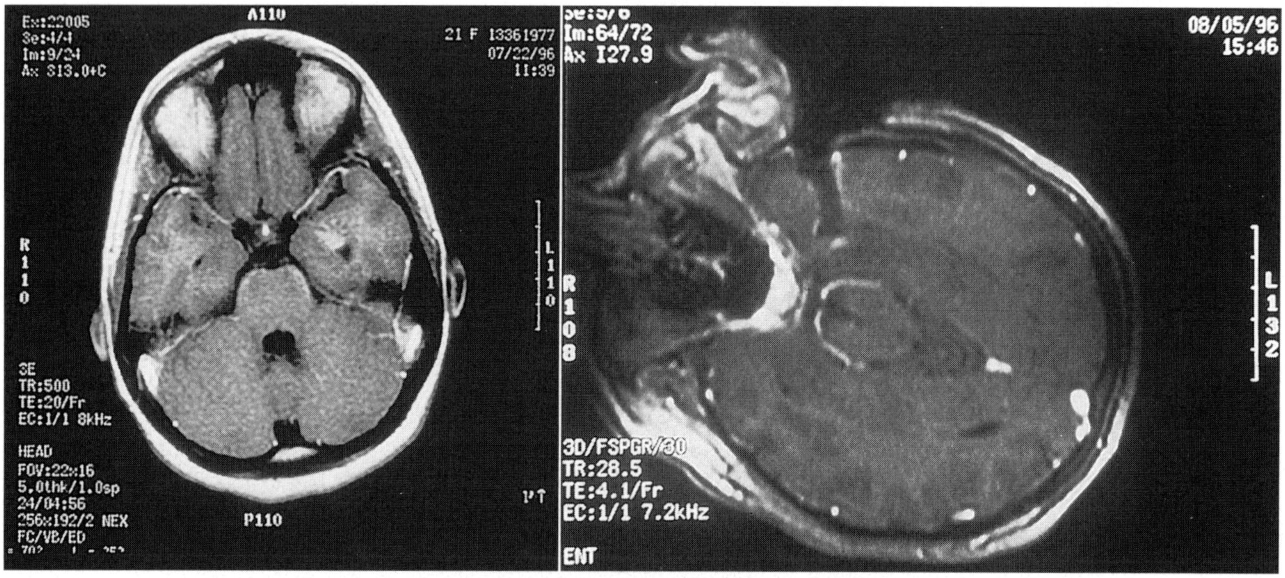

B

Fig. 3-15. A, Preoperative axial image from a 1.5-T magnetic resonance scanner, showing the mass and cyst in the left temporal lobe. **B**, T1-weighted, gadolinium-enhanced, intraoperative image acquired during the resection. (Courtesy of Thomas M. Moriarty, M.D. and Peter M. Black, M.D., Ph.D.)

phobics, and the MR-compatible equipment installed in the magnet room has led some institutions to use the system for general anesthesia cases. These examples show how original diagnostic applications have successfully exploited many features motivated by surgical applications. The diagnostic application potential of the system has not been exploited fully and may yield clinical information not attainable with present system configurations.

DISCUSSION

The development of an MR system optimized for guidance of minimally invasive surgical procedures has been motivated by a range of healthcare issues and enabled by various technological advancements. Cost pressures have been moving standard surgical procedures to minimally invasive procedures to reduce length of stay and the total cost of the procedure. Advances in computer technology, surgical instrumentation technology, MR compatibility of various clinical systems, and

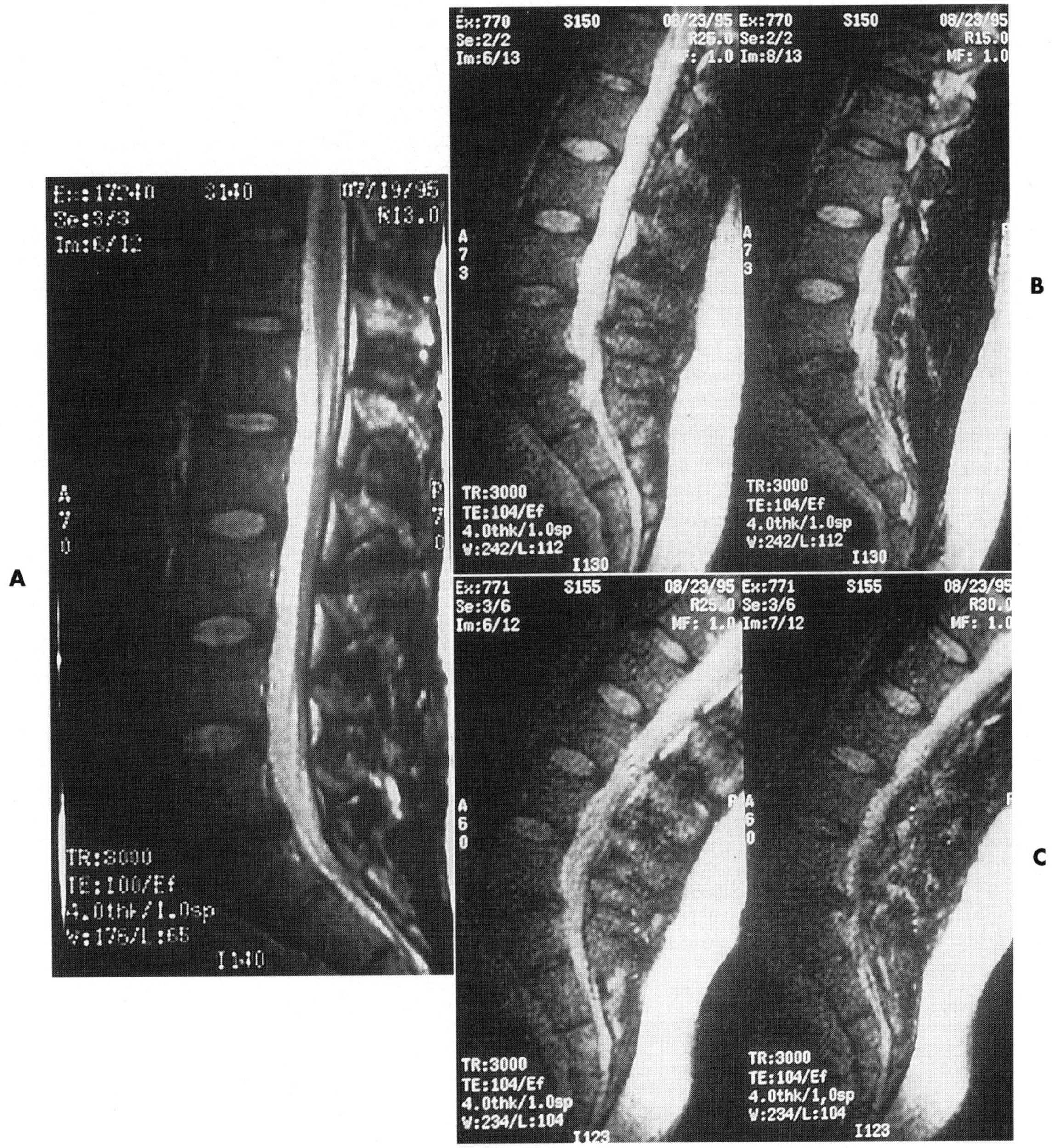

Fig. 3-16. A, A midsagittal T2-weighted image from a conventional 0.5-T scanner. **B** and **C**, T2-weighted midsagittal and right parasagittal loaded spine images in a sitting-neutral **(B)** and a sitting-extended **(C)** position. Notice the disk herniation with extension in the right parasagittal image. (**A** and **B**, Courtesy of Thomas M. Moriarty, M.D., Eric J. Woodard, M.D., and Amir A. Zamani, M.D.)

minimally invasive therapy contributed to the evolution of the field. The improved visualization possible with this intraoperative MR system will do more than enable the conversion of standard clinical procedures to minimally invasive procedures. It is anticipated that the system will enhance the safety and efficacy of today's procedures and facilitate the development of new procedures that have not been conceived.

The several sites around the world that have been working with these systems have produced more anecdotal reports on the advances and improved outcomes possible with the system. Publications detailing the improvements are available, the number of presentations about the system by international groups is growing, and the variety of procedures being done with the system is rapidly expanding. The rate of MR-compatible instrumentation and device development is constantly increasing as the demand for such instruments escalates and the instrument manufacturers more fully appreciate this developing market. These advances enable even more rapid development of new applications and cohesive multisite trials. As with most new technologies, reimbursement has lagged behind procedure development, but recent movement in this area has been encouraging.

Significant challenges remain. Formal outcomes studies that clearly delineate the advantages of the approach should be completed. Additional features to improve speed of procedures may be incorporated into the system. Enhanced integration and registration of preoperative images from many modalities with intraoperative images may further improve the operative use of the system. Improved imaging speed, contrast, and resolution may enable even more procedures than currently possible, allowing the physician to target smaller lesions in sites considered inoperable. More MR-compatible instruments are required to attempt procedures that cannot currently be done. These advances and many others will help usher in 21st Century medicine.

CONCLUSIONS

The design requirements of this system represented a marked departure from standard diagnostic MR system design, and a fresh approach was necessary to meet the challenge. All major components of the system—magnet, gradient, patient handling, RF, and computer—experienced a major redesign. Creative approaches used the latest technology and radical designs to make a quantum leap in MR system capabilities. Significant technologic advancements allowed designers to create a system with unparalleled patient access, a colocated imaging volume and working volume, interactive scan-plane prescription capabilities, and the ancillary functions required by a complete surgical team, all based on a standard MRI platform that can exploit subsequent advances in MR physics and technology. Many of these features may be found alone on other systems, but the combination of features is truly the strength of this unique system. This system has been designed to enhance the safety and quality of today's procedures and to provide a framework for the development of tomorrow's procedures. This system could foster the birth of a new modality and establish a new standard of care against which other systems will be measured.

REFERENCES

1. Hutchinson JMS, and others: A whole-body NMR imaging machine, *J Phys E Sci Instrum* 13:947, 1980.
2. Gronemeyer DHW, Seibel RMM, Kaufman L: Interventional MRI cracks device and design barriers, *Diagnostic Imaging International* Nov/Dec: 32, 1990.
3. Havens TJ, Smith RS: *Open architecture magnetic resonance imaging superconducting magnet assembly,* US patent #5696476.
4. Barber WD, Roemer PB, Rohling KW: *Open gradient coils for magnetic resonance,* US patent #5378989.
5. Repinski GA, Kinsey KE, Meyers CC: *Method for fabricating open MR magnet gradient coil,* US patent #5638595.

Chapter 4

A PROPOSED NEW MAGNET DESIGN FOR MR–GUIDED SURGERY AT 0.6 TESLA

Gordon Danby, John Linardos, Jevan Damadian, Jay Dworkin, Raymond V. Damadian

A new design concept has been proposed for a magnetic resonance imaging (MRI) magnet that will improve patient accessibility for MRI-guided surgery and minimally invasive therapy. The FONAR-360° MRI (FONAR Corporation, Melville, NY) uses a magnetic field strength of 0.6 T to provide the high resolution and imaging speed required to meet the demands of MR-guided surgery.[1]

DESIGN

Two magnetic poles are positioned at the center of a full-size room in this new design (Fig. 4-1). The walls and ceiling of the room provide an iron flux return to channel the magnetic field into the imaging volume where the patient is positioned. This design also minimizes the fringe magnetic field. The room dimensions are large enough to accommodate an entire surgical team. The ceiling height is a standard 8 feet, the room width is 14 feet, and the length is effectively unlimited. The iron-core vertical field electromagnet produces an imaging field strength of 0.6 T.

BENEFITS

This design has numerous benefits:

- The attending medical team will have improved access to the patient in a relatively magnetic field–free environment (Fig. 4-2).
- The surgical team can use much of the hardware now customary in standard operating rooms.
- Lateral decubitus positioning is possible (Fig. 4-3) because the vertical pole-to-pole gap dimension is 20 inches (51 cm). The increased imaging volume expands the range of potential MR-guided surgical applications.
- A special in-gap fully rotatable bed will allow the patient to be positioned at any height and any angle (Fig. 4-4) to meet the surgeon's specific needs and preferences during numerous procedures.
- The surgical team will be able to easily view in-room monitors and projection systems to reference the images, which are rapidly updated during the procedure (Fig. 4-5).

This design also uses a vertical magnetic field transverse to the patient axis (Fig. 4-6). From the earliest days of MRI, this magnetic field orientation allowed life-support and monitoring equipment to be placed next to the magnet because of the negligible fringe field (Fig. 4-7). The hazardous missile effect inherent in the solenoidal magnet design of typical superconducting MRI scanners (whereby loose ferromagnetic objects

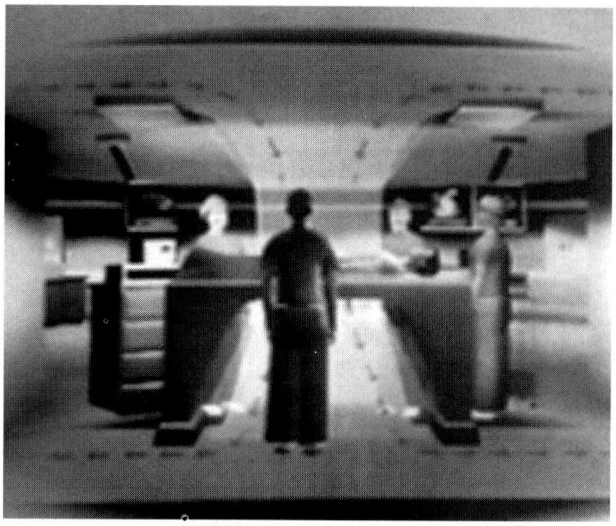

Fig. 4-1. Elevation view showing magnetic field lines.

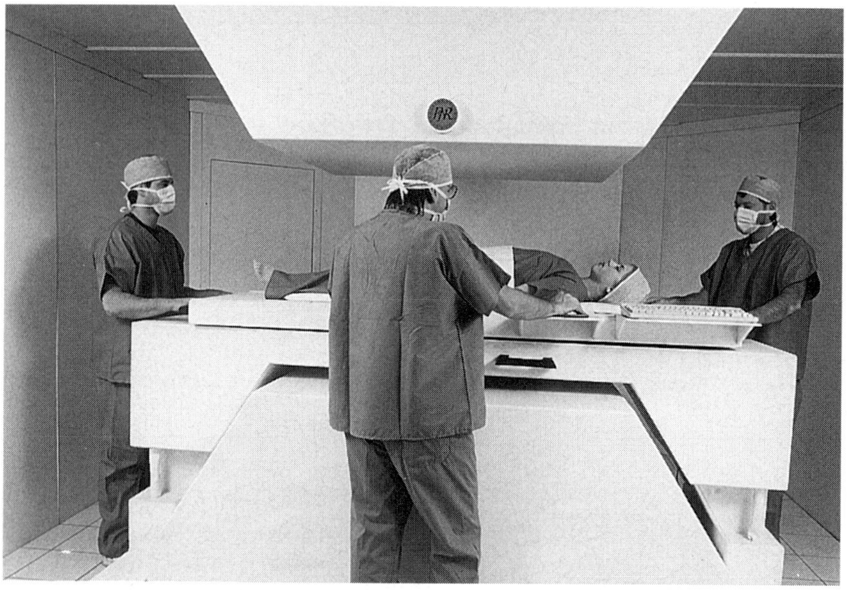

Fig. 4-2. Improved access for the surgical team.

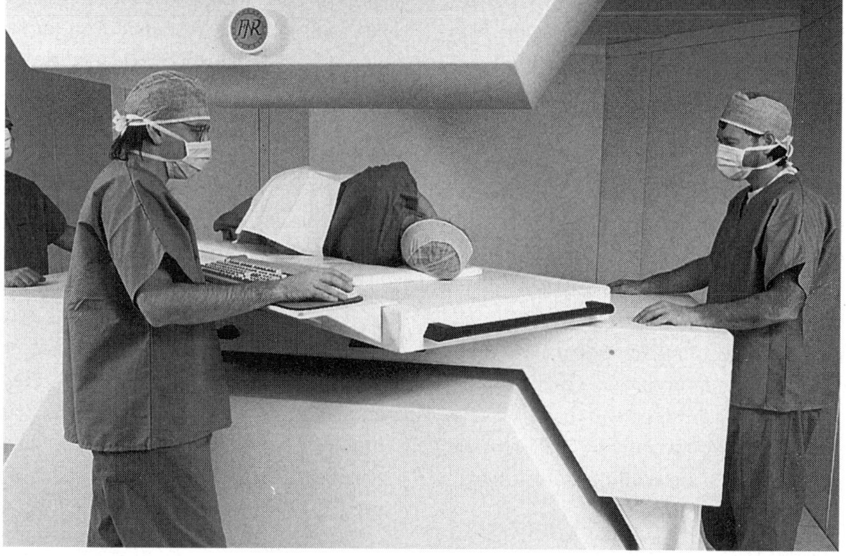

Fig. 4-3. Lateral decubitus positioning.

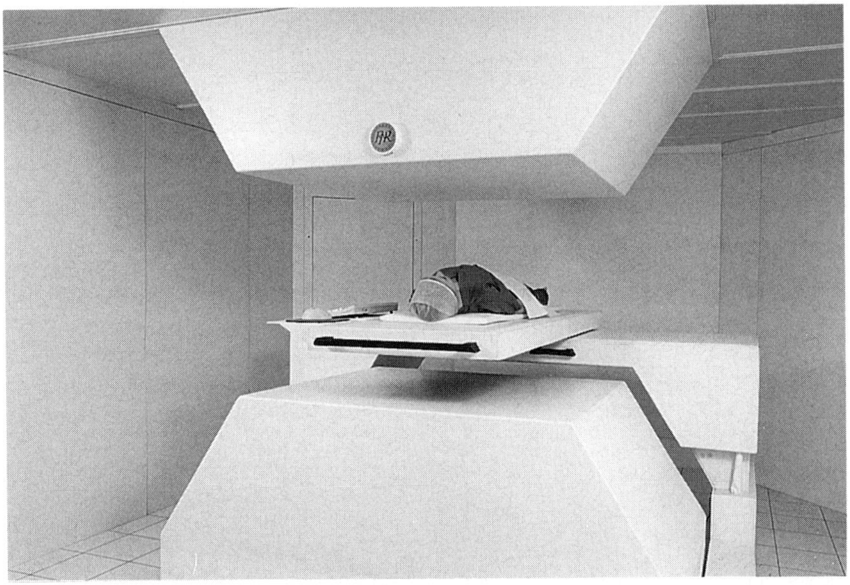

Fig. 4-4. In-gap fully rotatable patient bed.

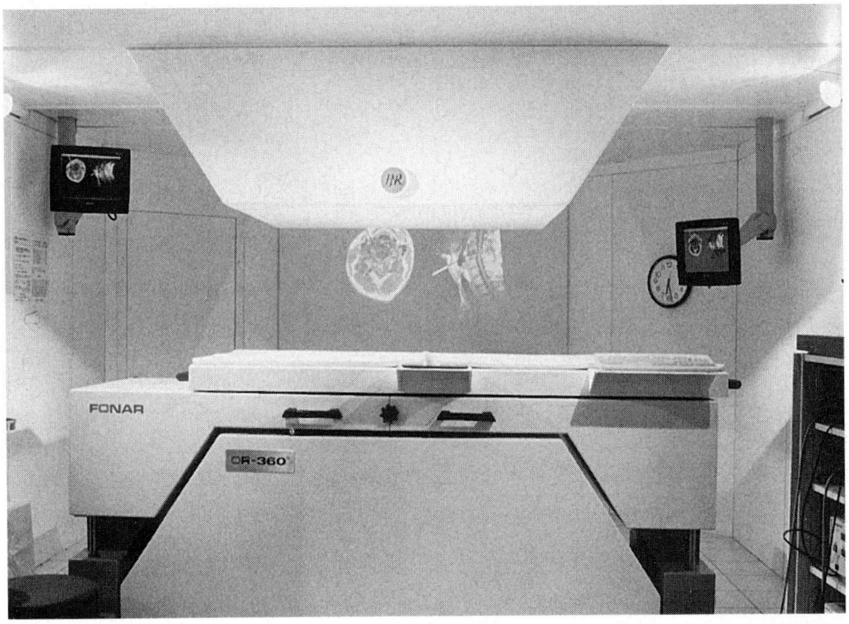

Fig. 4-5. Monitors and projection system for image visualization during procedures.

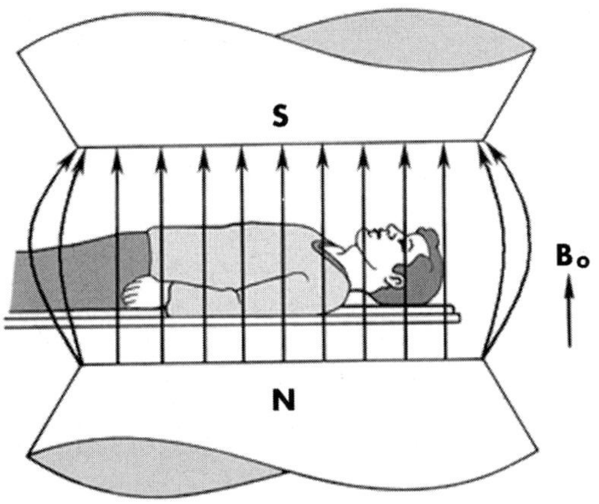

Fig. 4-6. Vertical magnetic field orientation.

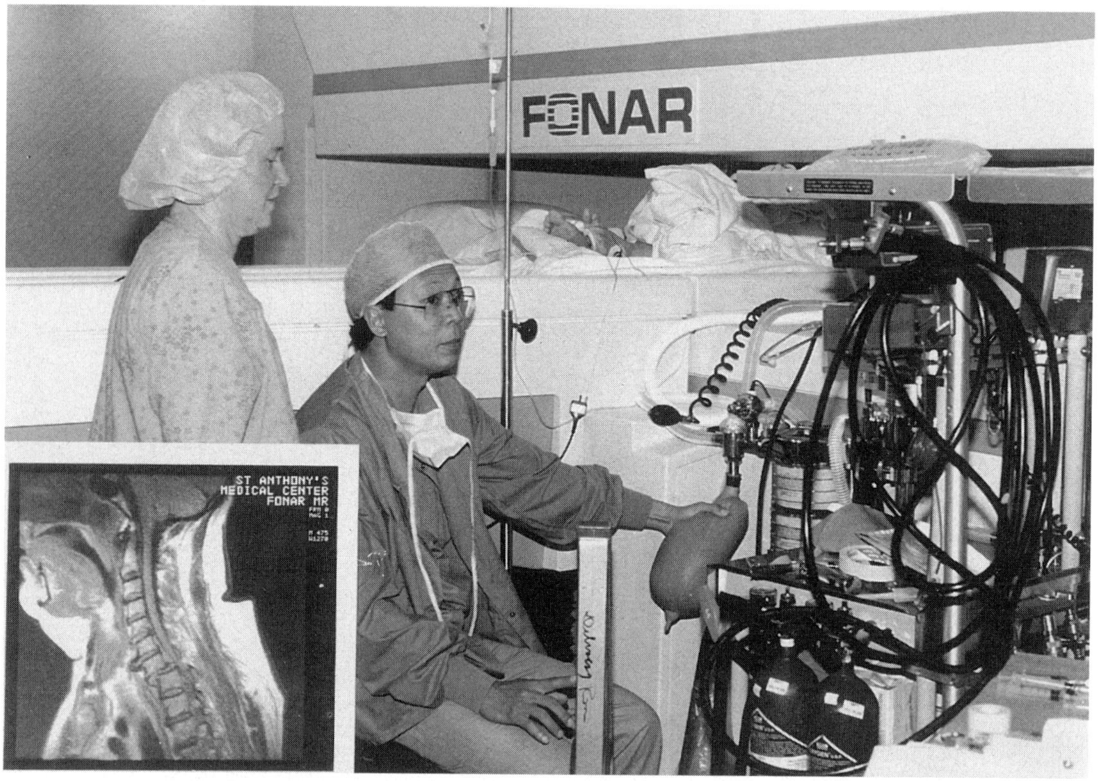

Fig. 4-7. Early open magnetic resonance imaging from the mid-1980s. (Courtesy of University of California, Los Angeles Medical Center. Inset Courtesy of St. Anthony's Medical Center, New York.)

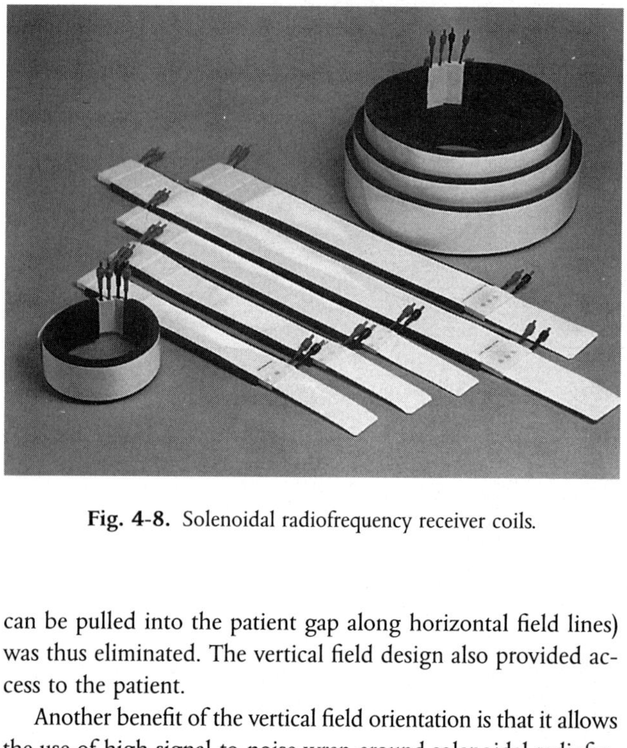

Fig. 4-8. Solenoidal radiofrequency receiver coils.

can be pulled into the patient gap along horizontal field lines) was thus eliminated. The vertical field design also provided access to the patient.

Another benefit of the vertical field orientation is that it allows the use of high signal-to-noise wrap-around solenoidal radiofrequency (RF) receiver coils.[2] Because patients are cylindrically symmetric, manufacturing coils with a wide range of circumferences provide high-performance RF receivers for nearly all anatomic MRI applications (Fig. 4-8). Any body part can be imaged with an optimal filling factor and a uniform signal intensity profile.[3] The patient surface area covered by the coils is also relatively small, so the surgeon will have increased flexibility in planning a target trajectory with MR-compatible surgical instruments. Specialized receiver coils can be constructed in an open fashion to facilitate MRI guidance (Fig. 4-9).

The new FONAR-360° design configuration is based on the capabilities of the 0.6-T QUAD™ 12000 Open MRI system (FONAR Corporation, Melville, NY) (Fig. 4-10). This state-of-the-art diagnostic MRI scanner, a recent generation iron-core vertical field electromagnet introduced in 1995, provides a large vertical gap and four-sided physician access to the patient.[4] The four-post construction in the magnet yields superior mechanical stability and uses symmetric flux coupling to achieve high field strength (0.6 T) with an open MR design.

The already substantial range of access to the patient for interventional procedures in the QUAD™ system is enhanced in the FONAR-360° design by moving the main magnet coils further from the pole surfaces and positioning them under the floor and above the ceiling of the operating room. However, many advantages of the QUAD™ MRI scanners exist in the FONAR-360° design:

- The gradients are constructed in a flat (planar) package that bolts to the surface of the immovable poles. This construction results in a dramatic reduction in the amount of

A

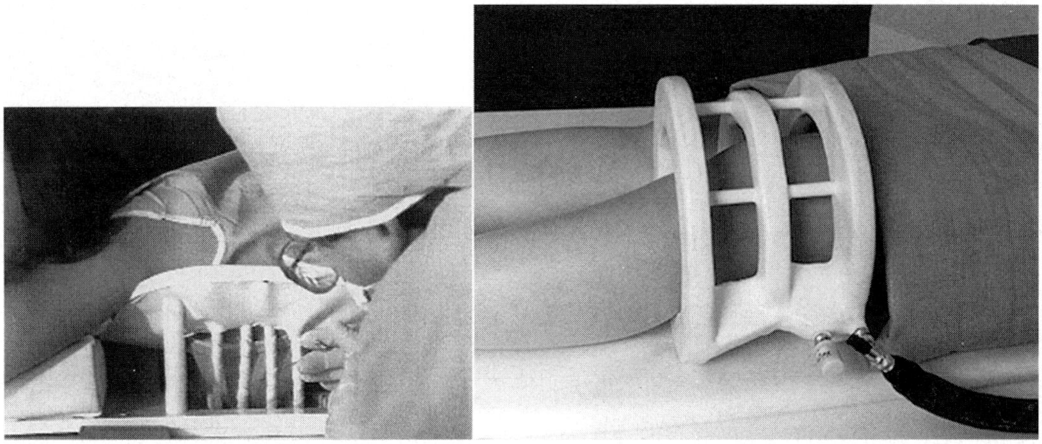

B

Fig. 4-9. **A,** Bilateral prone dedicated breast coil and **B,** knee coil.

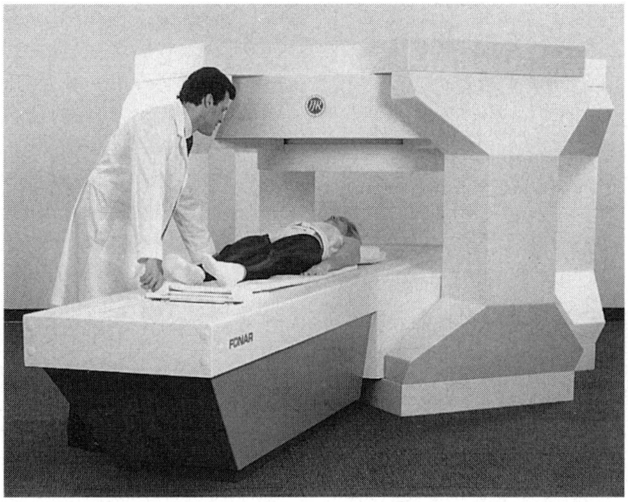

Fig. 4-10. 0.6-T QUAD™ 12000 MRI System (FONAR Corporation, Melville, NY).

A 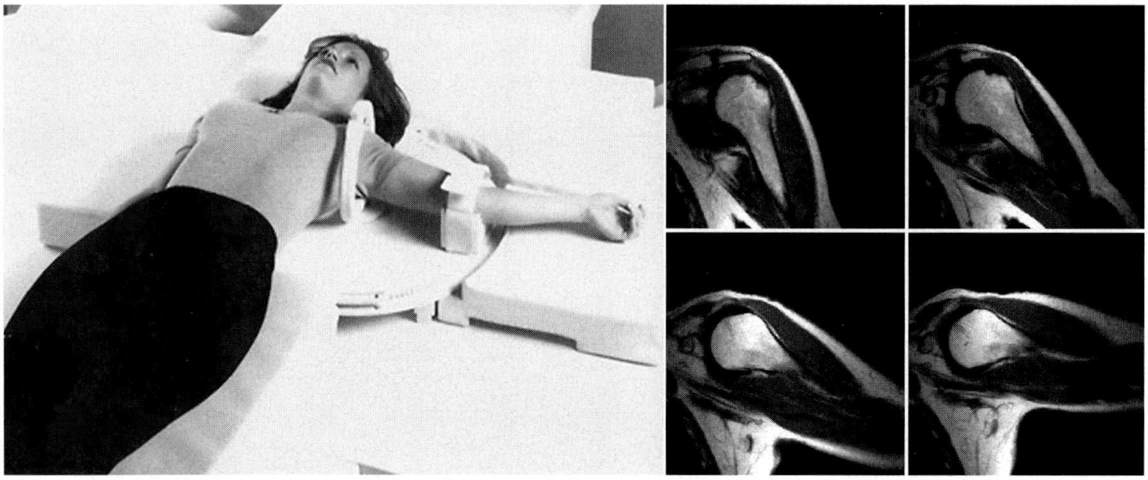 B

Fig. 4-11. Computer-controlled orthopedic fixture and resulting kinematic magnetic resonance imaging study. **A,** Device in place with patient. **B,** Resulting images.

acoustic noise, which would otherwise distract the patient and the MR interventionalist.

- A flat RF transmitter maximizes the available gap and the pole surface without restricting the placement of orthopedic fixtures for large range-of-motion computer-controlled kinematic studies (Fig. 4-11).
- An independent image display workstation using a 300-MHz Pentium II processor is integrated into a dual-screen technologist console (Fig. 4-12). The 1280 × 1024 pixel high-resolution display monitor can simultaneously display up to 20 (256 × 256) images. Advanced features include a mouse-controlled real-time continuous zoom and cine paging. The Windows NT operating system provides network compatibility and direct data transfer to satellite consoles. The workstation also supports interactive control of three-dimensional processing and advanced visualization techniques, such as surface renderings (Fig. 4-13) useful for surgical planning.

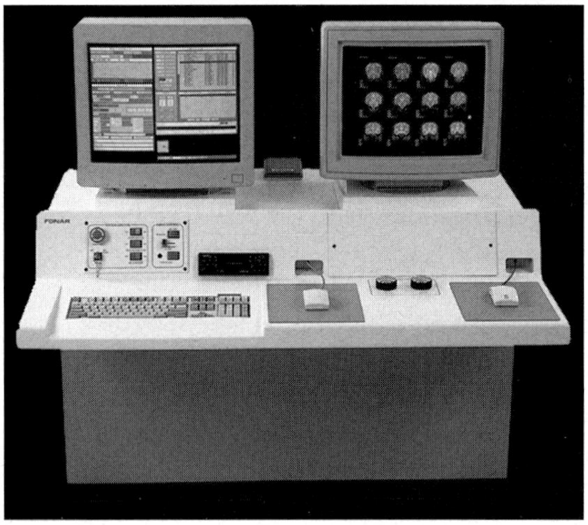

Fig. 4-12. Dual-screen technologist console.

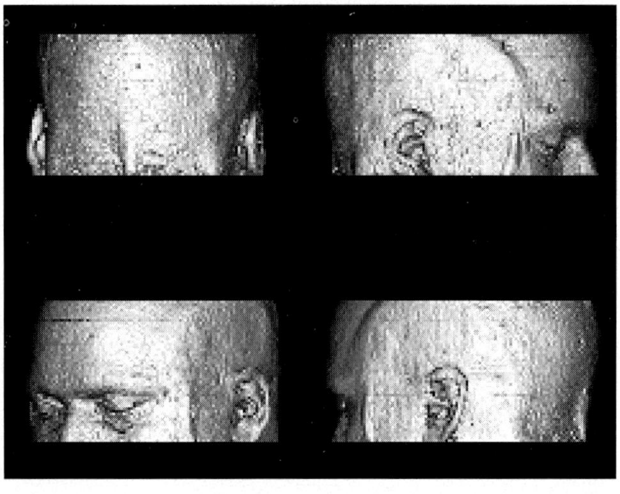

Fig. 4-13. Advanced visualization techniques useful for surgical planning include surface renderings calculated by segmenting a voxel data set.

SUMMARY

The realization of MR-guided surgery and minimally invasive therapy has been impeded by important physical limitations imposed by the designs of many current diagnostic open MRI systems. A new MRI design eliminates many restrictions and will provide the surgical team with improved patient accessibility.

REFERENCES

1. Krotz D: Interventional MR pricey, but occupies unique role, *Diagnostic Imaging* April, 1998.
2. Stark D: The argument for mid-field MRI, *Applied Radiology* February: 9, 1995.
3. Lufkin R, and others: Solenoid surface coils in MRI, *Am J Roentgenol* 146:409, 1986.
4. Pomeranz SJ: Rising to the challenge: a fresh look at open MR, *CMRS Vision* 2:5, 1996.

Chapter 5

HIGH-FIELD INTERVENTIONAL MR SYSTEM FOR NEUROLOGIC APPLICATIONS

Alastair J. Martin, Joop J. van Vaals

Magnetic resonance imaging (MRI) has become prominent over the past 15 years, principally as a result of its versatility and ability to discriminate soft tissue. Two-dimensional (2D) and three-dimensional (3D) acquisitions can be performed at arbitrary orientations and with many image contrasts. Additionally, MR has shown many advantages over anatomic mapping, including the ability to obtain angiographic data, perform quantitative flow measurements, assess functional parameters (e.g., perfusion, brain activation), perform localized spectroscopic analysis, and quantitatively assess temperature changes. This diversity in capabilities is not rivalled by any other imaging modality.

Although MR was originally targeted at neurologic applications, technical developments reducing MR's sensitivity to motion led to the development of abdominal, extremity, and even cardiac MR examinations. Areas previously considered inaccessible with MR (e.g., bone[1] and lung imaging)[2] are being pursued with some success, and MR is moving from strictly preoperative to intraoperative assessment.

Advantages

The capabilities that facilitated the growth of MR for diagnostic imaging make it attractive for interventional applications. The quality of data and breadth of MR capabilities are the driving forces behind the desire to use MR as a tool in interventional procedures. The success of interventional MR requires that it improve the efficiency or effectiveness of the therapy provided or that it allow procedures to be performed that would otherwise be impossible.[3] Economic considerations are more relevant to the former rather than the latter requirement.

Incorporation of MR into an interventional forum is sufficiently difficult and expensive that a clear clinical benefit (in terms of reduced morbidity, better prognosis, or shorter procedures) should be shown. The addition of an archive of intraoperative pictures is not justified if gains are only marginal in these areas. This chapter focuses on some early neurologic applications and assesses the value that interventional MR brings to each procedure (see below).

Another significant advantage of MR is that it does not require ionizing radiation. X-ray dose, although of minimal concern for many routine applications, can be of concern to patients undergoing long involved procedures.[4,5] The occupational dose accumulated by interventionists is also of concern. The principal safety concerns in interventional MR relate to projectiles in the static magnetic field and radiofrequency (RF) energy, switched magnetic fields, and acoustic noise exposure (see Chapter 10). Careful suite planning and monitoring minimize the potential for projectiles, and ear protection limits acoustic noise. Switched magnetic fields and RF exposure are limited by United States Food and Drug Administration (FDA) guidelines, and no significant health risk has been associated with this level of exposure. Thus, MR provides many diagnostic and therapeutic benefits in a manner that is safe to the patient and clinician.

System requirements

The ideal interventional MR scanner would provide the full capabilities of a state-of-the-art diagnostic scanner but would not encumber the interventionist or create a risk of high RF or switched magnetic field exposure. However, these desires are conflicting, and compromises must be made in some of these desired aspects. Of critical importance is the ability to obtain MR images with good tissue discrimination in a timely fashion. To achieve this goal, acceptable gradient linearity and static field homogeneity should be maintained over the imaging volume. Additionally, the raw signal-to-noise ratio (SNR) and pulse sequence capabilities of the scanner should permit high temporal resolution scanning with various image contrasts. Interactive control of the location and orientation of the scan plane may be required to efficiently guide and monitor the procedure.

Also, patient access should permit the interventionist to safely perform the procedure. When MR is not performed, it is implied that the patient should be easily removed from the scanner or that the scanner be sufficiently open to permit the full range of equipment and personnel to be brought to the patient. When intraoperative MR scanning is to be performed, a limited subset of equipment and personnel should typically be allowed access to the patient. An acceptable level of access depends on the procedure being performed and the expectations of healthcare providers. The physical configuration of the ideal interventional MR system is poorly defined; only when the clinical use of interventional MR is determined is the optimal system likely to be realized.

Finally, the MR environment should be compatible with the requirements of more conventional interventional suites. Sufficient space and access should be incorporated into the interventional MR suite to accommodate additional staff and equipment. Creation of a sterile environment within the suite should be possible, requiring appropriate ventilation and floor, wall, and ceiling construction. The suite should be equipped with a sufficient number of properly filtered power outlets and contain lighting comparable with that in an operating room.

IMPLEMENTATION

Numerous magnet designs, including "double-donut" and open "clam shell" magnets, have been proposed for interventional MR. These designs improve access to the patient while the patient is at isocenter. However, these systems operate with field strengths of 0.5 T or lower and may have significant constraints on basic specifications (e.g., homogeneity, maximum field of view, gradient strength, linearity). These features result in longer scan times, lower resolution, less SNR, increased image distortion, and potentially reduced functionality in areas such as fat suppression, diffusion imaging, functional imaging, temperature mapping, and real-time imaging. Thus, the full benefits of MR cannot be realized. Although this loss of functionality may be acceptable for some applications, for others the consequences of increased access may be too great. Many of the currently envisioned applications of MR, (e.g., temperature mapping during ablative therapies) do not require improved patient access. Additionally, because preintervention diagnostic scanning is typically performed on 1.5-T scanners, pre- and midintervention data can be difficult to properly mesh.

With these limitations in mind, an alternative approach that preserves the full range of MR functionality and maximizes patient access within these constraints should be investigated. A state-of-the-art high-field, short-bore, open-aperture scanner was selected as the foundation of a high-field interventional MR system. This system makes it possible to use, without limitations, the most advanced MR features (e.g., real-time interactive imaging, excellent MR angiography, functional assays such as brain activation and perfusion, MR thermometry). The high field strength and excellent gradient capabilities of this system ensure that scans will be of the highest quality in terms of spatial and temporal resolution and SNR. Alternative means of accessing the patient in a high-field system, including improved table mobility and remote control systems, can also be envisioned.

The MR system is combined with an angiography system to create a versatile research platform (Fig. 5-1). The duality of this hybrid system permits procedures that cannot be done without x-ray fluoroscopy or procedures in which the x-ray equipment can be used initially to validate the results obtained with MR guidance. Additionally, the x-ray system is a valuable alternative for physicians uncomfortable or unfamiliar with interventional MR.

The patient can be transported between the two systems in seconds by means of a floating table top. This shuttle system permits the patient to be rapidly removed from the magnetic field in emergency situations, in which the use of non–MR-compatible equipment may be necessary.

The magnetic resonance system

The MR system is based on a conventional Philips Gyroscan ACS-NT 1.5-T system (Philips Medical Systems, Best, The Netherlands) and is used with commercially available state-of-the-art sequences, such as echoplanar imaging (EPI) and GRASE. The main field magnet is actively shielded and produces a 5-G footprint that covers a peanut-shaped area with principal axis dimensions of 8.5 m and 4.75 m. The results re-

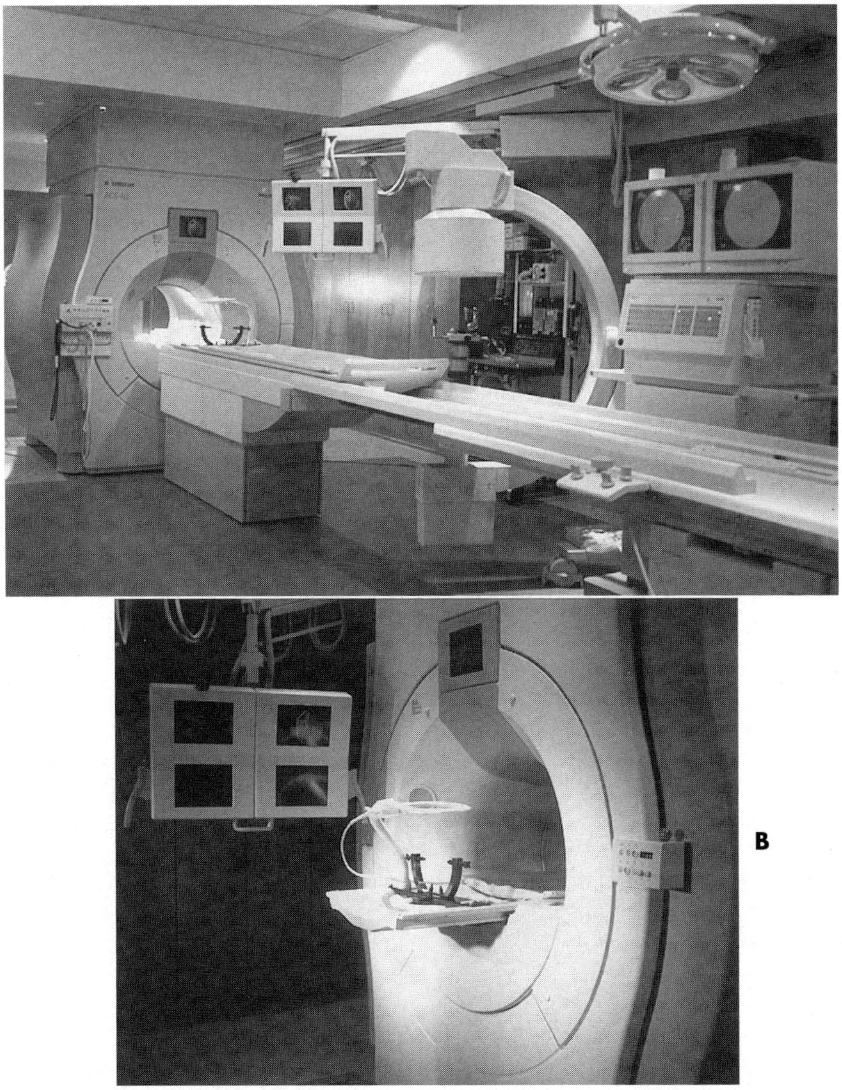

A

B

Fig. 5-1. The hybrid interventional magnetic resonance suite at the University of Minnesota. **A,** The suite is shown from the front, and the 1.5-T Gyroscan ACS-NT system (Philips Medical Systems, Best, The Netherlands) is visible in the background. The C-arm of the BV-212 x-ray angiography unit (Philips Medical Systems) is visible in the foreground and is positioned just outside the 5-G line of the scanner. The floating table top is visible on the continuous track between the MR unit and angiography table, and the ceiling-suspended liquid crystal display panel is also visible. **B,** The surgical pit at the rear of the magnet. The table extends 40 cm beyond the end of the scanner to improve access to the patient. The articulating arm of the liquid crystal display panel has been used to position the screens for maximal visibility for the neurosurgeon.

ported in this chapter were achieved with a gradient set capable of slew rates of 50 mT/m/sec and a rise-time of 0.3 msec to a maximum strength of 15 mT/m. These capabilities are realized in all three orthogonal directions, and the gradient exhibits less than a 1-mm deviation from the optimum over a 25-cm diameter spherical volume. An upgrade to a state-of-the-art gradient set capable of 23 mT/m and a rise-time of 0.2 msec was recently installed. The full strength and short rise time can be applied to any scan technique, including turbo spin-echo, EPI, and GRASE. There are no limitations with regard to duty cycle, double-oblique slice orientation, or nonstandard k-space sampling routes (e.g., radial, spiral). The total length of the MR system is 180 cm, with a bore diameter of 60 cm, which extends to 100 cm at the flared opening. The compact length and flared entries of this magnet provide adequate patient access for many procedures.

This system provides all of the imaging capabilities described above as desirable for interventional MR. No compromises have been made to the MR scanner, and thus the image quality and functional capabilities equal those of other diagnostic 1.5-T scanners. Real-time, interactive MR imaging (or MR fluoroscopy) has been implemented and allows on-the-fly manipulation of geometric and contrast parameters. Images are reconstructed and displayed immediately after acquisition at the console and at four MR-compatible liquid crystal display screens positioned next to the MR system. The liquid crystal display screens are attached to a flexible arm and can be moved freely along a ceiling-mounted rail system, allowing in-room viewing at the front and at the back of the magnet during interventional procedures at any location.

Interactive scanning can be performed with fast gradient or spin-echo methods (scan time per image, typically 1 to 3 sec), zoom-imaging[6,7] (typically 50 to 500 msec per image), or the radial scan technique.[8] The choice of pulse sequence depends on the desired image contrast, the required temporal resolution, and the acceptable extent of artifact. The high-field strength of the magnet, which produces greater susceptibility artifacts, often dictates the use of spin-echo–based sequences when instruments (e.g., a biopsy needle) are near the imaging volume. The interactive software is menu-driven and has been implemented on the MR console (Fig. 5-2). The software can be controlled from the MR console or within the MR suite via a remote control. Interactive scanning allows the operator to manipulate the scan plane arbitrarily in space and permits some control over image contrast. In-plane translation and rotation, through-plane movement, and scan planes of arbitrary obliquity can be achieved. For example, interactive scanning permits the operator to efficiently find scan planes containing needles. Display latency of the acquired images is approximately 100 to 200 msec, depending on the scan technique.

The radial scanning technique uses partially updated k-space[9] and reconstructs 23 256 × 256 images per second. Although the actual scan time to refresh all k-profiles is approximately 1 sec, the fast update rate mimics real-time imaging at a fluoroscopic rate. Radial scanning can be adapted for simultaneous imaging and catheter tracking, using a catheter equipped with an RF microcoil.[10] The position of the catheter is determined and displayed in real-time as a moving point in the image. The catheter position is also fed back to the scanner to automatically adjust the slice position and follow the catheter tip on-the-fly.

A temperature-mapping tool, based on the observed shift of the water resonance frequency with temperature, has also been implemented. The tool uses the shift of water resonance frequency (−0.01 ppm/°C) observed with gradient-recalled echo (GRE) scans[11, 12] and produces isotemperature contours that are visualized as color overlays on an anatomic reference image (Fig. 5-3). Up to three images can be monitored and updated

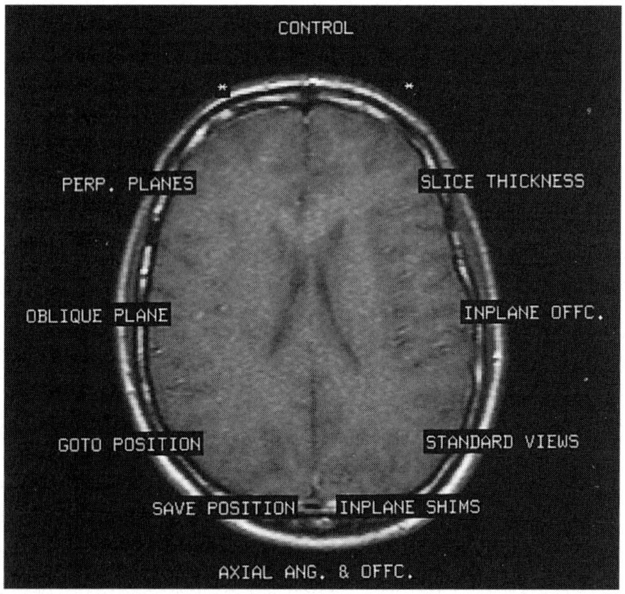

Fig. 5-2. The interactive menu is shown superimposed on a 3.3-sec T1-weighted turbo spin-echo fluoroscopic image. The menu appears on the operator's console and on the in-room liquid crystal displays. The menu can be controlled with the keyboard or mouse at the operator's console or with a remote control in the scan room. In-plane rotation and translation and through plane motion can quickly and easily be prescribed. Perpendicular views and arbitrary oblique views can also be performed. For gradient-recalled echo scans, the flip angle can be adjusted to modify image contrast. Desirable slice orientations can be saved and used to prescribe scan planes for subsequent acquisitions.

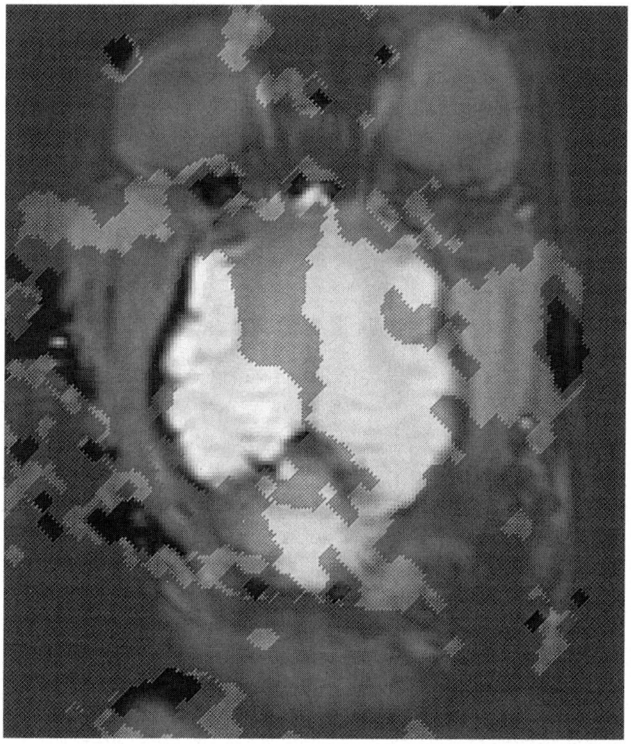

Fig. 5-3. An example of magnetic resonance (MR) thermometry during brain hypothermia in a cat. The scan plane is approximately axial, and the orbits are visible toward the top of the image. Blood entering the cat's right carotid artery has been chilled and is preferentially cooling this hemisphere. Translucent color overlays are applied to the image to depict local temperature. Red-tinted tissue is warmer than 36° C, yellow-tinted tissue is 33° to 36° C, and blue-tinted tissue is 30° to 33° C. Temperatures less than 30° C have no color overlay, revealing the underlying grey-scale MR image. See Color Plate 1.

with temperature-specific color overlays. The temperature contours can be updated as often as once every 2 sec, although longer gradient echo scans can be incorporated for more accurate thermometry.

Several other investigational techniques (e.g., advanced diffusion, perfusion imaging) and catheter tracking methods are also being implemented and under evaluation.

The angiography system

The BV-212 mobile x-ray C-arm (Philips Medical Systems) has a 31-cm image intensifier and can be used for fluoroscopy, digital subtraction angiography, and road mapping in maximal opacification mode. To prevent image distortion in the residual field of about 3 to 4 G at the working position, additional metal screening has been applied. This approach allows operation of the image intensifier within normal homogeneity specifications. Because the total aluminum equivalent of the MR table top positioned on the conventional angiography table at the BV-212 position exceeds the standard, the BV-212 cannot be operated with the table positioned between the patient and the image intensifier. Because this set-up is rarely needed, the consequences of this limitation for the functionality of the system are minimal.

Room requirements and ancillary equipment

The interventional MR suite needs sufficient room to house the MR imaging and angiography equipment, the operating room and anesthesia staff, and ancillary equipment. The interventional suite at the University of Minnesota (see Fig. 5-1) measures 10.5 × 5.25 m and represents the lower end of desirable room dimensions. Room ventilation is important when anesthesia gases are used to maintain a safe and sterile environment. The MR suite should be kept at positive pressure relative to connecting rooms, and air should recirculate approximately 25 times per hour. A substantial number of appropriately shielded power outlets, with emergency back-up power, is required to meet the multifaceted requirements of this type of suite. Room lighting should be substantially enhanced over that in conventional MR suites, and ceiling-mounted operating room lights may be required over the surgical field. An MR-compatible fiberoptic headlight system may be desired by the interventionist and vacuum ports for in-suite suction are necessary for many applications.

Anesthesia and patient monitoring are integral components of an interventional MR suite. Commercially available MR-compatible anesthesia systems are commonly found in conventional MR suites. When possible, the anesthesia equipment should be supplied with air, oxygen, and nitrous oxide via in-suite gas lines to minimize the number of gas canisters in the room. Patient monitoring within the MR suite can be challenging because the equipment represents a source of RF noise. FDA-approved MR-compatible patient monitoring equipment, including cardiac rhythm, respiration, end-tidal carbon dioxide, and invasive blood pressure, is commercially available. This equipment provides the anesthetist with many of the monitoring capabilities commonly found in conventional operating rooms. In-room display of patient waveforms should be customized to the MR environment because cathode ray tube monitors are not permitted within the suite. Appropriately shielded liquid crystal display monitors, however, are a proven alternative to CRT.

A wide range of other MR-compatible equipment is necessary to provide therapy within an MR suite. The tightly shielded footprint of the ACS-NT magnet permits non–MR-compatible equipment to be used relatively close to the scanner, but care must be taken that these devices are not moved to dangerous areas. As the field of interventional MR grows, MR-compatible equipment will become more readily available and less expensive. Currently, however, this equipment can be hard to find and may exhibit varying degrees of MR compatibility. Surgical instruments are available from several vendors and are typically constructed with titanium or 300-grade stainless steel. Stainless steel instruments have the same feel as conventional surgical instruments, whereas titanium instruments are much lighter. Stainless steel instruments, however, have varying degrees of MR compatibility, which may change after prolonged exposure to a strong magnetic field.

Patient immobilization is critical for neurosurgic intervention. To maintain ease of patient motion, immobilization should be performed by attaching the patient to the table top. Providing the immobilizing frame does not exceed bore dimensions, this approach permits full patient transport capabilities and allows accurate repositioning after such movements. A modified version of the Malcolm-Rand head frame (Composite Manufacturing, San Clemente, Calif) has been customized to the Philips table top (Fig. 5-4) and provides this functionality. Full integration of more complete stereotactic devices is also being

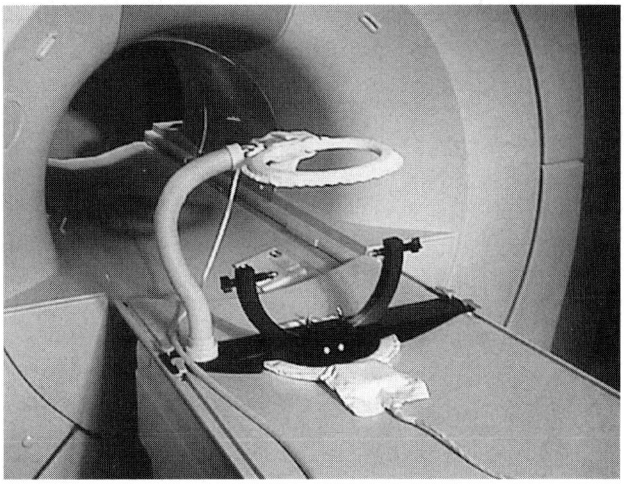

Fig. 5-4. The modified Malcolm-Rand head frame (Composite Manufacturing, San Clemente, Calif) is mounted to the floating magnetic resonance table top. The frame is made of carbon fiber and is attached to the table via dove-tailed grooves that run along the lateral sides of the table. Also shown integrated into the frame are the two phased array surface coils that are used as open head coils.

pursued by several vendors. A Bipolar cautery device (Codman, Randolph, Mass) has been developed and tested for use in the fringe field of a high-field magnet. Other areas of development include MR-compatible craniotomes and MR-compatible microscopes.

Finally, a very practical aspect of the room relates to access restrictions, which affect the sterility of the room and the safety of those within the magnetic field. A multitude of personnel (up to 10 persons) with varying degrees of knowledge about MR will enter the suite. A unique uniform can identify personnel who are members of the interventional MR team. At the University of Minnesota, these uniforms are teal-colored surgical scrubs; they do not have pockets and, therefore, reduce the likelihood of ferromagnetic objects being accidentally brought into the suite.

NEUROLOGIC APPLICATIONS

Of all possible applications of interventional MR, guidance of neurosurgical and neuroradiologic procedures may offer the greatest benefit. The excellent tissue discrimination capabilities of MR, including diffusion-weighted imaging, can be coupled with MR angiography, perfusion, and brain activation mapping to produce comprehensive data before, during, and after intervention.

Guided biopsy

The aim of any biopsy procedure is to, in a minimally invasive fashion, obtain tissue samples for pathologic evaluation. The use of imaging technologies to help guide these procedures has greatly enhanced the clinician's ability to target lesions safely and accurately. Although MR clearly provides the best discrimination of most brain lesions, the use of this modality is essentially limited to preoperative seeding of framed or frameless stereotactic devices. Thus, interaction of the biopsy device with tissue is simulated rather than directly imaged. As a result, the accuracy of these techniques is less than ideal and, in the case of framed stereotaxy, may require long set-up times before needle insertion.

The use of MR to guide a biopsy in real-time, as is frequently done with computed tomography and ultrasound (US), offers some significant advantages. The excellent contrast provided by MR in the brain can be coupled with a real-time view of the needle within the lesion, thereby guaranteeing the accuracy of the procedure. Additionally, fusing overlays of vessels or highlighting other sensitive structures in the volume may reduce the risk of complications from the procedure. Increased clinician confidence in the obtained biopsy samples should result in an increased number of patients, and because postbiopsy scans can immediately be performed to rule out hemorrhage, earlier release of patients.

Ideally, the surgeon has unencumbered access to the patient at the isocenter of the magnet during biopsy needle placement. Although cylindrical magnets do not permit this access, several alternative methods can be envisioned. Biopsies performed at the University of Minnesota use a freehand approach, in which the neurosurgeon judges the desired needle orientation based on geometric information in MR scans acquired immediately before needle insertion. This procedure is performed at the rear of the magnet (Fig. 5-5), and the initial needle insertion is conservative. Scan updates of the needle position are acquired by briefly rolling the patient back to isocenter; in this manner, the approach to the tumor can be monitored (Fig. 5-6). Interactive scanning is used to position the imaging slice through the needle and to switch between orthogonal views. Orthogonal views along the needle track are important to ensure that the needle is appropriately positioned. In one view, the extent of artifact surrounding MR-compatible instruments can erroneously depict the needle within a lesion (Fig. 5-7).

As discussed, complete understanding of needle artifact and of the artifact's form in different scans is crucial to proper interpretation of interventional MR data.[13–16] This understanding is especially important at high-field strength, which enhances susceptibility artifacts. At low-field, the opposite problem arises because too little artifact may be produced on spin-echo–based images. At 1.5 T, the extent of artifact surrounding available titanium biopsy needles reduces positional accuracy on GRE sequences, even when high bandwidth readouts are used. Figure 5-8 shows the extent of artifact on a GRE sequence and compares it with a corresponding turbo spin-echo scan. In this case, the needle is running approximately 20° from the B_o axis, and the artifact produced on the GRE scan is significantly more coarse than on the turbo spin-echo scan. The ball-shaped tip on the turbo spin-echo image is anticipated when the needle is oriented in the same general direction as B_o[17], and the position of the needle tip is at the geometric center of this artifact. In situations in which the biopsy needle is essentially colinear with B_o, or when small low-profile needles are used, the needle track can be difficult to detect on turbo spin-echo scans, even when using high-field systems. In these situations, GRE scans are useful for

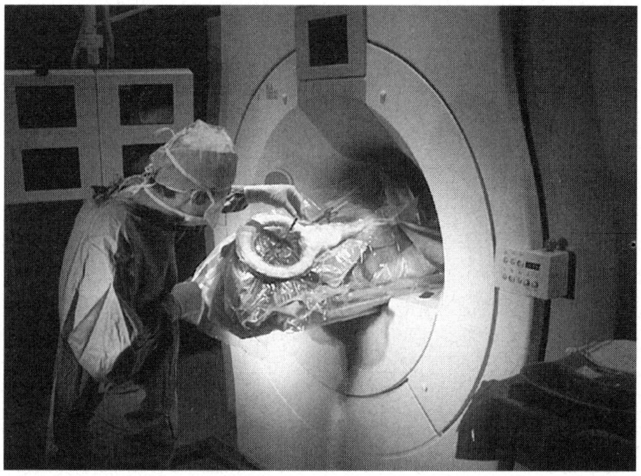

Fig. 5-5. The patient's head is extending out the back of the magnet, and the neurosurgeon is positioning the biopsy needle. Positional updates can be obtained by sliding the patient to the magnet center and rescanning.

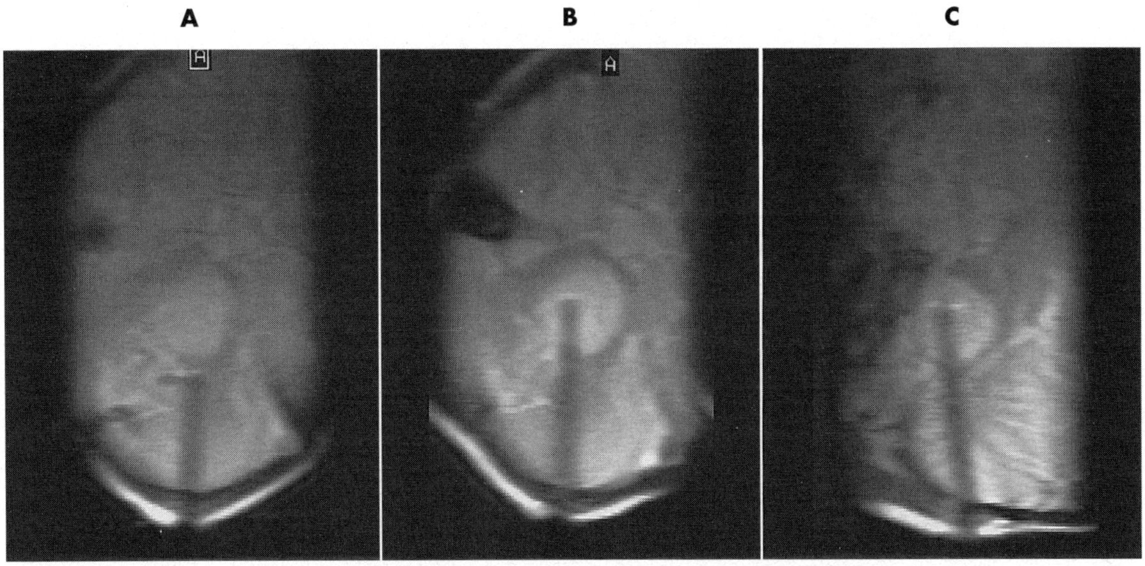

Fig. 5-6. T2-weighted lolo, or zoomed imaging, interactive scans (acquisition time, 0.5 sec) acquired in real-time show the approach of a biopsy needle to a brainstem lesion in a 2.5-year-old girl. **A**, The initial, conservative freehand approach, which is essentially an axial view of the brain. **B** and **C**, Axial and sagittal views, respectively, of the biopsy needle in the lesion. (Courtesy of C.L. Truwit and W.A. Hall, University of Minnesota.)

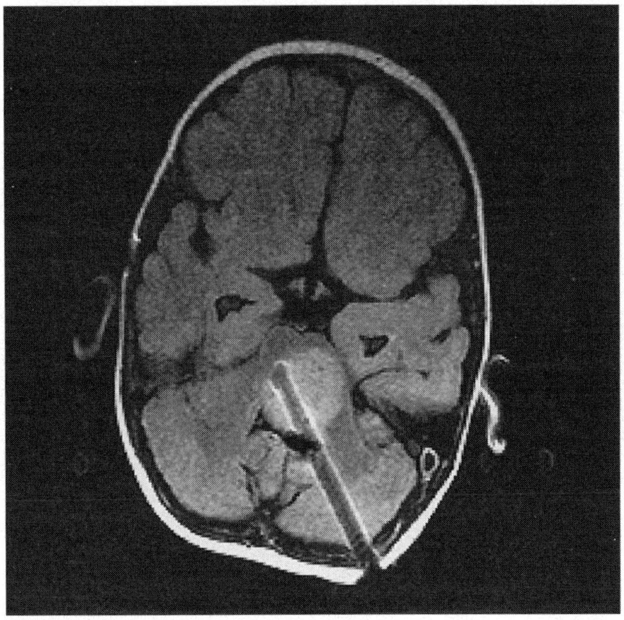

Fig. 5-7. Turbo-FLAIR image of the patient shown in Figure 5-5. This image appears to indicate that the needle is positioned within the lesion, although the needle is actually on the superior margin of the lesion, and only the artifact from the needle extends to this scan plane. (Courtesy of C.L. Truwit and W.A. Hall, University of Minnesota.)

coarse positioning; subsequent turbo spin-echo scans more accurately depict the true needle position. GRE scans are also useful for highlighting vessels, whereas spin-echo–based scans, in general, provide better anatomic maps and lesion conspicuity.

Often, the portion of the lesion to be biopsied is only visible on contrast-enhanced MR scans. The production of rapid T1-weighted spin-echo scans is technically challenging because long echo trains cannot be tolerated. This limitation places stringent demands on the switching times of gradients and places a practical limit on the temporal resolution that can be achieved. Figure 5-9 shows such a lesion, in which an enhancing rim is evident on a cyst that developed after radiation management of a brain tumor. This type of lesion is not easily biopsied with techniques using "old" imaging data because substantial brain shift may occur once the cyst has been punctured. The interactive pulse sequence had the following para-

A

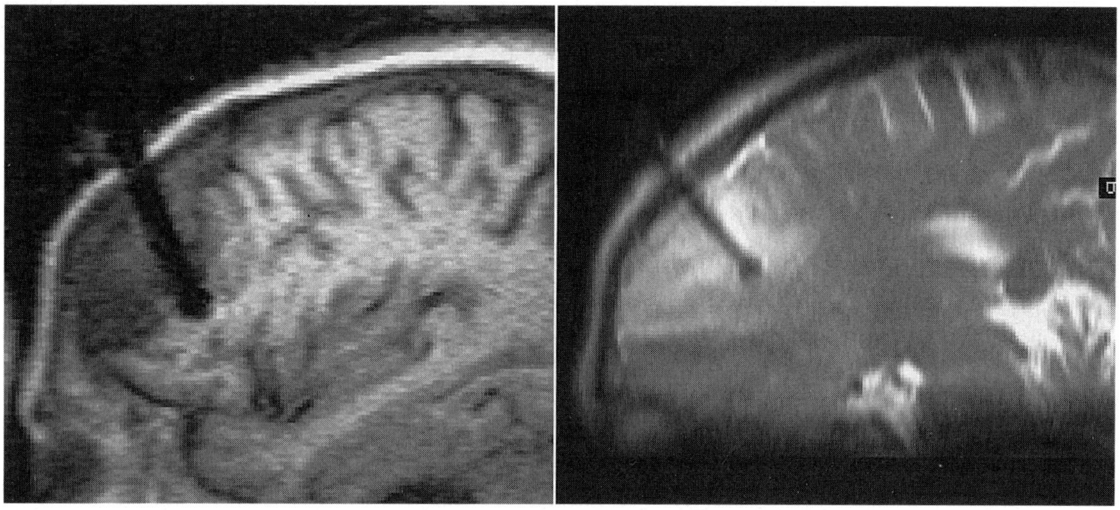

B

Fig. 5-8. The extent of artifact surrounding a titanium biopsy needle in a frontal lobe lesion. **A**, T1-weighted gradient-recalled echo acquisition (acquisition time, 6 sec) and **B**, T2-weighted spin-echo acquisition (acquisition time, 0.5 sec). The needle is oriented approximately 20° from B_o, and the scan plane is approximately sagittal. (Courtesy of C. Pozza and E. Nussbaum, University of Minnesota.)

A

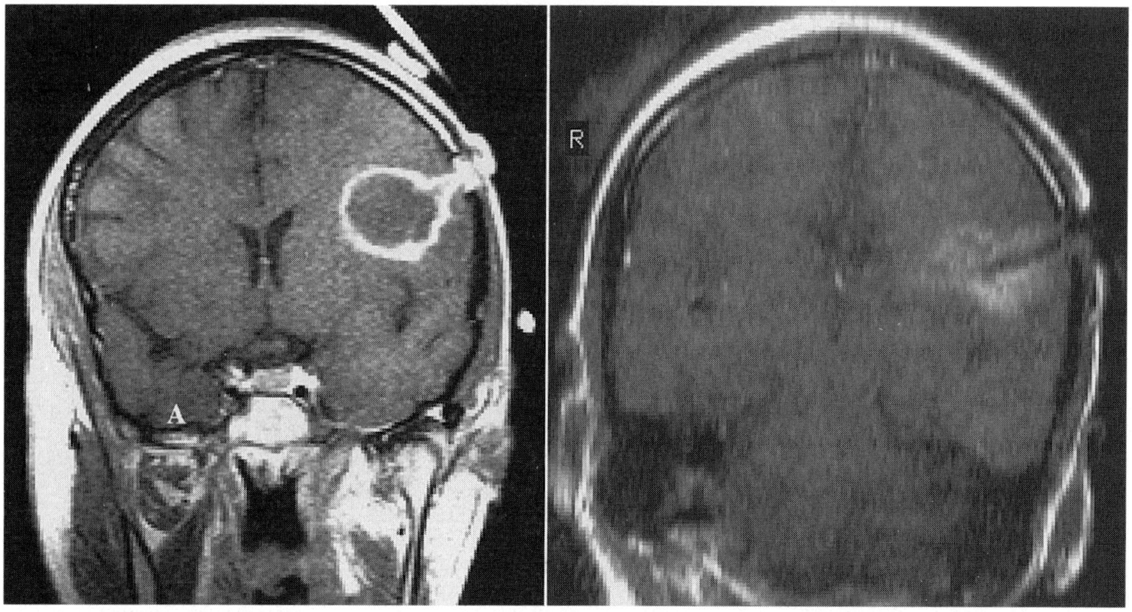

B

Fig. 5-9. Biopsy performed on a patient who previously had a tumor resected and who had undergone radiotherapy. The enhancing portion of the lesion is visible in **A**, before biopsy (conventional T1-weighted scan; time, 1 min, 14 sec and **B**, during interactive scanning after the central cystic component was drained and while the biopsy needle was in place. (Courtesy of C.L. Truwit and W.A. Hall, University of Minnesota.)

meters: echo time/repetition time, 20/300 msec; turbo factor, 11; matrix, 256 × 128; scan time, 1.5 sec. The interactive software permits determination of the needle path within seconds, and orthogonal views can be updated with a temporal resolution equivalent to the scan time.

The freehand approach to biopsies, with patient repositioning to isocenter for imaging updates, is relatively inefficient, and thus alternative methods within the confines of a short-bore cylindrical magnet are being developed. The clinician can reach isocenter but may need help appropriately directing the needle. A positioning device mounted to the skin or skull may support the biopsy needle at the appropriate angle and allow the physician to slowly insert the needle while monitoring its progress in the in-room liquid crystal displays. More automated remote control systems for needle alignment and needle insertion are being pursued.

Monitored tumor resection

The access requirements of an MR system when monitoring a tumor resection are typically less stringent than those of biopsies. The role of MR in these procedures is to assess surgical progress at discrete time intervals. These time intervals can be minutes or, more commonly, hours apart, and thus the necessity for the patient to be at isocenter throughout the surgery is minimal. With the spatial constraints placed on the surgeon by even the most open interventional MR systems, extraction of the patient from the magnet between scans may be desirable.

MR monitoring of tumor resection is expected to improve clinical outcomes as a result of its ability to detect residual tumor that a surgeon might otherwise not resect. A recent study indicated that while, on average, neurosurgeons thought they had removed 90% of a tumor on the first attempt, only 50% of the tumor had, on average, been removed.[18] A high field system with appropriate table top mobility offers some distinct advantages in this area. The improved image quality at 1.5 T over lower field systems provides higher sensitivity for detection of residual tumor. Another advantage is the ability to directly compare pre-, mid-, and postprocedure scans at identical locations without sophisticated image fusion technology. Once the patient's head is immobilized in a head frame, images can be obtained repeatedly at the same spatial and anatomic locations (Fig. 5-10) by returning the floating table top to its original location. The floating table top is designed to permit the patient to be moved back and forth between the MR and angio table locations within seconds, and allows repositioning at the magnet isocenter with mm accuracy. Because preresection scans are almost always performed at 1.5 T, there is no difficulty comparing "old" data with the surgical updates. This consistent depiction of the tissue provides the radiologist with an optimal set of data from which to attempt to distinguish residual tumor from tissue changes that may arise from the procedure.

MR also provides the possibility of performing more sensitive procedures with more precision by incorporating data over and above anatomic mapping. In brain surgery, it is critically important to avoid blood vessels and areas of functional importance (e.g., those responsible for motor skills or speech). MRA, venography and brain activation scans provide this functional data and indicate the proximity of these centers to the lesion

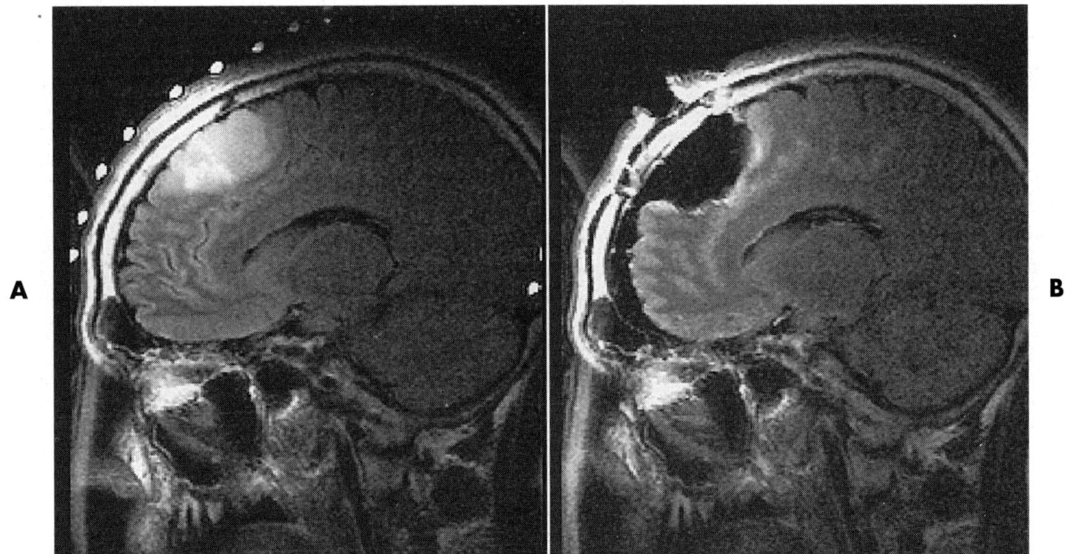

Fig. 5-10. Sagittal views of a low-grade glioma acquired immediately **A**, before and **B**, after initial resection of the tumor. Scan plane alignment is excellent, and residual tumor on the posterior margin of the resection cavity was identified and subsequently removed. A grid marker system that helps define the location and size of craniotomy that is required is visible on the preresection scan. The images are turbo-FLAIR acquisitions with a scan time of 2 min. (Courtesy of C.L. Truwit and W.A. Hall, University of Minnesota.)

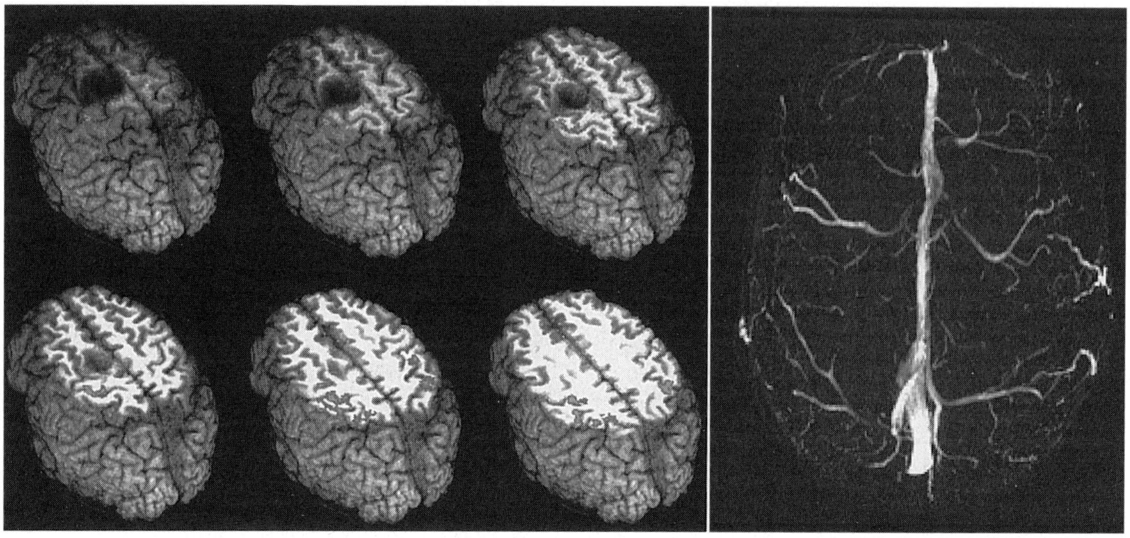

Fig. 5-11. A brain activation map **A**, during a finger tapping exercise and **B**, a venogram obtained before tumor resection. Similar brain activation maps were acquired for toe and tongue motion. These studies revealed a vein overlying the lesion and the close proximity of the motor strip to the lesion. However, overlap of the motor cortex with the lesion was not apparent, and thus full resection was possible. See Color Plate 2. (Courtesy of C.L. Truwit, University of Minnesota.)

(Fig. 5-11). Blood vessels maps are also useful as landmarks for the neurosurgeon once the brain has been exposed. The net effect of this additional data is to: (1) allow the neurosurgeon to appropriately place and minimize the size of the craniotomy flap; (2) determine an optimal trajectory to the lesion through normal brain parenchyma; and (3) permit as complete a resection of the tumor as possible without compromising sensitive neurologic tissue.

Ablation therapy

Ablation techniques are used to destroy tissue with heat (laser, RF, microwave, focused US), cold (cryogens), or chemical (ethanol) means. Although qualitative and quantitative monitoring of ablation therapy is essential in most situations, no established gold standard adequately provides this information. US is occasionally used to monitor ablation procedures, although it requires that an acoustic window be available. Also, US cannot view beyond the ice ball in cryogen ablations and cannot obtain reliable and quantitative measures of heat deposition in thermal ablation. MR may be important for monitoring any ablation technique. The water resonance frequency and T_1 relaxation time of tissue are temperature-dependent, and MR is sensitive to many phase transitions that may occur as a result of temperature changes. Additionally, MR can measure physical parameters (e.g., diffusion), which also correlate with temperature.

Temperature-dependent contrast changes in MR images are primarily determined by T_1 changes. These changes are tissue-dependent and can vary 0.2 to 1.2%/° C.[19] Thus, although this method is simple and easy to use with fast T1-weighted scans, caution is required when interpreting the results.[20] Diffusion is very sensitive to temperature variations because the diffusion constant changes by about 2.4%/° C. However, this technique is rather insensitive in terms of SNR[21–23] and, because it detects motion at a molecular level, may not perform well in moving tissue.

The proton chemical shift method is currently preferred and is potentially the most accurate method of MR thermometry.[20,24,25] The Larmor frequency of spins changes by approximately −0.01 ppm/° C; although this change is very small, it can be measured accurately at 1.5 T using GRE sequences. The technique is much less effective at lower field strengths. Phase images are subtracted from a baseline image, and temperature changes are inferred from this phase difference. This measured temperature difference can be used to place color overlays on anatomic images depicting the location and degree of tissue heating (Fig. 5-12). However, this method has limitations. Because the technique measures small phase changes and is based on subtraction of two temporally distinct images, it is not an absolute temperature measure and can be corrupted by bulk tissue motion. For neurologic applications, in which brain motion is relatively small, these concerns are less of an issue. Changes in the resonance frequency of fat, however, are very small in the relevant temperature window and cannot be detected. Thus, in fatty tissue, fat saturation may be necessary to avoid corruption of the derived temperature maps. Also, at high temperatures, slight changes of the local susceptibility of tissue reduces temperature accuracy,[25,26] and vessels may add flow artifacts.

Endovascular intervention

The justification for MR-guided vascular interventions arises from MR's ability to couple soft-tissue information with vascular mapping and the desire to avoid high radiation exposure during complex endovascular procedures. The ability to simultaneously visualize vascular structures and tissue (e.g., tumor,

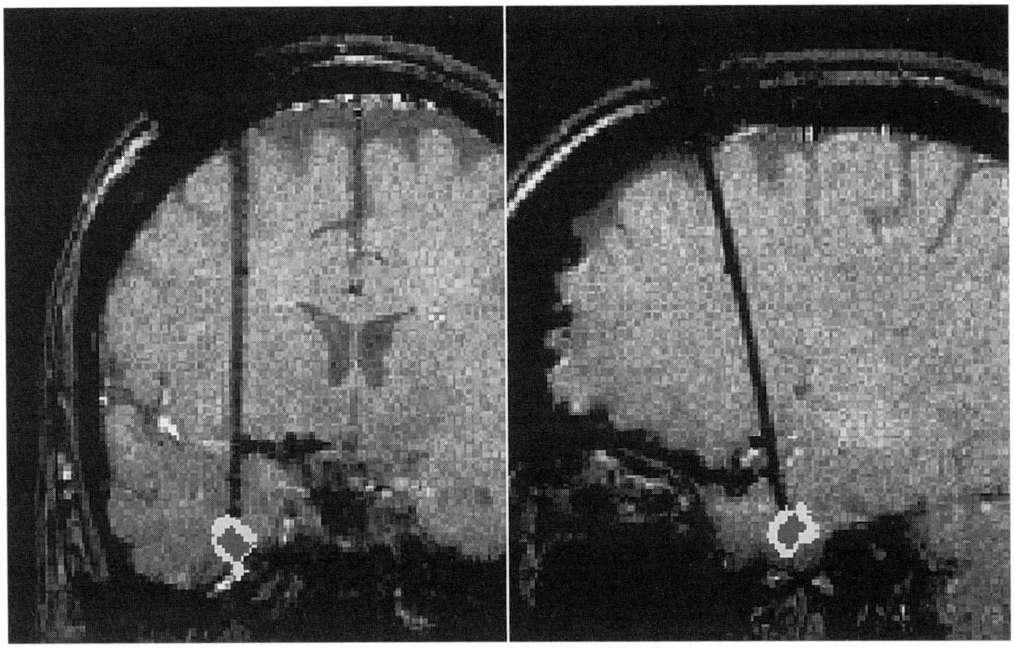

Fig. 5-12. Laser ablation of a deep brain astrocytoma was monitored with magnetic resonance thermometry. Scan planes approximating **A**, coronal and **B**, sagittal views show the laser track, and the color overlay indicates the region experiencing temperature rise. See Color Plate 3. (From Stollberger R, and others: Temperature monitoring of interstitial thermal tissue coagulation using MR phase images, *J Magn Reson Imaging* 8:188, 1998.)

atherosclerotic plaque, the thrombosed portion of an aneurysm) will provide new and potentially valuable clinical information. MR also exhibits the ability to acquire 3D volumes in arbitrary orientations, and thus no restrictions exist with respect to view orientation. Although the elimination of x-ray dose is not the primary drive to develop MR-guided vascular interventions, it is relevant for some procedures. Notably, management of brain aneurysms or arteriovenous malformations with fluoroscopic guidance typically requires high-dose radiation. In these areas and others, MR guidance may offer safety advantages over x-ray techniques.

Possible applications, in addition to aneurysm and arteriovenous malformation guidance, include highly accurate stent placement, monitored angioplasty or atherectomy, and diagnosis and management of ischemic stroke. Resolution, speed, and SNR will be at a premium. High-field strength, therefore, is considered imperative for MR-guided endovascular interventions to be clinically successful. It is necessary for real-time catheter guidance, high spatial resolution anatomic interrogation, and many functional parameters, (e.g., perfusion, quantitative flow, spectroscopy) that are not available with alternative modalities. Successful implementation of endovascular interventions will also rely heavily on the quality on the MR angiogram that can be obtained. Optimal angiography requires high-field and maximum gradient performance capabilities. Recent developments in contrast-enhanced angiography[27–29] have shown great promise and should continue to improve with the emergence of blood-pool contrast agents.

The hybrid interventional MR suite permits initial catheter and guidewire manipulations to be performed with the aid of the x-ray fluoroscopic unit. This ability is particularly advantageous at the early stages of MRI catheter tracking as a back-up option and as a method of confirming MR results. Patient movement between the angiography unit and the MR scanner is easily performed with the floating table top without danger of dislocating the catheter tip. Several approaches to MR catheter tracking have been proposed and include active,[30,31] passive,[32] and applied field inhomogeneity schemes.[33] All are currently under evaluation on the hybrid interventional MR system. (See Chapter 44.)

Passive visualization catheters are closest to clinical reality because they rely solely on susceptibility effects for visualization. As a result, they do not represent the same safety risk as other catheter visualization approaches. Realization of a safe catheter suitable for human use is therefore easier to accomplish. The first human has been scanned with a passive dysprosium-doped catheter,[34] and preliminary clinical work on diabetic patients with dialysis fistulas is beginning at the University of Utrecht, The Netherlands.

Active visualization catheters incorporate one or more RF microcoils and require multiple projection measurements to determine 3D spatial coordinates. Real-time imaging with continuous updates of catheter position requires efficient integration of scanning and positional measurements. Radial scanning efficiently couples these requirements, provided the radial scan line rotates by approximately 90° between measurements. The two in-plane spatial coordinates of the microcoils can be determined from these measurements, with only the positional measurement orthogonal to the scan plane requiring an additional step.[35] The frequency at which this additional step is performed can be set by the operator at any integer number of radial steps. A significant advantage of active catheters is that the positional information obtained can be used as feedback to the MR scanner, allowing automatic tracking of the scan plane containing the catheter.

The field inhomogeneity type of catheter creates a local field disturbance by application of a small direct current through a wire loop in the catheter. This loop produces a small magnetic field that disturbs the static magnetic field close to the catheter. The major advantage of the technique is that, by adjusting the current flowing in the wire loop, a variable magnitude of field inhomogeneity can be created. This feature allows full freedom in defining a desired scan technique because the extent of the artifact around the catheter can be customized. Similarly, the artifact can be set high for tranversing large vessels and adjusted arbitrarily to a small level for fine vessel manipulations. The effect can be removed completely for scans in which the current catheter position is not relevant or may obscure the anatomy to be visualized.

Each method of catheter visualization has advantages and disadvantages. The catheter tracking coil will likely be chosen by the specific application that it is to fulfill. The techniques are not necessarily mutually exclusive, and combinations of active and passive approaches may also prove beneficial.

Stroke therapy

Stroke is the third leading cause of death[36] and is a major cause of prolonged disability. Recent developments in acute stroke therapy have shown the potential benefits of early detection and management.[37,38] These studies indicated the presence of a therapeutic window of approximately 3 to 6 hr postictus, during which brain cells with reduced blood supply may be saved. These cells are thought to exist in a state of "electrical failure" rather than "energy failure." They may return to normal function once adequate circulation is restored. Beyond this therapeutic window, the affected brain tissue is irrevocably damaged, and therapy will produce no benefit and may lead to unnecessary complications. The necessity for immediate management of stroke has led to community awareness programs focusing on the concept of a "brain attack."[39] These programs parallel the need for immediate clinical attention associated with myocardial infarctions and have led to earlier presentation of stroke patients.

Stroke can be hemorrhagic or ischemic; each is managed differently. Approximately 80% of strokes are ischemic and may benefit from dissolution of the blood clot responsible for the stroke. Patients with hemorrhagic stroke do not benefit from clot-busting therapies. Thus, suspected stroke patients should initially be screened to differentiate the two types. Screening is typically performed by computed tomography, although MR may be equally capable of differentiating the two conditions. In ischemic stroke, the clinician should decide if clot-busting drugs (e.g., urokinase, tissue plasminogen activator) are warranted. These drugs may be administered intravenously or intra-arterially. Intra-arterial delivery may reduce complications as a result of localization of the anticoagulant to the affected site rather than systematically.[40,41] Intra-arterial delivery does, however, require arterial catheterization. The FDA has approved intravenous delivery of

A

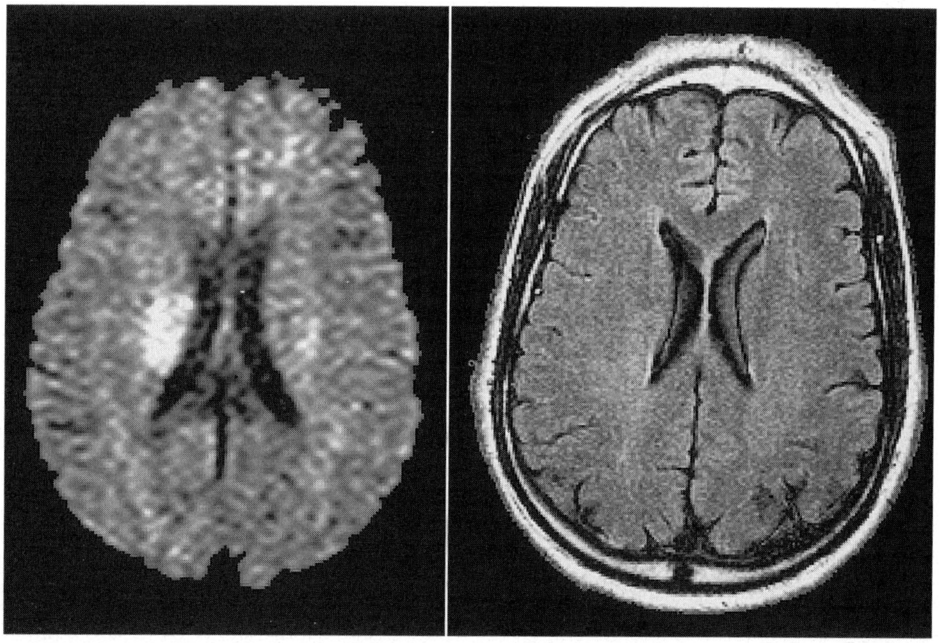

B

Fig. 5-13. **A**, Diffusion-weighted (b = 1000 s/mm^2) and **B**, turbo-FLAIR images of a patient approximately 3 to 4 hr postictus. The lesion, which is the hyperintensity on the diffusion-weighted image, extended from the posterior insular cortex to the posterior limb of the internal capsule to the corona radiata and caudate body. The lesion was not visible on turbo-FLAIR or other conventional scans at this time. (Courtesy of C.L. Truwit, University of Minnesota.)

tissue plasminogen activator provided the stroke is nonhemorrhagic and is less than 3 hr old. This 3-hr time interval is arbitrarily based on the potential benefits of the therapy outweighing the potential side effects on a population-wide scale. Indeed, some patients may benefit from therapy after this time interval, and others will not respond even within the 3-hr limit. MR may be a diagnostic tool that can identify salvageable brain tissue, irrespective of the time after stroke onset. MR may also be used to monitor therapy and minimize the dose of clot-busting drug that is required to restore patency to the affected vessels.

Delineation of affected tissue in the hyperacute stages of stroke is challenging because conventional MR and computed tomography scans are not sensitive to initial cellular changes and may take up to 24 hr before they reveal the developing lesion. Diffusion-weighted MR imaging[42] and perfusion imaging based on first pass of a bolus of contrast agent[43] have shown sensitivity to stroke within hours of onset. Diffusion scans are thought to delineate tissue that is not recoverable (Fig. 5-13), whereas perfusion analysis reveals areas of compromised circulation (Fig. 5-14). Therefore, the portion of the lesion

A

B

C

D

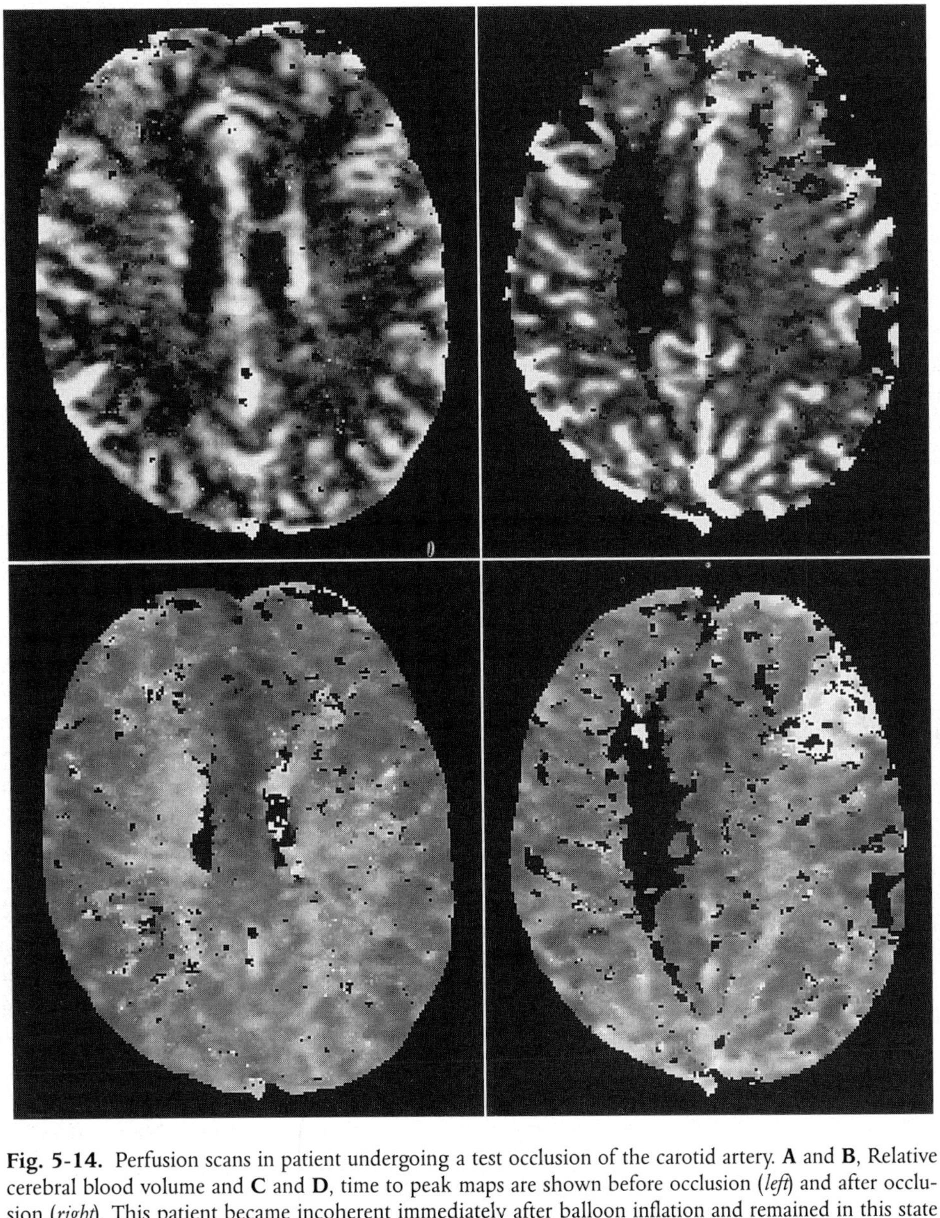

Fig. 5-14. Perfusion scans in patient undergoing a test occlusion of the carotid artery. **A** and **B**, Relative cerebral blood volume and **C** and **D**, time to peak maps are shown before occlusion (*left*) and after occlusion (*right*). This patient became incoherent immediately after balloon inflation and remained in this state even after the balloon was deflated. Perfusion magnetic resonance imaging performed 40 min after the event revealed the vascular deficit responsible for clinical manifestations. Watershed vascular territories on the patient's right side (the occluded side) show signal black-out on the cerebral blood volume and time to peak maps. This finding is indicative of very low perfusion levels because no passage of contrast agent is perceptible. On the contralateral side, delayed perfusion is noted in the frontal lobe (bright, wedge-shaped region on the time to peak map). These symptoms resolved within 24 hours, and no residual lesion was evident on conventional magnetic resonance scans. (Courtesy of C.L. Truwit, University of Minnesota.)

delineated with perfusion analysis that is external to the diffusion-weighted image–identified lesion may represent salvageable tissue. This ischemic penumbra is thought to have sufficient collateral circulation to prevent its immediate death but insufficient circulation to sustain the tissue indefinitely. This ischemic penumbra is likely to benefit from re-establishment of circulation via clot-busting therapy.

The role of the hybrid interventional MR and x-ray angiography suite is to provide a forum in which a complete diagnostic and therapeutic work-up can be efficiently performed on patients in the hyperacute stages of stroke. Initial scanning using turbo-FLAIR and T_2* sensitive GRE scans can rule out hemorrhagic stroke, possibly removing the need for an initial computed tomography scan. Diagnostic determination of the presence of salvageable tissue may be revealed by subsequent diffusion and perfusion MR scans. This information, along with the medical history and current neurologic status of the patient, can lead to an appropriate therapy. If intra-arterial administration of clot-busting agents is considered, MR angiography, with possible x-ray angiography as back-up, can determine the location and extent of vessel blockage. The angiography unit is also necessary to guide the catheter to the affected site. Fine positioning of the catheter may be performed with MR or x-ray scanning. Regardless of how the clot-busting agent is delivered, perfusion MR may be used to detect improvements in cerebral circulation. Incremental dosing with immediate perfusion MR follow-up may permit lower concentrations of clot-busting agents, which may decrease the incidence of hemorrhage, a common complication associated with these agents.

The use of MR to monitor and guide patients presenting with hyperacute ischemic stroke remains an area of clinical research. Although diffusion-weighted imaging is an early detector of stroke lesions, the role of perfusion MR is less clear. Technical improvements are required for quantitative, rather than relative, measures of cerebral blood volume and flow. Reliable detection of the ischemic penumbra after stroke requires these data before these techniques can have widespread clinical use.

Future applications

As interventionists become more familiar with intraoperative MR scanning and interventional MR techniques are improved, interventional MR will tend to be used to guide increasingly sensitive and challenging neurologic procedures. This use will require an appropriately designed interventional MR suite and software that can efficiently fuse functional and anatomic MR scan updates, with immediate display and feedback capabilities.

Pallidotomy is an initial application that requires targeting of smaller and more sensitively placed brain structures. Pallidotomy involves lesioning a portion of the globus pallidus to relieve motor dysfunction in persons with Parkinson's disease who no longer respond to drug therapy.[44] The globus pallidus is a deep-brain structure near the optic tract and internal capsule. It is often targeted with a stereotactic frame and microelectrode guidance.[45] The latter relies on measurement of potentials after neuronal stimulation in awake and responding persons. This process can be very time-consuming and costly, and some ambiguity surrounds the ultimate probe position when the lesion is to be created. MR has been used to confirm retrospectively the position of the lesion[45] but has not been used to guide the approach to the globus pallidus. Interventional MR can reduce operating time and increase the precision and accuracy of lesion placement. These advances should make the pallidotomy safer and more available to persons with Parkinson's disease.

Many other applications in functional neurosurgery and endovascular and other minimally invasive therapies can be envisioned. Interventional MR should first, however, show precision and accuracy in its preliminary applications before clinical acceptance for more sensitive neurologic therapies is pursued under MR guidance.

CONCLUSIONS

The development of interventional MR is at a very early stage, and many clinical applications have to be explored. Additionally, because the field is in a state of substantial flux, definitive studies of outcome, efficacy, and economic viability may be premature. Thus, many of interventional MR's potential benefits are difficult to quantify. Regardless, interventional MR is used to augment many interventions and has shown benefits to the patient, physician, and healthcare system.

The rationale for performing these procedures at 1.5 T was based on optimal MR functionality, which has paid off both in terms of clarity of MR data and increased clinician confidence. The use of a standard state-of-the-art 1.5-T scanner also has significant economic benefits in that it may be used for diagnostic scans when not being used for interventions. The design of a comprehensive interventional MR suite, with MR and x-ray imaging capabilities, efficient patient transport, and the possibility of performing surgery outside or within the fringe field of the magnet, greatly reduced the inertia surrounding the shifting of interventional procedures to a new environment. Limited patient access associated with a closed-bore scanner is acceptable for some applications (e.g., tumor resections, ablative therapies) but somewhat cumbersome for others (e.g., biopsies). Steps have been taken to overcome access limitations during biopsies by implementing remote control and positioning devices.

Numerous neurologic interventional procedures are done routinely in the interventional MR suite. Brain biopsies under interventional MR guidance have improved clinician confidence in the biopsy sample and shortened patient stays after the procedure. MR-monitored tumor resection has consistently shown regions of residual tumor after initial resection. In brain biopsies and tumor resection, the interventional MR suite also permits screening for hemorrhage before closure. The high-field strength permits reliable and quantitative temperature measures for monitoring ablative therapy. MR guidance of endovascular interventions has shown promise, although more research is required. The role of the interventional MR suite in the management of hyperacute stroke has shown great promise but also requires further investigation.

Although the clinical niche of interventional MR and the associated economic and medical benefits are not well-defined, an abundance of indications warrant continued development. Of critical importance for the field is the ongoing communication between technical developers and clinicians. Only through the judicious use of technology will interventional MR produce improved patient outcomes and economic justification.

REFERENCES

1. Jara H, and others: High resolution variable flip angle 3D MR imaging of trabecular microstructure in vivo, *Magn Reson Med* 29:528, 1993.
2. Albert MS, and others: Biological magnetic resonance imaging using laser-polarized ^{129}Xe, *Nature* 370:199, 1994.
3. Lufkin RB: Interventional MR imaging, *Radiology* 197:16, 1995.
4. Bieze J: Radiation exposure risks haunt interventionalists, *Diagn Imag* 8:68, 1993.
5. Wagner LK, Eifel PJ, Geise RA: Potential biological effects following high x-ray dose interventional procedures, *J Vasc Interv Radiol* 5:71, 1994.
6. Feinberg DA, and others: Inner volume MR imaging: technical concepts and their application, *Radiology* 156:743, 1985.
7. van Vaals JJ, and others: *Local Look (LoLo): zoom-fluoroscopy of a moving target.* In Proceedings of the first meeting of the Society of Magnetic Resonance, Dallas, 1994. *J Magn Reson Imaging* 4:38.
8. Rasche V, and others: Continuous radial data acquisition for dynamic MRI, *Magn Reson Med* 34:754, 1995.
9. Riederer SJ, and others: MR fluoroscopy: technical feasibility, *Magn Reson Imaging* 8:1, 1988.
10. Rasche V, and others: Catheter tracking using continuous radial MRI, *Magn Reson Med* 37:963, 1997.
11. Hindman JC: Proton resonance shift of water in the gas and liquid states, *J Chem Phys* 44:4582, 1966.
12. Ishihara Y, and others: A precise and fast temperature mapping using water proton chemical shift, *Magn Reson Med* 34:814, 1995.
13. Ludeke KM, Roschmann P, Tischle R: Susceptibility artifacts in NMR imaging, *Magn Reson Imaging* 3:329, 1985.
14. Bakker CJG, and others: Susceptibility artifacts in 2DFT spin-echo and gradient-echo imaging: the cylinder model revisited, *Magn Reson Imaging* 22:539, 1993.
15. Ladd ME, and others: Biopsy needle susceptibility artifacts, *Magn Reson Med* 36:646, 1996.
16. Lewin JS, and others: Needle localization in MR guided biopsy and aspiration: effects of field strength, sequence design and magnetic field orientation, *Am J Roentgenol* 166:1337, 1996.
17. Liu H, Martin AJ, Truwit CL: Interventional MRI at high field (1.5T): needle artifacts, *J Magn Reson Imaging* 8:214, 1998.
18. Albert FK, and others: Early postoperative magnetic resonance imaging after resection of malignant gliomas: residual tumor and its influence on regrowth and prognosis, *Neurosurgery* 34:45, 1994.
19. Stollberger R, and others: Temperaturmapping mittels MR-imaging am Beispiel der Laserkoagulation von Gehirngewebe, *Biomed Tech (Berlin)* 57:209, 1994.
20. Young IR, and others: Modeling and observation of temperature changes in vivo using MRI, *Magn Reson Med* 32:358, 1994.
21. LeBihan D, Delannoy J, Levin RL: Temperature mapping with MR imaging of molecular diffusion: application to hyperthermia, *Radiology* 171:853, 1989.
22. Delannoy J, and others: Noninvasive temperature imaging using diffusion MRI, *Magn Reson Med* 19:333, 1991.
23. Souza SP: *Uncertainties in temperature mapping via diffusion imaging.* In *Proceedings of the 11th meeting of the Society of Magnetic Resonance in Medicine,* Berlin, 1992, Society of Magnetic Resonance.
24. Vitkin IA, and others: Magnetic resonance imaging of temperature changes during interstitial microwave heating: a phantom study, *Med Phys* 24:269, 1997.
25. de Poorter J: Noninvasive MRI thermometry with the proton resonance frequency method: study of susceptibility effects, *Magn Reson Med* 34:359, 1995.
26. Young IR, and others: An evaluation of the effects of susceptibility changes on the water chemical shift method of temperature measurements in human peripheral muscle, *Magn Reson Med* 36:366, 1996.
27. Prince MR, and others: Dynamic gadolinium-enhanced three-dimensional abdominal MR arteriography, *J Magn Reson Imaging* 3:877, 1993.
28. Prince MR, Grist TM, Debatin JF: *3D contrast MR angiography,* Berlin, 1997, Springer-Verlag.
29. Kouwenhoven M: Contrast-enhanced MR angiography, methods limitations and possibilities, *Acta Radiol Suppl* 412:57, 1997.
30. Ackerman JL, and others: *Rapid 3D tracking of small RF coils.* In *Proceedings of the 5th annual meeting of the Society of Magnetic Resonance in Medicine,* Montreal, 1986, Society of Magnetic Resonance.
31. Dumoulin CL, Souza SP, Darrow RD: Real-time position monitoring of invasive devices using magnetic resonance, *Magn Reson Med* 29:411, 1993.
32. Bakker CJG, and others: Visualization of dedicated catheters using fast scanning techniques with potential for MR-guided vascular interventions, *Magn Reson Med* 36:816, 1996.
33. Glowinski A, and others: Catheter visualization using locally induced, actively controlled field inhomogeneities, *Magn Reson Med* 38:253, 1997.
34. Bakker CJG, and others: MR-guided endovascular interventions: susceptibility-based catheter and near-real-time imaging technique, *Radiology* 202:273, 1997.
35. Rasche V, and others: Catheter tracking using continuous radial MRI, *Magn Reson Med* 37:963, 1997.
36. American Heart Association: *Stroke facts,* Dallas, 1992, American Heart Association.
37. Ginsberg MD, Pulsinelli WA: The ischemic penumbra, injury thresholds, and the therapeutic window for acute stroke, *Ann Neurol* 36:553, 1994 (editorial).
38. Hossman K-A: Viability threshold and the penumbra of focal ischemia, *Ann Neurol* 36:557, 1994.
39. Camarata PJ, Heros RC, Latchaw RE: Brain attack: the rationale for treating stroke as a medical emergency, *Neurosurgery* 34:144, 1994.
40. Higashida RT, and others: Interventional neurovascular techniques in the treatment of stroke: state-of-the-art therapy, *J Intern Med* 237:105, 1995.
41. Barnwell SL: *Thrombolytic therapy for acute stroke: indications, technique, and results.* In *Proceedings, SCVIR 22nd annual scientific meeting,* Washington DC, *J Vasc Interv Radiol* 8 (suppl):28, 1997.
42. LeBihan D, and others: Diffusion MR imaging: clinical applications, *Am J Roentgenol* 159:591, 1992.
43. Kucharczyk J, and others: Contrast-enhanced perfusion-sensitive MR imaging in the diagnosis of cerebrovascular disorders, *J Magn Reson Imaging* 2:241, 1993.
44. Sutton JP, and others: Ventroposterior medial pallidotomy in patients with advanced Parkinson's disease, *Neurosurgery* 36:1112, 1995.
45. Kopyov O, and others: Microelectrode-guided posteroventral medial radiofrequency pallidotomy for Parkinson's disease, *J Neurosurg* 87:52, 1997.
46. Lehman RM, and others: Peri- and postoperative magnetic resonance imaging localization of pallidotomy, *Stereotact Funct Neurosurg* 62:61, 1994.

Chapter 6

ENDOVASCULAR COILS FOR INTERVENTIONAL MRI

Gregory C. Hurst

Although magnetic resonance imaging (MRI) applications are dominated by neurologic and orthopedic studies, the greater potential medical significance of cardiovascular imaging has been appreciated since the earliest days of biomedical nuclear magnetic resonance (NMR) and MRI. More than a decade ago, a catheter NMR probe was shown to localize and improve the signal-to-noise ratio (SNR) of P31 MR spectra from *in vivo* canine heart muscle.[1] One early survey and prospectus of cardiovascular MRI proposed that a catheter probe might be useful for direct *in vivo* visualization of atherosclerotic disease.[2]

To date, results from catheter probes have been limited to *ex vivo* samples and *in vivo* animal models. However, the interest and progress demonstrated by several different research groups offers hope for their use in research of cardiovascular wall disease or in human clinical application.

DEVICE DESIGN

Table 6-1 gives a summary, in reverse chronologic order, of various catheter NMR probe designs. This chapter describes, in forward chronological order, the progression of endovascular probe development.

Conductor patterns

Early concepts of catheter probes for wall imaging[3,4] derived from inside-out NMR machines designed for oil well logging.[5] The opposed solenoid conductor pattern (Fig. 6-1), first used to provide the homogeneous polarizing B_o field for borehole NMR, was adapted to provide a sensitive yet homogeneous receiver coil for viewing the arterial wall. This concept of the intravascular coil design problem assumes a relatively large lumen relative to the vessel wall, which may be appropriate for looking at very early stages of atherosclerosis but is not appropriate when the vessel is heavily occluded (or blocked completely).

The opposed solenoid catheter provides relatively homogeneous response in the axial plane between the solenoids, but the region of coverage along the axis of the solenoids is limited. An alternative conductor pattern, a sine coil, has been declared superior to opposed solenoid catheters for overall homogeneity.[6]

Several recent studies have presented designs that are much less demanding of arterial lumen "real estate" and thus are potentially more practical for studying occluded arteries. One novel approach locates an expandable probe in a vein appropriately adjacent to the artery of interest (Fig. 6-2).[7]

Other ideas have led to probes that are potentially or actually small enough for cardiac catheterization. Rubinson and Boska[8] showed a receiver probe with a diameter of only 2 mm, which was built by removing a section of shield from a coaxial

Table 6-1. Selected catheter probe designs

Conductor pattern	Tuning and coupling controls	Major innovations, conclusions	Reference/Year
Loopless dipole antenna	Coax balancing transformer; coax to remote tune and match	Highly miniature, highly flexible, highly homogeneous	Ocali and Atalar,[9] 1997
Shorted parallel wires (transmission line)	Capacitor network to coax line	Highly miniature, highly flexible	Atalar and others,[10] 1997
Loop on an inflatable balloon	Coax to remote tune and match	Balloon occlusion to reduce flow artifact	Quick and others,[14] 1997
Expanding loop	Twisted pair to remote tune and match	Intravenous approach to adjacent arteries	Martin and others,[7] 1996
Shorted coax	Untuned, remote tune and match	Readily miniaturized, flexible	Rubinson and Boska,[8] 1995
Opposed solenoids	Capacitor network to coax	Bullet tip to reduce flow artifact	Martin and Henkelman,[13] 1994
Opposed solenoids and long open saddle	Tuning capacitors near coil	Saddle better for S/N and large field of view	Burl and others,[18] 1993
Sine, loop, Golay, solenoid, opposed solenoid	Not specified	Best longitudinal and axial homogeneity with sine coil	McDonald and others,[6] 1993
Loop	Partial tune and match capacitors at coil to coax to remote tune and match	Signal-to-noise ratio improvement similar to opposed solenoid	Kandarpa and others,[19] 1993
Opposed solenoid	Capacitors tune and match coil to coax	Signal-to-noise ratio improvement similar to report below	Martin and others,[3] 1992
Opposed solenoid, center return, loop, others	Single fixed tuning capacitor with field effect transistor at coil	Miniature adaptation of opposed solenoid; tenfold S/N increase over surface coil	Hurst and others,[4] 1992
Loop	Coax to remote tune and match	First catheter nuclear magnetic resonance probe	Kantor and others,[1] 1984

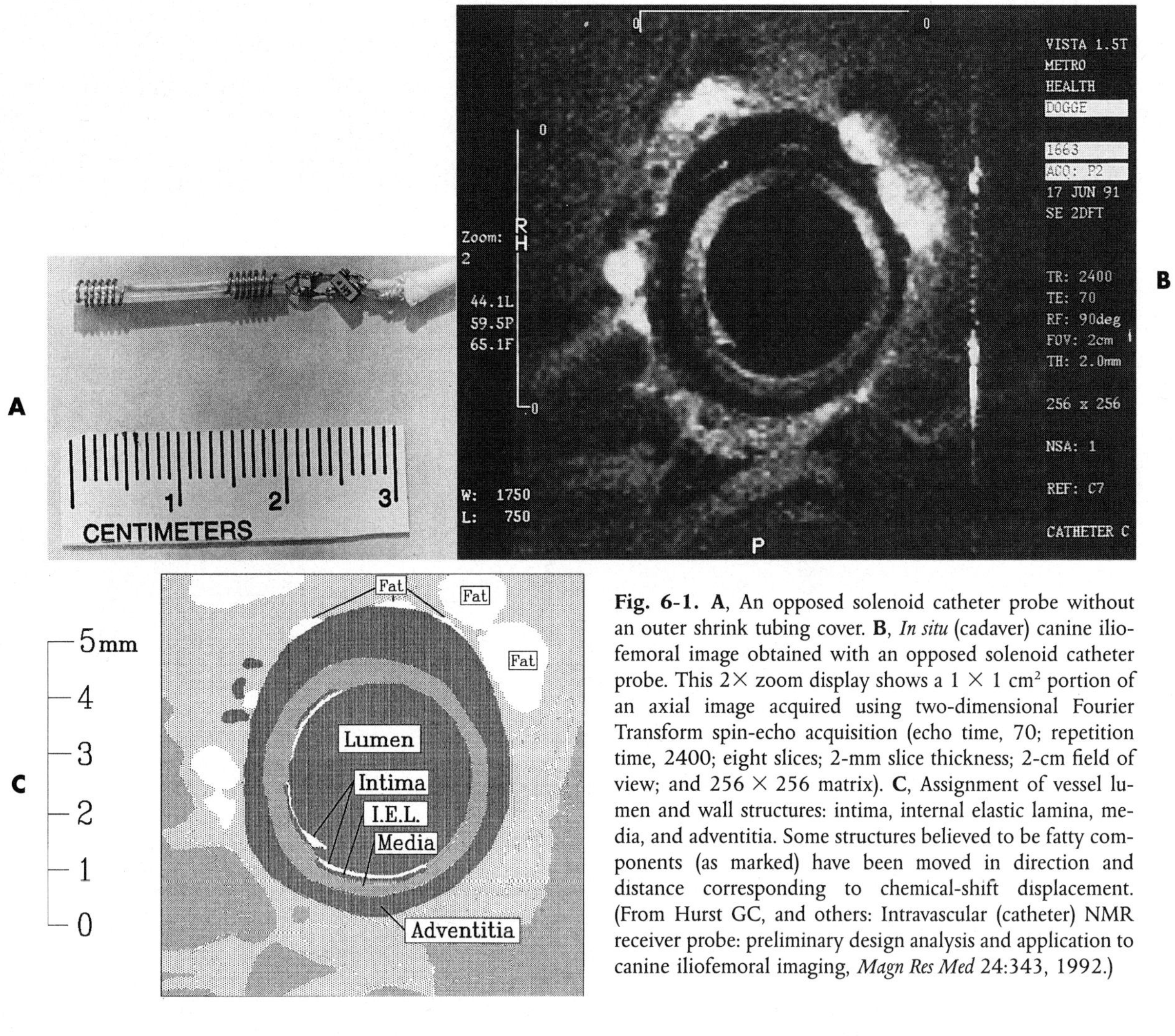

Fig. 6-1. A, An opposed solenoid catheter probe without an outer shrink tubing cover. **B**, *In situ* (cadaver) canine iliofemoral image obtained with an opposed solenoid catheter probe. This 2× zoom display shows a 1 × 1 cm^2 portion of an axial image acquired using two-dimensional Fourier Transform spin-echo acquisition (echo time, 70; repetition time, 2400; eight slices; 2-mm slice thickness; 2-cm field of view; and 256 × 256 matrix). **C**, Assignment of vessel lumen and wall structures: intima, internal elastic lamina, media, and adventitia. Some structures believed to be fatty components (as marked) have been moved in direction and distance corresponding to chemical-shift displacement. (From Hurst GC, and others: Intravascular (catheter) NMR receiver probe: preliminary design analysis and application to canine iliofemoral imaging, *Magn Res Med* 24:343, 1992.)

cable. The "loopless" design of Ocali and Atalar[9] is based on a dipole antenna, rather than a closed-loop inductor as is conventionally used to detect the magnetic field induced by the NMR sample. This design, which has been miniaturized to fit inside a 4-F sheath, offers excellent homogeneity over a large target area, mechanical flexibility, and easy coupling without large component circuitry. Another novel design from Atalar and others,[10] which is also realized in a long, thin, flexible package, is based on two parallel conductors having one end electrically shorted (Fig. 6-3).

Tuning, matching, and coupling schemes

A recent text summarized and illustrated tuning and coupling schemes used for internal MRI coils.[11] A recent journal article provided electrical diagrams and summarized and analyzed tuning and matching networks generally used for MR probes.[12]

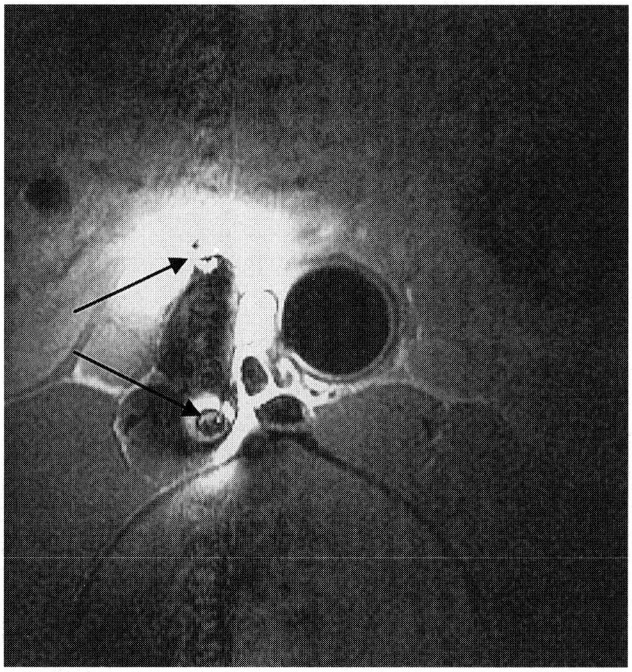

Fig. 6-2. A fast spin-echo image acquired with an intravenous coil in a living swine. The aorta is situated to the right of the coil, and the medial layer of the artery wall can be seen. The positions of the inductive elements of the coil are marked with arrows. Scan parameters include 50-mm field of view; 2-mm slice thickness; 1-mm skip; 256 × 224 matrix; echo time, 18 msec; cardiac gating with repetition time, 1791 msec (two R-R cycles); echo train length, 4; four averages; and superior and inferior saturation slabs. This is one of 12 images acquired in 6 minutes, 56 seconds. (From Martin AJ, and others: An expandable intravenous RF coil for arterial wall imaging, *J Magn Reson Imaging* 8:226, 1998.)

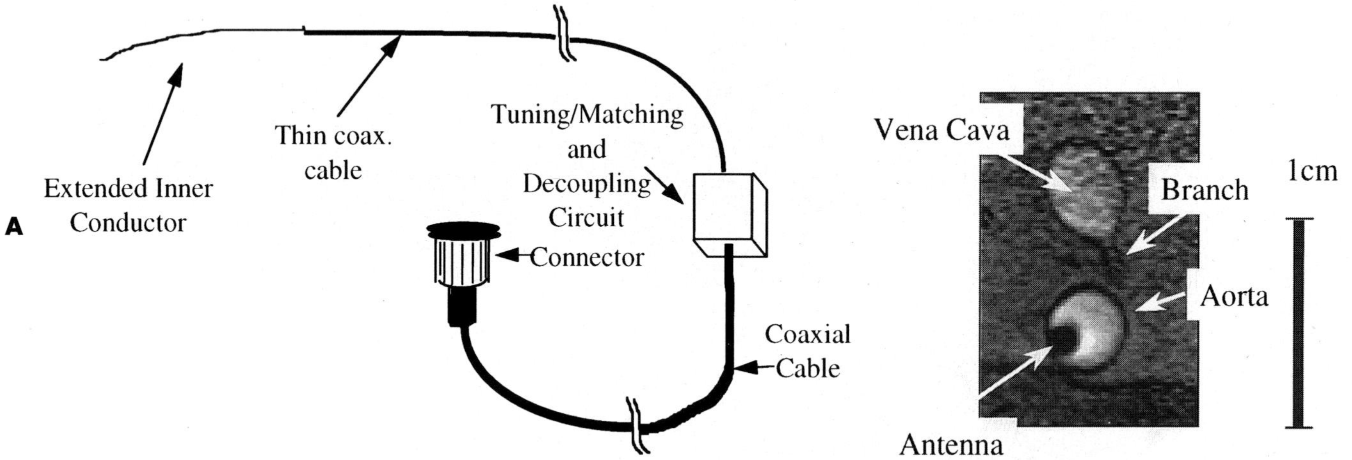

Fig. 6-3. A, Loopless catheter antenna design made from a thin coaxial cable with an extended inner conductor. Catheter antennae as small as 1.5 F (0.5-mm diameter) have been designed with this approach. **B**, Image using a loopless catheter antenna inserted via the femoral artery into a rabbit prepared using a high-cholesterol diet and aortic injury using a balloon catheter. Imaging parameters are 40-mm field of view; 3-mm slice thickness; 256 × 256 matrix; echo time, 3.2; repetition time, 9.9; eight excitations; and CINE, 8 frames. (Schematic and image courtesy of Ergin Atalar, and others: Department of Radiology and Radiological Science, Johns Hopkins University, Baltimore.)

The coupling scheme for the loopless antenna probe is straightforward and has been well described.[9]

Mechanical devices for suppressing motion artifacts

Early studies showed serious blurring and ghosting problems, which were attributed to blood flow or vessel motion.[4] Martin and Henkelman[13] implemented a bullet tip to centrally locate an endovascular coil and restrict its range of motion. They found substantially reduced ghosting and blurring, with further motion artifact reduction provided by saturation pulses (Fig. 6-4). Quick and colleagues[14] constructed a coil on the surface of a balloon catheter, such that the inflated balloon occludes flow in the vessel during imaging, and produced remarkably artifact-free images in living animals (Fig. 6-5).

SUMMARY OF EXPERIMENTAL RESULTS

Table 6-2 summarizes the vessel wall structures that have been visualized using intravascular-type probes, together with the imaging machine used and the subject. Most researchers have used clinical imaging machines, presumably in hopes of eventual use in humans or because these systems were the most available. Dogs, pigs, and rabbits have been used; the appropriateness and limitations of these animal models are well known.[15]

CHALLENGES AND FUTURE DIRECTIONS

The prototype catheter coils need to be substantially modified for use at the relatively low-operating frequencies of the open MR imaging systems currently associated with interventional applications. For conventional detectors (e.g., loops,

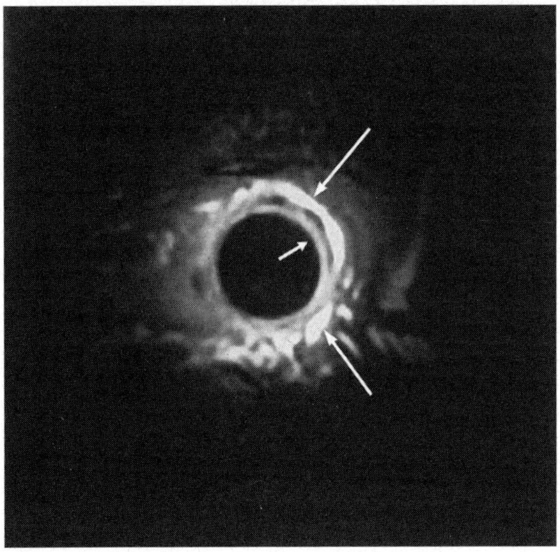

Fig. 6-4. Intravascular coil image of a swine at the level of the kidneys. Image parameters include 80-mm field of view; 3-mm slice thickness; 256 × 256 matrix; echo time, 15 msec; cardiac gating with repetition time, 904 msec; magnification, 2× ; and two averages for a total imaging time of 7 minutes, 42 seconds. The coil had the stabilizing tip placed on its end, and a saturation pulse was applied superior to the imaging plane. Fat deposits are seen around the periphery of the artery *(long arrows)*, and layering within the artery wall is evident (*short arrow*). (From Martin AJ, Henkelman RM: Intravascular MR imaging in a porcine animal model, *Magn Reson Med* 32:224, 1994.)

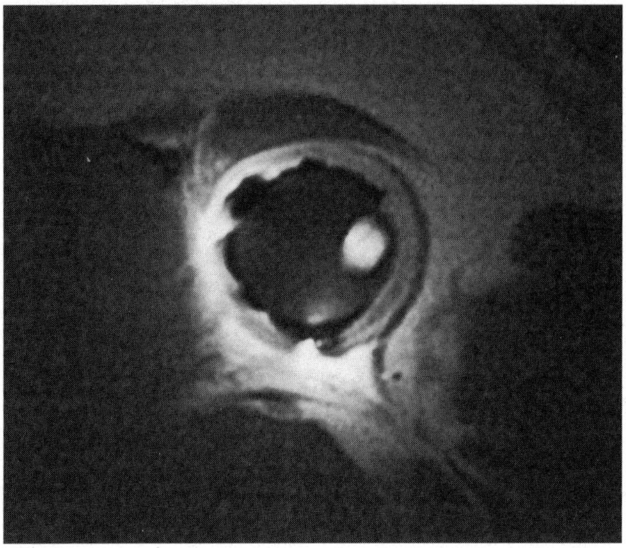

Fig. 6-5. Intravascular coil image of the aorta of a Watanabe hereditary hyperlipedic rabbit. Image parameters include 30 × 15-mm field of view; 4-mm slice thickness; 256 × 96 matrix; echo time, 20 msec; repetition time, 400 msec; six excitations; acquisition time, 3 minutes, 54 seconds. (Courtesy of Harald H. Quick, Gesine G. Zimmerman, Jorg F. Debatin: Department of Radiology, University Hospital, Zurich.)

Table 6-2. Vessel wall structures seen using catheter probes

Imaging system, field strength	Subjects and vessels	Findings	Reference/Year
Clinical, 1.5 T	*In vivo* rabbit aorta	Wall thickening, calcification	Quick and others,[14] 1997
Clinical, 1.5 T	*Ex vivo* human aorta	Wall layers	Atalar and others,[10] 1997
	In vivo rabbit aorta	Lumen and wall layers	
	In situ dog circumflex coronary artery	Water and lipid spectral peaks	
Clinical, 1.5 T	*In vivo* pig aorta	Wall layers	Martin and Henkelman,[13] 1994
Research (30-cm bore), 1.9 T	*Ex vivo* human popliteal arteries	Intimal hyperplasia, medial calcification, focal plaque	Kandarpa and others,[19] 1993
Clinical, 1.5 T	Dog cadaver, iliac artery	Wall layers (intima, media, adventitia)	Martin and others,[3] 1992

opposed solenoids), probe size will be problematic because lower frequency requires more space to accommodate the necessary larger capacitance. With the loopless antenna, impedance (and noise resistance) is a function of the antenna length,[9] such that the optimal length may be impractical at lower frequencies.

Design issues are not particularly meaningful without a defined application to give context to technical performance. For example, the vessel size and the structure of interest should be defined to give meaning to analysis of SNR relative to probe size. Thus, intravascular ultrasound[16,17] may prove beneficial by helping define applications of vessel wall visualization.

These interesting and progressively better results and the overwhelming significance of cardiovascular disease should motivate further development.

REFERENCES

1. Kantor HL, Briggs RW, Balaban RS: In-vivo 31P NMR measurements in canine heart using a catheter coil, *Circ Res* 55:261, 1984.
2. Wesbey GE, and others: Magnetic resonance applications in atherosclerotic vascular disease, *Cardiovasc Intervent Radiol* 8:342, 1986.
3. Martin AJ, Plewes DB, Henkelman RM: MR imaging of blood vessels with an intravascular coil, *J Magn Reson Imaging* 2:421, 1992.
4. Hurst GC, and others: Intravascular (catheter) NMR receiver probe: preliminary design analysis and application to canine iliofemoral imaging, *Magn Reson Med* 24:343, 1992.
5. Jackson JA, Burnett LJ, Harmon JF: Remote (inside-out) NMR. III. Detection of nuclear magnetic resonance in a remotely produced region of homogeneous magnetic field, *J Magn Reson Imaging* 41:411, 1980.
6. McDonald GG, Chwialkowski M, Peshock RM: *Performance comparison of several coil geometries for use in catheters,* Proceedings of the 1993 Meeting of the Radiological Society of North America.
7. Martin AJ, and others: *An expandable intravenous RF coil for imaging the artery wall,* Proceedings of the ISMRM Annual Meeting, 1996.
8. Rubinson KA, Boska M: NMR imaging with shorted coaxial line probes, *Magn Reson Imaging* 13:291, 1995.
9. Ocali O, Atalar E: Intravascular magnetic resonance imaging using a loopless catheter antenna, *Magn Reson Med* 37:112, 1997.
10. Atalar E, and others: High resolution intravascular MRI and MRS using a catheter receiver coil, *Magn Reson Med* 1997.
11. Hurst GC, Misic GJ: *Coils for insertion into the human body.* In *Encyclopedia of NMR,* Chichester, England, 1996, John Wiley & Sons.
12. Viohl I, Gullberg GT: Tuning and matching networks for MR imaging and spectroscopy, *J Magn Reson Imaging* 4:627, 1994.
13. Martin AJ, Henkelman RM: Intravascular MR imaging in a porcine animal model, *Magn Reson Med* 32:224, 1994.
14. Quick HH, and others: In vivo high resolution intravascular imaging with a single loop receiver coil, Proceedings of the 1997 Meeting of the ISMRM.
15. Averbook A, White GH, Wilson SE: *Atherosclerosis and arteriosclerosis: human pathology and experimental animal methods and models,* Boca Raton, Fla, 1989, CRC Press.
16. Cavaye DM, White RA: *Intravascular ultrasound imaging,* 1993, Raven Press.
17. Hodgson JM, Sheehan HM, editors: *Atlas of intravascular ultrasound,* 1994, Raven Press.
18. Burl M, Young IR, Hajnal JV: *Performance of small internal coils for MRI,* Proceedings of the ISMRM Annual Meeting, 1993.
19. Kandarpa K, and others: Prototype miniature endoluminal MR imaging catheter, *J Vasc Interv Radiol* 4:419, 1993.

Chapter 7

MR–COMPATIBLE INSTRUMENTS FOR INTERVENTIONAL MRI

Andreas Melzer, Dieter Stoeckel, Martin Busch, Martin Deli, Armin Schmidt, Karl Kipfmüller, Dietrich Grönemeyer, Rainer M.M. Seibel

Interventional magnetic resonance imaging (MRI) has made significant progress in recent years. Although the new open magnets have stimulated this progress significantly, interventions can also be performed in closed MR units, shown more than 10 years ago.[1] In open and closed configurations, the physical nature of MRI is governing the application of instruments and electric equipment within or near the magnet.

Specific materials and processing are required to provide MR-compatible instruments that are adequately represented in an MRI scan. High emission (radiofrequency [RF]) from electric equipment, particularly near the Larmor frequency of the MRI scanner, can severely reduce the image quality (Fig. 7-1). Shielding and electronic filters are helpful but can be difficult to use and expensive. Many devices and ancillary equipment can be placed outside the MR suite. Electric transmission and control of the device can be achieved via glass fiberoptic coupling. In addition, the acquisition system can be used to control electric equipment that emits problematic frequencies so that the devices are switched on and off during the acquisition. Specific application of pulsed energy can used to control the acquisition, similar to gating or electrocardiographic (ECG) triggering.

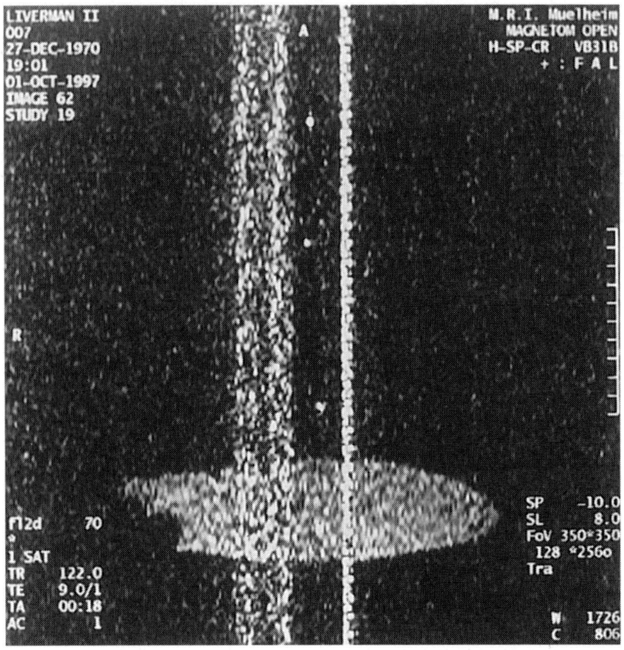

Fig. 7-1. Magnetic resonance (MR) image acquisition (Magnetom Open, Siemens, Erlangen, Germany) during an MR-guided neuroendoscopic procedure using an incompatible radiofrequency system.

This chapter deals with the instruments and equipment required for MR-guided interventions and surgery.[2–4]

PRINCIPLES OF MAGNETIC RESONANCE COMPATIBILITY

Various terms describe the possible use of instruments and ancillary equipment during MR-guided procedures. The term *MR compatibility,* when referring to instruments used in the magnet room or incorporated in the body and displayed within the image plane, is not clearly defined. To avoid misunderstanding, only one major classification should be used for these tools. However, because of this ambiguity and because instrumentation is more or less inappropriate, classification of MR compatibility is preliminary.

Two levels of MR compatibility should be considered: instruments and devices that can be used near the magnet (level 1) and devices that are fully MR compatible and can be used in the image plane and during acquisition (level 2). The following principles of MR compatibility are incomplete and reflect only initial experiences with MR guidance.

- Any instrument moved into the MR suite should be nonmagnetic and not attracted by the magnetic field.
- Two levels of MR compatibility can be recognized: level 1—nonmagnetic; and level 2—MR compatible.
- All instruments and devices to be used in an MR suite should be classified as level 1 or 2 and approved according to the magnet type.
- Level 2 devices can be used in the RF cabin during acquisition. They are nonmagnetic but can cause susceptibility artifacts when used within the image plane.
- MR-compatible instruments should be labeled according to the MR system for which they can be used. The label should include the brand name, the manufacturer of the magnet, and the sequence type with the respective artifact size.
- An instrument used near the magnet but not during acquisition should be nonmagnetic.
- An implant present in the magnetic field during acquisition should not cause major artifacts that alter the images.
- An instrument in the image plane but outside the body should not cause relevant distortion of the magnetic field.
- An implant that is in the image plane and the field of view (FOV) should not cause relevant distortion of the magnetic field and should feature an adequate visualization or artifact.

ARTIFACT SIZE

Material, magnet field strength, angle of the instrument to the magnet field B_o, and sequence type are key factors for determining artifact size. These parameters cannot simply be changed during the procedure. FOV, read-out direction, bandwidth, and echo time (TE) are secondary influences on the artifact size and allow adjustment during the procedure. The appropriate size of the artifact depends on the procedure and the anatomic region of the volume of interest; it can be influenced by modification of the above-mentioned parameters.

Any instrument requires adequate display on the MRI to allow control of its position at any time. If the instrument diameter is less than 1 mm, visualization of the tool may be difficult. A 256 $\times$ 256 matrix gradient-recalled echo (GRE) and an FOV of 256 mm lead to a pixel size of 1 mm; an instrument with an artifact size of 1 mm can just be visualized. An artifact with a 1:1 relation to the instrument size is not optimal in all cases. Targets and volumes of interest within a body having T_1-weighted low-intensity structures (e.g., bone, air, liver, liquid) impede the visibility of the dark grey artifacts. Thus, for interventions in these areas, cannulas with larger artifacts are essential for the procedure. Based on clinical experience, 2 to 3 mm is the minimum useful artifact size. A size of 3 to 5 mm allows initial localization of the instrument in a larger FOV. Abdominal interventions are usually performed with a 350-mm FOV.

Sequence types influence artifact size and orientation (Fig. 7-2). Artifacts appear larger in GRE. Because higher field systems allow the use of turbo GREs and are more sensitive to susceptibility differences, the artifact of an instrument is larger. Therefore, each interventional device requires evaluation for each field strength. If the instrument diameter decreases, the artifact should become smaller so that a 3-mm instrument is displayed with an artifact size of 3 mm. If the diameter is greater than 3 mm, the instrument should be displayed in 1:1 ratio (Tables 7-1 and 7-2).

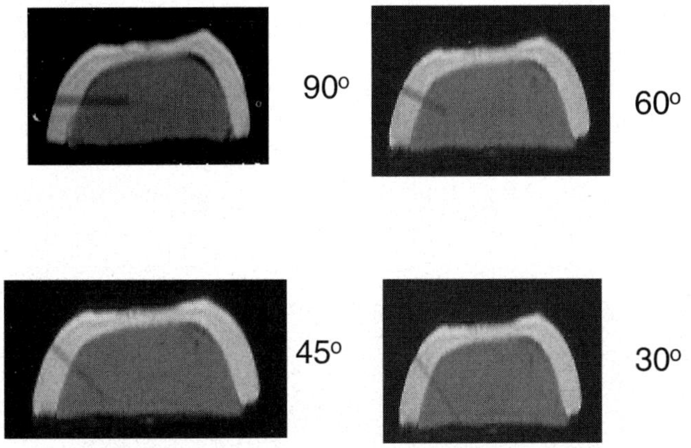

Fig. 7-2. Influence of B_0 angle to an artifact size of a 20-G titanium needle in a magnetic resonance phantom.

Table 7-1. Artifact sizes of 0.2-T, 90° to B_0, spin-echo puncture cannulas*

Instrument diameter	Material	Artifact size
22 G ≈ 0.6 mm	Stainless steel	1 mm with stylet, not visible without stylet
20 G ≈ 0.8 mm	Stainless steel	1 mm with stylet, 1 mm without stylet
18 G ≈ 1 mm	Stainless steel	2 mm with stylet, 1 to 2 mm without stylet
22 G	Titanium grade 4	Difficult to see with stylet, difficult to see without stylet† 1 mm with stainless steel stylet
20 G	Titanium grade 4	1 mm with stylet, is not visible and thus cannot be measured
18 G	Titanium grade 4	2 mm with stylet, >2 mm without stylet
16 G ≈ 1.2 mm	Titanium grade 4	2 to 3 mm with stylet, side-cut biopsy‡
14 G ≈ 1.6 mm	Titanium grade 4	3 mm with stylet, side-cut biopsy‡

*Magnet/Sequence—0.2-T Magnetom Open/rectangular field of view, 350-mm spin-echo, 30 sec; repetition time, 300 sec; echo time, 30 sec; flip angle 90.
†22-G Titanium can be recommended only in combination with a stainless steel stylet.
‡Stylet cannot be removed.

Table 7-2. Artifact sizes of 0.2-T, 90° to B_0, gradient echo puncture cannulas*

Instrument diameter	Material	Artifact size
22 G ~ 0.6 mm	Stainless steel	3 mm with stylet, 2 mm without stylet, 2 mm with titanium stylet
20 G (0.8 mm)	Stainless steel	4 mm with stylet, 3 mm without stylet
18 G (1 mm)	Stainless steel	6 mm with stylet, 4 mm without stylet
22 G	Titanium grade 4	2 mm with stylet, > 2 mm without stylet†, 3 to 4 mm with stainless steel stylet
20 G	Titanium grade 4	3 mm with stylet, 2 to 3 mm without stylet
18 G	Titanium grade 4	4 mm with stylet, 3 mm without stylet
16 G (1.2 mm)	Titanium grade 4	4 to 5 mm with stylet, side-cut biopsy‡
14 G (1.6 mm)	Titanium grade 4	5 to 6 mm with stylet, side-cut biopsy‡

*Magnet/sequence—0.2-T fast low-angle shot, two-dimensional (2D) gradient echo, rectangular field of view 350 mm, fast imaging with steady state precision.
†Very difficult to see. 22-G titanium can be recommended only in combination with a stainless steel stylet.
‡Stylet cannot be removed.

MAGNETIC RESONANCE–COMPATIBLE MATERIALS

Ferromagnetic materials cannot be used for MR instruments. The magnetic field distortion is so extensive that imaging is impossible. Stainless steel has the best mechanical properties for most interventional instruments. Iron-free alloys with high nickel content and nonmagnetic characteristics are appropriate for smaller interventional instruments of up to 1 mm in diameter (Fig. 7-3).

Some types of brass, aluminum, and copper are MR compatible and lead only to a 1:1-sized artifact. However, their biocompatibility is inappropriate for intracorporeal application. Mechanical characteristics of these alloys are insufficient for

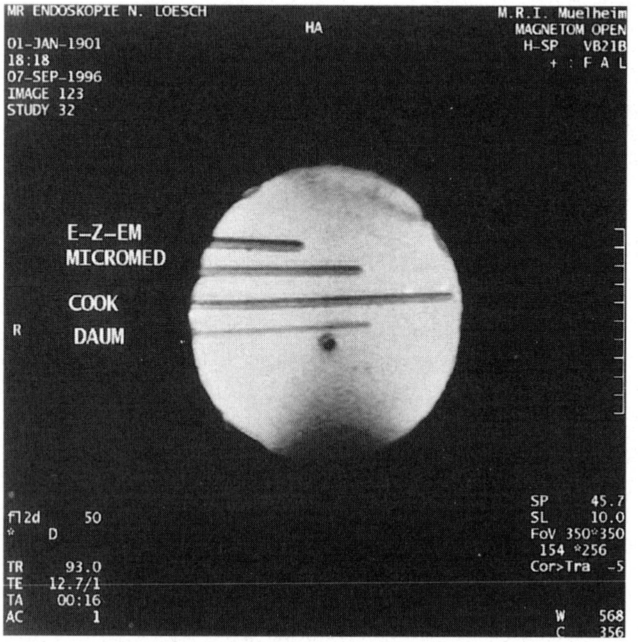

Fig. 7-3. An artifact of different needle materials (20 G).

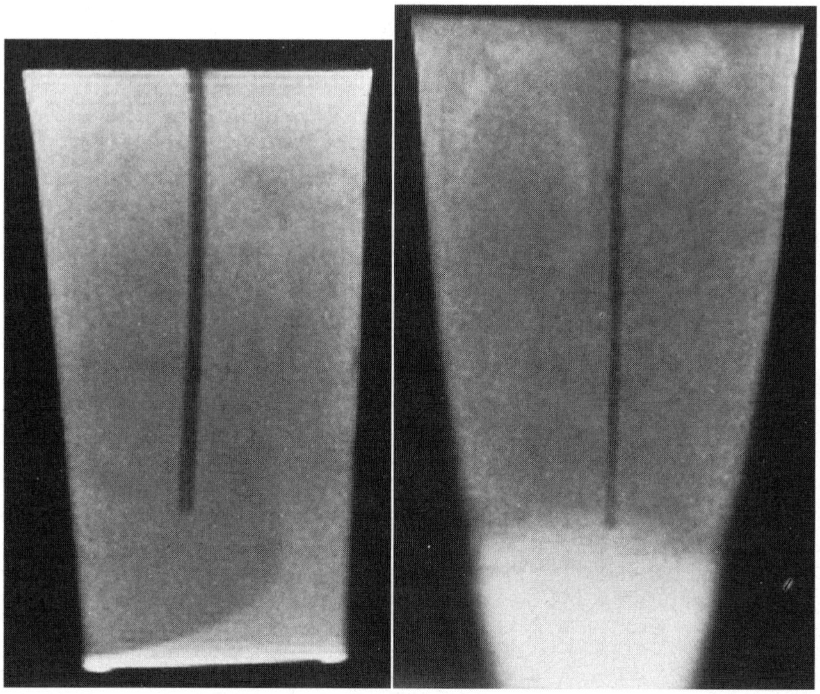

Fig. 7-4. Samples of catheter tubing.

smaller instruments, such as cannulas, forceps, and baskets (see Tables 7-1 and 7-2). Nonmagnetic stainless steel, titanium alloys, and nickel-titanium are more suitable.[5]

Various MR-compatible ceramics are available. Ceramics that were recently improved with zirconium oxide and aluminum oxide (increased elasticity, improved machining) are useful for special purposes in interventional instruments. One neurosurgical skull frame made from zirconium oxide ceramic is fully MR compatible.

Synthetic materials have excellent MR compatibility provided that the plastic does not contain para- or ferromagnetic substances for coloring. Information about the content of new catheters and balloons is often proprietary but is sometimes known (Fig. 7-4). Material that is to be used under MR guidance should be tested for compatibility.

MECHANISM OF THE MAGNETIC RESONANCE ARTIFACT

Items with different magnetic susceptibility than the tissue create a susceptibility artifact. Distortion of the magnetic field caused by paramagnetism decreases the relaxation time (TR) of the protons near the instrument. Thus, the signal is not detected in the respective TE. The center of a titanium probe is signal-free, but a signal-intensive zone is located in the periphery (Fig. 7-5). This peripheral shining can be interpreted as a T1 effect similar to the signal enhancement of gadolinium. This effect is not seen in GRE images. In theory, the bright shadow can be used to find an instrument that has been moved out of the image plane. However, in 250 clinical cases, no positive correlation was noted because the fast spin-echo in breathhold technique does not provide adequate image quality.

PUNCTURE NEEDLES WITH ADJUSTABLE ARTIFACT SIZE

Many interventional procedures require T1- and often T2-weighted spin-echo and turbo–spin-echo control images. Because these sequences are not very sensitive to susceptibility, instruments smaller than 1 mm cannot be detected. If the needle trajectory is in the direction of the magnet B_0 field, the artifact becomes small and often invisible. For these drawbacks to be overcome the artifact size can be adjusted by simply using different mandrins. Titanium or nonmagnetic stainless cannulas with mandrins or stylets allow different materials to be introduced (Fig. 7-6). Synthetic stylets are beneficial for the insertion of cannulas larger than 18 G, artifact-sensitive sequences, and high-field systems and for precise placement of smaller cannulas. Titanium stylets should be used for puncture with medium-sized cannulas and for insertion into difficult areas with low signal intensity, such as the paravertebral region. Small cannulas less than 20 G require nonmagnetic stainless steel to provide optimal visibility of artifacts. Smaller titanium needles (<20 G) should be equipped with a stainless steel stylet.

A B

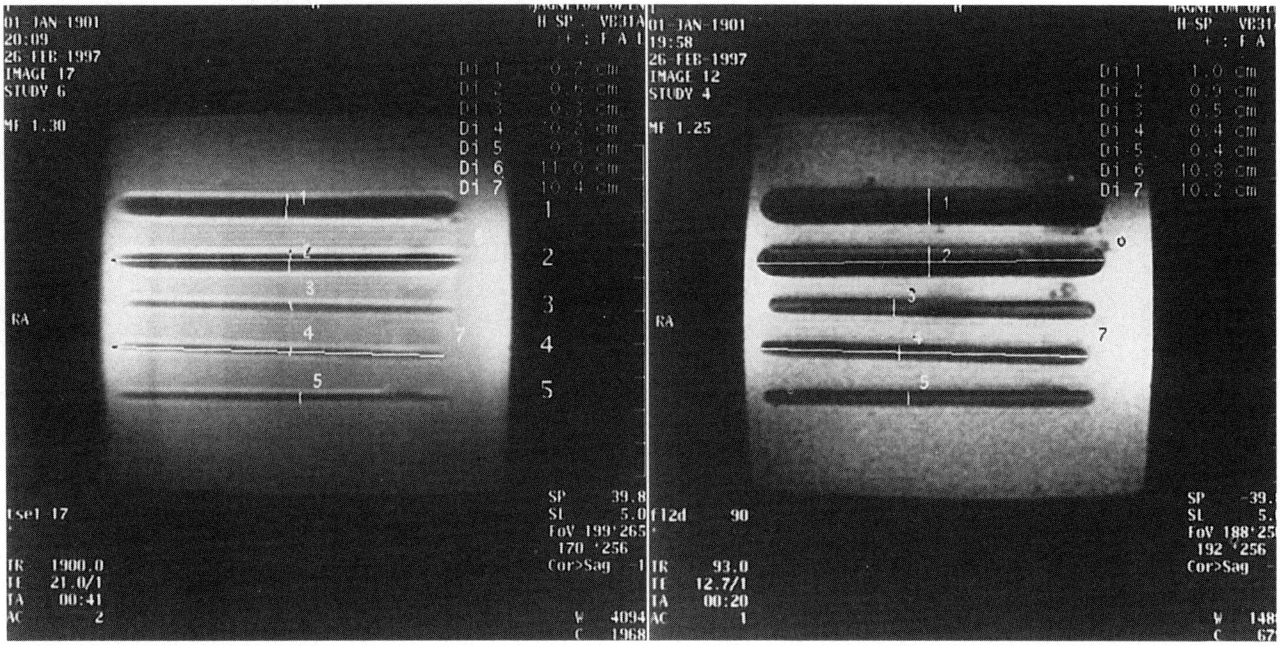

Fig. 7-5. Signal characteristic of a titanium artifact in T1-weighted sequences: **A,** Spin-echo and **B,** gradient echo.

A

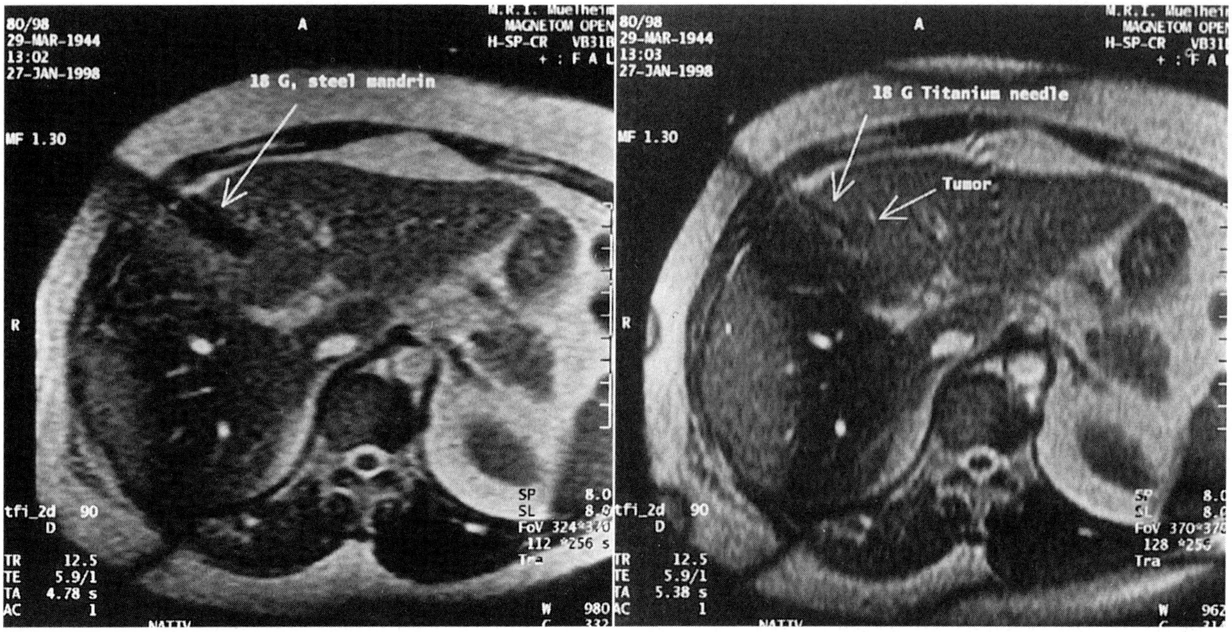

B

Fig. 7-6. Artifact appearance of a titanium 13-G cannula with a stylet made of **A,** stainless steel, and **B,** titanium during a liver biopsy.

PUNCTURE NEEDLES

MR-compatible cannulas have been available for many years in sizes of 22 G, 100 m, and 150 mm. Excellent nonmagnetic stainless steel needles are available from E-Z-EM (Lufkin Needle). The authors found only the 22-G stainless steel needles (Cook, Bjaevetskov, Denmark) useful for punctures and for procedures such as periradicular therapy ($N =$ 185), ethanol lumbar sympathectomy ($N = 18$), intratumoral ethanol injections ($N = 10$), and local pain management ($N =$ 20). For larger needles, which overextend the artifact, titanium needles were developed (Daum Medical, Schwerin, Germany). Magnetic susceptibility and artifact size render these cannulas superior to stainless steel items (Tables 7-1 and 7-2). The relatively rough surface and the risk of kinking are drawbacks of titanium cannulas.

Needles made from Nitinol (nickel titanium, Naval Ordnance Laboratory) do not kink permanently because of superelasticity. The needles allow a puncture around the corner (Fig. 7-7). The sharpness is excellent and entails a particular advantage. If the sharp tip of a Nitinol needle touches bone, no kinking occurs.

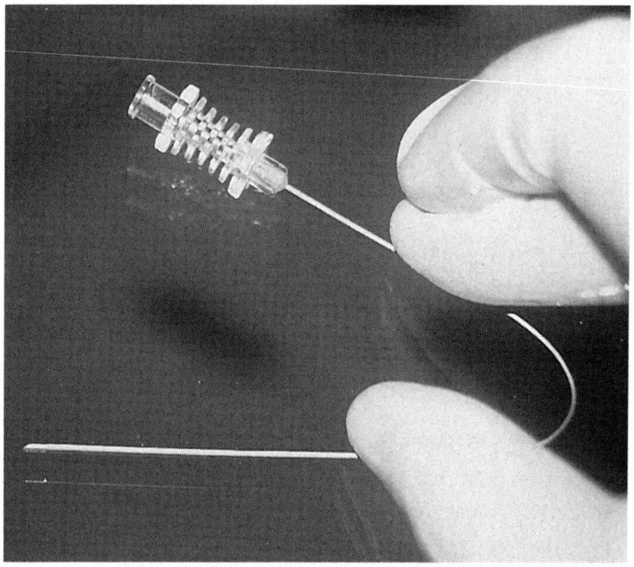

Fig. 7-7. A superelastic 22-G cannula provides puncture over a finger.

NEEDLES FOR CELL ASPIRATION AND CORE BIOPSY

The authors prefer aspiration full-core biopsy using a modified titanium Menghini cut cannula (Daum Medical, Schwerin, Germany). This cannula comes with different stylets to control artifact size. For core biopsy, a standard aspiration handle for 20-ml syringes is used.

An automatic biopsy needle that features a lightweight spring-loaded gun is available from Daum Medical. According to tests, an MR-compatible spring has been included in the handle (Fig. 7-8).

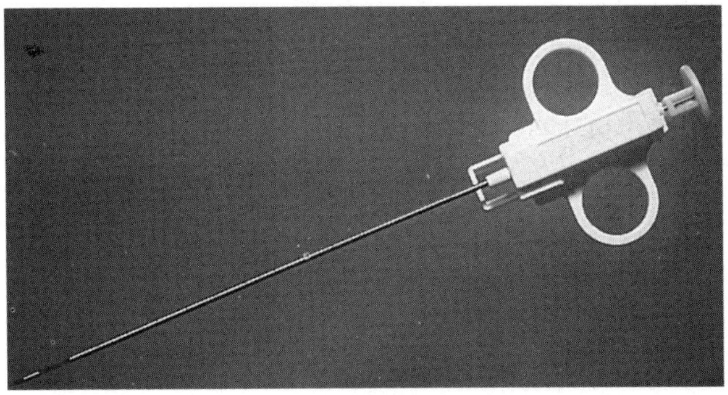

Fig. 7-8. A spring-loaded biopsy gun (Daum Medical, Schwerin, Germany).

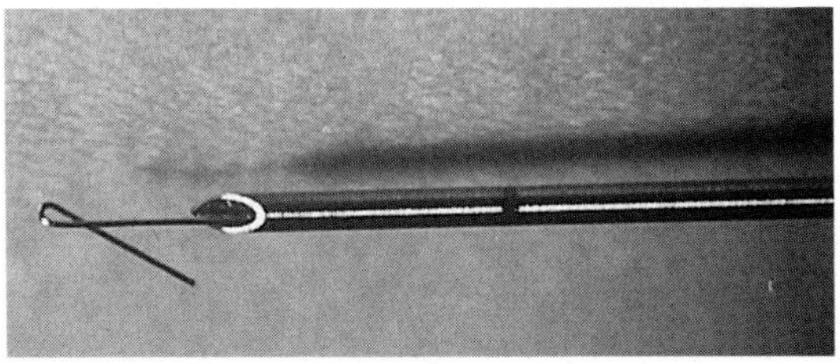

Fig. 7-9. A magnetic resonance–compatible tumor localizer (Daum Medical, Schwerin, Germany).

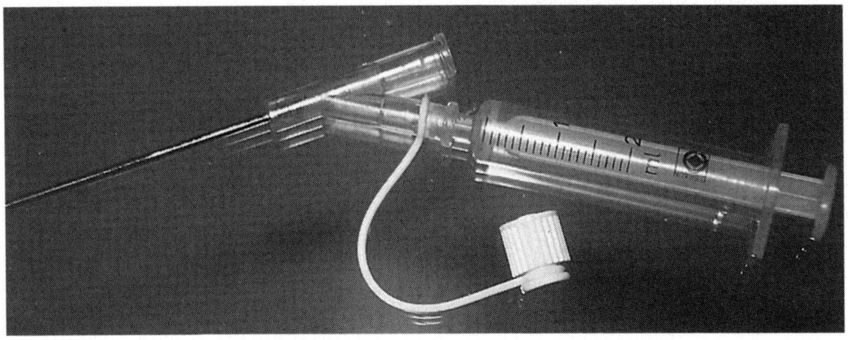

Fig. 7-10. New puncture needles have been equipped with a Y-shaped Luer-Lock to facilitate connection of devices such as syringes or introduction of laser fibers within the narrow gap of magnet (Daum Medical, Schwerin, Germany).

CANNULAS FOR NEUROLOGIC INTERVENTIONS

Interventional procedures in the central nervous system require specially designed cannulas that provide mounting in the magnet bore. Two neurosurgical groups have developed prototypes that allow their use under MRI. MRI-compatible neurocannulas by Pilling and Weck (Fort Washington, Penn) are available in Europe. Basically, the important aspects are the same as for other interventional instruments. The distal end requires adequate visibility and an artifact size that allows precise placement. The exterior elements for fixation to the skull should not interfere with imaging but can have an artifact. Thus, titanium, ceramic, and plastic are preferable materials. NeuroGate (Daum Medical, Schwerin, Germany), an interventional needle holder, comprises a ball-socket joint in a base that is screwed directly into the skull.

TUMOR LOCALIZER

Tumor localizers should meet requirements similar to those of other MR tools. The device, including the insertion cannula, should be MR compatible, and the marker should be visible in MR mammography sequences. Presence of a controlled artifact or appearance of the marker is desirable to allow better differentiation within the surrounding tissue. A simple tumor localizer has been evaluated together with DAUM that incorporates a nonmagnetic stainless steel wire in a titanium 20-G needle (Fig. 7-9). Both adequately localize lesions. Other MR-compatible markers are available from Cook and from Mitek (MamaLock).

DEFLECTABLE CANNULAS

Current open magnets feature spatial limitations for human access. To help overcome limited access capabilities, various technologies (e.g., Y Luer-Lock, deflectable cannulas and instruments) have been developed.

The Y-shaped twin Luer-Lock permits syringes and other devices to be connected in a variable angle (Fig. 7-10). Introduction of catheters, endoscopes, or laser fibers during the procedure is also facilitated.

Based on examinations of the material and former experiences with superelastic nitinol, two sizes of deflectable cannulas have been developed. Nitinol has the characteristics of thermal and stress-induced shape memory. The thermal shape memory entails a shape recovery on heating above a certain temperature threshold between 0° and 100°. Below the Austenite finish temperature, the material allows plastic deformation (up to 10%) with a low elastic module. Because the Austenite finish temperature can be set to a specific temperature (i.e., room or body temperature), the material properties change. Above the Austenite finish temperature, the material can be constrained up to 10%, and it elastically recovers its shape when deconstrained. The load required for deformation is relatively constant. This so-called plateau effect creates several excellent and unique features for instruments and other devices. Self-expanding stents, guide wires, catheters, vena cava filters, and in particular endoscopic instrumentation benefit from the superelastic shape memory of Nitinol.[5]

The deflectable cannula SmartGuide (Daum Medical, Schwerin, Germany) comprises a straight outer sleeve and a superelastic internal precurved cannula that is constrained when introduced into the sleeve. When advanced the internal cannula gradually recovers its initial shape, whereby a curved puncture is achieved (Fig. 7-11). From the practical clinical point-of-view, this feature has two significant benefits. (1) It enables a more convenient and safer approach to the operative volume, whereby important anatomic structures (e.g., vessels) can be passed. (2) It increases the accessible volume in accordance with the radius of the curvature of the internal cannula, which is important for biopsies and intratumoral management. In combination with the Y Luer-Lock, the limited vertical access within the magnet gap has been overcome to some extent.

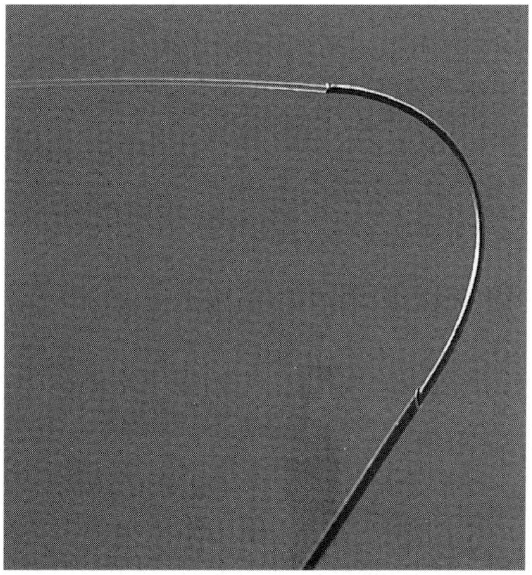

Fig. 7-11. A superelastic deflectable cannula provides puncture around the corner.

FLEXIBLE SHEATH AND CATHETERS

Various commercially available catheters of different sizes and materials have been evaluated. All materials and synthetic catheters tested feature a more or less 1:1 artifact. Because of the many catheter types, items of interest for a particular procedure should be tested. Catheters marked with platinum and gold rings are MR compatible provided that appropriate tools have been used for marking the rings. Other materials for MR marking are titanium and nickel alloys. In the plating of catheter material with superparamagnetic iron oxide, a thin film of iron oxide leads to excellent marking with minimal risk to the patient because the particles are clinically used as superparamagnetic contrast agents. Endorem (Guerbet, Aulnay-Sous-Bois, France) was dissolved in acrylic and painted on the catheter. Modification of the concentration allows the artifact size to be modulated.

ANGIOPLASTY BALLOON CATHETER

Balloon catheters require the same features as standard catheters to be MR compatible. Usually only the marking rings can interfere with MR (Fig. 7-12). The major aspect of using dilation balloons relates to balloon filling. Visibility is only achieved if the characteristics of the filling agent significantly differ from the signals of the surrounding tissue or liquid. Saline, superparamagnetic iron oxide, and gadolinium solutions (1 mmol/l up to pure gadolinium) have been evaluated as filling agents. The choice of the filling material depends on the application. If the balloon is used in vessels for percutaneous transluminal angioplasty and is controlled by MR angio

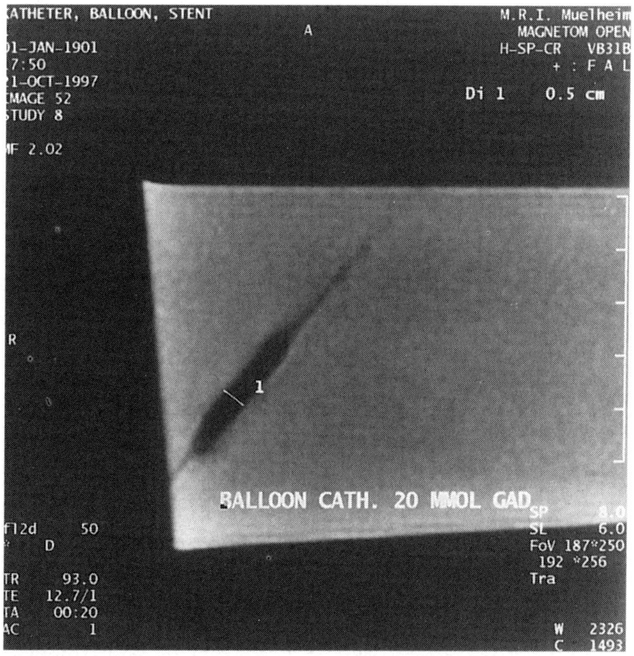

Fig. 7-12. Magnetic resonance–compatible angioplasty balloon catheter filled with gadolinium contrast agent.

time-of-flight sequences, filling with a gadolinium solution of 50 mmol/l saline is required; a higher concentration does not lead to significant differences in signal intensity. If the balloon is controlled by T1-weighted spin-echoes or GREs, the filling should be gadolinium at no more than 4 mmol/l concentration to provide the highest intravascular contrast. For assessment of the vascular wall to be optimal (which is impossible in low-field open systems), filling with saline is appropriate. By washing out the different solutions, it is possible to modulate the signal intensity and the image size of the balloon, which varies from 1:1 for pure saline and 2 to 4 mmol/l gadolinium concentration filling up to 1:3 with 1:10 Endorem solution. Gadolinium filling at 50 mmol/l should be useful in cases in which T1 hyperintensive structures are surrounding the balloon (i.e., dilation of strictures).

ANCILLARY EQUIPMENT

Most electrical devices should be placed outside the RF cabin of the magnet. RF generators and laser or high-power light sources may require costly modification to become MR compatible. In-room MR compatibility can, in some cases, be achieved by using special pass filters that eliminate the respective Larmor resonance frequencies. However, the sensitivity of MR units and the variance of open and closed magnets with their different RF systems make general RF compatibility very difficult. Thus, for each magnet, special adaptation is required. For the purpose of RF ablation, it is possible to switch the RF device on and off during image acquisition. This ability, however, requires a kind of triggering or synchronization between the RF generator and the acquisition system. Control of the RF unit should be provided, and transmission should be done by optic coupling to avoid interaction with the MR system. Interruptions of the RF application can reduce effective heating of tissue.

ECG triggering can provide the MR system with a similar signal characteristic to control the acquisition. The RF generator should have a pulsed application and a transceiver that provides the ECG signal. In view of costs and effectiveness of tissue ablation, RF techniques are superior to laser techniques. Laser, however, has no electric connection to the patient, which makes it technologically safer. Conventional laser generators disturb the image acquisition and need to be placed outside the cabin. Dornier (Germering, Germany) provides 600- and 400-U bare fibers up to 10 m (Fig. 7-13). Diode laser may be used inside the MR suite.

Cold-light generators

Siemens (Erlangen, Germany) has developed a low-power halogen light source with no interference with the imaging system. This light source can be used only for illumination of the external operating field within the magnet gap. Endoscopy requires xenon light because of its brightness and better color temperature.

The light source CLV 20 (Olympus, Tokyo, Japan) (Fig. 7-14) can be used in the MR suite if it is placed on the floor near the magnet. However, this position is unacceptable in terms of safety. To avoid this drawback, a 10-m light cable has been developed with full MR compatibility. It can be used throughout the procedure; even when the light cable is within the image plane, it does not cause artifacts. Two types are available having 3.5- and 5-mm light transmission. The light source can be placed inside the RF cabin and does not interfere with imaging.

Light intensity is adjusted through the camera control unit, which can be connected to the light source via a coaxial cable. Placement of the camera unit outside the magnet is preferable because RF emissions cannot be eliminated completely. The cable connection between the control unit and the chip camera can transmit RF energy and should thus be shielded.

In-room video display

Interventional MRI requires an MR-compatible in-room monitor with standard image quality. For the use of fluoro-like sequences, immediate observation of the intraoperatively gathered images is mandatory for a safe approach.

Video projectors are possible, but the image may have reduced quality. In addition, they cannot be displaced easily and two may be required. The beam can be interrupted by equipment or by assistants.

Cathode ray tube monitors cannot be used near the magnetic field because the image becomes distorted. Standard liquid crystal display monitors do not have adequate resolution and grey shades. Analog thin-film technology active matrix monitors provide excellent MRI scans. A 14-inch 1024 × 768 line display has been modified and electrically shielded. An ultrathin metal net in front of the screen is used to eliminate

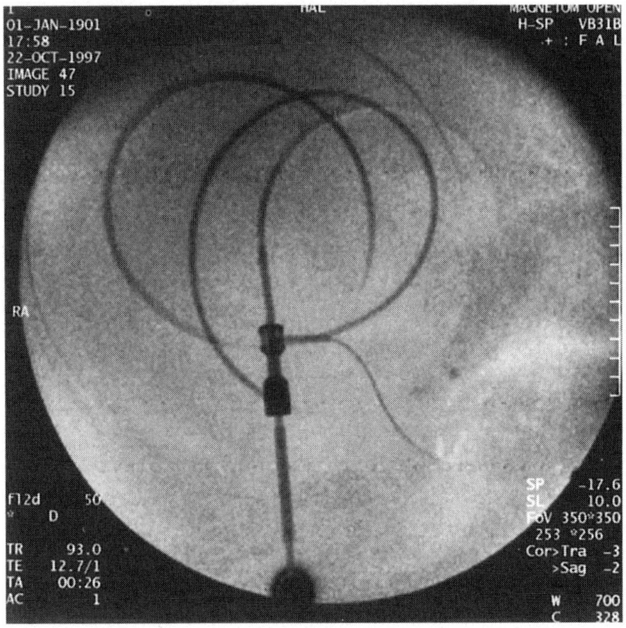

Fig. 7-13. A magnetic resonance–compatible bare fiber for neodymium: yttrium-aluminum-garnet laser application.

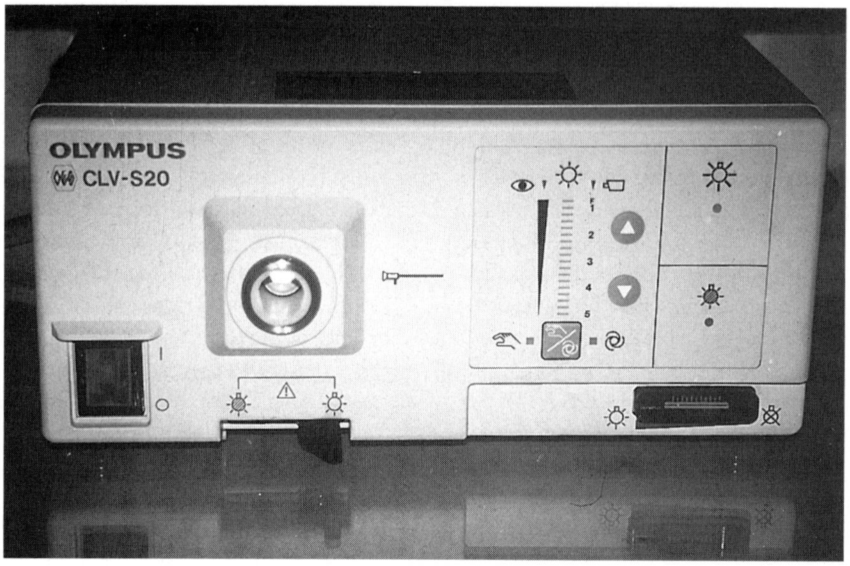

Fig. 7-14. The light source CLV 20 (Olympus, Tokyo, Japan) can be used in the magnetic resonance (MR) radiofrequency cabin in combination with an MR-compatible 10-m light cable.

high-frequency emission, and specially developed electric circuits are necessary to provide resistance of the display to the magnetic field. The first prototype, developed by Pritzel (Prutting, Germany) and Siemens (Erlangen, Germany), was tested during various *in vitro* interventions and was then clinically approved (Fig. 7-15). Further development and improved display technology led to an excellent image that fulfills the diagnostic requirements of MRI. The console should be moved carefully because the rear ground wheels are not fully rotating and the socket is too small and thus unstable. An MR-compatible trackpad mouse that can be handled under sterile conditions is being developed by Siemens.

Endoscopes

Rigid rod lens endoscopes contain stainless steel elements and have a stainless steel outer tube. These components create large artifacts, which impede intra-MR application. The rod lens design has recently been perfected to provide autoclavable optics. Replacement of materials and modification of processing techniques are required to achieve optics with adequate reliability, durability, and biocompatibility. In more than 100 hours of imaging, all components of MR-compatible endoscopes were evaluated after a standardized sequence protocol (Box 7-1).

Full MR compatibility (level 1) was established for endoscopes, which often remain within the imaging plane during acquisition to allow correlation of endoscopic and tomographic image.

Material examinations revealed adequate alloys and design principles of MRI-compatible endoscopes. The 4-, 5-, and 10-mm telescopes with straight and 30° view optics cause an artifact equal to the diameter of the scope. The first series of endoscopes was released in June, 1998. MRI-compatible lengthened light cables for a cold-light source are placed out-

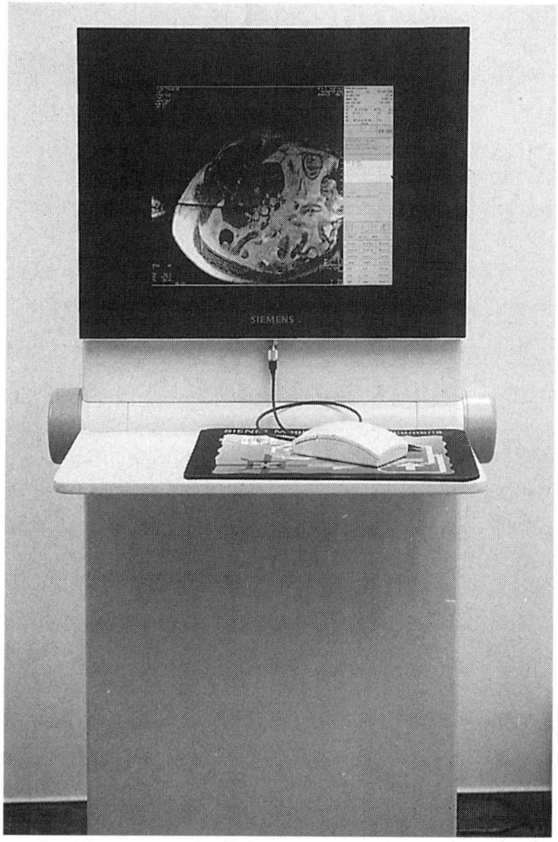

Fig. 7-15. The analogous thin-film technology active matrix screen of the magnetic resonance–compatible in-room console provides excellent image quality for endoscopy (Siemens, Erlangen, Germany; Pritzel, Prutting, Germany).

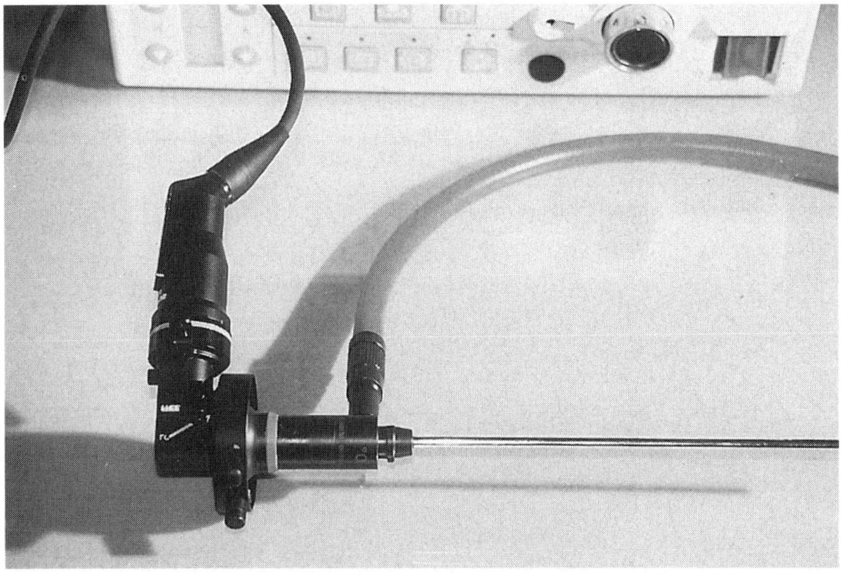

Fig. 7-16. Magnetic resonance–compatible camera and endoscope (Olympus Winter & Ibe, Hamburg, Germany).

Box 7-1. Test protocol of magnetic resonance compatibility

Water container (350-mm diameter) with 10° to 20° saline with 2-mmol/gadolinium.
Field of view, 350 body small coil
Field of view, 200 multipurpose large coil for smaller items
Matrix 256 × 256
Fast low-angle shot, two-dimensional; repetition time, 92 sec; 7 slice thickness 8 mm; echo time, 12 sec
Fast imaging with steady state precession, two-dimensional; slice thickness 8 mm; repetition time, 32 sec; echo time, 12 sec

side the MR unit and a one chip camera (OTV 5) (Olympus Winter & Ibe, Hamburg, Germany) has also been developed (Fig. 7-16). The first experimental applications have been promising. No significant alterations of the MRI scan, the endoscopic image, or the electronic camera system have been noted, but some RF artifacts need to be eliminated.

Videoendoscopic monitoring

Although image quality is less than that of the standard cathode ray tube system, liquid crystal display flat screens are marketed for endoscopy. In a comparison test of a standard digital thin-film technology screen and a high-resolution endoscopy monitor (Sony, black matrix), the active thin-film technology matrix display incorporated in the in-room console from Siemens is the only adequate flat screen available for endoscopy. An additional in-room monitor is used for experimental endoscopic procedures. Siemens is preparing a multimedia console with Red Green Blue and other video-input interfaces. A future development is video-inlet technology, whereby the endoscopic image can be overlaid on the MRI scan and further manipulated to provide optimal tomographic information on the operative volume.

Trocars and cannulas

For operative laparo-endoscopic procedures to be enabled within or close to the magnet, trocars and cannulas are required; they feature adequate operative functions and appropriate representation on the MRI scan. MRI compatibility of trocars and cannulas was evaluated *in vitro.* In terms of cannula sleeves, several disposable items made from synthetic, (i.e., MR-compatible) materials are available.

However, the trocars are usually produced from hardened stainless steel and are ferromagnetic, which preclude their use in the MRI suite. Some disposable trocars are produced from aluminum alloy and are fully MRI compatible. Because most disposable trocars are sharp and have so-called safety shield mechanisms, their use requires care and experience. Only blunt and cone-shaped trocars should be applied. The most suitable access tool seems to be the Step system (Innerdyne, Sunnyvale, Calif).[6] The Veress needle that comes along with the Step system can be modified to an MRI-compatible self-made item.

The Step system allows relatively atraumatic and safe access to the abdominal cavity. Prior puncture with the MR-compatible Veress needle and initial insufflation can be performed under MR fluoroscopic control, whereby the insufflation and distention of the abdominal wall can be observed. Retroperitoneal access can be performed with conventional balloon dissectors.[7] The GSI system (General Surgical Innovations, Portola Valley,

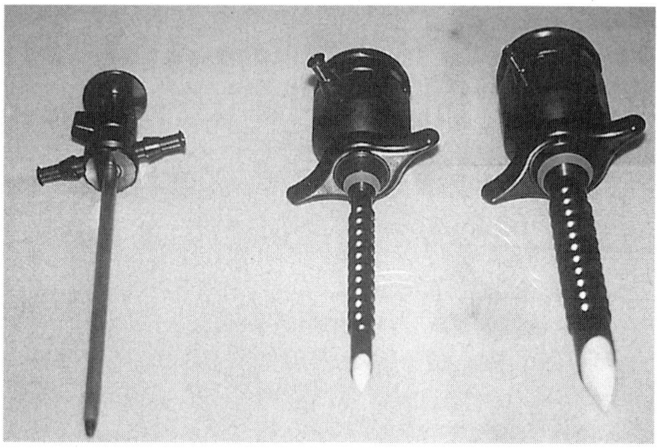

Fig. 7-17. Magnetic resonance (MR)–compatible trocars and cannulas for MR-guided laparo-endoscopic surgery (Olympus Winter & Ibe, Hamburg, Germany).

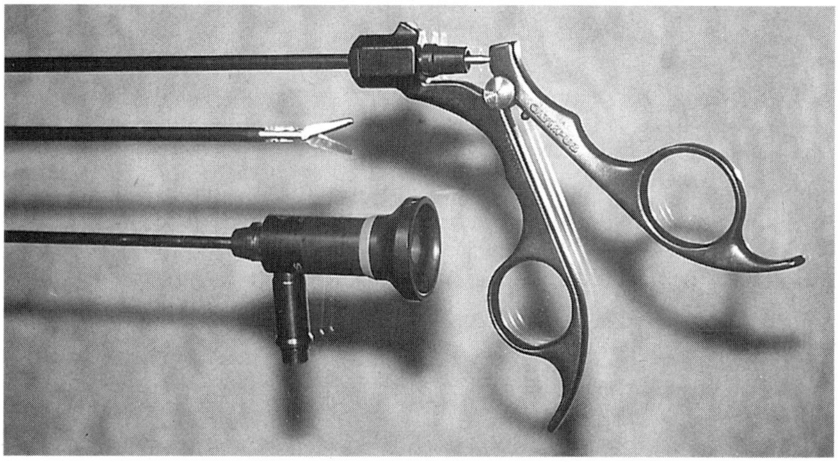

Fig. 7-18. Magnetic resonance (MR)–compatible 5-mm scissors and forceps for MR-guided endoscopic surgery (Olympus Winter & Ibe, Hamburg, Germany).

Calif) is appropriate. The balloon should be filled with 2 to 3 mmol/l of gadolinium or saline contrast agent. Thus, the dissection procedure can be observed under MR fluoroscopic control.

Olympus Winter & Ibe (Hamburg, Germany) has prepared two types of trocars in 5 and 10 mm. One version has blunt conical trocars, and the other has ceramic pointed sharp trocars (Fig. 7-17).

SURGICAL INSTRUMENTS

For MRI compatibility to be achieved in endoscopic instruments (e.g., probes, hooks, forceps, scissors), extensive research is necessary because the hinge complex of handles and jaws excludes the use of synthetic materials. Ceramics, although MRI compatible, are too expensive and difficult to machine. Olympus Winter & Ibe has produced prototypes of MR-compatible titanium instruments (5-mm scissors and forceps) (Fig. 7-18). Because titanium has poor mechanical properties and the small hinges and mechanical articulation have hysteresis and wearing, a substitution of the hinge complex has been developed.[8] The 10-times higher elasticity of nitinol versus stainless steel provides wide opening of the jaws (Fig. 7-19) and a relatively constant load on grasping of tissues of different thickness and elas-

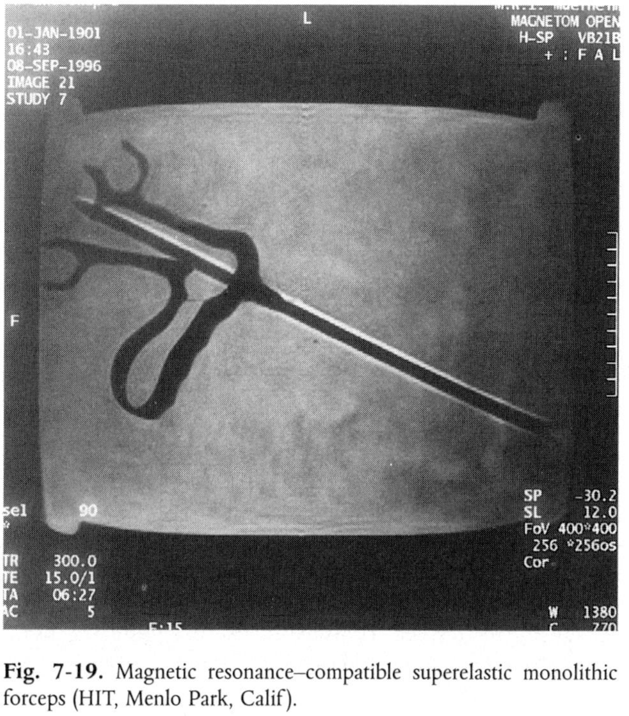

Fig. 7-19. Magnetic resonance–compatible superelastic monolithic forceps (HIT, Menlo Park, Calif).

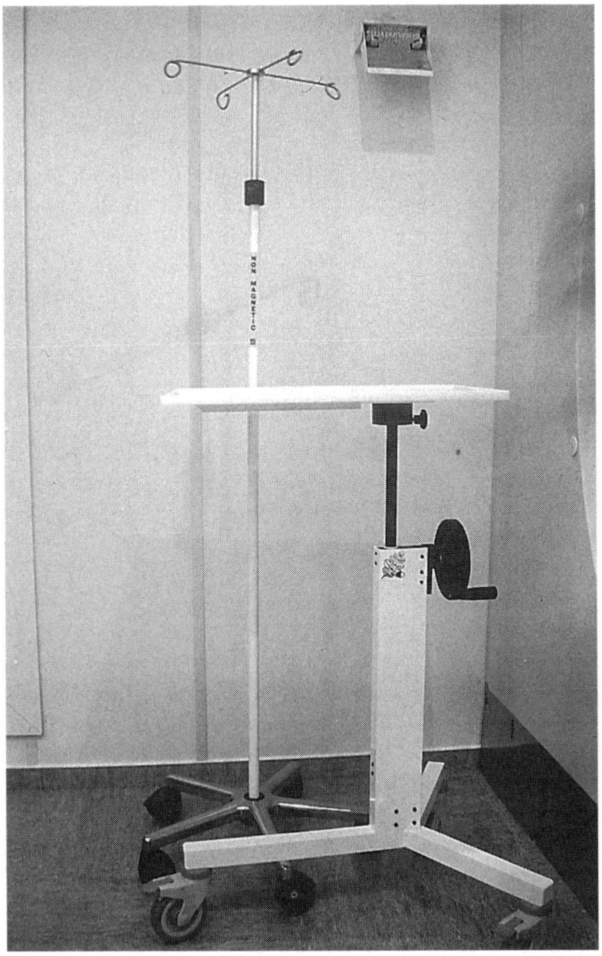

Fig. 7-20. Magnetic resonance–compatible instrumentation table (Veenstra, Joure, The Netherlands).

ticity. Because the action of the jaws is not transmitted via articulation but by direct compression of the jaws at the distal end through the advancing tube, clamping load increases on closing, and a ratchet locking mechanism is unnecessary. A monolithic handle provides variable handling position and improves the ergonomics.

IN-ROOM FURNITURE

Operative procedures require instrument tables, charts, waste bins, chairs, and other equipment. Usually, these items are made from stainless steel and are thus not MR compatible. A table made from wood is MR compatible and can fit into the interior of the suite. However, the wood absorbs water and limits adequate disinfection if the surface is scratched. Some researchers are collaborating with Veenstra (Joure, The Netherlands) to develop fully MR-compatible in-room furniture. Veenstra produces various devices, such as intravenous stands, small and large instrumentation tables, trolleys, waste bins, and other items (Fig. 7-20). All items are made from nonmagnetic components and can thus be used in closest proximity even to high-field magnets and high-field systems.

FUTURE OF MAGNETIC RESONANCE INSTRUMENT GUIDANCE

Current techniques of MR guidance require improvement of the instrument display. Visualization of interventional devices that include automatic slice orientation can be active and passive. Early results are promising, but extensive further research is necessary.[9]

Interactive magnetic resonance slice orientation

During MRI-guided procedures, orientation of the image plane and the interventional tool should be aligned precisely. If the instrument moves out of the sliced time, intensive search is necessary to find it again. Inadvertent movements of the patient during the insertion can lead to frequent loss of the instrument artifact within the image plane.

Active instrument navigation consists of the following components: RF-shielded infrared optical tracking systems with three charged coupled devices, cameras, light-emitting diodes, and a workstation for processing data. These cameras are placed according to the magnet gap and the position of the instrument handle. Multiple light-emitting diodes are attached to a handle that connects to the interventional or surgical instrument and a set of light-emitting diodes mounted at the magnet. The position information is sent to the MR unit and matched with the coordinates of the magnet. The position of the instrument is continuously traced (60 Hz), and the data are processed and transmitted to the MR control unit. The instrument is displayed on the MR screen to match the previous instrument position or to update the scan plane orientation during fluoroscopic mode (Fig. 7-21).

Images can be generated in alignment or perpendicular to the distal tip of instrument. The image plane orientation can be changed and redefined without moving the instrument itself, which ensures constant control of a surgical instrument during movement. Further light-emitting diodes can be attached to the patient or the table so that the navigation system can be used for other MR-guided procedures. Unattended curvature or bending of the instrument can lead to a distortion of the position of the instrument tip.[10]

Tip tracking

A miniature RF coil at the tip of an instrument can acquire local proton spin signals. The signal source representing the tip of the instrument can be localized within the coordinate system of the magnetic field and thus within the human body.[11,12] This technique has been evaluated experimentally and is known as *tip tracking* (see Chapter 16). If the instrument is moved, the position of the signal moves accordingly and can be traced. The current approach of tip tracking by Dumoulin[13] includes the need of an additional workstation to compute the 30 coordinates of the coil and to display the position as a moving symbol in two planes of a morphologic previously acquired road

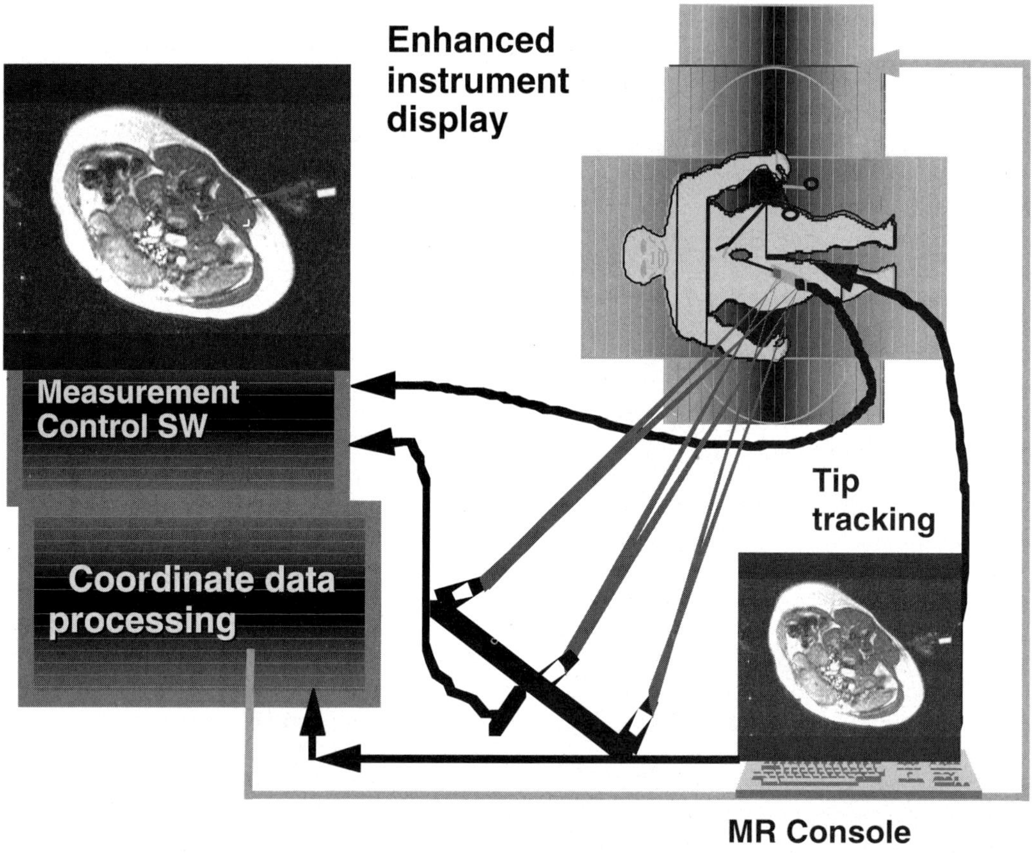

Fig. 7-21. Interactive slice orientation by means of an optoelectronic navigation system.

map MRI scan. Thus, direct on-line control is impossible. Online tip tracking allows direct display of the instrument's signal in a complete MRI scan, whereby interactive slice orientation in axial or perpendicular position in accordance to the instrument can be obtained. Thus, the same function as with an optolectronic navigation is achieved. Tip tracking provides spatial information independent of bending of the instrument.

A new technique has been developed in collaboration with the Case Western University, Cleveland, Ohio, to image the tip of an interventional device, such as a cannula or catheter, during an MRI-guided interventional procedure, whereby real-time imaging and tip localization are achieved. This technique enables localization within a single fluoroscopic mode sequence, unlike that done with other techniques.[13–15] New phase-read keyhole data in combination with a true fast imaging with steady state precision sequence provide a near real-time frame rate.[16] The catheter tip image data acquisition is separated by one repetition from the standard coil spin detection. Localization and superimposition of the two images with minimum spatial error are achieved. Misalignment problems associated with patient movement, which may occur between acquisition of the anatomic reference and device localization image data, can be avoided. Feasibility of this technique has been proved in an animal trial (Fig. 7-22).

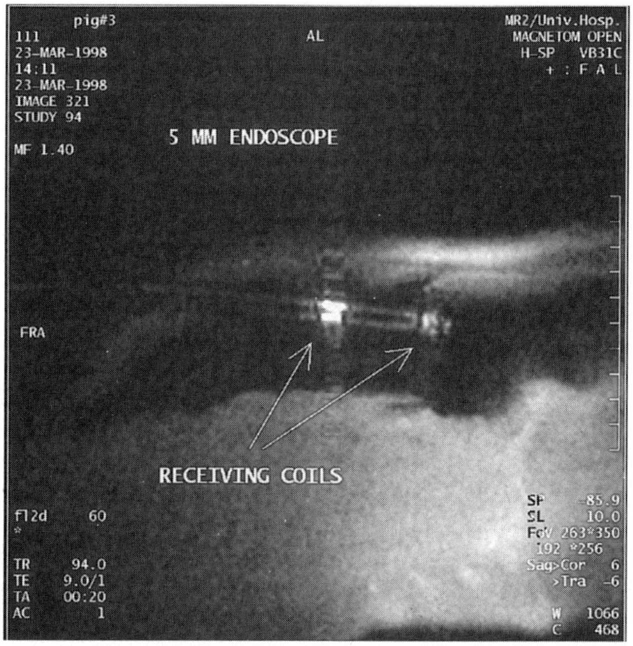

Fig. 7-22. A magnetic resonance image of a tip tracking laparoscope with attached micro coil introduced into the abdominal cavity of a pig.

REFERENCES

1. Lufkin R, Teresi L, Hanafee W: New needle for MR-guided aspiration cytology of the head and neck, *Am J Roentgenol* 149:380, 1987.
2. Melzer A, and others: Methodology, technological prerequisites and preliminary clinical results of interventions in a horizontal open MRI unit, *Proceedings ISMRM* 96, 2:897, 1996.
3. Melzer A, and others: Technology and principles of tomographic image guided interventions and surgery, *Surg Endosc* 11:946–956, 1997.
4. Melzer A, and others: Prerequisites for magnetic resonance 1996 image-guided interventions and endoscopic surgery, *Minimally Invasive Therapy and Allied Technologies* 5:255, 1996.
5. Duerig TW, Melton KN, Stoeckel D: *Engineering aspects of shape memory alloys,* New York, 1990, Butterworth-Heinemann.
6. Melzer A, and others: Ports, trocars/cannulae and other access techniques, *Seminars in Laparoscopy* 2:170, 1995.
7. Melzer A, Buess G, Cuschieri A: *Instruments and alled technologies.* In Cuschieri A, Buess G, Perissat J. editors: *Operative manual for endoscopic surgery,* Berlin-Heidelberg, 1994, Springer.
8. Melzer A, Stoeckel D: Performance improvement of surgical instrumentation through the use of Ni-Ti materials, *Proceedings SMST* 94:401, 1995.
9. Busch M, and others: Active tip tracking as a control method for the positioning of medical instruments during MR-guided interventional procedures, *Proc Int Soc Magn Reson Med* 1922, 1997.
10. Silverman SG, and others: Interactive MR-guided biopsy in an open configuration MR imaging system, *Radiology* 197:175, 1995.
11. Davis CP, and others: Ultra-high-speed MR imaging, *European Radiology* 6:297, 1996.
12. Leung DA, and others: Real-time biplanar needle tracking for interventional MR imaging procedures, *Radiology* 197:485, 1995.
13. Dumoulin CL, Souza SP, Darrow RD: Real-time position monitoring of invasive devices using magnetic resonance, *Magn Reson Med* 29:411, 1993.
14. Leung DA, and others: Intravascular MR tracking catheter, *Am J Roentgenol* 164:1265, 1995.
15. Wildermuth S, Leung DA, Debatin JF: MR imaging-guided intravascular procedures: initial demonstration in a pig model, *Radiology* 202:578, 1997.
16. Bornstedt A, and others: Turbo accelerated asymmetric phase read keyhole (PHREAK) imaging as a method for fast and high contrast MR-guided intervention, *Proc ESMRMB* #260, 1996.

Chapter 8

SITE PLANNING FOR INTERVENTIONAL MR

Andreas Staubert, Christian R. Wirtz, Volker M. Tronnier

Based on years of extensive scientific research and application to clinical diagnostic imaging, magnetic resonance (MR)-guided interventional procedures are becoming routine in tumor management. The potential impact of interventions (e.g., biopsy, minimally invasive surgery) on radiology and oncology is significant.[1–3] For example, the control of destructive energy deposition for tumor management is one of the most challenging and exciting methods in image-guided interventions.[4–6] The advantages of MR imaging justify full integration of diagnostic and therapeutic tools within a single system. These advantages include good spatial resolution with excellent soft-tissue discrimination; sensitivity to blood flow, perfusion, and temperature; lack of ionizing radiation; ability to image in any orientation; and recent development of fast and ultrafast imaging techniques, which permit rapid repeated imaging.[7,8]

This combination of diagnostics and therapy requires highly sophisticated technology and a multidisciplinary team of interventional radiologists, surgeons, radiotherapists, oncologists, engineers, and physicists. It also requires that the surgical theater or interventional radiological procedure room be well thought out.[9–12]

Besides quality assurance, which is essential in image-guided surgery, maximum use of the site should be secured to reduce costs compared with conventional procedures.[13] Furthermore, an effective change from inpatient management to an outpatient basis is possible, which may reduce healthcare costs worldwide. For these reasons, thorough site planning is essential to ensure that necessary space and services for every application are available. Moreover, further evolution of diagnostic and interventional procedures should be anticipated because of continued research, technical development, and improved system performance. The possibility for future extensions should be considered at the time of initial site planning.

A complete survey of the requirements (e.g., scanner, room design, additional hardware, software, surgical instruments, technical services) requires that site planning for interventional magnetic resonance imaging (MRI) be divided into three parts (Fig. 8-1):

- Normal requirements for MRI
- Additional requirements inside the radiofrequency (RF) cabin of the scanner
- Additional requirements outside the RF cabin of the scanner

NORMAL REQUIREMENTS FOR MAGNETIC RESONANCE IMAGING

Unlike traditional radiologic procedures, interventional procedures involving MR scanners require that the surgeon be more intimately involved with the technical machinery providing the imaging information. Because more interventional sites will probably be installed in different surgical departments (in-

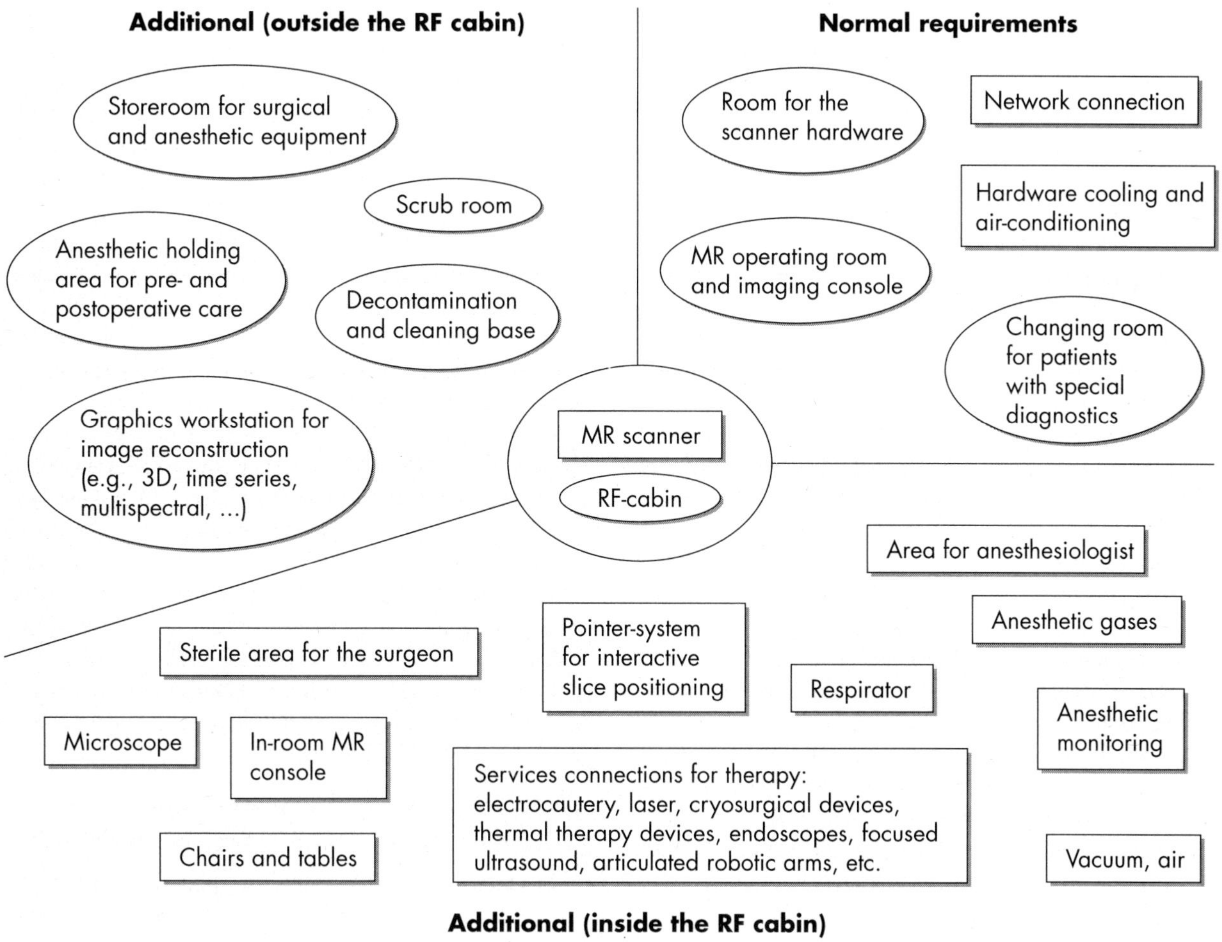

Fig. 8-1. The technical requirements *(open squares)* and space *(open circles)* needed for an interventional magnetic resonance site.

volving radiologists, surgeons, and anesthesiologists in the planning process), this chapter summarizes the normal components of an MR imaging system.

MRI requires a strong, static magnetic field that is highly uniform over the imaging field of view (FOV)[14] to achieve alignment of many magnetic moments in the examination region. Magnet configurations that produce these fields can be divided in three groups according to field strength: low (0.05 to 0.20 T), middle (about 0.5 T), and high ($\geq$1.0 T). To assess the influence of the field strength on the induced magnetization and thus on image quality, physical and clinical aspects should be considered.

Stronger magnetic fields lead to higher signal-to-noise and contrast-to-noise ratios in the images because the induced magnetization in the probe increases linearly with field strength.[15] However, the chemical shift artifact between fat and water and the increase of the T1 relaxation times with higher fields work in such a way that the scaling of these ratios corresponds only with the square root of the field strength.[15,16] Therefore, the decrease of T1 relaxation times in low-field scanners positively influences image quality, especially for very fast imaging techniques, which are important in image-guided surgery.

Besides the physical definition, clinical aspects of image quality versus field strength should be discussed. Different studies compare scanners with 0.5 T and 1.5 T with respect to different diagnostic indications (e.g., various neurologic conditions,[17] focal hepatic lesions[18]). If the scan time and the other scan parameters are constant, the difference between the diagnostic yield for the examined disease categories with the two different scanners is not significant. Another study[19] compared the ultralow field strength of 0.064 T with 1.5 T, with different scan parameters, in various neurologic conditions and showed that the sensitivity of the ultralow field scanner is slightly lower. These studies suggest that larger field strength does not guarantee acceptable diagnostic quality with MRI. Furthermore, the overall system performance of an MR scanner for interventional MRI depends on magnet design and on the degree to which essential imaging and therapeutic features can be integrated.

Magnets for MRI are principally designed based on laws of physics, requirements of technical and practical design (e.g., field strength, gradient performance, patient access), and economic considerations. After the introduction of MRI into clinical diagnostic use, superconducting magnets using a long cylindrical coil integrated in a cryostat, with fields between 0.5 and 1.5 T, had become standard. Because of limited patient access in the tube, several open magnet configurations were developed in the late 1980s. The technical design of these magnets changed from the cylindrical coil to Helmholtz's configuration, which consists of two ringed coils, allowing free access to the imaging FOV between the coils. The coils are oriented vertically or horizontally. If the coils are vertical, the physician can stand in the vertical gap during the procedure.[7] If the coils are horizontal, the physician operates in a sitting position and has lateral access to the patient.[8]

The open magnet design not only allowed for several different geometric configurations, but also brought about different technical ways of producing the magnetic field.[10] Besides normal- and high-temperature superconducting magnets, permanent and resistive magnets are also frequently used (Table 8-1). The differences in the coil material and associated technology mainly determine the price for an MR scanner. Depending on the magnet technology (superconducting or resistive magnets), additional costs incurred for electrical power and the cooling of the magnets should be taken into account.

Because every MR scanner must be located in an RF cabin, which shields it from unwanted external RF, site planning should determine whether all steps of the interventional or surgical procedure can be carried out inside the scanner. In the case of horizontally arranged coils, patient access is vertically restricted, and the patient is often moved temporarily out of the scanner during the intervention. This approach requires that the RF cabin be large enough to start or continue the operation adjacent to the scanner without moving the patient off of the scanner table. The size of the RF cabin and the vertical distance to the lower and higher floors of the building are also influenced by the location of the 5-G line of the magnetic field, which restricts the safety control area for the installation of conventional electronic systems in the operation facility.

Close to the RF cabin, two additional rooms are needed for the basic MRI site. The operator room with the MRI console should be located next to the RF cabin and should have an RF-shielded window or cameras to ensure two-way audiovisual communication between the operator and the surgeon during intervention. Another room contains the electronics of the MR scanner, with power supplies for the magnet and the gradients, RF amplifier and receiver, spectrum analyzer, control unit, and imaging workstations. For special MR applications, such as echoplanar imaging (EPI) or a second RF channel, additional space is required or should be reserved for possible later use. This room and the RF cabin should be supplied with a powerful and reliable air-conditioning system to prevent overheating of the electronics, gradients, and coils and to prevent any breakdown of the system during the procedure.

Changing or waiting rooms for the patients are required in a conventional MR site. These rooms may be less necessary for an interventional site because the patients often enter lying on a bed through the preoperative holding area. On the other hand, the unique design of some open systems allows functional musculoskeletal studies or imaging in a standing or sitting position, which makes the scanner very interesting for unusual diagnostic studies. This capability is particularly important because the number of open MRI scanners is limited in one hospital and the access of normal diagnostic patients could help to increase the relative use of the site.

ADDITIONAL REQUIREMENTS INSIDE THE RADIOFREQUENCY CABIN OF THE SCANNER

In contrast to purely diagnostic applications, image-guided interventions performed inside the scanning facility require several additional devices to be located near the scanner. Special MR-compatible technology is often required, particularly in the presence of strong magnetic fields when metal instruments and electronic devices are used. MR diagnostic staff has to be retrained for interventional work because they were initially taught to protect the RF cabin from any nonimaging devices.

Almost every electronic device transmits electromagnetic waves and should be shielded by RF cages (Faraday cages) to avoid additional noise in the MR images. This approach is not only important for electronics that generate RF in the range of

Table 8-1. Advantages and disadvantages of different magnet technologies

Magnet type	Advantages	Disadvantages
Permanent	No current and no cooling required for magnetic field Lower cost	Heavy magnet No turning off of the magnetic field in case of emergency
Resistive	Fast turning off of the magnetic field in case of emergency	Heavy magnet Water cooling and stable current required for magnetic field
Normal- and high-temperature superconducting	Lower weight Higher field strength possible	Slow turning off of the magnetic field (risk of quenching) in case of emergency Very high costs of superconducting coils Special cooling techniques required (cryogens, temperatures less than 20 K)

the resonance frequency of the scanner because the receiving system of the scanner is also quite sensitive to lower or higher harmonics of the transmitted frequencies. The shielding of AC power cables may also be necessary.

Vice versa, the functionality of the additional electronic devices should not be influenced by the RF signals or the magnetic field of the scanner. Even when the field is less than 5 G, which is normally safe for integrated electronic elements, disturbances remain because of the residual magnetic field. For example, normal computer monitors cannot be used in this range because they are sensitive to even lower magnetic fields and will be disturbed by any movement of the monitor in the magnetic stray field; in this case, a liquid crystal display monitor is used. To ensure the correct functionality, careful test measurements with phantoms should be performed before using new electronic devices during an interventional procedure.

To avoid loss of information, transmission of data in the immediate vicinity of the high magnetic field should occur via glass fiber rather than ordinary wires.

Several materials are usable for interventional procedure devices (Table 8-2). These materials should be nonmagnetic, but if they are also used in the surgical field, the materials' ability to be sterilized and their influence on susceptibility artifacts in the MR image should be considered. These circumstances require the redesign of most commonly used surgical instruments, which are constructed of mainly ferromagnetic materials or stainless steel; these elements cause large susceptibility artifacts if used in or near the FOV. The concept of moving the patient out of the magnet before, during, or after the surgical procedure can partially avoid the problem of a complete redesign of all surgical devices and instruments but requires sufficient free space in the RF cabin or in an adjacent operating room.[20]

The primary devices for anesthetic management during surgery (e.g., an MR-compatible patient monitoring system, a respirator inside the RF cabin) are commercially obtainable (see Chapter 9). Additionally, service connections should be provided for anesthetic gases, and a supply of the most important anesthetic drugs and accessories should be kept inside the RF cabin. Several nonmagnetic attachments (e.g., a seat and a table for the anesthesiologist, a cupboard for drugs and accessories, an infusion-stand) are also needed.

Because the sterile operating area in and near the FOV is defined by the magnet design, the working area for the surgeon, assistant, and scrub nurse differs for every scanning system, and therefore no standard arrangement, similar to that in a normal operating environment, can be described. Site planning should thus consider the different demands and devices needed to perform interventional procedures during MR image guidance:

- The design and location of chairs and tables depend mainly on the operating position. Ergonomic solutions are important to find because access to the patient is restricted and sometimes not very comfortable.
- RF transmit-receive coils placed over the region of interest play an important role in image quality. Normally, the standard coils for the imaging system cannot be used intraoperatively because they are not sterilizable or block surgical access. Thus, development of RF coils dedicated to the different interventional applications is important.
- To ensure online access to the images, one or more additional MR monitors should be installed near the surgeon. To permit the input of data to the MR system by the surgeon (e.g., choosing sequences, modifying parameters, writing documentation notes), there should be access to a sterilizable input device.

Table 8-2. Nonmagnetic materials used for interventional magnetic resonance imaging devices

Material	Characteristics or properties	Examples
Wood	Inexpensive Easy to work with	Specialized furniture (e.g., chair, shelf) Paneling for larger devices
Plastic	Inexpensive Easy to produce Many types for different applications and requirements Small or no magnetic resonance artifacts	Single-use surgical instruments (e.g., clamp, aspirator) Attachments for furniture (e.g., knob, roller) Paneling for smaller devices
Ceramic	Very stable Heat insensitive (steam sterilizable) Very precise manufacturing possible Small magnetic resonance artifacts	Biopsy or other cannula Head fixation Surgical instruments (e.g., scalpel, scissors)
Aluminum	Light Easy to work with Heat insensitive (steam sterilizable)	Attachments for furniture or paneling (e.g., screws, rods)
Titanium	Light Easy to work with Heat insensitive (steam sterilizable) Harder than aluminum Biocompatible, implantable	Surgical instruments (e.g., retractors, aspirators, microforceps, curettes, scissors) Accessories for implantation (e.g., sheets, screws)

- Interactive localization and control of image orientation are needed to use the three-dimensional (3D) information for accurate definitions of targets and entry trajectories. Thus, a 3D pointer device[7,21,22] should be integrated into the MR system.
- The most obvious role of MRI is in controlling various ablative thermal therapy methods (e.g., interstitial laser therapy,[23,24] RF heating,[5] cryosurgery,[25,26] focused ultrasound surgery,[27] ethanol therapy[28,29]) or in monitoring the delivery of drugs. Other therapeutic devices may include endoscopes[30] or, in the future, articulated robotic arms. Dedicated service connections and space should be available in the RF cabin and in the operating field.
- Other common service connections, which are necessary in an interventional suite but not in a normal RF cabin, are vacuum, air, suction containers, patient-heating devices, uninterruptable power supplies, and computer network connections.

ADDITIONAL REQUIREMENTS OUTSIDE THE RADIOFREQUENCY CABIN OF THE SCANNER

To complete the requirements for a functioning site for interventional MR, the combination of surgery and diagnostics may require additional rooms. The standard rooms needed at every operational site should also be integrated into the interventional site:

- Anesthetic holding area for pre- and postoperative care
- Storeroom for surgical and anesthetic equipment
- Scrub rooms
- Decontamination and cleaning base for the room and the equipment
- Locker rooms and passage to the operational site

Further, space next to the MR console may accommodate one or more graphics workstations for data processing and image reconstruction. During interventional procedures, many image data should be analyzed online. For example, 3D reconstruction[31] and segmentation of the acquired images into tissue classes[32,33] are often necessary to appreciate the anatomy, define the tumor volume, and provide sufficient information for surgical planning. Real-time image processing is also necessary if segmentation and subsequent 3D visualization are used to construct virtual reality, within which free navigation and manipulation are allowed.[9] Furthermore, during the application of different therapeutic methods to destroy or diminish tumors controlled by MR, these images should be processed and visualized by computer systems.[4,6,34] The correction of artifacts[35–37] is another application for online computing because the magnetic susceptibility of human tissues and of instruments introduced into the imaging field results in geometric image distortions,[38,39] which may interfere with interventional procedures.

CONCLUSIONS

In specially designed sites, it is possible to integrate tumor detection, image-guided biopsy, and tumor management combined with intra- and postoperative monitoring. Image-guided surgery has many advantages, including the integration of diagnosis and therapy (e.g., increased surgical success, reduced costs). The surgeon or therapeutic interventional radiologist, however, is responsible for ensuring the safety of the patient and support staff working near high magnetic fields with many electrical devices. The design of the imager and the planning of the interventional site need careful consideration to accomplish the best results for the patient, establish good working conditions for the staff, achieve a high throughout, prevent accidents, and meet all regulations from local or state regulatory bodies.[40,41]

REFERENCES

1. Kormos D, Piraino DW: Image-guided surgery attains clinical status, *Diag Imag* 9:77, 1994.
2. Bieze J: Interventional MRI moves from dream to reality, *Magn Reson Med* 3:22, 1994.
3. Lufkin R: MRI asserts potential in interventional care, *Diagn Imag* 3:119, 1990.
4. Farahani K, and others: Hyperacute thermal lesions: MR imaging evaluation of development in the brain. *Radiology* 196:517, 1995.
5. Schwarzmaier H, Kahn T: Magnetic resonance imaging of microwave induced tissue heating, *Magn Reson Med* 33:729, 1995.
6. Anzai Y, and others: Preliminary experience with MR-guided thermal ablation of brain tumors, *Am J Neuroradiol* 16:39, 1995.
7. Schenck JF, and others: Superconducting open-configuration MR imaging for image-guided therapy, *Radiology* 195:805, 1995.
8. Lenz GW, Dewey C: *An open MRI system used for interventional procedures: current research and initial clinical results.* In *Proceedings, computer assisted radiology,* Heidelberg, Germany, 1995, Springer.
9. Jolesz FA, Shtern F: The operating room of the future, *Invest Radiol* 27:326, 1992.
10. Grönemeyer D, and others: Equipment configuration and procedures: preferences for interventional microtherapy, *Digit Imaging* 9:81, 1996.
11. Moriarty TM, and others: Magnetic resonance imaging therapy: intraoperative MR imaging, *Neurosurgery* 7:323, 1996.
12. Riederer SJ: The future technical development of MRI, *Magn Reson Imaging* 1:52, 1996.
13. Bieze J: Image guidance lowers costs, risks of surgery, *Diagn Imaging* 4:53, 1994.
14. Thomas SR: *Magnets and gradient coils: types and characteristics.* In Bronskill MJ, and others, editors: *The physics of MRI: medical physics,* New York, 1993, American Institute of Physics, Monograph no. 21.
15. Rutt BK, Lee DH: The impact of field strength on image quality in MRI, *Magn Reson Imaging* 1:57, 1996.
16. Hoult DI, Chen CN, Sank VJ: The field dependence of NMR imaging, *Magn Reson Med* 3:722, 1986.
17. Jack CR, and others: Field strength in neuro-MR imaging: a comparison of 0.5 T and 1.5 T, *Comput Assist Tomogr* 14:505, 1990.
18. Steinberg HV, Alarcon JJ, Bernadino ME: Focal hepatic lesions: comparative MR imaging at 0.5 and 1.5 T, *Radiology* 174:153, 1990.
19. Orrison WW Jr, and others: Comparison of CT, low-field-strength MR imaging, and high-field-strength MR imaging, *Radiology* 181:121, 1991.
20. Tronnier VM, and others: Intraoperative diagnostic and interventional magnetic resonance imaging in neurosurgery, *Neurosurgery* 40:891, 1997.
21. Lewin JS, and others: A *clinical trial of interactive MRI for diagnostic procedure guidance on a C-arm system: progress update.* In *Proceedings, ISMRM, 5th scientific meeting,* Vancouver, 1997.
22. Busch MHJ, and others: *Active tip tracking as a control method for the positioning of medical instruments during MR-guided interventional procedures.* In *Proceedings, ISMRM, 5th scientific meeting,* Vancouver, 1997.
23. Vogl TJ, and others: Recurrent nasopharyngeal tumors: preliminary clinical results with interventional MR imaging-controlled laser-induced thermotherapy, *Radiology* 196:725, 1995.

24. Kahn T, and others: MRI-guided interstitial Nd:YAG laser phototherapy of cerebral neoplasms, *J Comput Assist Tomogr* 18:519, 1994.
25. Hong J, and others: MR imaging assisted temperature calculations during cryosurgery, *Magn Reson Imaging* 7:1021, 1994.
26. Matsomoto R, and others: MR monitoring during cryotherapy in the liver: predictability of histologic outcome, *Magn Reson Imaging* 3:770, 1993.
27. Cline HE, and others: Focussed US system for MR imaging-guided tumor ablation, *Radiology* 194:731, 1995.
28. Bartolozzi C, and others: Hepatocellular carcinoma: CT and MR features after transcatheter arterial embolization and percutaneous ethanol injection, *Radiology* 191:123, 1994.
29. Sironi S, and others: Small hepatocellular carcinoma treated with percutaneous ethanol injection: unenhanced and gadolinium-enhanced MR imaging follow-up, *Radiology* 192:407, 1994.
30. Scholz M, and others: MRI-guided endoscopy in the brain: a feasability study, *Minim Invasive Neurosurg* 39:33, 1996.
31. Bedell BJ, Narayana PA, Johnston DA: Three-dimensional MR image registration of the human brain, *Magn Reson Med* 35:384, 1996.
32. Vinitski S, and others: Improved intracranial lesion characterization by tissue segmentation based on a 3D feature map, *Magn Reson Med* 37:457, 1997.
33. Alfano B, and others: Unsupervised, automated segmentation of the normal brain using a multispectral relaxometric magnetic resonance approach, *Magn Reson Med* 37:84, 1997.
34. Matsumoto R, and others: Tissue temperature monitoring for thermal interventional therapy: comparison of T_1-weighted MR-sequences, *Magn Reson Imaging* 4:65, 1994.
35. Irarrazabal P, and others: Inhomogeneity correction using an estimated linear field map, *Magn Reson Med* 35:278, 1996.
36. Beuf O, and others: Magnetic resonance imaging for the determination of magnetic susceptibility of materials, *J Magn Reson* B112:111, 1996.
37. Nauta HJW: Error assessment during "image guided" and "imaging interactive" stereotactic surgery, *Comput Med Imaging Graph* 18:279, 1994.
38. Lüdeke KM, Römschmann P, Tischler R: Susceptibility artifacts in MR imaging, *Magn Reson Imaging* 3:329, 1985.
39. Czervionke LF, and others: Magnetic susceptibility artifacts in gradient-recalled echo MR imaging, *Am J Neuroradiol* 9:1145, 1988.
40. Shellock FG, Kanal E: *Magnetic resonance bioeffects, safety, and patient management,* New York, 1994, Raven.
41. Shellock FG, Morisoli S, Kanal M: MR procedures and biomedical implants, materials, and devices: 1993 update *Radiology* 189:587, 1993.

Chapter 9

ANESTHETIC MANAGEMENT FOR INTRAOPERATIVE MRI

Heinrich Polarz, Angela M. Browne, Eike Martin

When confronted with the management of a patient during magnetic resonance imaging (MRI) the anesthesiologist should be aware of the required conditions under which anesthesia can be applied and monitored in an uninterrupted and safe manner.

These preconditions are as follows:

- No unsecured ferromagnetic material should be in the imaging room.
- Monitoring equipment should pose no risk to the patient.
- The MRI unit should not degrade the monitoring equipment.
- The monitoring equipment should not reduce the quality of the image caused by electromagnetic interference.[1–3]

Interactions between the monitoring equipment and MRIs should be definitively excluded.[4–6] In particular, anesthetic equipment and methods should not interfere with image quality. Likewise, the strong magnetic fields generated during imaging should not interfere with proper functioning of anesthetic equipment. Electronic or mechanical components that do not fulfill these requirements should be exchanged or shielded.

In the strong magnetic field, metal implants are prone to torque, and heating may result from induced currents. Objects containing ferromagnetic materials (e.g., scissors, glasses, stethoscopes, laryngoscopes) may also be propelled within strong magnetic fields. Likewise, because magnetic strips may be disrupted, credit cards, check-cashing cards, and identity cards should be deposited outside the imaging room.

PATIENT EXCLUSION CRITERIA

Patients with electronic, magnetic, or mechanically active implants may be adversely affected by the induced magnetic and radiofrequency fields. In general, artificial pacemakers are an absolute contraindication to MRI. The pacer may be inactivated or reprogrammed by the electromagnetic forces. In addition, induced voltage across the pacer leads can induce local overheating and tissue damage. Likewise, deleterious effects may be induced in internal defibrillators and implanted dosing pumps.

The presence of a Swan-Ganz catheter is also an exclusion criterion in MRI. Most modern heart valves are not ferromagnetic and do not present a problem. However, older valves have been associated with dysfunction during imaging. To avoid any risk, only patients with valves of biologic or nonferromagnetic material should be admitted to these procedures.

Glass eyes should be removed before the procedure. Nonferromagnetic hip prostheses and similar materials are not problematic because they are predominantly made of nonferromagnetic material and securely anchored in place.

Whether cosmetic tattooing and permanent eye make-up with dyes containing ferromagnetic material should be a contraindication to MRI is debatable; reports have been made of local tissue sensitivity. The safety of MR imaging among pregnant patients and staff is unproven. Patients with metal shrapnel from traumatic injuries and those with intestinal stoma with metal closures should be excluded from MRI.

In general, any material that is neither magnetic nor metallic may undergo MRI techniques. (See Chapter 10 for a full discussion of this area.)

MAGNETIC FIELDS

Problems with anesthetic equipment may result from the strong magnetic fields produced.[7] This field strength wanes with distance from the magnet. Points with similar Gauss values are joined, constituting so-called Gauss lines. Similar to isobar markings on a weather chart, Gauss lines reveal in which magnetic field strength a given point lies (Fig. 9-1).

It should be emphasized that the delineation of these Gauss lines is individually programmed by the manufacturer of the magnet; therefore, Gauss lines are unique to each imaging unit. Gauss lines of interest to the anesthesiologist include 5 G (0.5 mT), 200 G (20 mT), and 30 G (3 mT). The ventilator should be placed outside the 200-G line, and the remaining equipment (e.g., pulse oximeter, capnometer, blood pressure monitor, infusion pumps) should be placed outside the 30-G line. The safety zone for patients with electromagnetic implants (e.g., pacemakers, internal defibrillators, artificial hearts) is approximately delineated by the 5-G line.

MONITORING

What monitoring is necessary to ensure safety for the patient during MRI? Monitoring of vital functions can be undertaken only with instruments and equipment that do not contain ferromagnetic materials and do not otherwise interfere with the proper functioning and image quality of the unit.[8,9] The anesthesiologist should have available electrocardiography (ECG), pulse oximetry, capnography, oscillometric blood pressure monitoring, and invasive blood pressure monitoring.

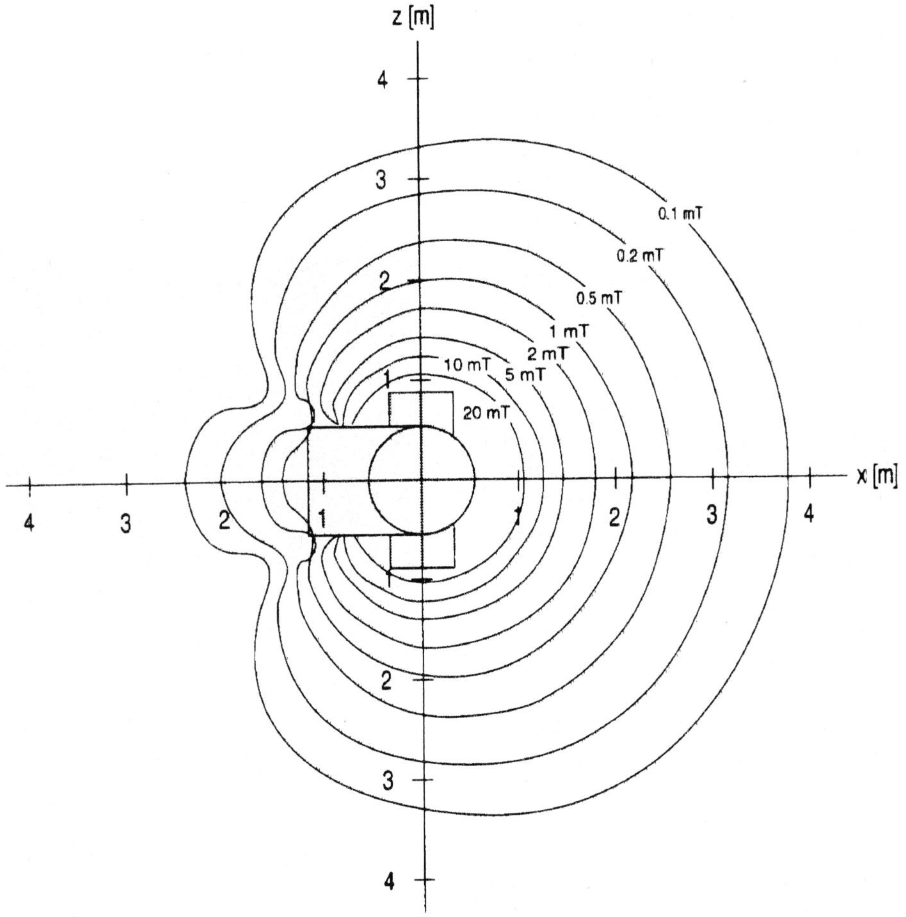

Fig. 9-1. The magnetic field relative to the magnetic field center.

Electrocardiographic monitoring

Particular attention should be paid to the placement of nonferromagnetic electrodes to ensure accurate monitoring. Some physicians use carbon fiber electrodes. Ideally, these electrodes should be placed near the magnetic field, and interelectrode distance should be as short as possible.[8] Further signal distortion may result from voltage induction across individual leads. For this reason, nonmetallic leads are used and are placed parallel to each other to avoid induction and possible overheating with local thermal injury.[6]

Streaming blood, acting as an electrical conductor, may give rise to ECG signal changes within the magnetic field. As a result, ECG is of little diagnostic value during MRI. Artifacts are common and may mimic ECG changes seen in pericarditis and hyperkalemia.

Pulse oximetry

Pulse oximetry facilitates continuous monitoring of pulse and oxygen saturation and is particularly valuable during MRI. Pulse oximetry is based on the absorption and refraction characteristics of oxygenated hemoglobin to calculate the arterial oxygen saturation. The relation between transmission of light of two wavelengths (660 and 940 nm) is used as the basis for this calculation.

Normally, the pulse oximetry sensor contains two diodes and a photocell connected to a monitor via a cable. The sensor and cable act as potent active and passive interference sources. To avoid interference, the diode and the sensor are shielded in a special unit and are connected via a fiberoptic light conductor. The loss of light intensity inherent in using such conductors is compensated for by the pulse oximeter. Placement of the sensor clip should be done with care because the slightest displacement may result in complete signal loss.[8,10,11] Fiberoptic transmission is the only continuous, interference-free mode of signal transmission.

Capnometry

End-expiratory capnography is possible only with sidestream sampling and a long sampling line. The obtained values may be used only as an approximation and for trend monitoring. This use is particularly important with high-frequency ventilation.[8] The carbon dioxide concentration in the expiratory gas is measured by infrared spectroscopy.

Retrospective analysis has shown that 3% of critical incidents could have been avoided using capnography alone and 35% using pulse oximetry. The combination of both monitors could have avoided more than 50% of all recorded critical incidents. Thus, both of these parameters are very valuable in ensuring patient safety during anesthesia; they should be used for this purpose during MRI.

Blood pressure monitoring

No specific problems are associated with noninvasive blood pressure monitoring, provided that the equipment used is deployed at the specified distance and the cuff contains no metallic components. In invasive monitoring, the pressure transducer should be relatively near the patient. All electrical components should be meticulously shielded.[12]

MONITORING UNIT

An integrated, purpose-built monitor for use during MRI cannot be surpassed in ensuring continuous, uninterrupted monitoring (Fig. 9-2). Such a unit (Bruker Maglife, Bruker Medical, Ettlingen, Germany) combines a monitoring unit for MRI, an additional screen for use in the control room external to the magnet, and hardware and software for connection to a personal computer.

Artifact reduction and safety are ensured by shielded leads, sensors, and electrodes. The electric circuitry is enclosed by a Faraday cage, and the unit is consequently shielded from the changing electromagnetic fields. Sensitivity and accuracy of the measured parameters are provided for by the use of fiberoptic data transmission.

VENTILATION

Provision of a completely reliable ventilator during MRI is an absolute requirement. An ideal ventilator contains no ferromagnetic material, is pneumatically regulated, and provides appropriate ventilation for all age groups.[13] A Servo 900 C (Siemens, Erlangen, Germany) fulfills these requirements, and the alarm limits allow for tightly controlled ventilation parameters. It is equipped with a flow meter and an isoflurane vaporizer. The reliability of the vaporizer is unaffected by the magnet. The ventilator is connected via wall outlets in the imaging room to a central gas supply, and approximately 4 m of tubing connects the patient to the ventilator. The ventilator should be

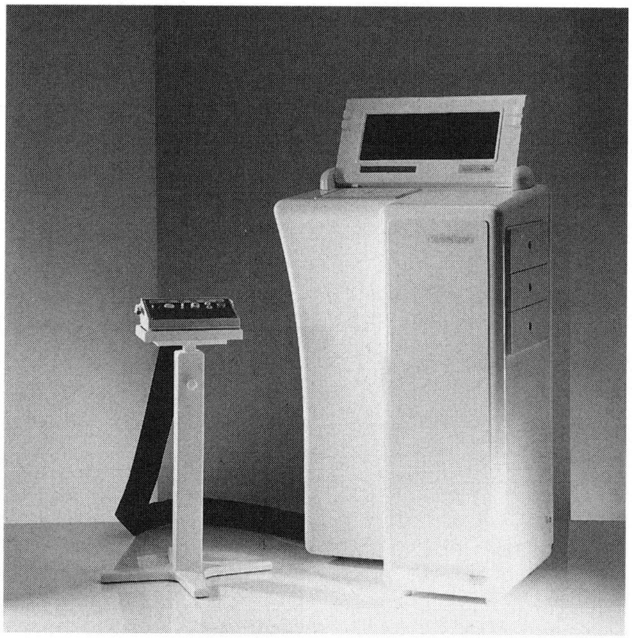

Fig. 9-2. Monitoring unit (Bruker Maglife, Bruker Medical, Ettlingen, Germany).

placed outside the 200-G line. When the magnetic field strength is greater than 20 mT, the following may occur:

- The generating pressure manometer may give a false value.
- Ventilator pressure, alveolar pressure, and expiratory minute volume may be inaccurate.
- Mechanical dysfunction of the inspiratory and expiratory valve may occur.

The ventilator should be thoroughly checked if it appears to have been within a magnetic field greater than 20 mT.

ANESTHETIC TECHNIQUE

The anesthetic technique is of little consequence in relation to MRI. All techniques (inhalation, balanced, total intravenous, regional anesthesia) are possible. When the necessary monitoring is available, anesthesia for MRI is not associated with higher morbidity than that in any other clinical circumstances.

REFERENCES

1. Menon DK, and others: Magnetic resonance for the anaesthetist, *Anaesthesia* 47:240, 1992.
2. Zorab JSM: A general anaesthesia service for magnetic resonance imaging, *Eur J Anaesthesiol* 12:387, 1995.
3. Hoishouser BA, Hinshaw DB, Shellock FG: Sedation, anesthesia, and physiologic monitoring during MR imaging: evaluation of procedures and equipment, *J Magn Reson Imaging* 3:553, 1993.
4. Nixon C, and others: Nuclear magnetic resonance: its implications for the anaesthesist, *Anaesthesia* 41:131, 1986.
5. Patteson SK, Chesney JT: Anesthetic management for magnetic resonance imaging: problems and solutions, *Anesth Analg* 74:121, 1992.
6. Stephen BC: Anesthesia in the interventional magnetic resonance imaging unit, Boston, 1994, Workshop Society of Magnetic Resonance.
7. Schenck JF, and others: Superconducting open-configuration MR: imaging system for image-guided therapy, *Radiology* 195:805, 1995.
8. Peden CJ, and others: Magnetic resonance for the anaesthetist, *Anaesthesia* 47:508, 1992.
9. Jorgensen NA, and others: Patient monitoring during MRI, *Anesth Analg* 72:S130, 1991.
10. Bashein G, Syrovy G: Burns associated with pulse oximetry during magnetic resonance imaging, *Anesthesiology* 75:382, 1991.
11. Kanal E, Shellock FG: Patient monitoring during clinical MR imaging, *Radiology* 185:623, 1992.
12. Taber KH, and others: Invasive pressure monitoring of patients during magnetic resonance imaging, *Can J Anaesth* 40:1092, 1993.
13. Sury MRJ, Johnstone G, Bingham RM: Anaesthesia for magnetic resonance imaging of children, *Paediatric Anaesthesia* 2:61, 1992.

Chapter 10

SAFETY ISSUES FOR INTERVENTIONAL MRI

Frank G. Shellock

During magnetic resonance imaging (MRI), a patient is exposed to three forms of electromagnetic radiation: a static magnetic field, gradient magnetic fields, and radiofrequency (RF) electromagnetic fields. Each form may cause significant bioeffects if applied at sufficiently high exposure levels. During interventional MRI, the MR healthcare worker is exposed to the same types of electromagnetic fields; however, the exposure level is more intermittent and chronic.

Numerous investigations have been conducted to identify potentially adverse bioeffects of MRI.[1–83] Although investigation has not determined the presence of any substantial or unexpected hazards,[1–83] the data are not comprehensive enough to presume absolute safety. In addition to bioeffects related to exposure to the electromagnetic fields used for MRI, several areas are of concern for the healthcare worker with respect to the use of interventional MRI. However, virtually no effort has been made to investigate the bioeffects specifically related to the use of interventional MRI.

This chapter discusses the safety and bioeffects of static, gradient, and RF electromagnetic fields with an emphasis on the data that pertain to MRI. It provides an overview of other safety considerations pertaining to the use of interventional MRI.

BIOEFFECTS OF STATIC MAGNETIC FIELDS

General bioeffects

Few data address the effects of static magnetic fields on humans. Vyalov[84,85] performed some of the original investigations on humans exposed to static magnetic fields ranging from 0.0015 to 0.3500 T (i.e., workers involved in the permanent magnet industry). He reported headache, chest pain, fatigue, vertigo, loss of appetite, insomnia, itching, and other more nonspecific ailments.[84,85] Exposure to other potentially hazardous environmental working conditions (e.g., elevated room temperature, airborne metallic dust, chemicals) may have been partially responsible for these symptoms. Because this investigation lacked an appropriate control group, determination of a correlation between the exposure to the static magnetic field and the reported abnormalities is difficult. More scientific studies have not substantiated many of these findings.[86–89]

MR healthcare workers involved in interventional MRI are chronically exposed to relatively high-intensity static magnetic fields. Research is warranted to determine possible effects associated with these electromagnetic environmental conditions.

Temperature effects

Reports in the literature are conflicting regarding the effect of static magnetic fields on body and skin temperatures of mammals, including humans. Some reports indicate that static magnetic fields increase or both increase and decrease tissue temperature depending on the orientation of the organism in the static magnetic field,[19,66] whereas others indicate that static magnetic fields have no effect on skin and body temperatures.[55,61,88,90]

None of the investigators who identified a specific static magnetic field effect on temperatures proposed a plausible mechanism for this response, nor has this experimental work been supported by subsequent studies. In addition, investigations that reported static magnetic field–induced skin or body temperature changes used laboratory animals with labile temperatures or measurement instrumentation likely affected by the static magnetic fields.[19,66]

Several investigations indicated that exposure to a high static magnetic field does not alter skin and body temperatures.[55,61,90] These studies were performed using a special fluoroptic thermometry system shown to be unaffected by high-intensity static magnetic fields. Therefore, skin and body temperatures in humans are believed to be unaffected by exposure to static magnetic fields of up to 1.5 T.[55,61] Healthcare workers involved in the interventional MRI have not reported any unusual temperature-related sensations.

Electric induction and cardiac effects

Induced biopotentials may be seen during exposure to static magnetic fields. They are caused by blood, a conductive fluid, flowing through a magnetic field. The induced biopotential is exhibited by an augmentation of T-wave amplitude and by other nonspecific waveform changes apparent on the electrocardiogram (ECG) at static magnetic field strengths as low as 0.1 T.[86,91,92]

The increase in T-wave amplitude directly relates to the intensity of the static magnetic field, such that at low static magnetic field strengths the effects are not as predominant as those at higher field strengths. The effect on the T-wave is thought to be most marked when the blood flows through the thoracic aortic arch. This T-wave amplitude change can be significant enough to falsely trigger the RF excitation during cardiac-gated MRI.

Other portions of the ECG may also be altered by the static magnetic field; these alterations vary with the placement of the recording electrodes. Alternate lead positions can be used to attenuate the static magnetic field–induced ECG changes to facilitate cardiac-gated studies.[93] Once the patient is no longer exposed to the static magnetic field, the ECG voltage abnormalities revert to normal. Because no circulatory alterations appear to coincide with these ECG changes, biologic risks are not believed to be associated with exposure to static magnetic fields of up to 2 T.[86,91,92]

Neurologic effects

Theoretically, electrical impulse conduction in nerve tissue may be affected by exposure to static magnetic fields. However, this area in the bioeffects literature contains inconclusive information. Some studies have reported remarkable effects on the function and structure of portions of the central nervous system associated with exposure to static magnetic fields, whereas others have failed to show any significant changes.* Further investigations of potential unwanted bioeffects are needed because of the relative lack of clinical studies in this field that directly apply to MRI. Exposure to static magnetic fields of up to 2 T does not appear to significantly influence bioelectric properties of neurons in humans.[97–99]

In summary, there is no unrefuted evidence of irreversible or hazardous biologic effects related to acute, short-term exposures of humans to static magnetic fields of strengths up to 2 T. However, as of 1997, several 3- and 4-T whole-body MR systems were operating at various research sites around the world. In at least one study, healthcare workers and volunteers exposed to a 4-T MR system experienced vertigo, nausea, headaches, a metallic taste, and magnetophosphenes (visual flashes).[50] Considerable research is required to study the mechanisms responsible for these bioeffects and to determine possible means, if any, to counterbalance them.

Most interventional MRI procedures are using static magnetic fields of 0.5 T or less. Therefore, any associated bioeffects

*Refs. 14, 20, 34, 68, 69, 76-79, 94-99.

should be attenuated because the exposure is related to mid- or low-strength static magnetic fields.

BIOEFFECTS OF GRADIENT MAGNETIC FIELDS

MRI exposes humans to rapid variations of magnetic fields caused by transient application of magnetic field gradients during the imaging sequence. Gradient magnetic fields can induce electrical fields and currents in conductive media (including biologic tissue) according to Faraday's law of induction. The potential for interaction between gradient magnetic fields and biologic tissue is inherently dependent on the fundamental field frequency, the maximum flux density, the average flux density, the presence of harmonic frequencies, the waveform characteristics of the signal, the polarity of the signal, the current distribution in the body, and the electrical properties and sensitivity of the particular cell membrane.[97–99]

For animals and humans, the induced current is proportional to the conductivity of the biologic tissue and to the rate of change of the magnetic flux density.[98–101] In theory, the largest current densities will be produced in peripheral tissues (i.e., at the greatest radius) and will linearly diminish toward the body's center.[98–101] The current density will be enhanced at higher frequencies and magnetic flux densities and will be further accentuated by a larger tissue radius with a greater tissue conductivity. Current paths are affected by differences in tissue types, such that tissues with low conductivity (e.g., adipose, bone) will change the pattern of the induced current.

Bioeffects of induced currents can be caused by the power deposited by the induced currents (thermal effects) or by the direct effects of the current (nonthermal effects). In MRI, thermal effects caused by switched gradients are negligible and are not believed to be clinically significant.[96,98,99]

Possible nonthermal effects of induced currents are stimulation of nerve or muscle cells, induction of ventricular fibrillation, increased brain mannitol space, epileptogenic potential, stimulation of visual flash sensations, and bone healing.[98–103] The threshold currents required for nerve stimulation and ventricular fibrillation are much higher than the estimated current densities induced under routine clinical MRI conditions.[96–100]

The production of magnetophosphenes is one of the most sensitive physiologic responses to gradient magnetic fields.[96–99] Magnetophosphenes are supposedly caused by electrical stimulation of the retina and are completely reversible with no associated health effects.[96–99] These magnetophosphenes have been elicited by current densities of approximately 17 $\mu A/cm^2$, whereas currents required for the induction of nerve action potentials require approximately 3000 $\mu A/cm^2$, and those required for ventricular fibrillation induction of normal cardiac tissue are 100 to 1000 $\mu A/cm^2$.[96] Although no cases have been reported for fields of 1.95 T or less, magnetophosphenes have been reported in volunteers working around a 4-T research system.[50] In addition, a metallic taste and symptoms of vertigo, which appear to be reproducible, are associated with rapid motion within the static magnetic field of these 4-T systems.[50]

Time-varying, extremely low-frequency magnetic fields have been associated with multiple effects, including clustering and altered orientation of fibroblasts, increased mitotic activity of fibroblast growth, altered deoxyribonucleic acid (DNA) synthesis, and reduced fentanyl-induced anesthesia.[49,64,99] Possible effects in other organisms, including humans, have also been mentioned.[99] Although no studies conclusively show carcinogenic effects from exposure to magnetic fields of various intensities and durations, several reports suggest that an association between the two is possible.[104–106]

BIOEFFECTS OF RADIOFREQUENCY ELECTROMAGNETIC FIELDS

General bioeffects

RF radiation can generate heat in tissues as a result of resistive losses. Therefore, the main bioeffects associated with exposure to RF radiation relate to the thermogenic qualities of this electromagnetic field.[96–99,107–116] Exposure to RF radiation may also cause athermal, field-specific alterations in biologic systems that are produced without a significant increase in temperature.[108–114] This topic is somewhat controversial because of assertions that electromagnetic fields produce cancer and developmental abnormalities and of the concomitant ramifications of such effects.[108–114]

A report from the United States Environmental Protection Agency claimed that the evidence on this issue is sufficient to show a relationship between low-level electromagnetic field exposures and the development of cancer.[106] No specific studies have addressed the potential athermal bioeffects of MRI. Beers[113] thoroughly reviewed this topic, particularly as it pertains to MRI.

Regarding RF power deposition, investigators have typically quantified exposure to RF radiation by determining the specific absorption rate.[108–112,116–119] Specific absorption rate is the mass normalized rate at which RF power is coupled with biologic tissue (in W/kg). Measurements or estimates of specific absorption rate are not trivial, particularly in humans; several methods are available to determine this parameter for RF energy dosimetry.[108–112,119]

The specific absorption rate produced during MRI is a complex function of numerous variables, including the frequency (determined by the strength of the static magnetic field), type of RF pulse (i.e., 90° or 180°), repetition time, pulse width, type of RF coil, volume of tissue within the coil, resistivity of the tissue, and configuration of the anatomic region imaged.[96–99] The increase in tissue temperature caused by exposure to RF radiation depends on the patient's thermoregulatory system (e.g., skin blood flow, skin surface area, sweat rate).[97–99]

The efficiency and absorption pattern of RF energy are mainly determined by the physical dimensions of the tissue in relation to the incident wavelength.[108–112] Therefore, if the tissue size is large relative to the wavelength, energy is predominantly absorbed on the surface; if it is small relative to the wavelength, there is little absorption of RF power.[108–112] Because of this relationship between RF energy and physical dimensions, studies designed to investigate the clinical effects of exposure to RF radiation during MRI require tissue volumes and anatomic shapes similar to those of humans. Of note, no laboratory animal sufficiently mimics or simulates the thermoregulatory system or responses of humans. Thus, results obtained in laboratory animal experiments cannot simply be scaled or extrapolated to humans.[110–112,119]

Magnetic resonance imaging and exposure to radiofrequency energy radiation

Little quantitative data were available on thermoregulatory responses of humans exposed to RF radiation before MRI. The few studies that existed did not directly apply to MRI because they examined thermal sensations or therapeutic applications of diathermy, usually involving only localized regions of the body.[108–110,114]

Several recent studies of RF power absorption during MRI yielded useful information about tissue heating in humans.* During MRI, tissue heating results primarily from magnetic induction with a negligible contribution from the electric fields, so heating is greatest at the surface of the body and approaches zero at the center of the body. Predictive calculations and measurements in laboratory phantoms and humans exposed to MRI support this pattern of temperature distribution.[58–60,115,116]

Although one study of MRI reported significant temperature increases in internal organs,[65] it was conducted on anesthetized dogs and is unlikely to apply to nonanesthetized adults because of differences in physical dimensions and themoregulatory systems. However, these data may have important implications for the use of MRI in pediatric patients, who are typically sedated or anesthetized for MRI examinations.

An investigation using fluoroptic thermometry probes unaffected by electromagnetic fields[117] showed that humans exposed to MRI at specific absorption rates up to 4 W/kg have no statistically significant increases in body and skin temperature. However, these temperature changes were not believed to be clinically hazardous.[62] Additional studies are needed, however, to assess physiologic responses of patients with conditions that may impair thermoregulatory function (e.g., elderly patients; patients with underlying health conditions such as fever, diabetes, cardiovascular disease, and obesity; and patients taking medications that affect thermoregulation such as calcium blockers, β blockers, diuretics, or vasodilators) before subjecting them to MRI procedures that require high specific absorption rates.

Temperature-sensitive organs

Certain human organs that have reduced capabilities for heat dissipation (e.g., testis, eye) are particularly sensitive to elevated temperatures. Therefore, these are primary sites of potential harmful effects if RF radiation exposures during MRI are excessive. Laboratory investigations have shown detrimental effects on testicular function (i.e., reduction or cessation of spermatogenesis, impaired sperm motility, degeneration of seminiferous tubules) caused by RF radiation-induced heating from exposures sufficient to raise scrotal or testicular tissue temperatures up to 38° to 42° C.[118]

Scrotal skin temperatures (i.e., an index of intratesticular temperature) were measured in volunteers undergoing MRI at a whole-body averaged specific absorption rate of 1.1 W/kg.[63] The largest change in scrotal skin temperature was 2.1° C, and the highest temperature recorded was 34.2° C.[63] These temperature changes were below the threshold known to impair testicular function. However, excessive heating of the scrotum during MRI can exacerbate certain preexisting disorders associated with increased scrotal or testicular temperatures (e.g., acute febrile illnesses, varicocele) in oligospermic patients, and it may lead to temporary or permanent sterility.[63] Therefore, additional studies are needed to investigate these issues, particularly if patients are scanned at higher whole-body averaged specific absorption rates than those previously evaluated.

Dissipation of heat from the eye is slow and inefficient because of its relative lack of vascularization. In animal studies, acute near-field exposures of RF radiation to the eyes or head were shown to be cataractogenic as a result of the thermal disruption of ocular tissues if the exposure is of a sufficient intensity and duration.[108,110] Sacks and others[53] found no discernible effects with MRI of the eyes of rats using exposures that exceeded typical clinical imaging levels. However, these data may not be acceptable to extrapolate to humans considering the coupling of RF radiation to the anatomy and tissue volume of eyes in rats (compared with those in humans).

Corneal temperatures have been measured in patients undergoing MRI of the brain using a send-receive head coil at local specific absorption rates up to 3.1 W/kg.[59] The largest corneal temperature change was 1.8° C, and the highest temperature measured was 34.4° C. Because the temperature threshold for RF radiation-induced cataractogenesis in animals was shown to be 41° to 55° C for acute near-field exposures, clinical MRI using a head coil did not appear to be capable of causing thermal damage in ocular tissue.[59] The effect of MRI at higher specific absorption rates and the long-term effects of MRI on ocular tissues remain to be determined.

Radiofrequency radiation and "hot spots"

Theoretically, RF radiation hot spots caused by uneven distribution of RF power may arise whenever current concentrations are produced in association with restrictive conductive patterns. RF radiation hot spots are suggested to generate thermal hot spots under certain conditions during MRI. Because RF radiation is mainly absorbed by peripheral tissues, thermography has been used to study the heating pattern associated with MRI at high whole-body specific absorption rates.[57] This study showed no evidence of surface thermal hot spots related to MRI of humans. The thermoregulatory system apparently responds to the heat challenge by distributing the thermal load, smearing the surface temperatures. However, internal thermal hot spots may develop from MRI.[59]

*Refs. 28, 56-60, 62, 63, 65.

Radiofrequency radiation and interventional magnetic resonance imaging procedures

No studies have addressed possible RF-induced heating in healthcare workers involved in interventional MRI procedures. Because the static magnetic fields associated with interventional MR systems are at mid- or low-field levels, the related thermogenic capabilities of the RF electromagnetic radiation exposures should not present risks to healthcare workers. However, the use of certain medical devices (e.g., instruments made from conductive materials, electronically activated instruments) may create conditions whereby RF energy or gradient field-induced currents cause unusual concentrations of electromagnetic fields that, in turn, generate excessive heat. Therefore, the aforementioned situations may warrant a cautious approach before assuming absolute safety.

MAGNETIC RESONANCE IMAGING AND ACOUSTIC NOISE

The acoustic noise produced during MRI represents a potential risk to patients. Acoustic noise is associated with activation and deactivation of electrical current that induces vibrations of the gradient coils. This repetitive sound is enhanced by higher gradient duty cycles and sharper pulse transitions. Acoustic noise is thus likely to increase with decreases in section thickness, field of view (FOV), repetition times, and echo times.

Gradient magnetic field–related noise levels measured on several commercial MR scanners were in the range of 65 to 95 dB, which is within the safety guidelines recommended by the United States Food and Drug Administration (FDA) and other governmental agencies.[107] However, some reports found that acoustic noise generated during MRI caused patient annoyance, interference with oral communication, and reversible hearing loss in patients who did not wear ear protection.[9,120] In a recent study, 43% of patients undergoing MR imaging without earplugs experienced temporary hearing loss.[9] Furthermore, significant gradient coil–induced noise may produce permanent hearing impairment in patients particularly susceptible to the damaging effects of relatively loud noises.[9,120]

The safest and least expensive means of preventing problems associated with acoustic noise during clinical MRI is to encourage the routine use of disposable earplugs.[9,120,121] The use of hearing protection avoids the potential temporary hearing loss associated with clinical MRI.[9,120,121] MR-compatible headphones that significantly muffle acoustic noise are also commercially available.

An acceptable alternative strategy for reducing sound levels during MRI is to use an antinoise or destructive interference technique that reduces noise and permits better patient communication.[122] This technique consists of a real-time Fourier analysis of the noise emitted from the MR system.[122] A signal is produced that has the same physical characteristics but opposite phase than the sound generated by the MR system. The opposite-phase signals are then combined, resulting in a cancellation of the repetitive noise while allowing other sounds (e.g., music, voice) to be transmitted to the patient.[122] A recent investigation showed no significant degradation of image quality with MR systems that use this antinoise method.[122] Although this technique has not found widespread clinical application, it has considerable potential for minimizing acoustic noise and its associated problems.

Healthcare workers in the field of interventional MRI are subjected to acoustic noise caused by the operation of MR systems that may be at levels comparable with those experienced by patients. These persons should wear protective hearing devices to minimize stress-related noise.

INVESTIGATIONS OF MAGNETIC RESONANCE IMAGING SAFETY AND BIOEFFECTS

Many investigations have specifically studied the potential safety and bioeffects of MRI.[1–83] The results of these studies have been predominantly negative, supporting the widely held view that no significant health risks are associated with the use of this imaging modality. Experiments that yielded positive results identified possible nonspecific biologic responses, determined short-term biologic changes that were not considered to be deleterious, or found bioeffects that required further substantiation.

The dosimetric aspects of the exposures to static, gradient, or RF electromagnetic fields varied and include those that exceeded clinical exposures, simulated clinical exposures, or involved low-level chronic exposures. In certain cases, the effects of only one electromagnetic field used for MRI were evaluated. Theoretically, the combination of static, gradient, and RF electromagnetic fields may produce unusual or unpredictable bioeffects unique to MRI.

Window effects are often present with respect to biologic changes that occur in response to electromagnetic radiation. Window effects are biologic changes associated with a specific spectrum of electromagnetic radiation that are not observed at levels below or above this range.[108,119] Field strength and frequency windows have been reported in the literature.[108,119] Virtually all experiments on MRI biologic effects have been performed at specific windows, and the results cannot be assumed to apply to all of the various field strengths or frequencies used for clinical MRI.

Various biologic systems were used for these experiments. As mentioned, because the coupling of electromagnetic radiation with biologic tissues depends on subject size, anatomic factors, duration of exposure, sensitivity of the involved tissues, and many other variables, results from animal studies may not be extrapolated or directly applicable to humans or to clinical use of MRI. Therefore, the results of these studies should be interpreted with caution.

ELECTRICALLY, MAGNETICALLY, OR MECHANICALLY ACTIVATED IMPLANTS AND DEVICES

The United States FDA requires labeling of MR systems to indicate that the device is contraindicated for persons with electrically, magnetically, or mechanically activated implants because electromagnetic fields produced by the MR system may interfere with the operation of these devices.[107] Therefore, patients and healthcare workers with internal cardiac pacemakers, implantable cardiac defibrillators, cochlear implants, neurostimulators, bone-growth stimulators, implantable electronic drug infusion pumps, and other similar devices that could be adversely affected by the electromagnetic fields used for MRI should not be examined by this imaging technique.[120,123–126] Prior *ex vivo* testing of certain implants and devices may indicate that they are MR compatible.

The risks of having persons with cardiac pacemakers in the MR environment relate to the possibility of movement, reed switch closures or damage, programming changes, inhibition, reversion to an asynchronous mode of operation, electromagnetic interference, and induced currents in lead wires.[120,123,124,126] At least one patient with a pacemaker was scanned by MRI without incident.[125] In one case, a patient who was not pacemaker dependent underwent MRI by having the pacemaker disabled during the procedure.[125] Although this patient sustained no apparent discomfort and the pacemaker was not damaged, this type of maneuver should not be routinely performed in patients with pacemakers because of the potential risks. At least one patient with a pacemaker died of MRI-related complications.[99]

Of particular concern is that pacemaker lead wires or other similar intracardiac wire configurations could act as an antenna in which the gradient or RF electromagnetic fields may induce sufficient current to cause fibrillation, a burn, or another potentially dangerous event.[99,120,123,124,126] Because of this theoretically deleterious and unpredicted effect, patients with residual external pacing wires, temporary pacing wires, Swan-Ganz thermodilution catheters, or any other internally or externally positioned conductive wires or devices should not undergo MRI because of the possible risks.[99,120,127]

Some cochlear implants use a relatively high field strength cobalt samarium magnet in conjunction with an external magnet to align and retain an RF transmitter coil on the patient's head, whereas other cochlear implants are electronically activated.[128] Consequently, MRI is absolutely contraindicated in persons with cochlear implants because of the possibility of injury or damage to or alteration of the implant.

Implants involving magnets (e.g., dental implants, magnetic sphincters, magnetic stoma plugs, magnetic ocular implants) may be demagnetized, necessitating surgery to replace the damaged implant, and should thus be removed before MRI if possible.[128–130] Otherwise, MRI should not be performed in a patient with an electrically, magnetically, or mechanically activated implant or device unless the implant or device has been previously shown to be unaffected by the magnetic and electromagnetic fields used for MRI.[120]

METALLIC IMPLANTS, MATERIALS, AND FOREIGN BODIES

MRI is contraindicated in patients with certain ferromagnetic implants, materials, or foreign bodies, primarily because of the possibility of movement or dislodgement of these objects.[97–99] Box 10-1 lists examples of implants and devices that may be problematic in MRI. Other causes of these problems include induction of electrical current in the object, excessive heating of the object, and misinterpretation of an artifact produced by the presence of the object as an abnormality.[97,99,131–134] These latter situations, however, occur infrequently or are insignificant compared with movement or dislodgement of a ferromagnetic implant or foreign body by the magnetic fields of the MR system.

Numerous investigations have evaluated the ferromagnetic qualities of various metallic implants, materials, or foreign bodies by measuring deflection forces or movements associated with the static magnetic fields used by MRI.[134–153] These studies were conducted to determine the relative risk of movement or dislodgement when performing MRI in a patient with a metallic object.

Various factors require evaluation when establishing the relative risk of performing an MR procedure in a patient with a ferromagnetic implant, material, device, or foreign body.

These factors include the strength of the static and gradient magnetic fields, the relative degree of ferromagnetism of the object, the mass of the object, the geometry of the object, the location and orientation of the object in situ, and the length of time the object has been in place.[98,99] Each factor should be considered before a patient with a ferromagnetic object enters the electromagnetic environment of the MR system.

Aneurysm and hemostatic clips

Many aneurysm clips but no vascular clips are ferromagnetic. Therefore, only persons with nonferromagnetic aneurysm clips or previously tested hemostatic clips should be exposed to the magnetic fields used for MRI.

Carotid artery vascular clamps

Each carotid artery vascular clamp evaluated for ferromagnetism exhibited deflection forces. However, only the Poppen-Blaylock clamp (Codman, Randolph, MA) was contraindicated in persons undergoing MRI because of its significant ferromagnetism. Other carotid artery vascular clamps are believed to be safe for MRI because of the minimal deflection forces relative to their use in in vivo application (i.e., the deflection forces are insignificant and, therefore, significant movement or dislodgement of the implant is unlikely).

Dental devices and materials

Various dental devices and materials have been tested for ferromagnetism. Although many have shown deflection forces, only a few are magnetically activated devices, which pose a possible risk to persons undergoing MRI.

Heart valves

Many commercially available heart valve prostheses have been tested for ferromagnetism. Most displayed measurable deflection forces; however, these deflection forces were relatively insignificant compared with those exerted by the beating heart.

Box 10-1. Metallic implants, materials, and objects that are potential risks for patients undergoing magnetic resonance imaging

Aneurysm clips

Drake (DR14, DR 24), Edward Weck, Triangle Park, NJ
Drake (DR16), Edward Weck
Drake (301 SS), Edward Weck
Downs multi-positional (17-7PH)
Heifetz (17-7PH), Edward Weck
Housepian
Kapp (405 SS), V. Mueller
Kapp curved (404 SS), V. Mueller
Kapp straight (404 SS), V. Mueller
Mayfield (301 SS), Codman, Randolph, Mass
Mayfield (304 SS), Codman
McFadden (301 SS), Codman
Pivot (17-7PH), V. Mueller
Scoville (EN58J), Downs Surgical, Decatur, Ga
Sundt-Kees (301-SS), Downs Surgical
Sundt-Kees Multi-Angle (17-7PH), Downs Surgical
Vari-Angle (17-7PH), Codman
Vari-Angle Micro (17-7PM SS), Codman
Vari-Angle Spring (17-7PM SS), Codman

Carotid artery vascular clamp

Poppen-Blaylock (SS), Codman

Dental devices and materials

Palladium clad magnet,* Parkell Products, Farmindale, NY
Titanium clad magnet,* Parkell Products
Stainless steel clad magnet,* Parkell Products

Intravascular coils, stents, and filters

Gianturco embolization coil,† Cook, Bloomington, Ind
Gianturco bird nest IVC filter,† Cook
Gianturco zig-zag stent,† Cook
Gunther IVC filter,† Cook
New retrievable IVC filter,† Thomas Jefferson University, Philadelphia, Pa
Palmaz endovascular stent,† Ethicon, Sommerville, NJ

Ocular implants

Fatio eyelid spring/wire†
Retinal tack (SS-martensitic), Western European

Otologic implants

Cochlear implant (3M/House)
Cochlear implant (3M/Vienna)
Cochlear implant, Nucleus Mini 22-channel, Cochlear, Englewood, Colo
McGee piston stapes prosthesis (platinum/17Cr-4Ni SS), Richards Medical, Memphis, Tenn

Pellets, bullets, shrapnel, and other ammunition‡

BB's, Daisy
BB's, Crosman
Bullet, 7.62 × 39 mm (copper, steel), Norinco
Bullet, 0.380 inch, (copper, nickel, lead), Geco
Bullet 0.45 inch, (steel, lead), North America Ordnance
Bullet, 9 mm, (copper, lead), Norma

Penile implants

Penile implant, OmniPhase, Dacomed, Minneapolis, Minn

Miscellaneous

Cerebral ventricular shunt tube, connector (type unknown)
Swan-Ganz catheter,§ Thermodilution, American Edwards, Irvine, Calif
Tissue expander with magnetic port,† McGhan Medical, Santa Barbara, Calif

*The potential for significant injury to the patient is minimal. However, performing magnetic resonance imaging in a patient with one of these devices may be uncomfortable or may damage the implant.
†Ferromagnetic coils, filters, and stents typically become firmly incorporated into the vessel wall several weeks after placement. They are unlikely to become dislodged by magnetic forces after a suitable time has passed.
‡The relative risks of performing magnetic resonance imaging in patients with pellets, bullets, or shrapnel relate to whether the ammunition is positioned near a vital structure.
§Although no magnetic deflection is associated with the Swan-Ganz thermodilution catheter, catheter melting has been reported in one patient undergoing magnetic resonance imaging. Therefore, this catheter is considered a contraindication.
SS—Stainless steel.

Therefore, persons with heart valve prostheses may safely undergo MRI.

Intravascular coils, filters, and stents

Less than half of the intravascular coils, filters, and stents tested were ferromagnetic.[145,152] These ferromagnetic devices are usually attached firmly into the vessel wall approximately 4 to 6 weeks after introduction.[152] Therefore, they are unlikely to become dislodged by attraction from magnetic forces in MRI. Persons with intravascular coils, filters, or stents that may not be properly positioned or firmly held in place should not undergo MRI.

Ocular implants

Various ocular implants have been evaluated for ferromagnetism. The Fatio eyelid spring and retinal tack (made from martensitic stainless steel) displayed measurable deflection forces. Although the associated deflection forces are unlikely to cause movement or dislodgement of these implants, a person with one of these implants may be uncomfortable or may sustain a minor injury during MRI.

Orthopedic implants, materials, and devices

Most orthopedic implants, materials, and devices tested for ferromagnetism are made of nonferromagnetic materials. Therefore, persons with these orthopedic implants, materials, and devices may be imaged safely by MRI. The Perfix interference screw for reconstruction of the anterior cruciate ligament, although made of ferromagnetic material, does not pose a hazard to persons undergoing MRI because of the significant force that holds the screw in place, *in vivo.* However, the resulting imaging artifact precludes diagnostic assessment of the knee using MRI.

Otologic implants

Cochlear implants are a contraindication for MRI. Besides being attracted by static magnetic fields, these implants are electronically or magnetically activated. Only one otologic implant has associated deflection forces. This implant, the McGee stapedectomy piston prosthesis (Richards Medical, Memphis, Tenn) made of platinum and chromium-nickel alloy stainless steel, was made on a limited basis during mid-1987 and was recalled by the manufacturer. Persons with this otologic implant were warned to not undergo MRI.

Pellets, bullets, shrapnel, and other ammunition

Most of the pellets and bullets previously tested for ferromagnetism are made of nonferromagnetic materials.[143,145] Ferromagnetic ammunition typically comes from foreign countries or is used by the military. Shrapnel usually contains various amounts of steel and therefore presents a potential hazard for MRI. Furthermore, because pellets, bullets, and shrapnel may be contaminated with ferromagnetic materials, they are relative contraindications for MRI. Persons with these foreign bodies should be regarded individually with respect to whether the ammunition is near a vital neural, vascular, or soft-tissue structure. The location may be assessed by careful history-taking and by plain-film radiography.

Penile implants and artificial sphincters

One penile implant displayed significant deflection forces. Although this implant, the OmniPhase (Dacomed, Minneapolis, Minn) is unlikely to cause serious injury to a person undergoing MRI, it does cause discomfort. Therefore, this implant is a relative contraindication for MRI. Artificial sphincters made of nonferromagnetic materials have been tested. However, at least one artificial sphincter has a magnetic component; persons with this device should not undergo MRI.

Vascular access ports

Two vascular access ports showed measurable deflection forces, but these forces were insignificant relative to the *in vivo* application of these implants.[142] Therefore, MRI can be safely performed in a patient with one of these previously tested vascular access ports. However, patients with a vascular access port that is programmable or electronically activated should not undergo MRI.

Miscellaneous

Various other metallic implants, materials, and foreign bodies have been tested for ferromagnetism. The cerebral ventricular shunt tube connector (type unknown) and magnetically activated tissue expander exhibited deflection forces that may pose a risk during MRI. An O-ring washer used as a vascular marker also showed ferromagnetism, but the deflection force was minimal relative to *in vivo* use of this device.

All contraceptive diaphragms tested for ferromagnetism displayed significant deflection forces. However, MRI patients with these devices did not complain of any sensation related to movement of these objects. Therefore, scanning persons with diaphragms is not considered physically hazardous.

According to the Society for Magnetic Resonance Imaging Safety Committee,[120] persons with electrically, magnetically, or mechanically activated or electrically conductive devices should not undergo MRI unless the device was previously shown (i.e., usually by *ex vivo* testing procedures) to be unaffected by the electromagnetic fields used for clinical MRI and unless injury to the individual is impossible. During screening for MRI, persons with these devices should be identified before examination and before exposure to the electromagnetic fields used for this imaging technique. Many implants, materials, devices, and other foreign bodies have not been evaluated for MRI compatibility, which may be encountered in the clinical setting. Persons with previously untested devices should not undergo MRI.

SCREENING PATIENTS WITH SUSPECTED METALLIC FOREIGN BODIES

All persons with a history of metallic foreign bodies (e.g., slivers, bullets, shrapnel), should be carefully screened before MRI. The relative risk of exposing these persons to the magnetic fields of MRI depends on the ferromagnetic properties of the object, the geometry and dimensions of the object, and the strength of the static and gradient magnetic fields of the MR system. Also important are the strength with which the object is fixed within the tissue and whether it is positioned in or adjacent to a potentially hazardous site of the body (e.g., a vital neural, vascular, or soft-tissue structure).

A person with an intraocular metallic foreign body who undergoes the static magnetic field of MRI is at risk for significant eye injury. One person who experienced a vitreous hemorrhage, resulting in blindness, underwent MRI on a 0.35-T scanner; during the procedure, an occult intraocular metal fragment measuring 2.0×3.5 mm became dislodged.[154] This incident emphasizes the importance of adequately screening persons with suspected intraocular metallic foreign bodies before MRI.

Intraocular metallic fragments as small as $0.1 \times 0.1 \times 0.1$ mm have been detected using standard plain-film radiography.[155] Although thin slice (i.e., ≤ 3 mm) computed tomography (CT) can detect metallic foreign bodies as small as approximately 0.15 mm, a metallic fragment of this size is unlikely to become dislodged during MRI, even with a static magnetic field up to 2.0.[155] In animal studies, metallic intraocular fragments ranging from 0.1 × 0.1 × 0.1 mm to 3.0 × 1.0 × 1.0 mm have been examined to determine if they were moved or dislodged during exposure to a 2.0-T MRI system.[155] Only the largest fragment (3.0 × 1.0 × 1.0 mm) rotated, but it did not cause any discernible damage to the ocular tissue.[155] Therefore, plain-film radiography may be used to identify or exclude an intraocular metallic foreign body that may be a potential hazard to the person undergoing MRI.[120]

Persons with a high suspicion of having an intraocular metallic foreign body (e.g., metal workers exposed to metallic slivers with a history of an eye injury) should undergo plain-film radiography of the orbits to rule-out the presence of a metallic fragment before exposure to the static magnetic field. If a person with a suspected ferromagnetic intraocular foreign body has no symptoms, and plain-film series of the orbits does not show a radiopaque foreign body, the risk of performing MRI is minimal.[120]

Using plain-film radiography to search for metallic foreign bodies is a sensitive and relatively inexpensive means of identifying persons who are unsuitable for MRI. It can also be used to screen out persons that may have metal fragments in other potentially hazardous sites of the body.[120]

Each MRI site should establish a standardized policy for screening persons with suspected foreign bodies. The policy should include guidelines as to which persons require work-up by radiographic procedures and the specific procedure to be performed (i.e., number and type of views, position of the anatomy); each case should be considered individually. These precautions should be taken for all persons referred for MRI using any type of MR system regardless of field strength, magnet type, and the presence or absence of magnetic shielding.[120]

PERFORMING MAGNETIC RESONANCE IMAGING DURING PREGNANCY

Although MRI is not believed to be hazardous to the fetus, only a few investigations have examined the teratogenic potential of this imaging modality. By comparison, many studies have examined the possible hazards of ultrasound during pregnancy, and controversy still exists concerning the safe use of this non-ionizing radiation imaging technique.

Most early studies conducted to determine possible unwanted bioeffects during pregnancy showed negative results.* More recently, one study examined the effects of MRI on mice exposed during midgestation.[22] No gross embryotoxic effects were observed; however, crown-rump length decreased.[22] In another study performed by Tyndall and Sulik,[73] exposure to the electromagnetic fields used for a simulated clinical MRI examination caused eye malformations in a genetically prone mouse strain. Therefore, the electromagnetic fields used for MRI appear to be able to produce developmental abnormalities.

*Refs. 17, 22, 26, 31, 41, 47, 82.

Various mechanisms can produce deleterious bioeffects with respect to the developing fetus and the use of electromagnetic fields during MRI.* In addition, cells undergoing division, as in the case of the developing fetus during the first trimester, are highly susceptible to damage from different physical agents. Therefore, because of the limited data available, MRI should be used with caution in pregnant women.

The current guidelines of the FDA require labeling of MRI devices to indicate that the safety of MRI of the fetus and the infant "has not been established."[107] In Great Britain, the National Radiological Protection Board in 1983 specified that "it might be prudent to exclude pregnant women during the first three months of pregnancy."[108]

According to the Safety Committee of the Society for Magnetic Resonance Imaging[120] (and recently the American College of Radiology), MRI is indicated for use in pregnant women if other nonionizing forms of diagnostic imaging are inadequate or if the examination provides important information that would otherwise require exposure to ionizing radiation (i.e., x-ray, CT). Pregnant women should be informed that clinical MRI during pregnancy has produced no deleterious effects to date. However, as noted by the FDA, the safety of MRI during pregnancy has not been proved.[107]

Women who are pregnant or suspect they are pregnant should be identified before undergoing MRI to assess the risks versus the benefits of the examination. Because the general population has a spontaneous abortion rate greater than 30% during the first trimester of pregnancy, particular care should be exercised with the use of MRI during the first trimester because of associated potential medicolegal implications relative to spontaneous abortions.

MAGNETIC RESONANCE IMAGING AND CLAUSTROPHOBIA, ANXIETY, AND PANIC DISORDERS

Claustrophobia and various other psychologic reactions, including anxiety and panic disorders, may occur in as many as 5% to 10% of persons undergoing MRI. These complications originate from several factors, including the restrictive dimensions of the interior of the scanner, the duration of the examination, the gradient-induced noises, and the ambient conditions within the bore of the scanner.[156–164] No prior comparison on the incidence of claustrophobia in persons undergoing MR procedures in mid- and low-field open MR systems versus conventional MR systems substantiates the fact that a more open configuration improves individual tolerance.

Adverse psychologic responses to MRI are usually transient. However, in one report, two persons with no prior history of claustrophobia tolerated MRI with great difficulty and had persistent claustrophobia that required long-term psychiatric management.[157] Because adverse psychologic responses to MRI typically delay or require cancellation of the examination, several techniques have been developed to avert these problems.[120,156–164] These techniques include the following:

*Refs. 86, 88, 89, 102, 108, 109, 118.

1. The patient should be informed about the specific aspects of the MRI examination, including the expected level of gradient-induced noise, the internal dimensions of the scanner, and the length of the examination.
2. An appropriately screened relative or friend can remain with the patient during the procedure.
3. Headphones with calming music can decrease the repetitive noise created by the gradient coils.
4. Physical or verbal contact with the patient should be maintained throughout the examination.
5. The patient should be placed in a prone position with the chin supported by a pillow. In this position, the patient can visualize the opening of the bore and thus alleviate the "claustrophobic" feeling. An alternative method is to place the patient feet-first instead of head-first into the scanner.
6. Use of scanner-mounted mirrors or mirror or prism glasses within the scanner allows the patient to see out of the scanner.
7. A large light at either end of the scanner will decrease the anxiety of being in a long, dark enclosure.
8. The patient should be blindfolded and unaware of the close surroundings.
9. Relaxation techniques (e.g., controlled breathing, mental imagery,[165] and hypnotherapy) have been shown to reduce MRI-related claustrophobia and anxiety.
10. Psychologic desensitization techniques can be used before MRI examination.

Several investigators recently attempted to compare the effectiveness of some of the above mentioned techniques in reducing MRI-induced anxiety or claustrophobia.[158,159,162] One study showed that obtaining detailed information about the MRI procedure and using relaxation exercises reduced the anxiety level in patients before and during MRI. A similar reduction in anxiety could not be shown in persons given only information or stress reduction counseling. Relaxation methods also significantly decrease anxiety during other medical procedures.

In the interventional MRI setting, patients will likely be sedated or anesthetized during most of the procedures. Therefore, problems related to claustrophobia and anxiety are nonexistent.

MONITORING PATIENTS DURING INTERVENTIONAL MAGNETIC RESONANCE IMAGING

Monitoring a patient's physiologic state during interventional MRI is necessary to ensure the safe performance of the procedure. Conventional monitoring equipment was not designed to operate in the MRI environment where static, gradient, and RF electromagnetic fields can adversely affect the operation of these devices. MR-compatible monitors that have been developed consider the problems related to the presence of the electromagnetic fields used for MRI.[166–174] Table 10-1 lists examples of monitoring equipment and other support devices that have been used successfully in the MRI environment.

Every physiologic parameter that can be obtained under normal circumstances in the intensive care unit or operating room can be monitored during interventional MRI, including heart rate, systemic blood pressure, intracardiac pressure, end-tidal carbon dioxide, oxygen saturation, respiratory rate, skin blood flow, and temperature.[167–174] In addition, MR-compatible ventilators are available for patients who require ventilatory support.

Monitors that contain ferromagnetic components (i.e., transformers, outer casings) can be strongly attracted by mid- and high-field MR systems, posing a serious hazard to patients and possible damage to the MR system. Because the intensity of standard static magnetic field decreases as the third power of the distance from the magnet, placing the monitor a suitable distance from the MR system is sufficient to protect the operation of the device and prevent it from becoming a potential projectile.[171,174] If monitoring equipment is not placed in a permanently fixed position, instructions should be given to all appropriate personnel regarding the hazards of moving this equipment too close to the MR system.[171,174]

In addition to being influenced by the static magnetic field, monitors may be adversely affected by electromagnetic interference from the gradient and RF pulses from the MR system.[171,174] In these instances, increasing the length of the patient-monitor interface and positioning the equipment outside the RF-shielded room (e.g., the control room) will enable the monitor to operate properly. It is usually necessary to position all monitors with cathode ray tubes at a location in the magnetic fringe field such that the display is not bent or distorted.

Certain monitors emit spurious electromagnetic noise that can result in moderate to severe imaging artifacts.[171,174] These monitors can be modified to work during MRI by adding RF-shielded cables, using fiberoptic transmission of the signals (which is becoming increasingly the method of choice in the MRI environment), or using special outer casing. Also, special filters may be added to the monitor to inhibit electromagnetic noise.

Of further concern is the fact that some monitoring equipment can be potentially harmful to patients if special precautions are not followed.[171,174–177] A primary source of adverse MR system and physiologic monitor interactions has been the patient-monitor interface, which usually requires a conductive cable or other device. The presence of a conductive material in the immediate MR system area is a safety concern because of the potential for monitor-related burns. For example, an anesthetized patient sustained a third-degree burn of the finger associated with the use of a pulse oximeter during MRI.[176] Investigation of this incident revealed that the cable leading from the pulse oximeter to the finger probe may have been looped during MRI and the gradient or RF magnetic fields induced sufficient current to exorbitantly heat the finger probe, resulting in the burn.[176] This problem may also occur with the use of ECG lead wires or any other cables that may be looped or form a conductive loop that contacts the patient.

Table 10-1. Examples of magnetic resonance–compatible monitors and ventilators*

Device and manufacturer	Function
MR-Compatible Pulse Oximeter Invivo Research, Inc. Orlando, FL	Oxygen saturation, heart rate
MRI Fiber-optic Pulse Oximeter Nonin Medical Inc. Plymouth, MN	Oxygen saturation, heart rate
MR-Compatible Pulse Oximeter Patient Monitoring System Magnetic Resonance Equipment Corp. Bay Shore, NY	Oxygen saturation, heart rate
Omega 1400 Invivo Research, Inc. Orlando, FL	Blood pressure, heart rate
Omni-Trak 3100 MRI Vital Signs Monitor Invivo Research, Inc. Orlando, FL	Heart rate, electrocardiogram, oxygen saturation, respiratory rate, gas exchange, blood pressure
MR Equipment Vital Signs Monitor Model 6500 Bay Shore, NY	Heart rate, electrocardiogram, oxygen saturation, respiratory rate, gas exchange, blood pressure
Laserflow Blood Perfusion Monitor Vasomed, Inc. St. Paul, MN	Cutaneous blood flow
Medpacific LD 5000 Laser-Doppler Perfusion Monitor Medpacific Corporation Seattle, WA	Cutaneous blood flow
Respiratory Rate Monitor, Models 515 and 525 Biochem International Waukesha, WI	Respiratory rate, apnea
MicroSpan Capnometer 8800 Biochem International Waukesha, WI	Respiratory rate, end-tidal carbon dioxide, apnea
Fluoroptic Thermometry System, Model 3000 Luxtron Santa Clara, CA	Temperature
Omni-Vent, Series D Columbia Medical Marketing Topeka, KS	Ventilator
Ventilator, Models 225 and 2500 Monaghan Medical Corporation Plattsburgh, PA	Ventilator
Anesthesia Ventilator Ohio Medical Madison, WI	Ventilator
Infant Ventilator MVP-10 Bio-Med Devices, Inc. Madison, WI	Ventilator
Ohmeda Excel MRI Anesthesia Delivery System Ohmeda, Inc. Madison, WI	Delivery of gas anesthesia
Siemens-Elema Model 900C Iselin, NJ	Ventilator

*These devices may require modifications to make them magnetic resonance compatible and none of them should be positioned closer than 8 feet from the entrance of the bore of a 1.5-T magnetic resonance system. Also, monitors with metallic cables, leads, probes, or other similar patient interfaces may cause mild-to-moderate imaging artifacts if placed near the imaging area of interest. Consult the manufacturers for additional information related to compatibility with specific magnetic resonance systems.

Monitoring blood pressure

Noninvasive blood pressure monitors typically use the oscillometric technique, which uses a pressure transducer connected to a pressure cuff via a pneumatically filled hose. Certain monitors (i.e., Omega 1400, In-vivo Research Laboratories Inc., Broken Arrow, Okla) have adjustable audible and visual alarms and a strip-chart recorder.

Occasionally, cuff inflation tends to disturb lightly sedated patients, especially pediatric patients, causing them to move and distort the MRI. For this reason, the noninvasive blood pressure monitor may not be optimal for obtaining vital signs in all patient groups. Direct pressure monitoring of systemic or intracardiac pressures, if necessary, can be accomplished using a plastic fiberoptic pressure transducer.

Monitoring respiratory rate, oxygenation, and gas exchange

Monitoring of respiratory parameters during MRI of sedated or anesthetized patients is particularly important because the drugs used for these procedures may produce complications of respiratory depression. Therefore, as a standard of care, a pulse oximeter, capnograph, or capnometer should always be used to monitor patients who are sedated or anesthetized during MRI.

The respiratory monitors used on sedated pediatric or adult patients (i.e., the model 515 Respiration Monitor and model 8800 Capnometer, Biochem International, Waukesha, Wis) are relatively inexpensive and can be modified during MRI by simply lengthening the plastic tubing interface to the patient. Thus, the monitors can be placed at least 8 feet from the unshielded MRI system.

Pulse oximeters are used to record oxygen saturation and heart rate. Commercially available modified pulse oximeters using hard wire cables have been previously used to monitor sedated and anesthetized patients during MRI and the recovery period with moderate success. These pulse oximeters tend to work intermittently during MRI because of interference from the gradient or RF electromagnetic fields. In certain instances, patients have been burned, presumably as a result of excessive current being induced in inappropriately looped conductive cables attached to the patient probes of the pulse oximeters.[175–177]

Various fiberoptic pulse oximeters are available for use during interventional MR procedures.[178] Using fiberoptic technology to obtain and transmit physiologic signals from patients undergoing MRI does not have any associated MRI-related electromagnetic interference. A patient cannot be burned using this fiberoptic monitor during MRI because there are no conductive pathways formed by any metallic materials.

Monitoring cutaneous blood flow

Cutaneous blood flow can be monitored during MRI by means of the laser-Doppler velocimetry technique. This noninvasive measurement technique uses laser light that is delivered to and detected from the region of interest by flexible, graded-index fiberoptic light wires. Doppler broadening of laser light scattered by moving erythrocytes within the tissue is analyzed in real-time by an analogue processor that is indicative of instantaneous blood velocity and the effective blood volume and flow. A small circular probe can be attached to the patient on any available skin surface. Areas with a relatively high cutaneous blood flow (e.g., hand, finger, foot, toe, ear) yield the best results.

Hard-copy tracings obtained by laser-Doppler velocimetry can be used to determine the patient's heart rate, respiratory rate, and cutaneous blood flow. An audible signal may be activated to permit the operator to hear blood flow changes during monitoring. This technique of continuous physiologic monitoring is easily tolerated and is thus particularly useful when there is concern about disturbing a sedated patient.

Monitoring heart rate

Monitoring the ECG during MRI is typically required for cardiac imaging, for gating to reduce imaging artifacts from the physiologic motion of cerebrospinal fluid in the brain and spine, and for determining the patient's heart rate. Artifacts caused by the static, gradient, and RF electromagnetic fields may severely distort the ECG, making determination of cardiac rhythm during MRI extremely difficult and unreliable. Although sophisticated filtering techniques can be used to attenuate the artifacts from the gradient and RF fields, the static magnetic field augments the T-wave, as mentioned, and other nonspecific waveform changes that are proportional to the strength of the field, which cannot be easily counterbalanced.

In some instances, static magnetic field–induced augmented T-waves have a higher amplitude than the R-waves, resulting in false triggering and inaccurate determination of beats per minute. ECG artifacts can be minimized during MRI by using special filters, using ECG electrodes with minimal metal, selecting lead wires with minimal metal, twisting or braiding the lead wires, and using special lead placements.[173]

The previously mentioned pulse oximeters may also be used to accurately record heart rate during MRI examinations. These devices have probes that may be attached to the finger, toe, or ear lobe of the patient.

MEDICAL DEVICES DEVELOPED FOR USE IN INTERVENTIONAL MAGNETIC RESONANCE IMAGING

Various vendors, prompted by the recommendations and requests from MR users, have recognized the need for developing specialized equipment and medical devices to facilitate the performance of interventional MRI procedures. *Ex vivo* testing and evaluation are required to show the safe use and operation of these instruments and devices before applying them in the MRI environment.[179–182] The test procedures include an assessment of magnetic field attraction, heating, induced current (for certain devices), and artifacts using standardized techniques.[179–182] Medical devices can then be characterized with respect to compatibility with the electromagnetic fields of MRI. Appendix 10A lists the vendors for various instruments and devices for interventional MRI procedures.

REFERENCES

1. Adzamli IK, Jolesz FA, Blau M: An assessment of blood-brain barrier integrity under MRI conditions: brain uptake of radiolabeled Gd-DTPA and In-DTPA-IgG, *J Nucl Med* 30:839, 1989.
2. Barber BJ, and others: Thermal effects of MR imaging: worst-case studies in sheep, *Am J Roentgenol* 155:1105, 1990.
3. Bartels MV, and others: Magnetresonanztomographie und Sicherheit: Elektroenzephalographische und neuropsychologische Befunde vor und nach MR-Untersuchungen des Gehirns, *Fortschr Rontgenstr* 145:383, 1986.
4. Besson J, and others: Cognitive evaluation following NMR imaging of the brain, *J Neurol Neurosurg Psychiatry* 47:314, 1984.
5. Bore PJ, and others: Are quenches dangerous? *Magn Reson Imaging* 3:112, 1986.
6. Bourland JD, and others: *Physiologic indicators of high MRI gradient-induced fields.* In *Book of abstracts,* Berkeley, Calif, 1990, Society of Magnetic Resonance in Medicine.
7. Brody AS, and others: Induced alignment of flowing sickle erythrocytes in a magnetic field: a preliminary report, *Invest Radiol* 20:560, 1985.
8. Brody AS, and others: Preservation of sickle cell blood flow patterns during MR imaging: an in vivo study, *Am J Roentgenol* 151:139, 1988.
9. Brummett RE, Talbot JM, Charuhas P: Potential hearing loss resulting from MR imaging, *Radiology* 169:539, 1988.
10. Budinger TF, and others: Physiological effects of fast oscillating magnetic field gradients, *J Comput Assist Tomogr* 15:909, 1991.
11. Carson JJL, and others: Time-varying fields increase cytosolic free Ca2 in HL-60 cells, *Am J Physiol* 259:C687, 1990.
12. Cohen MS, and others: Sensory stimulation by time-varying magnetic fields, *Magn Reson Med* 14:409, 1990.
13. Cooke P, Morris PG: The effects of NMR exposure on living organisms: II. A genetic study of human lymphocytes, *Br J Radiol* 54:622, 1981.
14. Doherty JU, and others: Changes in cardiac excitability and vulnerability in NMR fields, *Invest Radiol* 20:129, 1985.
15. Fischer H: Physiological effects of fast oscillating magnetic field gradients, *Radiology* 173:382, 1989.
16. Garber HJ, and others: MRI gradient fields increase brain mannitol space, *Magn Reson Imaging* 7:605, 1989.
17. Geard CR, and others: Magnetic resonance and ionizing radiation: a comparative evaluation in vitro of oncogenic and genotoxic potential, *Radiology* 152:199, 1984.
18. Gore JC, and others: An assessment of the safety of rapidly changing magnetic fields in the rabbit: implications for NMR imaging, *Magn Reson Imaging* 1:191, 1982.
19. Gremmel H, Wendhausen H, Wunsch F: Biologische Effekte statischef Magnetfelder bei NMR-Tomographie am Menschen, *Wiss, Radiologische, Klinik, Christian-Albrechts-Universitat zu Kiel* 1983.
20. Gulch RW, Lutz O: Influence of strong static magnetic fields on heart muscle contraction, *Phys Med Biol* 31:763, 1986.
21. Hammer BE, and others: *In vivo measurement of RF heating in Capuchin monkey brain.* In *Book of abstracts,* Berkeley, Calif, 1991, Society of Magnetic Resonance in Medicine.
22. Heinrichs WL, and others: Midgestational exposure of pregnant balb/c mice to magnetic resonance imaging, *Magn Reson Imaging* 6:305, 1988.
23. Hong CZ, Shellock FG: Short-term exposure to a 1.5 Tesla static magnetic field does not effect somato-sensory evoked potentials in man, *Magn Reson Imaging* 8:65, 1989.
24. Innis NK, and others: Behavioral effects of exposure to nuclear magnetic resonance imaging II. Spatial memory tests, *Magn Reson Imaging* 4:281, 1986.
25. Jehenson P, and others: Change in human cardiac rhythm by a 2 Tesla static magnetic field, *Radiology* 166:227, 1988.
26. Kay HH, Herfkens RJ, Kay BK: Effect of magnetic resonance imaging on *Xenopus Laevis* embryogenesis, *Magn Reson Imaging* 6:501, 1988.
27. Keltner JR, and others: Magnetohydrodynamics of blood flow, *Magn Reson Med* 16:139, 1990.
28. Kido DK, and others: Physiologic changes during high field strength MR imaging, *American Journal of Neuroradiology* 8:263, 1987.
29. LaPorte R, and others: Magnetic resonance imaging (MRI) effects on rat pineal neuroendocrine function, *Brain Res* 506:294, 1990.
30. McRobbie D, Foster MA: Cardiac response to pulsed magnetic fields with regard to safety in NMR imaging, *Phys Med Biol* 30:695, 1985.
31. McRobbie D, Foster MA: Pulsed magnetic field exposure during pregnancy and implications for NMR foetal imaging: a study with mice, *Magn Reson Imaging* 3:231, 1985.
32. Messmer JM, and others: Exposure to magnetic resonance imaging does not produce taste aversion in rats, *Physiol Behav* 40:259, 1987.
33. Montour JL, Fatouros PP, Prasad UR: Effect of MR imaging on spleen colony formation following gamma radiation, *Radiology* 168:259, 1988.
34. Muller S, Hotz M: Human brainstem auditory evoked potentials (BAEP) before and after MR examinations, *Magn Reson Med* 16:476, 1990.
35. Niemann G, and others: Influence of magnetic resonance imaging on somatosensory potential in man, *J Neurol* 235:462, 1988.
36. Ngo FQH, Blue JW, Roberts WK: The effects of a static magnetic field on DNA synthesis and survival of mammalian cells irradiated with fast neutrons, *Magn Reson Med* 5:307, 1987.
37. Osbakken M, Griffith J, Taczanowsky P: A gross morphologic, histologic, hematologic, and blood chemistry study of adult and neonatal mice chronically exposed to high magnetic fields, *Magn Reson Med* 3:502, 1986.
38. Ossenkopp KP, and others: Exposure to nuclear magnetic imaging procedure attenuates morphine-induced analgesia in mice, *Life Sci* 37:1507, 1985.
39. Ossenkopp KP, and others: Behavioral effects of exposure to nuclear magnetic resonance imaging. I. Open-field behavior and passive avoidance learning in rats, *Magn Reson Imaging* 4:275, 1986.
40. Papatheofanis FJ, Papthefanis BJ: Short-term effect of exposure to intense magnetic fields on hematologic indices of bone metabolism, *Invest Radiol* 24:221, 1989.
41. Peeling J, and others: Biological effects of magnetic fields on the nemtode *Panagrellus* redivivus, *Magn Reson Imaging* 6:655, 1988.
42. Prasad N, and others: *Delayed tumor onset following MR imaging exposure.* In *Book of abstracts,* Berkeley, Calif, 1990, Society of Magnetic Resonance in Medicine.
43. Prasad N, and others: *Effects of 4.5 T MR exposure on mouse testes and epididymes.* In *Book of abstracts,* Berkeley, Calif, 1990, Society of Magnetic Resonance in Medicine.
44. Prasad N, and others: Effect of nuclear resonance on chromosomes of mouse bone marrow cells, *Magn Reson Imaging* 2:37, 1984.
45. Prasad N, and others: Effects of MR imaging on murine natural killer cell cytotoxicity, *Am J Roentgenol* 148:415, 1987.
46. Prasad N, and others: The effect of 2.35-T MR imaging on natural killer cell cytotoxicity with and without interleukin-2, *Radiology* 175:251, 1990.
47. Prasad N, and others: Safety of 4-T MR imaging: a study of effects of developing frog embryos, *Radiology* 174:251, 1990.
48. Prasad N, Wright DA, Forster JD: Effect of nuclear magnetic resonance on early stages of amphibian development, *Magn Reson Imaging* 1:35, 1982.
49. Prato FS, and others: Attenuation of morphine-induced analgesia in mice by exposure to magnetic resonance imaging: separate effects of the static, radiofrequency and time-varying magnetic fields, *Magn Reson Imaging* 5:9, 1987.
50. Redington RW, and others: *MR imaging and bio-effects in a whole body 4.0 Tesla imaging system.* In *Book of abstracts,* Berkeley, Calif, 1988, Society of Magnetic Resonance Imaging.
51. Reid A, Smith FW, Hutchinson JMS: Nuclear magnetic resonance imaging and its safety implications: follow-up of 181 patients, *Br J Radiol* 55:784, 1982.
52. Roschmann P: Human auditory system response to pulsed radiofrequency energy in RF coils for magnetic resonance at 2.4 to 170 MHz, *Magn Reson Med* 21:197, 1991.

53. Sacks E, and others: The effects of nuclear magnetic resonance imaging on ocular tissues, *Arch Ophthalmol* 104:890, 1986.
54. Schwartz JL, Crooks LE: NMR imaging produces no observable mutations or cytotoxicity in mammalian cells, *Am J Roentgenol* 139:583, 1982.
55. Shellock FG, Schaefer DJ, Gordon CJ: Effect of a 1.5 T static magnetic field on body temperature of man, *Magn Reson Med* 3:644, 1986.
56. Shellock FG, Crues JV: Temperature, heart rate, and blood pressure changes associated with clinical MR imaging at 1.5 T, *Radiology* 163:259, 1987.
57. Shellock FG, and others: Thermal effects of high-field (1.5 Tesla) magnetic resonance imaging of the spine: clinical experience above a specific absorption rate of 0.4 W/kg, *Acta Radiol Suppl* 369:514, 1986.
58. Shellock FG, Gordon CJ, Schaefer DJ: Thermoregulatory responses to clinical magnetic resonance imaging of the head at 1.5 Tesla: lack of evidence for direct effects on the hypothalamus, *Acta Radiol Suppl* 369:512, 1986.
59. Shellock FG, Crues JV: Corneal temperature changes associated with high-field MR imaging using a head coil, *Radiology* 167:809, 1986.
60. Shellock FG, Crues JV: Temperature changes caused by clinical MR imaging of the brain at 1.5 Tesla using a head coil, *American Journal of Neuroradiology* 9:287, 1988.
61. Shellock FG, Schaefer DJ, Crues JV: Effect of a 1.5 Tesla static magnetic field on body and skin temperatures of man, *Magn Reson Med* 11:371, 1989.
62. Shellock FG, Schaefer DJ, Crues JV: Alterations in body and skin temperatures caused by MR imaging: is the recommended exposure for radiofrequency radiation too conservative? *Br J Radiol* 62:904, 1989.
63. Shellock FG, Rothman B, Sarti D: Heating of the scrotum by high-field-strength MR imaging, *Am J Roentgenol* 154:1229, 1990.
64. Shivers RR, and others: Magnetic resonance imaging temporarily alters blood-brain barrier permeability in the rat, *Neurosci Lett* 76:25, 1987.
65. Shuman WP, and others: Superficial and deep-tissue increases in anesthetized dogs during exposure to high specific absorption rates in a 1.5-T MR imager, *Radiology* 167:551, 1988.
66. Sperber D, Oldenbourg R, Dransfeld K: Magnetic field induced temperature change in mice, *Naturwissenschaften* 71:100, 1984.
67. Stick VC, and others: Beeinflussen starke statische magnetfelder in der NMR-tomographie die gewebedurchblutung? *Fortschr Rontgenstr* 154:326, 1991.
68. Stojan L, Sperber D, Dransfeld K: Magnetic-field-induced changes in the human auditory evoked potentials, *Naturwissenschaften* 75:622, 1988.
69. Sweetland J, and others: The effect of magnetic resonance imaging on human cognition, *Magn Reson Imaging* 5:129, 1987.
70. Teskey GC, and others: Exposure to time varying magnetic fields associated with magnetic resonance imaging reduces fentanyl-induced analgesia in mice, *Bioelectromagnetics* 9:167, 1988.
71. Tesky GC, and others: Survivability and long-term stress reactivity levels following repeated exposure to nuclear magnetic resonance imaging procedures in rats, *Physiol Chem Phys Med NMR* 19:43, 1987.
72. Thomas A, Morris PG: The effects of NMR exposure on living organisms. I. A microbial assay, *Br J Radiol* 54:615, 1981.
73. Tyndall DA, Sulik KK: Effects of magnetic resonance imaging on eye development in the C57BL/6J mouse, *Teratology* 43:263, 1991.
74. Tyndall DA: MRI effects on the tertogenicity of X-irradiation in the C57BL/6J mouse, *Magn Reson Imaging* 8:423, 1990.
75. Vogl T, and others: Influence of magnetic resonance imaging on human body core and intravascular temperature, *Med Phys* 15:562, 1988.
76. Von Klitzing L: Do static magnetic fields of NMR influence biological signals, *Clin Phys Physiol Meas* 7:157, 1986.
77. Von Klitzing L: Static magnetic fields increase the power intensity of EEG of man, *Brain Res* 483:201, 1989.
78. Von Klitzing L: A new encephalomagnetic effect in human brain generated by static magnetic fields, *Brain Res* 540:295, 1991.
79. Weiss J, and others: Bio-effects of high magnetic fields: a study using a simple animal model, *Magn Reson Imaging* 8:166, 1990.
80. Willis RJ, Brooks WM: Potential hazards of NMR imaging: no evidence of the possible effects of static and changing magnetic fields on cardiac function of the rat and guinea pig, *Magn Reson Imaging* 2:89, 1984.
81. Withers HR, Mason KA, Davis CA: MR effect on murine spermatogenesis, *Radiology* 156:741, 1985.
82. Wolff S, and others: Tests for DNA and chromosomal damage induced by nuclear magnetic resonance imaging, *Radiology* 136:707, 1980.
83. Yamagata H, and others: *Evaluation of dB/dt thresholds for nerve stimulation elicited by trapezoidal and sinusoidal gradient fields in echo-planar imaging.* In *Book of abstracts,* Berkeley, Calif, 1991, Society of Magnetic Resonance in Medicine.
84. Vyalov AM: Magnetic fields as a factor in the industrial environment, *Vestn Ross Akad Med Nauk* 8:72, 1967.
85. Vyalov AM: *Clinico-hygenic and experimental data on the effect of magnetic fields under industrial conditions.* In Kholodov Y, editor: *Influence of magnetic fields on biological objects,* Moscow, 1971, Joint Publications Research Service (Translated).
86. Barnothy MF: *Biological effects of magnetic fields,* vols 1 & 2, New York, 1964, Plenum Press.
87. Persson BR, Stahlberg F: *Health and safety of clinical NMR examinations,* Boca Raton, Fla, 1989, CRC Press.
88. Tenforde TS: *Magnetic field effects on biological systems,* New York, 1979, Plenum Press.
89. Michaelson SM, Lin JV: *Biological effects and health implications of radiofrequency radiation,* New York, 1987, Plenum Press.
90. Tenforde TS: Thermoregulation in rodents exposed to high-intensity stationary magnetic fields, *Bioelectromagnetics* 7:341, 1986.
91. Beischer DE, Knepton J: Influence of strong magnetic fields on the electrocardiogram of squirrel monkey (Saimiri sciures), *Aerospace Medicine* 35:939, 1964.
92. Tenforde TS, and others: Cardiovascular alterations in Macaca monkeys exposed to stationary magnetic fields: experimental observations and theoretical analysis, *Bioelectromagnetics* 4:1, 1983.
93. Dimick RM, and others: Optimizing electrocardiographic electrode placement for cardiac-gated magnetic resonance imaging, *Invest Radiol* 22:17, 1987.
94. Abdullakhozhaeva MS, Razykov SR: Structural changes in central nervous system under the influence of a permanent magnetic field, *Bulletin of Experimental Biology and Medicine* 102:1585, 1986.
95. Hong CZ: Static magnetic field influence on human nerve function, *Arch Phys Med Rehabil* 68:162, 1987.
96. Budinger TF: Nuclear magnetic resonance (NMR) in vivo studies: known thresholds for health effects, *J Comput Assist Tomogr* 5:800, 1981.
97. Shellock FG, Crues JV: MRI: safety considerations in magnetic resonance imaging, *MRI Decisions* 2:25, 1988.
98. Shellock FG: Biological effects and safety aspects of magnetic resonance imaging, *Magn Reson Q* 5:243, 1989.
99. Kanal E, Talagala L, Shellock FG: Safety considerations in MR imaging, *Radiology* 176:593, 1990.
100. Reilly JP: Peripheral nerve stimulation by induced electric currents: exposure to time-varying magnetic fields, *Med Biol Eng Comput* 27:101, 1989.
101. Bernhardt J: The direct influence of electromagnetic fields on nerve and muscle and muscle cells of man within the frequency range of 1 Hz to 30 MHz, *Radiat Environ Biophys* 16:309, 1979.
102. Adey WR: Tissue interactions with nonionizing electromagnetic fields, *Physiol Rev* 61:435, 1981.
103. Watson AB, Wright JS, Loughman L: Electrical thresholds for ventricular fibrillation in man, *Med J Aust* 1:1179, 1973.
104. Modan B: Exposure to electromagnetic fields and brain malignancy: a newly discovered menace? *Am J Ind Med* 13:625, 1988.
105. Brown HD, Chattopadhyay SK: Electromagnetic-field exposure and cancer, *Cancer Biochem Biophys* 9:295, 1988.
106. Pool R: Electromagnetic fields: the biological evidence, *Science* 249:1378, 1990.

107. The United States Food and Drug Administration: Magnetic resonance diagnostic device: panel recommendation and report on petitions for MR reclassification, *Federal Register* 53:7575, 1988.
108. NCRP Report No. 86: *Biological effects and exposure criteria for radiofrequency electromagnetic fields,* Bethesda, Md, 1986, National Council on Radiation Protection and Measurements.
109. Erwin DN: Mechanisms of biological effects of radiofrequency electromagnetic fields: an overview, *Aviat Space Environ Med* 59(suppl):A21, 1988.
110. Gordon CJ: *Thermal physiology.* In *Biological effects of radiofrequency radiation.* Washington DC, EPA-600/h8-830-026A.
111. Gordon CJ: Normalizing the thermal effects of radiofrequency radiation: body mass versus total body surface area, *Bioelectromagnetics* 8:111, 1987.
112. Gordon CJ: Effect of radiofrequency radiation exposure on thermoregulation, *ISI Atlas of Science, Plants and Animals* 1:245, 1988.
113. Beers J: Biological effects of weak electromagnetic fields from 0 Hz to 200 MHz: a survey of the literature with special emphasis on possible magnetic resonance effects, *Magn Reson Imaging* 7:309, 1989.
114. Coulter JS, Osbourne SL: Short wave diathermy in heating of human tissues, *Archives of Physical Therapy* 17:679, 1936.
115. Bottomley PA, Edelstein WA: Power disposition in whole body NMR imaging, *Med Phys* 8:510, 1981.
116. Bottomley PA, and others: Estimating radiofrequency power disposition in body NMR imaging, *Magn Reson Med* 2:336, 1985.
117. Wickersheim KA, Sun MH: Fluoroptic thermometry, *Medical Electronics* Feb: 84, 1987.
118. Berman E: *Reproductive effects.* In *Biological effects of radiofrequency radiation,* Washington DC, 1984, EPA 600/8-83-026A.
119. Michaelson SM, Lin JC: *Biological effects and health implications of radiofrequency radiation,* New York, 1987, Plenum Press.
120. Shellock FG, Kanal E: Policies, guidelines, and recommendations for MR imaging safety and patient management, *J Magn Reson Imaging* 1:97, 1991.
121. Hurwitz R, and others: Acoustic analysis of gradient-coil noise in MR imaging, *Radiology* 173:545, 1989.
122. Goldman AM, Grossman WE, Friedlander PC: Reduction of sound levels with antinoise in MR imaging, *Radiology* 173:549, 1989.
123. Hayes DL, Holmes DR, Gray JE: Effect of a 1.5 Tesla nuclear magnetic resonance imaging scanner on implanted permanent pacemakers, *J Am Coll Cardiol* 10:782, 1987.
124. Gangarosa RE, and others: Operational safety issues in MRI, *Magn Reson Imaging* 5:287, 1987.
125. Alagona P, and others: Nuclear magnetic resonance imaging in a patient with a DDD pacemaker, *PACE Pacing Clin Electrophysiol* 12:619, 1989.
126. Edelman RR, Shellock FG, Ahladis J: *Practical MRI for the technologist and imaging specialist.* In Edelman RR, Hesselink J, editors: *Clinical magnetic resonance imaging,* Philadelphia, 1990, WB Saunders.
127. ECRI: *Health devices alert: a new MRI complication?* 1988, ECRI.
128. Dormer KJ, and others: The use of rare-earth magnet couplers in cochlear implants, *Laryngoscope* 91:1812, 1981.
129. Shellock FG: Ex vivo assessment of deflection forces and artifacts associated with high-field MRI of ``mini-magnet" dental prostheses, *Magn Reson Imaging* 7(suppl 1):IT-03, 1989.
130. Liang MD, Narayanan K, Kanal E: Magnetic ports in tissue expanders: a caution for MRI, *Magn Reson Imaging* 7:541, 1989.
131. Lund G, and others: Tattooing of eyelids: magnetic imaging artifacts, *Ophthalmic Surg* 17:550, 1986.
132. Sacco DA, and others: Artifacts caused by cosmetics in MR imaging of the head, *Am J Roentgenol* 148:1001, 1987.
133. Jackson JG, Acker JD: Permanent eyeliner and MR imaging, *Am J Roentgenol* 149:1080, 1987.
134. Pusey E, and others: Magnetic resonance imaging artifacts: mechanism and clinical significance, *Radiographics* 6:891, 1986.
135. Buchli R, Boesiger P, Meier D: Heating effects of metallic implants by MRI examinations, *Magn Reson Med* 7:255, 1988.
136. Davis PL, and others: Potential hazards in NMR imaging: heating effects of changing magnetic fields and RF fields on small metallic implants, *Am J Roentgenol* 137:857, 1981.
137. Shellock FG, Crues JV: High-field MR imaging of metallic biomedical implants: an in vitro evaluation of deflection forces and temperature changes induced in large prostheses, *Radiology* 165:150, 1987.
138. Shellock FG, Crues JV: High-field MR imaging of metallic biomedical implants: an ex vivo evaluation of deflection forces, *Am J Roentgenol* 151:389–392, 1988.
139. Dujovny M, and others: Aneurysm clip motion during magnetic resonance imaging: in vivo experimental study with metallurgical factor analysis, *Neurosurgery* 17:543, 1985.
140. Shellock FG, and others: Ex vivo evaluation of 9 different ocular and middle-ear implants exposed to a 1.5 Tesla MR scanner, *Radiology* 177:271, 1990.
141. Shellock FG, Schatz CJ: High-field strength MRI and otologic implants, *AJNR* 12:279, 1991.
142. Shellock FG, Meeks T: Ex vivo evaluation of ferromagnetism and artifacts for implantable vascular access ports exposed to a 1.5 T MR scanner, *J Magn Reson Imaging* 1:243, 1991.
143. Teitelbaum GP, and others: Metallic ballistic fragments: MR imaging safety and artifacts, *Radiology* 175:855, 1990.
144. Shellock FG: MR imaging of metallic implants and materials: a compilation of the literature, *Am J Roentgenol* 151:811, 1988.
145. Shellock FG, Curtis JS: MR imaging and biomedical implants, materials, and devices: an updated review, *Radiology* 180:541, 1991.
146. Holtas S, and others: Comparison of MR imaging and CT in patients with intracranial aneurysm clips, *AJNR* 9:891, 1988.
147. Huttenbrink KB, Grobe-Nobis W: Experimentelle untersuchungen und theoretische betrachtungen uber das verhalten von stapes-metall-prothesen im magnetfeld eines kernspintomographen, *Laryngologicie, Rhinologie, Otologie* 66:127, 1987.
148. Becker R, and others: MR imaging in patients with intracranial aneurysm clips, *AJNR* 9:885, 1988.
149. Randall PA, and others: Magnetic resonance imaging of prosthetic cardiac valves in vitro and in vivo, *Am J Cardiol* 62:973, 1988.
150. Romner B, and others: Magnetic resonance imaging and aneurysm clips, *J Neurosurg* 70:426, 1989.
151. Augustiny N, and others: MR imaging of large nonferromagnetic metallic implants at 1.5 T, *J Comput Assist Tomogr* 11:678, 1987.
152. Teitelbaum GP, Bradley WG, Klein BD: MR imaging artifacts ferromagnetism, and magnetic torque of intravascular filters, stents, and coils, *Radiology* 166:657, 1988.
153. Yuh WTC, and others: *Extrusion of a magnetic eye implant after MR examination: a potential hazard to the enucleated eye.* In *Book of abstracts,* 1991, American Society of Neuroradiology.
154. Kelly WM, and others: Ferromagnetism of intraocular foreign body causes unilateral blindness after MR study, *AJNR* 7:243, 1986.
155. Williams S, and others: Ferrous intraocular foreign bodies and magnetic resonance imaging, *Am J Ophthalmol* 105:398, 1988.
156. Flaherty JA, Hoskinson K: Emotional distress during magnetic resonance imaging, *N Engl J Med* 320:467, 1989.
157. Fishbain DA, and others: Long-term claustrophobia following magnetic resonance imaging, *Am J Psychiatry* 145:1038, 1988.
158. Quirk ME, and others: Anxiety in patients undergoing MR imaging, *Radiology* 170:463, 1989.
159. Quirk ME, and others: Evaluation of three psychological interventions to reduce anxiety during MR imaging, *Radiology* 173:759, 1989.
160. Hricak H, Amparo EG: Body MRI: alleviation of claustrophobia by prone positioning, *Radiology* 152:819, 1984.
161. Weinreb JC, and others: Magnetic resonance imaging: improving patient tolerance and safety, *Am J Roentgenol* 143:1285, 1984.
162. Klonoff EA, Janata JW, Kaufman B: The use of systematic desentization to overcome resistance to magnetic resonance imaging (MRI) scanning, *J Behav Ther Exp Psychiatry* 17:189, 1986.

163. Granet RB, Gelber LJ: Claustrophobia during MR imaging, *N J Med* 87:479, 1990.
164. Phelps LA: MRI and claustrophobia, *Am Fam Physician* 42:930, 1990.
165. McGuinness TP: Hypnosis in the treatment of phobias: a review of the literature, *Am J Clin Hypn* 26:261, 1984.
166. Karlik SJ, and others: Patient anesthesia and monitoring at a 1.5 T MRI installation, *Magn Reson Med* 7:210, 1988.
167. Barnett GH, Ropper AH, Johnson KA: Physiological support and monitoring of critically ill patients during magnetic resonance imaging, *J Neurosurg* 68:244, 1988.
168. Dunn V, and others: Mechanical ventilation during magnetic resonance imaging, *Magn Reson Imaging* 3:169, 1985.
169. McArdle CB, and others: Monitoring of the neonate undergoing MR imaging: technical considerations, *Radiology* 159:223, 1986.
170. Roth JL, and others: Patient monitoring during magnetic resonance imaging, *Anesthesiology* 62:80, 1985.
171. Shellock FG: Monitoring during MRI: an evaluation of the effect of high-field MRI on various patient monitors, *Medical Electronics* Sept:93, 1986.
172. Shellock FG: Monitoring sedated patients during MRI, *Radiology* 177:586, 1990 (letter).
173. Wendt RE, and others: Electrocardiographic gating and monitoring during NMR imaging, *Magn Reson Imaging* 6:89, 1988.
174. Holshouser BA, Hinshaw DB, Shellock FG: *Sedation, anesthesia, and physiologic monitoring during MRI.* In Hasso AN, Stark DO, editors: *Catagorical course syllabus: spine and body magnetic resonance imaging,* 1991, American Roentgen Society.
175. Kanal E, Applegate GR: *Thermal injuries/incidents associated with MR imaging devices in the US: a compilation and review of the presently available data.* In *Book of abstracts,* 1990, Society for Magnetic Resonance Imaging.
176. Shellock FG, Slimp G: Severe burn of the finger caused by using a pulse oximeter during MRI, *Am J Roentgenol* 153:1105, 1989.
177. Kanal E, Shellock FG: Burns associated with clinical MR examinations, *Radiology* 175:585, 1990.
178. Shellock FG, Myers SM, Kimble K: Monitoring heart rate and oxygen saturation during MRI with a fiber-optic pulse oximeter *Am J Roentgenol* 158:663, 1992.
179. Shellock FG: *Guide to MR procedures and metallic objects: update 1997,* New York, 1997, Lippincott-Raven Press.
180. Moscatel M, Shellock FG, Morisoli S: Biopsy needles and devices: assessment of ferromagnetism and artifacts during exposure to a 1.5 Tesla MR system, *J Magn Reson Imaging* 5:369, 1995.
181. Shellock FG, Shellock VJ: Ceramic surgical instruments: evaluation of MR-compatibility at 1.5 Tesla, *J Magn Reson Imaging* 6:954, 1996.
182. Shellock FG, Shellock VJ: MR-compatibility of an endoscope designed for use in interventional MR imaging procedures, *Am J Roentgenol* (in press).

APPENDIX 10A

VENDORS OF MEDICAL PRODUCTS USED FOR INTERVENTIONAL MRI PROCEDURES

AESCULAP
1000 Gateway Boulevard
Southern San Francisco, CA 94080
PRODUCT(S): General surgical instruments
CATALOG OR SPECIAL ITEMS:
MR-compatible surgical instruments
CONTACT: Haio F. Fauser
New Business Development Manager
Phone: 800-282-9000 or 415-876-7000

AESCULAP AG
AM Aesculap-Platz
PO Box 40
78501 Tuttlingen/Germany
Phone: 49-74-61-95-2801
Fax: 49-74-61-95-2600

BIP
AM Brand 1,
D-82299 Tuerkenfeld, Germany
PRODUCTS: Core biopsy gun
CONTACT: Norbert Heske
Phone: 49-81-93-6026 or 49-81-93-6548

COGENT LIGHT
26145 Technology Drive
Santa Clarita, CA 91355-1137
PRODUCT(S): Headlight, light sources
CONTACT: Richard B. Davies
Phone: 805-294-2989 or 800-294-2989 ext. 101
Fax: 805-294-2904

COOK MEDICAL
PO Box 489
Bloomington, IN 47402
PRODUCT(S): Needles, biopsy guns, catheters
CONTACT: John DeFord, PhD
Product Development Manager
Phone: 812-339-2235 or 800-346-2686
Fax: 812-339-5369
Customer Service: 800-457-4500

CRYOMEDICAL SCIENCES
1300 Piccard Drive, Suite L105
Rockville, MD 20850
PRODUCT(S): Cryotherapy equipment
CONTACT: John Baust
Vice President of Research and Development
Phone: 301-417-7070
Fax: 301-417-7077
INTERNATIONAL CONTACT: John Baust
B&K Medical (German distributor)
Phone: 49-5143-93227
Fax: 49-5143-93228

CUDA PRODUCTS
6000 Powers Avenue
Jacksonville, FL 32217
PRODUCT(S): Adaptors for the light source to the endoscope
CATALOG OR SPECIAL ITEMS: Olympus C-0200, Wolff C-0201, ACMI C-0202
Phone: 904-737-7611
Fax: 904-733-4832

DAUM CORPORATION
UMBC Technology Center
1450 South Rolling Road
Baltimore, MD 21227
PRODUCT(S): Needles
Phone: 410-455-5786
Fax: 410-455-5787
Email: info@daum.de or medinfo@daum.de
INTERNATIONAL CONTACT: Wolfgang Daum, President

Daum GmbH Deutschland
Hagenower Strasse 73
D-19061 Schwerin
Phone: 49-385-6344-344
Fax: 49-385-6344-152

DORNIER MEDIZINLASER GMBH
Industriestrasse 15
82110 Germering, Germany
PRODUCTS: MR-compatible laser-delivery-systems and various MR-compatible applicators for laser-inducted thermotherapy
CONTACT: Wolfgang Illich
Development Engineer
Phone: 49-89-84108-133
Fax: 49-89-84108-745
Email: wolfgang.illich@domedtech.de
Dr. Werner Rother
Sales Manager
Phone: 49-89-84108-640
Fax: 49-89-84108-552
Email: werner.rother@domedtech.de

E-Z-EM, INC
717 Main Street
Westbury, NY 11590
PRODUCT(S): Lufkin 22 gauge cytology biopsy needles;
MRI histology biopsy needles; MRI core biopsy guns, 14 and 18 gauge; MRI lesion-marking systems (20-gauge needle with Kopans style localization wire);
CONTACT: Andy Zwarun, Vice President
Phone: 516-333-8230 ext. 304
Fax: 516-333-8278
E-mail: anzwar@worldnet.att.net
INTERNATIONAL CONTACT: Germany: Edwin Schneider (Guerbet)
Phone: 49-6196-7620
Fax: 49-6196-79934
Switzerland: Christopher Jackson
Manager, Medilink
Phone: 41-91-972-8417
Fax: 41-91-972-8568

ELEKTA
8 Executive Park West, Suite 809
Atlanta, GA 30329
PRODUCT(S): Neurosurgical instruments
CATALOG OR SPECIAL ITEMS: Lumbar carbon fiber retractor, neuro 14G biopsy needle, Fukishima retractor arm blades
CONTACT: Kent Iverson
Operations General Manager
Phone: 800-535-7355 ext. 146 or 404-315-1225
Fax: 404-315-7850

ERBE ELEKTROMEDIZIN GMBH
Waldhoernlestrasse 17
72072 Tuebingen, Germany
General Phone Number: 49-7071-755-0

ERBE USA Inc.
2225 Northwest Parkway, Suite 105
Marietta, GA 30067
PRODUCT(S): Electrosurgical Equipment: ICC 350-MRI (MR-Compatible generator allowing mono- and bipolar operation), instruments and accessories; cryosurgery units
CONTACT: David Hartnett
Vice President of Marketing
Phone: 800-778-3723
Fax: 770-955-2577
INTERNATIONAL CONTACT: Martin Hagg
Vice President of Design & Engineering
Phone: 49-7071-755-249
Fax: 49-7071-755-549
E-mail: mhagg@erbe-med.de

GREATBATCH SCIENTIFIC
9645 Wehrle Drive
Clarence, NY 14031
PRODUCT(S): Batteries, lithium; endoscopes, rigid and flexible; endoscopic accessories; flashlights (including penlight); intubating laryngoscope sets; peripheral nerve stimulator
CATALOG OR SPECIAL ITEMS: Catalog items
CONTACT: Charles L. Mozeko
Manager, Interventional MR Products
Phone: 716-759-5659
Fax: 716-759-5654
Robert C. Rusin
Director, Sales and Distribution
Phone: 716-759-5656
Fax: 716-759-5654

GROUPE BRUKER ODAM
34, Rue de l'Industrie
Wissembourg, France 67160
PRODUCT(S): Patient monitoring
CONTACT: Laurent Sigrist
Secretaire General
Phone: 33-88-63-3606
Fax: 33-88-54-3632
Phone: 33-88-63-3600
Fax: 33-88-94-1282

INTERMETRO INDUSTRIES
651 North Washington Street
Wilkes-Barre, PA 18705
PRODUCT(S): Drug/storage carts
Phone: 717-825-2741
Fax: 717-825-2852
E-mail: www.intermetro.com

ITI MEDICAL TECHNOLOGIES
2452 Armstrong Street
Livermore, CA 94550
PRODUCT(S): Prototype biopsy needle
CONTACT: Roger W. Werne, PhD
Phone: 510-371-8305
Fax: 510-371-8222

IN-VIVO RESEARCH
12601 Research Parkway
Orlando, FL 32826
PRODUCT(S): Vital sign monitoring equipment capable of monitoring ECG, respiratory, invasive and noninvasive blood pressure, and temperature
CATALOG OR SPECIAL ITEMS: All products have been 510K cleared for MRI use and are standard catalog items
CONTACT: Amy Kilgore
Director of Marketing
Phone: 407-275-3220
Fax: 407-249-2022
INTERNATIONAL CONTACT: Sally Dugan
International Sales Manager

JOHNSON & JOHNSON ETHICON, INC.
US Route 22
PO Box 157
Somerville, NJ 08876
PRODUCT(S): Needles with sutures
CONTACT: Bill McJames
Phone: 908-218-2297
Fax: 908-218-2531

JOHNSON & JOHNSON PROFESSIONAL, INC.
(CODMAN DIVISION)
375 Paramount Drive
Raynham, MA 02767
PRODUCT(S): CMC3 irrigation bi-polar, Bookwalter arm and table post, Rhoton microsurgical, Hudson twist drill
CONTACT: Paula Papineau
Associate Product Director
Richard Van Zandt
Director of Instrumentation
Phone: 508-828-3228
Fax: 508-828-3065

LIFE INSTRUMENTS
14 Wood Road
Braintree, MA 02184
PRODUCT(S): Penfields, curettes, mini cobbs, Hudson twist drill, drill bits, periosteal elevators
CONTACT: Larry Foley
Phone: 781-849-0109 or 800-925-2995
Fax: 781-849-0128

LONE PEAK ENGINEERING
470 Lawndale Drive, Suite G
Salt Lake City, UT 84115
PRODUCT(S): Ceramic scissors C-124
CONTACT: Vickie Coombs
Phone: 801-466-5518
Fax: 801-466-5817

MAGNETIC RESONANCE EQUIPMENT CORPORATION
6 Washington Avenue
Bay Shore, NY 11706
PRODUCT(S): Patient monitors and patient communication and music systems
CATALOG OR SPECIAL ITEMS: Catalog items
CONTACT: John V. Plump
Phone: 516-243-3500
Fax: 516-243-3516

MAGNETIC Vision GMBH
Lochacher 6
CH-8630 Ruti, SWITZERLAND
PRODUCT(S): Neurosurgery drill, neurobiopsy needle guide, Dura hook, retractor
INTERNATIONAL CONTACT: Dr. Adriano Vigano
Phone: 41-55-260-1855
Fax: 41-55-260-1856
E-mail: AVigano@swissonline.ch

MEDILAS AG
Grindlenstrasse 3
Ch-8954 Geroldswil, Switzerland
PRODUCT(S): Drapes
INTERNATIONAL CONTACT: Markus Kleger
Phone: 41-1-748-4000
Fax: 41-1-748-0105

MEDRAD
1 Medrad Drive
Indianola, PA 15051
PRODUCT(S): Spectris MR injector (for injection of contrast media only, and explicitly not for drug or chemotherapy infusion)
Phone: 800-633-7237 or 412-967-9700
Fax: 412-767-4120
INTERNATIONAL CONTACT: Medrad Europe
Postbus 3084
NL-6202 N.B. Maastricht, The Netherlands
Phone: 31-43-358-5600
Fax: 31-43-365-0020
CONTACT: Brigette Palt/ra (Meditron)
Phone: 41-55-450-2121
Fax: 41-62-390-0315

MIDAS REX, L.P.
3001 Race Street
Fort Worth, TX 76111
PRODUCT(S): Pneumatic drills
CONTACT: Gary B. Gage
Director of Research and Development
Phone: 817-831-2604 or 800-433-7639
Fax: 817-834-4835

MÖLLER MICROSURGICAL
7 Industrial Park
Waldwick, NJ 07463
PRODUCT(S): Microscopes
CONTACT: Dick Montgomery
Vice President, Marketing & Sales
Phone: 201-251-9592
Fax: 201-251-9516
INTERNATIONAL CONTACT: Dr. Martin Schmidt, President
J.D. Möller Optische Werke GmbH
Rosengarten 10
PO Box 280
D-22880 Wedel/Germany
Phone: 04103-70-9333
Fax: 04103-70-9355

MR RESOURCES INC
P.O. Box 880
Gardner, MA 01440
PRODUCT(S): MR parts and accessories, stethoscopes
CATALOG OR SPECIAL ITEMS: Catalog items
CONTACT: Ann Cochran, Catalog Manager
Phone: 800-443-5486 or 978-632-7000

NORTH AMERICAN DRAEGER
3135 Quarry Road
Telford, PA 18969
PRODUCT(S): MRI anesthesia unit with electronic ventilator and monitoring system
CATALOG OR SPECIAL ITEMS:
Catalog items
CONTACT: Greg Sutherland
Product Manager
Phone: 800-462-7566

DATEX-OHMEDA
P.O. Box 7550
Madison, WI 53707-7550
PRODUCT(S): Anesthesia machines, vaporizers, breathing circuit
CATALOG OR SPECIAL ITEMS: Catalog items
CONTACT: Deb Schmaling
Marketing Product Manager for Excell
Phone: 800-345-2700 ext. 3357
Fax: 608-221-4384
E-mail: deb.schmalin@gohmeda.doc.com

OLYMPUS AMERICA
2 Corporate Center Drive
Melville, NY 11747
PRODUCT(S): Endoscopes, light sources, video systems
CONTACT: Gene Eldrige
Senior Design Engineer
Research and Development, Medical Instrument Division
Phone: 516-844-5467
Fax: 516-844-5442

OMI SURGICAL PRODUCTS
4900 Charlemar Drive
Cincinnati, OH 45227
PRODUCT: Mayfield skull clamp
CATALOG OR SPECIAL ITEMS: MR-compatible skull pins
CONTACT: Chuck Dinkler
Research and Development
Phone: 800-755-6381 or 513-561-2705
Fax: 513-561-0195

OMNIVENT
Topeka, KS
PRODUCT(S): Patient ventilation and ventilator monitors
CATALOG OR SPECIAL ITEMS: Both
CONTACT: Uma Aggarwal, President
Phone: 800-933-7902

PACIFIC SURGICAL INNOVATIONS, INC.
360 Industrial Road, Unit H
San Carlos, CA 94070
PRODUCT(S): Neurosurgical instruments
CATALOG OR SPECIAL ITEMS: Catalog items
CONTACT: Terry Johnston
Phone: 800-810-6610 or 650-802-6988
Fax: 650-802-0120

PENLON LTD
Radley Rd.
Abingdon
Oxfordshire, England OX14 3PH
PRODUCT(S): MR-compatible ventilator
Nuffield, Series 200
CONTACT: Craig Thompson
Marketing Manager
Phone: 44-1235-554-222
Fax: 44-1235-547-041

PFIZER-SCHNEIDER
Ackerstrasse 6
Switzerland CH-8180 Bolach
PRODUCT(S): Diagnostic catheters with MR tracking tips
CONTACT: Eugene Hofmann
Manager, Research and Development
Phone: 41-1-872-1111
Fax: 41-1-862-0504

PINA-VERTRIEBS AG
Langrietstrasse 17a
Neuhausen 2/Sh, Switzerland Ch-8212
PRODUCT(S): Surgical instruments, MR-compatible custom devices, implants, scissors
CATALOG OR SPECIAL ITEMS: MR-compatible scissors in any size and shape
INTERNATIONAL CONTACT: Axel Hoehn
Director of Sales and Marketing
Phone: 41-52-672-40-42
Fax: 41-52-672-40-48
Mobile: 49-171-349-41-19

GENZIME SURGICAL PRODUCTS
5175 South Royal Atlanta Drive
Tucker, GA 30084
PRODUCT(S): Titanium surgical instruments
CATALOG OR SPECIAL ITEMS: Catalog items
CONTACT: Customer Service Department
Phone: 800-367-7874
Fax: 770-934-4922
INTERNATIONAL CONTACT: Customer Service Department
Phone: 770-496-0952

SOMATEX
Postfach 420620
D-12066 Berlin Germany
PRODUCT(S): MR-compatible needles
CONTACT: Frank Kniep
Phone: 49-30-625-3046
Fax: 49-30-625-3047

STERILE CONCEPTS
5658 E. Port Blvd.
Richmond, Va 23231
PRODUCT(S): Custom healthcare procedure trays
CATALOG OR SPECIAL ITEMS: Supplies Brigham & Women's Hospital with the MRI biopsy pack (Order BX9123A)
Phone: 804-236-0260
Fax: 804-236-7255

STUDER MEDICAL ENGINEERING
Rundbuckstrasse 2
H-212 Neuhausen Switzerland
PRODUCT(S): Moeller microscopes and stands
CONTACT: Rudolf Hensler
Phone: 41-52-674-0878
Fax: 41-52-674-0879
Karl Weissbach
Mobile: 49-171-210-6812

role of compatibility QA is to determine the mutual compatibility of MRI and interventional instruments.

Several aspects of MR compatibility may be defined in interventional MRI. First, as a safety consideration for the patient and the operating staff, a device can only be considered compatible if it does not introduce any risk of becoming a projectile in the magnetic field environment of the MRI suite. Devices with a large portion of ferromagnetic components (e.g., iron) carry such a risk.

Second, the presence of the device within the field of view of imaging cannot produce significant amounts of susceptibility artifact. This artifact is produced at the interface of two materials having a significant difference in magnetic susceptibility, a physical property of elements that describes their ability of becoming magnetized in an external magnetic field.[14] Susceptibility artifacts appear as severe geometric and signal intensity distortions along the interface of two objects having a large susceptibility difference (Fig. 11-1). They are more prevalent on gradient echo images, on which no spin rephasing occurs, than on spin echo images. The artifacts are also proportional to the magnetic field strength and increase with the echo time.[15] Therefore, they are generally less problematic at low field strengths used in open configuration systems. In some situations, generally with the use of small interstitial probes, the susceptibility artifact generated by the probe helps in its identification in the image.[16]

The third aspect of MR compatibility pertains to electronic devices that are operational during MRI acquisition, such as anesthesia machines, patient monitoring systems, and surgical apparatus. Operation of electronic devices during imaging can lead to electromagnetic interference artifacts, which appear as zipper-like signal distortions in the phase-encoding direction across an image. For this reason, electromagnetic interference artifacts are also referred to as zipper artifacts. Depending on the interference bandwidth, the electromagnetic interference artifact may distort part or all of an image.

Clearly, all instruments used during interventional MR procedures should be MR compatible in all of these three aspects. Unlike imaging QA, which should be performed routinely, compatibility QA should be performed at least once for every new apparatus used in interventional MRI. Depending on the type of procedure, various instruments may be used. These instruments are divided into three categories: patient monitoring systems, surgical instruments, and therapeutic modalities.

Patient monitoring systems

Vital signs and anesthesia monitoring are performed during surgical and therapeutic operations. Use of conventional models almost invariably produces electromagnetic interference artifacts on MRI. Currently, several MRI-compatible vital sign-monitoring and anesthesia systems are available.

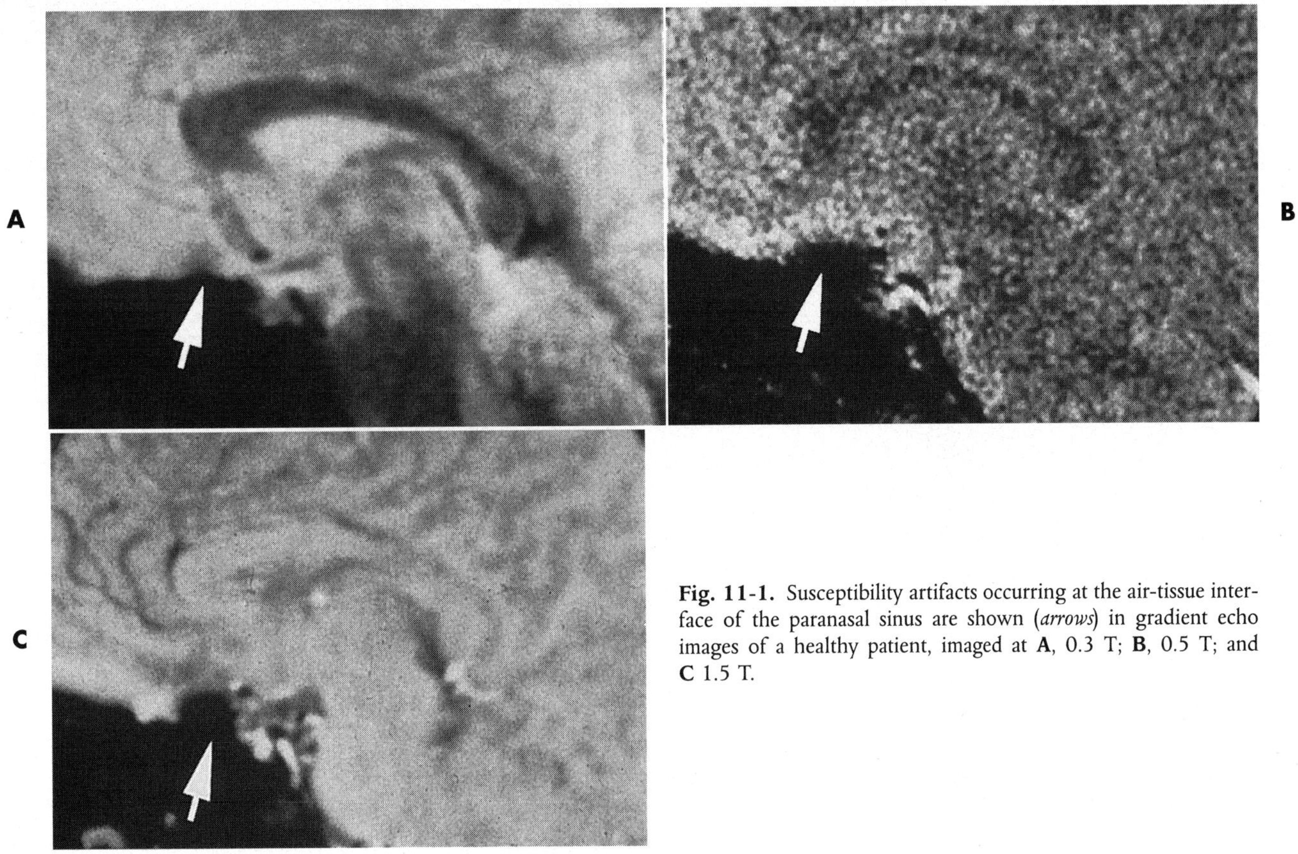

Fig. 11-1. Susceptibility artifacts occurring at the air-tissue interface of the paranasal sinus are shown (*arrows*) in gradient echo images of a healthy patient, imaged at **A**, 0.3 T; **B**, 0.5 T; and **C** 1.5 T.

Surgical instruments

Surgical instruments include scalpels, needles, catheters, biopsy devices, drill bits, and stereotactic frames. Devices such as needles and catheters may be tested for artifact production using a grid MR phantom[17] (Figs. 11-2 and 11-3). Although MR-compatible biopsy needles and stereotactic frames have been available for some time, some manufacturers (e.g., Micro-Surgical Techniques, Fort Collins, Colo) are beginning to produce ceramic and other MR-compatible surgical instruments, such as scalpels, scissors, tweezers, and drill bits.[18,19]

Therapeutic modalities

Thermal ablation devices, such as lasers, RF generators, focused ultrasound, and microwave probes, are sometimes used in

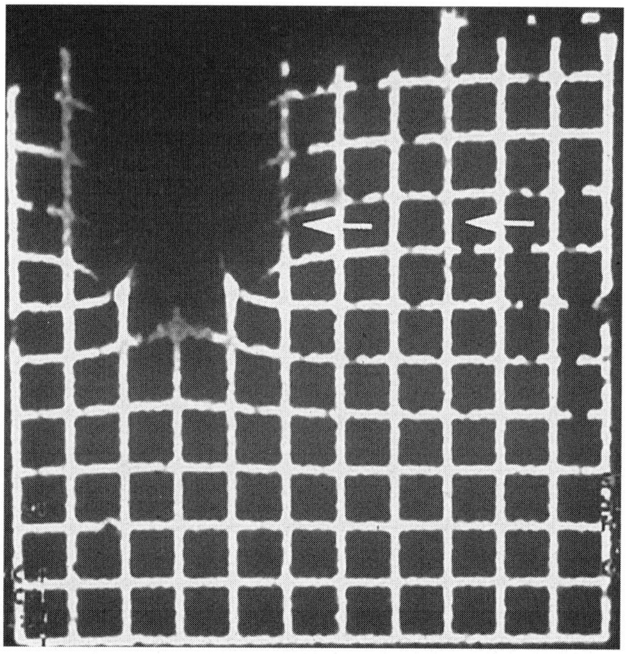

Fig. 11-2. Two 22-gauge biopsy needles in a quality assurance grid phantom are tested for artifact generation at 0.2 T. A conventional needle (*left arrow*) produced a significant amount of susceptibility artifact compared with a magnetic resonance–compatible needle (*right arrow*).

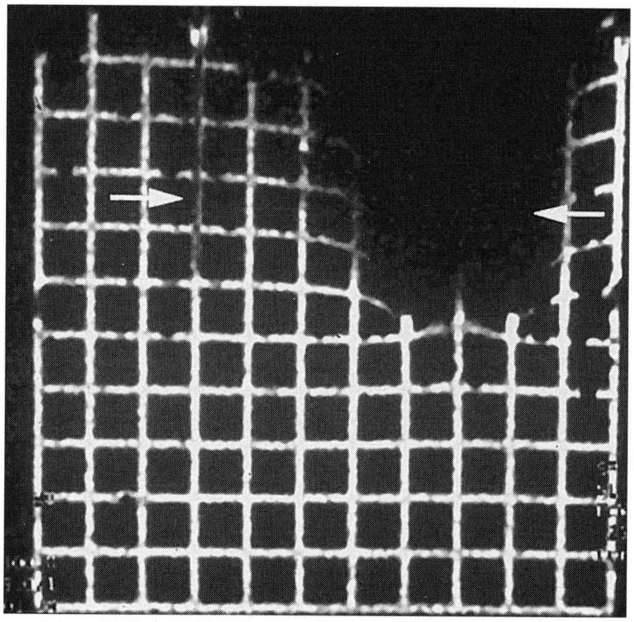

Fig. 11-3. Components of a micropuncture catheter showing various degrees of magnetic resonance (MR) compatibility at 0.2 T. Although the introducer sheath (*left arrow*) appears to be MR compatible, the guide wire (*right arrow*) produces a significant amount of susceptibility artifact.

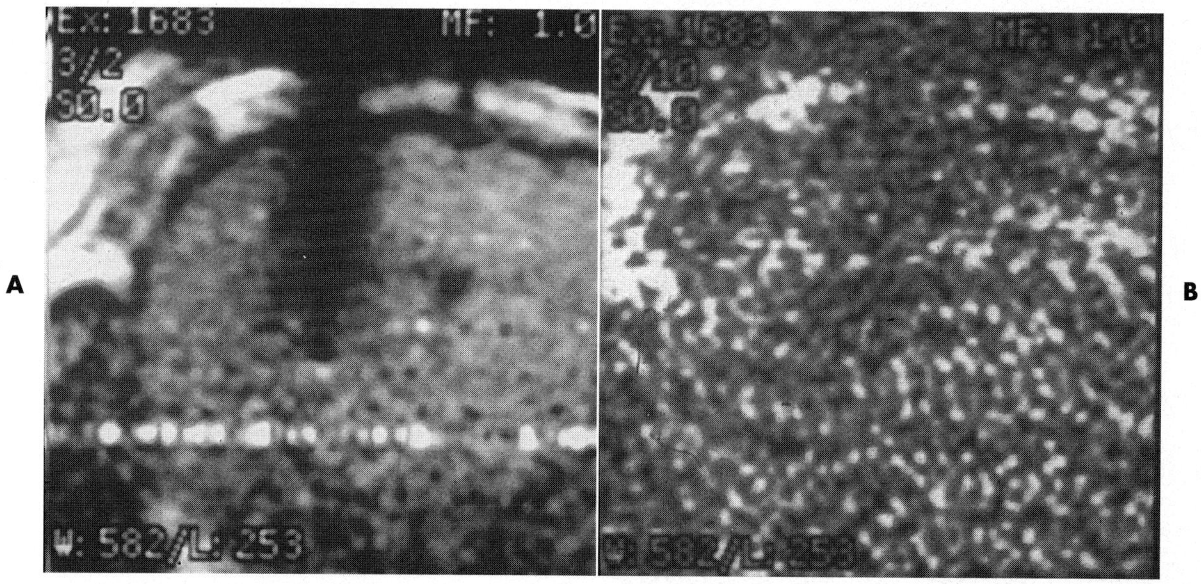

Fig. 11-4. Electromagnetic interference artifacts are produced intermittently during simultaneous operation of a radiofrequency generator and scanner. **A,** generator off; **B,** generator on.

interventional MR procedures. Although lasers and RF generators deposit energy through interstitial probes, focused ultrasound and microwave probes applied at the tissue surface concentrate their energy deposition locally in the target site. Lasers use fiberoptics to transmit laser energy to the target. Fiberoptics are nonconductive and nonferromagnetic. Therefore, they generally do not produce any image artifacts. However, in RF ablation, electrically conductive probes are used to conduct a current through the patient. For this reason, RF generators and probes are prone to producing susceptibility susceptibility and electromagnetic interference artifacts (Fig. 11-4).

SUMMARY

The advent of interventional MRI systems has created an interest in performing minimally invasive image-guided procedures. The operating magnetic field exerts a force on ferromagnetic surgical instruments brought into the interventional MRI suite. Furthermore, use of certain surgical or therapeutic instruments may introduce image artifacts, the magnitude of which may render an image or series of images useless for guidance purposes.

In general, any type of image artifacts—susceptibility, electromagnetic interference, and spatial nonlinearity artifacts—may be encountered in interventional MR procedures. A comprehensive interventional QA program should consist of routine imaging QA for basic and interventional pulse sequences, and QA for mutual compatibility of MR and interventional instruments.

REFERENCES

1. Price RR, and others: Quality assurance methods and phantoms for magnetic resonance imaging: report of AAPM nuclear magnetic resonance Task Group No. 1, *Med Phys* 17:287, 1990.
2. The American College of Radiology: Magnetic Resonance Imaging Accreditation Program, Reston, Va, 1996.
3. Farahani K, Lufkin RB: *MR planning for image based interstitial thermal therapy: interventional MRI workshop syllabus,* Berkeley, Calif, 1994, Society of Magnetic Resonance.
4. Van Vaals J, and others: Keyhole method for accelerating imaging of contrast agent uptake, *J Magn Reson Imaging* 3:671, 1993.
5. Jones RA, and others: K-space substitution: a novel dynamic imaging technique, *Magn Reson Med* 29:830, 1993.
6. Hu X, Parrish T: Field of view reduction for dynamic imaging, *Magn Reson Med* 31:691, 1994.
7. Parrish T, Hu X: Continuous update with random encoding (CURE): a new strategy for dynamic imaging, *Magn Reson Med* 33:326, 1995.
8. Matsumoto R, Oshio K, Jolesz FA: Monitoring of laser and freezing-induced ablation in the liver with T1-weighted MR imaging, *J Magn Reson Imaging* 2:555, 1992.
9. Cline HE, and others: MR temperature mapping of focused ultrasound surgery, *Magn Reson Med* 31:628, 1994.
10. De Poorter J, and others: Non-invasive MRI thermometry with the proton resonance frequency (PRF) method: in-vivo results in human muscle, *Magn Reson Med* 33:74, 1995.
11. Ishihara Y, and others: A precise and fast temperature mapping using water proton chemical shift, *Magn Reson Med* 34:814, 1995.
12. Cline HE, and others: Simultaneous magnetic resonance phase and magnitude temperature maps in muscle, *Magn Reson Med* 35:309, 1996.
13. Sinha S, and others: Phase imaging on a 0.2T MR scanner: application to temperature monitoring during ablation procedures, *J Magn Reson Imaging* 7:918, 1997.
14. Ludeke KM, Roschmann P, Tischler R: Susceptibility artifacts in NMR imaging, *Magn Reson Imaging* 3:329, 1985.
15. Farahani K, and others: Effect of field strength on susceptibility artifacts in magnetic resonance imaging, *Comput Med Imaging Graph* 14:409, 1990.
16. Lewin JS, and others: Needle localization in MR-guided intervention: effect of field strength, sequence design and magnetic field orientation, *Am J Roentgenol* 166:1337, 1996.
17. Farahani K, and others: Interventional MRI quality assurance phantom: design and application for screening of instruments, *Am J Roentgenol* 168:145, 1997.
18. Shellock FG, Shellock VJ: Ceramic surgical instruments: ex-vivo evaluation of compatibility with MR imaging at 1.5 T, *Magn Reson Med* 6:954, 1996.
19. Lenz G, Dewey C: *Study of new titanium alloy needles for interventional procedures.* In *Book of abstracts,* Berkeley, CA, 1995, Society of Magnetic Resonance.

Part **II**

INTERVENTIONAL MR–GUIDANCE TECHNIQUES

Chapter 12

PULSE SEQUENCES FOR *IN VIVO* TEMPERATURE MEASUREMENT USING MRI

Ian R. Young

Magnetic resonance imaging (MRI) is based on many parameters that depend on temperature; one or more of these parameters will likely be used for monitoring thermal therapies. This chapter explores some of the techniques that have been investigated and the methods by which they may be implemented. Many data are available about the use of these techniques in phantom studies, whereas relatively little has been published about their use in *in vivo* animal studies and even less about their use in humans.

The temperature-dependent parameters that have been most extensively investigated include T1, the diffusion coefficient (D), and the chemical shift of water. Parameters that have been considered include proton density (ρ), the relative shifts of spectral lines, and the relaxation behavior of various paramagnetic and chemical moieties are administered to the patient.

The first MRI temperature experiment used T1 in an animal study;[1] similar studies were later performed in humans.[2] Use of the diffusion coefficient was later proposed[3] and tested on humans.[4,5] Ishihara and others[6] improved early studies of water by Hindman[7] and showed how the temperature dependence of the chemical shift of the water peak could be exploited in imaging terms. De Poorter and others[8–10] laid much of the groundwork for this technique. Cady and others[11] investigated the same effect using spectroscopic studies in animal model systems and human neonates.[11]

The literature involves few animal and human studies but extensive studies on phantoms (including lumps of excised tissue). In other studies, the use of fluorocarbons[12] and the relaxation behavior of other systems (e.g., paramagnetic agents) have been considered as potential *in vivo* temperature scales. However, procedures that work well in model systems are frequently difficult in human tissue undergoing thermal stress.[13,14] This chapter describes in detail these problems in conjunction with the various techniques.

PERFORMANCE TARGETS FOR TEMPERATURE MEASUREMENT

The selection of appropriate and accurate targets for the spatial and temporal resolution of temperature maps is guided by the investigation of radiofrequency (RF) hyperthermia. This process is essentially slow, with relatively poor localization, so criteria have been developed emphasizing the need to spare adjacent healthy tissue. Recently, the criteria have been tightened because of the observation that prolonged (≥1 hour) exposure at 42° C is sufficient to damage tissue. The most recent parameters are:[15]

- Spatial localization—5 mm³ (i.e., an isotropic voxel with sides of 5 mm)
- Temporal resolution—10 sec (based on the requirement of methods such as focused ultrasound, which can deliver large quantities of energy to a very small volume very quickly)
- Temperature accuracy—0.5° C

One or more of these parameters can be relaxed for any thermal therapy strategy. For example, temporal resolution can be relaxed for RF hyperthermia, cryotherapy, or clinical strategies such as the use of hypothermia in the management of neonatal brain damage.[16] Spatial resolution is generally appropriate, except when the appropriate target is small (e.g., necrosis of individual blood vessels in regions where the rest of the tissue is healthy). For example, spatial localization is too loose when focused ultrasound having a potential target size of 1 mm³, is considered.[17] It can be tightened, if necessary up to 1 mm³, but this is likely to be at the expense of the other two factors.

MEASUREMENT OF TEMPERATURE USING T1

T1 is technically the least demanding technique used to measure temperature in MRI. In principle, the nuclear magnetization itself may be less awkward, but its coefficient of change (−0.32%/°C) is much smaller than that of water (approximately 1.3%°C), so in reality it is more difficult. (Note: In this chapter a negative sign means that a variable decreases as the temperature increases).

Apparent proton density variations arise directly from the Curie equation for nuclear paramagnetism:

$$M = \frac{N\gamma^2 h^2 I(I+1)}{3kT} B_o \qquad (1)$$

where M is magnetization, γ is Larmor constant, N is the number of spins, I is the quantum number, h is Planck's constant, k is Boltzman constant, T is absolute temperature, and B_0 is the applied field.

Measurement *in vivo* has suggested that the change in apparent proton density (proportional to magnetization) is significantly larger when the tissue is cooled.[13,14,18] A coefficient of about −1%/°C is often observed, suggesting that a change in the water in the tissue is probably due to some degree of edema formation. Figure 12-1 shows an experiment in which the calf muscle of a volunteer was placed between water pads, which were used to cycle its temperature. The figure plots proton density against temperature for two places in the leg—one directly under the cooling pads and the other at a muscle site removed from the pads themselves. Both points were at a depth of approximately 15 mm into muscle. If straight line fits to the data were calculated in both instances—though managing the two sides of the large hysteresis loop independently, the coefficients

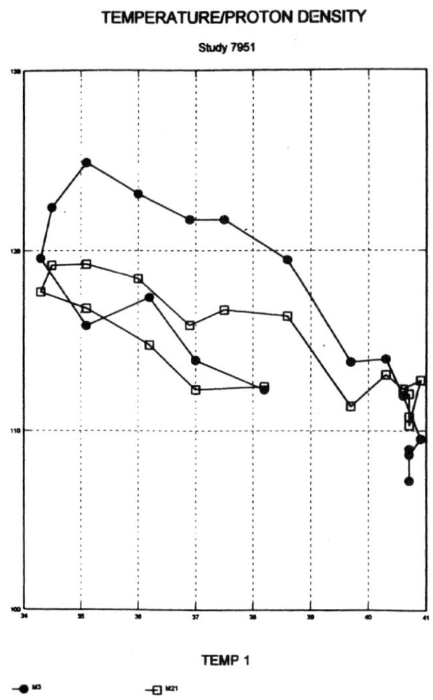

Fig. 12-1. Proton density versus temperature for an experiment in which the calf muscle of a volunteer was stabilized at a temperature of 37° C, and then reduced by pads containing chilled water before being returned to the starting temperature. Results from two locations are shown: one directly underneath one of the pads (*filled circles*), and the other at the top of the calf at a place removed from the pads (*empty squares*). (Reproduced from Young IR, and others: An evaluation of the effects of susceptibility changes on the water chemical shift method of temperature measurement in human peripheral muscle, *Magn Reson Med* 36:372, 1996. With permission.)

of temperature are approximately 2.2%/°C for the initial part of the loop (as the temperature falls) and 1.4%/°C for the part of the loop during recovery for the point under the pad. Away from the pads, the temperature characteristic is compatible with the Curie coefficient at all parts of the temperature cycle. During the earlier part of the temperature cycle, at the point under the pad, the abnormally large coefficient indicates that other effects are occurring, the most likely being development of edema.

Using T1 to measure temperature has been widely investigated in phantoms, in excised tissue, and, to a much lesser degree, in animals. Most investigators have found T1 to be a satisfactory strategy,[19-21] although these studies have not included humans. Because temporal and spatial resolutions are required, most investigations have used an initial long repetition time (TR), short echo time (TE) sequence (at a starting temperature A, with that latter being added as a subscript to any relevant parameter), followed by short TR sequences with the same TE in succession throughout the procedure (e.g., at temperature B). Spin-echo and gradient-recalled echo sequences have been used; attention has been given to saturating the spins properly in the short TR sequence because failure to do so can lead to significant errors in the measurements.[22]

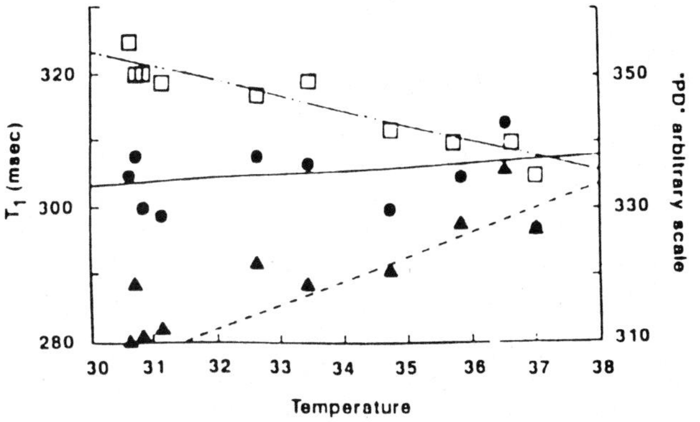

Fig. 12-2. Proton density (*empty squares, dash/dotted line*), T1 calculated from a long repetition time (TR) obtained at the start of the study and subsequent short TR measurements ($T1_R$) (*filled triangles, dotted line*), and T1 calculated from long and short TR data acquired at nominally the same temperatures ($T1_N$) (*filled circles, continuous line*) (Reproduced from Young IR, and others: Modeling and observation of temperature changes *in vivo* using MRI, *Magn Reson Med* 32:366, 1994. With permission.)

T1 is then calculated from:

(2)

$$\frac{S_B}{S_A} = \frac{P_B\left(1 - \exp\left(-\frac{TR_B}{T1_B}\right)\right)}{P_B\left(1 - \exp\left(-\frac{TR_A}{T1_A}\right)\right)}$$

where S_A and S_B are the respective signals from the two sequences. In both cases, TE is the same, and $T2_A = T2_B$ (T2 seems to have a relatively small temperature coefficient *in vivo*[4]). If ρ_B is assumed to be the same as ρ_A,

$$\frac{T1_B - T1_A}{T1_A}$$

can readily be calculated and related to temperature variations if the temperature coefficient is known.

However, the model is simplified, and can result in erroneous results (Fig. 12-2). This figure shows values of T1 measured *in vivo* in an experiment in which a volunteer's calf muscle was first cooled down then rewarmed. Tissue temperatures were measured using optical probes (Luxtron 300, Luxtron Inc, Santa Clara, Calif), one of which was implanted to a depth of 15 mm into muscle (under one of the water pads used to vary the temperature) near where the MR data were measured. Two sets of data for T1 are shown: $T1_R$ shows the values calculated as described, with one long TR "reference" data acquisition at normal temperature being used in the second equation; short TR data acquisitions were made throughout the temperature cycle, and such considerations (e.g., the possible temperature dependency of proton density) were ignored. $T1_N$ was obtained by acquiring long and short TR data at each temperature point, so any potential variables (e.g., proton density) should be nearly the same in both instances, even if they are strongly temperature dependent.

The differences are quite marked and are explained by the third curve, which uses the right-hand scale for values of the apparent proton density (on an arbitrary scale). The temperature coefficient of proton density substantially exceeds that predicted by the first equation, suggesting the presence of an increasing amount of edema. This finding is also suggested by changes in tissue size (as evaluated by planimetry[18]).

Young and others[13] point out a better representation of the signal changes (derived from a more rigorous model) as calculated from:

(3)

$$\frac{\sum_{m} S_{Br}}{\sum_{m} S_{Ar}} = \frac{\sum_{r=1}^{m} x_{nr}\,(1 - E_{1nBr})E_{2nr}\rho_{nr}}{\sum_{r=1}^{m} x_{nr}\,(1 - E_{1nAr})E_{2nr}\rho_{nr}}$$

where r is the temperature during acquisition of a pair of data sets, x_n is the fraction of tissue in the nth partial volume fraction of the tissue (thus, $T1_n$ and $T2_n$, are time constants); $x_n + \ldots + x_A \ldots + x_m = 1$ (for any temperature), and ρ_{nr} describes the nuclear magnetic resonance (NMR) signal of the nth component at the rth temperature and is likely temperature dependent. The fractions x_n are also temperature sensitive (e.g., when edema develops). m is unlikely to be less than three in any voxel (parenchymal muscle tissue, blood and lipid components) and could be more. This point includes only significant contributors to the voxel signal and excludes metabolites occurring only in millimolar concentrations. In the E notation $E_{1X} = \exp\left(-\frac{t_x}{T_1}\right)$, and so on. In general, the equation involves multiple unknown quantities, which result in approximations that determine the actual achievable accuracy of the temperature measurement.

Inversion recovery is a more sensitive method of observing T1 than is saturation recovery. The maximum sensitivity $\left(\frac{dS}{dT1}\right)$ for the sequence is obtained with a TR greater than 0, at which the normal magnetization is very small, and the signal-to-noise ratio is poor. The relationship for the inversion recovery sequence is well known:

(4)

$$S_{IR} = S_o\left(1 - 2\exp\left(-\frac{TI}{T1}\right) + \exp\left(-\frac{TR}{T1}\right)\right)\exp\left(-\frac{TE}{T2}\right)$$

where TI is inversion time. Maximum sensitivity is obtained when T1 approximates TI (i.e., when the signal is relatively small). In modern machines, with fast spin-echo or echoplanar imaging data acquisition, temporal resolution is not still a problem with this technique. Experimental data on the use of the approach *in vivo* are very limited, and the only results in the literature were obtained at very low field.[13]

Another possible variant of T1 measurement is to ally the measurement to the development of magnetization transfer contrast. Because Wolff and Balaban[23] first described this approach in the context of MRI, it has been extensively developed. In principle, it allows the measurement of T1 of the free water pool, which should behave very much like bulk water. The measurement is, however, not direct, and involves multiple experiments. The model used for the exchange process is shown in Figure 12-3. Some investigators believe this formulation is over-simplified, but the process has limited sensitivity, and further sophistication is unlikely to be justified by the data quality likely to be obtained *in vivo*.

In the practical experiment, the system is ideally irradiated substantially longer than 3T1 by an RF that is typically a few kilohertz away from the resonant frequency of the system as a whole and before the data are recovered in a conventional manner. This approach has the effect of saturating the very broad resonance characteristic of the protons forming the bound pool B (i.e., those in the large macromolecules in the cell structures). As protons in these large molecules exchange chemically or magnetically with those from the surrounding water, a new equilibrium is reached in which the apparent size of the free water pool A is reduced (from M_0 to M_T). The fractional reduction can be significant (30% to 40% in brain tissue, 40% to 50% in muscle[24]). The TR constant of the system appears shortened to T1.

The relation governing this process (neglecting T2-based decay during the formation of the echo at the center of the data acquisition) is:

$$M_t = M_{oASAT} + (M_o - M_{oASAT})\exp\left(-\frac{t}{T1_{ASAT}}\right) \tag{5}$$

where M_t is the magnetization measured after an off-resonance irradiation period t, M_{oASAT} is the observed magnetization after extended irradiation, and $T1_{ASAT}$ is the time constant. $T1_A$ (T1 of pool A in the absence of any others is likely to behave more like pure water than values observed from whole tissue) is given by:[25]

$$\frac{T1_A}{T1_{obs}} = \frac{M_o}{M_{oASAT}} \tag{6}$$

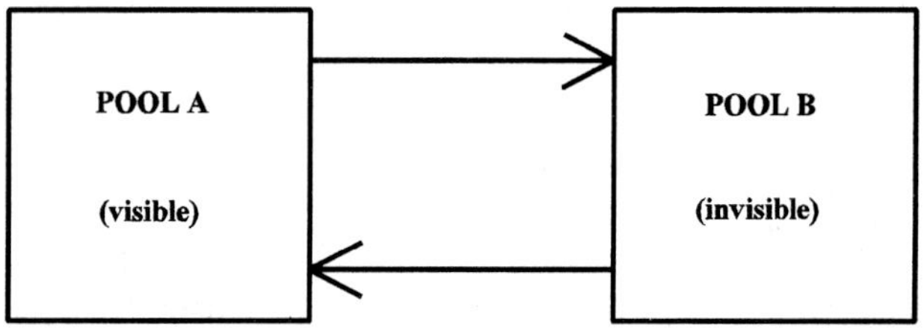

Fig. 12-3. This model is used to describe the exchange processes involved in magnetization transfer contrast. A two-pool model is used: Pool A is visible in the nuclear magnetic resonance experiment being performed, whereas pool B is not detected.

where $T1_{obs}$ is the value measured for the tissue without irradiation.

A series of experiments in which t is incremented until it is longer than $T1_{obs}$ or $T1_{ASAT}$ allow the measurement of the parameters needed to determine $T1_A$. Only one attempt has been made to use the experiment in the measurement of temperature.[13] Results were affected by substantial scattering, and the experiment was inconclusive. This study was, however, performed at 0.15 T; it may be useful to repeat the study on a higher field machine equipped with echoplanar imaging.[26] The time taken for data acquisition on the platform was so extended that only a very few data points could be obtained in any study before the patients' tolerance failed and the study had to be terminated.

TEMPERATURE MEASUREMENT USING THE DIFFUSION COEFFICIENT

Le Bihan, Delannoy, and Levin[3] first suggested using the dependency of the diffusion coefficient as a means of measuring temperature. The method is attractive in theory because the temperature coefficient for the diffusion of water is 2.2%/°C, which is significantly higher than that for T1. The method is, in principle, simple, based on the classic pulsed gradient spin-echo (PGSE) experiment of Stejskal and Tanner.[27] In Fig. 12-4, a pair of large gradient pulses is added on either side of the inverting pulse in an otherwise standard spin-echo experiment. The axis selected for the large diffusion-weighting gradient determines the direction along which the diffusion coefficient is measured.

The relationship governing the effect is:

$$M = M_o\left(1 - \exp\left(-\frac{TR}{T1}\right)\exp\left(-\frac{TE}{T2} - D\gamma^2G^2\delta^2\left(\Delta - \frac{\delta}{3}\right)\right)\right) \tag{7}$$

where δ is the effective duration of the gradient pulses (regarded as square), Δ is the time between their leading edges, G is the amplitude of the gradient pulses (assumed to be identical), and D is the diffusion coefficient.

Mimicking the same pattern as for T1, phantom data and calibrations are good. *In vivo* data are predicted to be much less acceptable for the reasons discussed below. The method is more demanding of machine performance than the measurement of T1, and less *in vivo* data are available. Hall and others[4] and Morvan and others[5] reported the only human studies, and little additional information is available.

Le Bihan and others[28] described the parameter they measured as the apparent diffusion coefficient D* in their original discussion of diffusion-weighted imaging, in which they developed the b notation. This was intended to reflect that tissue structure and parameters may cause variations in the expected diffusion coefficient, relative to its value in a homogeneous medium. The signal from any one PGSE diffusion experiment is then given by:

(8)

$$S = S_o\left(1 - \exp\left(-\frac{TR}{T1}\right)\right)\exp\left(-bD^\star - \frac{TE}{T2}\right)$$

where S_o is the fully recovered signal. Two data acquisitions (A and B), identical except for differences in the values of b would result in the relationship

(9)

$$\frac{S_A}{S_B} = \exp(b_B - b_A)D^\star$$

from which $D^\star$ can be obtained.

As Young and others[13] noted, both data acquisitions should be made at the same temperature to avoid artifacts caused by changes in the proton density as the tissue changes and as its temperature alters. Beyond this, a problem that has been discussed[13] but never shown is that, as the tissue swells and its effective structure alters, so will any anisotropy of the diffusion coefficient. Moseley and others[29] first showed the extent of the anisotropy in the diffusion of water molecules in white matter in the cat brain. Others subsequently evaluated the extent in the human brain[30] and muscle tissue.[31] The observed diffusion coefficient in any direction reflects the limitation to random progression imposed by cellular and structural boundaries in that direction. Any changes will affect the calibration of a temperature scale based on the diffusion coefficient. Diffusion in tissue is now accepted as a tensor quantity,[32] but the difficulty in determining how its variations relate to temperature is greater than assessing the variations using a scalar variable.

CHEMICAL SHIFT OF WATER

As an imaging experiment

Ishihara and others[6] were the first to suggest the possible application of the temperature dependence of the chemical shift of water described by Hindman[7] as a means of mapping temperature distributions *in vivo*. The coefficient is very small (approximately $-0.0108 \times 10^{-6}/°C$), but, using phase mapping, the problems can be overcome.[6] In principle, the method is very simple. In a gradient-recalled echo sequence, the data acquisition is delayed for sufficient time to allow the small resonant frequency variations caused by temperature alterations to develop sufficient phase changes. Differences between an initial and subsequent phase map show grey scale variations with enough sensitivity for the desired temperature performance to be achieved.

If the data acquisition has adequate TE then:

(10)

$$\phi_{TB} - \phi_{TA} = (f_B - f_A)TE = \gamma B_0 C(T_B - T_A)TE$$

where C is the coefficient of temperature shift, and ϕ_{TB} and ϕ_{TA} are the phase shifts at the two temperatures T_B and T_A. The explanation for the chemical shift of water with temperature is a change in the anisotropy of the electronic screening coefficient of the molecule. De Poorter and others[8] evaluated the behavior of water and lipid tissues and suggested that changes in the latter were caused by susceptibility variations, which contributed very little to the effects observed in water. They later emphasized[9] the importance of eliminating contributions from this source in practical studies and used the method *in vivo*.[10]

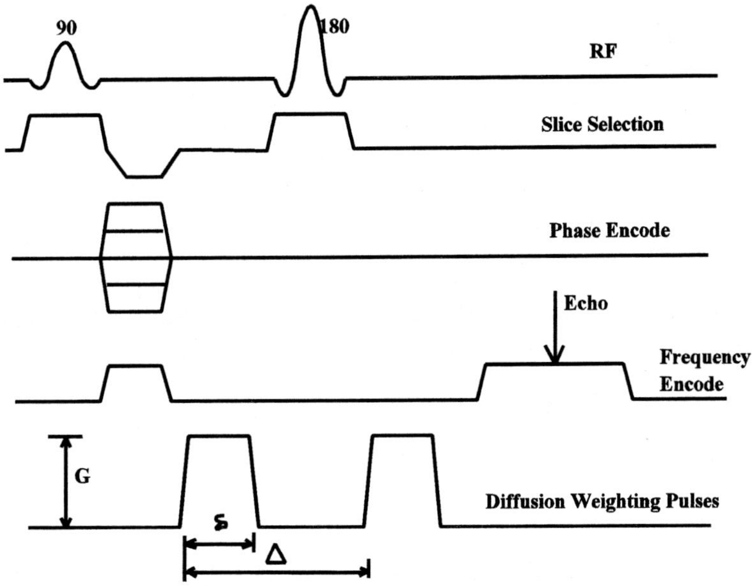

Fig. 12-4. Gradient profiles used in the pulsed gradient spin-echo experiment. The diffusion weighting gradients are shown on a separate line but can be included in any gradient profile or in any combination of gradient profiles. All three gradients can be excited to ensure some degree of independence from structural anisotropy, which means that the diffusion coefficient, as measured, appears to differ as the direction of diffusion weighting is changed.

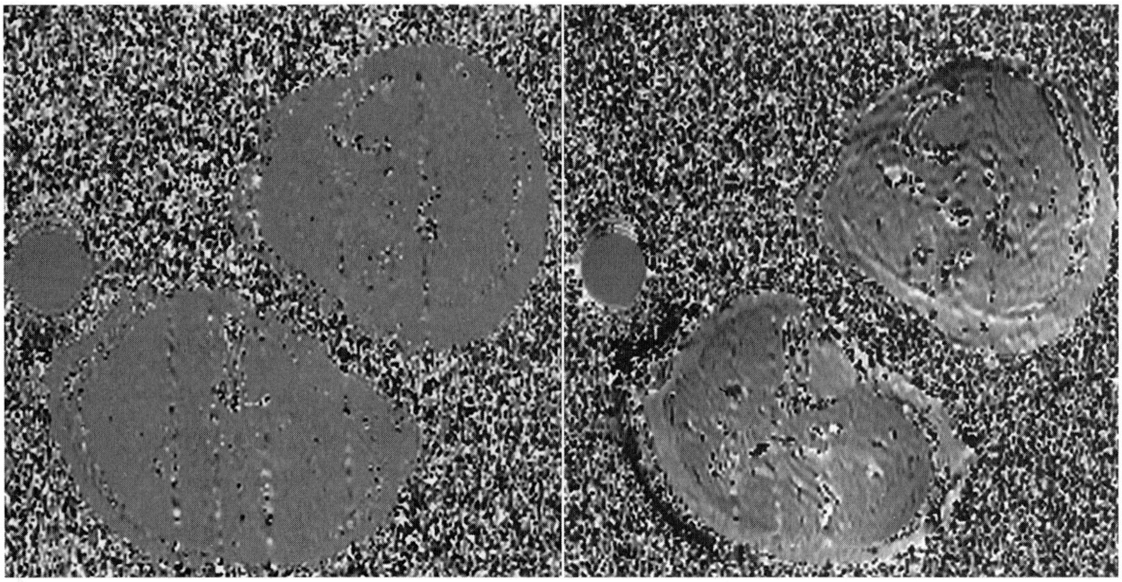

Fig. 12-5. Pair of phase maps illustrate how they alter as the temperature changes. These images were obtained at 1.0 T using a Picker HPQ (Cleveland, Ohio) scanner. The repetition time was 300 msec, and the echo time was 60 msec (giving a sensitivity of just less than 10°). Slice thickness was 10 mm, image matrix was 128 × 192, and field of view was 250 mm. The pads containing the cooling water can be seen on either side of the calf, and a reference phantom is also visible. **A**, Phase difference map obtained at the start of the study, between two data acquisitions obtained before temperature was altered. **B**, Phase difference maps obtained between the initial reference and about 30 minutes into a cooling cycle, when the muscle temperature beneath the pads had fallen by 5° to 6° C at a depth of approximately 10 mm into the tissue.

Young and others,[14] in other *in vivo* studies comparing chemical shift data with the results from implanted temperature sensors, found anomalies, which they attributed to susceptibility effects caused by alterations in the oxygenation of the tissue.[14] The required sensitivity of the experiment is such that great care is needed to make it work. Machine fields drift slowly, and eddy current and other residual effects can also cause errors. Reference phantoms can be used (with temperature monitoring) as a means of developing corrections. Figure 12-5 shows an initial phase difference map before a temperature change and one obtained later in a cooling cycle using water pads on either side of the calf of a volunteer.

As a spectroscopy experiment

Cady and others[10] used a spectroscopy experiment to provide an internal reference (or more than one reference) against which the shift in the water peak can be measured. Significant susceptibility effects affecting a region being studied should affect all similarly observed spectral components. Assuming that the spectral dispersion is small, relative chemical shift differences should reflect temperature changes if some lines in the spectrum have chemical shifts that do not depend on temperature.

Various metabolites meet this criterion.[10,33,34] Cady and others[10] used the PRESS sequence[35] (Fig. 12-6) to select a single voxel in phantom and animal model studies, using *N*-acetyl aspartate as the reference against which to measure changes in the chemical shift of the water peak. They showed that the temperature of some neonatal brains were as expected. Later, Corbett, Laptook, and Weatherall[36] confirmed these results in adults, whereas Young and others[37] investigated the relative stability of the creatine and choline peaks in human calf muscle and compared them with the chemical shift of water.

Spectroscopy has shown the most robust temperature scale *in vivo*. Its internal references eliminate many of the potential artifacts that can occur with other techniques. Its main problem is lack of sensitivity, meaning that temporal and spectral resolutions are low. Typical voxel dimensions range from 10 to 20 mm^3, and acquisition times last several minutes. Because thermal gradients in tissue can be substantial[14] and temperature changes with some ablation methods can occur very quickly,[17] the usefulness of this approach is limited. However, in principle, it can be used as a reference method for chemical shift imaging experiments and is applicable to slowly evolving methods such as hypothermia (which is being considered as a potential therapy in neonatal birth asphyxia).[16]

TEMPERATURE SCALES USING OTHER CHEMICAL MOIETIES

Many other systems have more or less complex temperature dependencies. Thus, the T1 values of various fluorocarbons and the relaxivities of various paramagnetic systems are strongly temperature sensitive. Very little has been done in these areas, and no human application has been reported.

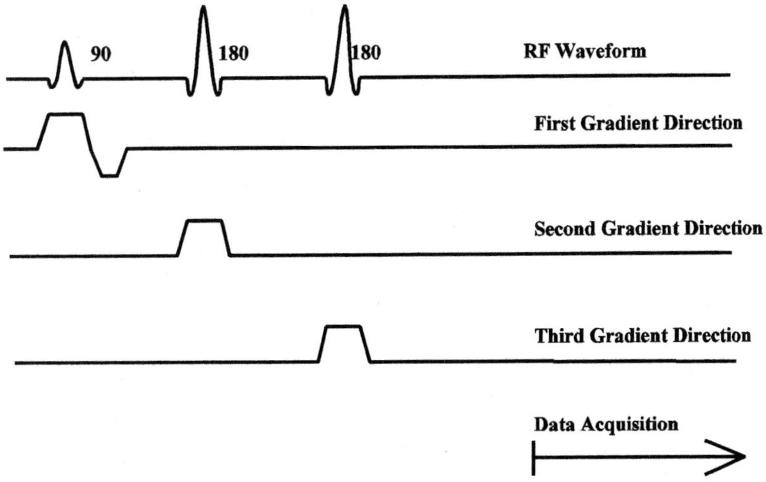

Fig. 12-6. The PRESS sequence used in the proton spectroscopy studies. The preceding water suppression procedure, which is normal in most proton spectroscopy, is limited or not used because the target in temperature measurement is to attenuate the water peak to a level where it can be handled at the same time as the very much smaller metabolite peaks that provide the references. Extending echo time is one method of accomplishing this goal and works effectively in muscle tissue (an echo time of 270 msec is typical).

Table 12-1. Region of interest tracking

	Equivalent temperature spread (°C)			
Region of interest*	No tracking	GT tracking	GET tracking	Registration (no tracking)
In muscle, near well-defined structure	1.7	11.7	5.5	2.8
In muscle, removed from structure	9.5	5.6	4.0	3.5
In muscle, very near a vessel	13.5	16.6	16.6	6.7
Near edge of muscle, close to fat	10.6	6.4	6.1	4.3
Mean	8.8	10.1	8.1	4.3
Standard deviation	4.4	4.1	5.0	1.5

*Results of attempts to track Regions of Interest as the tissue in which they are located shifts. Regions of Interest were 5 pixels in diameter (about 1 × 1 mm, slice thickness, 5 mm, data acquired at 1.5 T using a Picker prototype machine; echotime 20, msec; repetition time, 300 and 1500 msec). Values of T1 were converted to equivalent temperature changes using a temperature coefficient of 1.3%/°C.

Moreover, the fluorocarbon TR constants depend on the local dissolved oxygen concentration ($\rho(O_2)$) and on temperature. The relationship for T1 is as follows:

$$1/T1 = A + BT + C(\rho(O_2)) + D(T\rho(O_2)) \tag{11}$$

where the coefficients A, B, C, and D vary among spectral lines in a complex way. Mason, Shukla, and Antich[12] exploited these differences in their studies of how to use fluorocarbons for monitoring temperature and oxygenation *in vivo*. Again, sensitivity is a problem, and allied with the need to generate the data necessary to solve a set of simultaneous equations, it seems likely that the method will not be easy to apply in clinical practice.

No studies dependent on the temperature sensitivities of erythrocyte sedimentation rate systems have shown significant potential for *in vivo* temperature measurement.

REGION OF INTEREST TRACKING

The need for accuracy in the measurement of NMR parameters to achieve the necessary temperature precision is exacerbated by the tendency for tissue to shift under its own weight[38] and to swell when thermal stress is applied to it.[13,39,40] Thus, regions of interest originally selected for monitoring are no longer in the same place relative to the tissue structure and may include significantly different tissue structures (and chemical components) from those at the start.

Saeed and others[38,41] evaluated means of tracking the regions of interest in various circumstances, including using image registration as described elsewhere.[42] Table 12-1 shows a sample of results from the study described by Hajnal and others.[42] T1 data were calculated from pairs of images (using the combination of long and short TR acquisitions, calculated using the second equation, taken at 10-min intervals for 1 hr).

Tracking based on grey scale levels (GT tracking), on a combination of grey scale and edge data (GET tracking), and on registration is compared with data derived from a fixed region of interest. The results are expressed as equivalent temperature changes, using a T1 coefficient of 1.3%/°C. The spreads in these temperature values exceeded the target criterion, although they were, in reality, unchanged. This finding is a very powerful indication of how vulnerable thermal measurements are in humans.

CONCLUSIONS

Temperature measurement *in vivo* remains elusive relative to the desirable targets. To indicate regions where significant temperature change has occurred, MRI is likely to be applicable during thermal therapies. MRI may have an earlier clinical application when real temperature accuracy is needed but temporal and spatial resolutions are relatively unimportant. Some strategies (notably the chemical shift approaches and other studies dependent on spectroscopic resolution) will likely function best at higher fields, and the T1 approach will be preferable at lower fields. However, as suggested, this technique is prone to several artifacts, making ready application *in vivo* difficult. This problem should be resolved because interventional procedures for which temperature measurement may be needed are likely to be performed in machines operating at 0.5 T or less. Nevertheless, this topic is being actively researched, and substantial progress in development and applications is soon expected.

Acknowledgment

The author is grateful to the Medical Research Council and Picker International Inc. for their continuing support of the work that forms the background to this contribution. The author also thanks his colleagues in the Robert Steiner MRI Unit, Hammersmith Hospital, London, for much of the data and material used in this chapter.

REFERENCES

1. Parker DL, and others: Temperature distribution measurements in two-dimensional NMR imaging, *Med Phys* 10:321, 1983.
2. Dickinson RJ, and others: Measurements of changes in tissue temperature using magnetic resonance imaging, *J Comput Assist Tomogr* 10:468, 1986.
3. Le Bihan D, Delannoy J, Levin RL: Temperature mapping with MR imaging of molecular diffusion: application to hyperthermia, *Radiology* 171:853, 1989.
4. Hall AS, and others: Observation by MR imaging of *in vivo* temperature changes induced by radio frequency hyperthermia, *J Comput Assist Tomogr* 14:430, 1990.
5. Morvan D, and others: Simultaneous temperature and regional blood volume measurement in human muscle using an MRI fast diffusion technique, *Magn Reson Med* 29:371, 1993.
6. Ishihara Y, and others: A precise and fast temperature mapping using water proton chemical shift, *Magn Reson Med* 34:814, 1995.
7. Hindman JC: Proton resonance shift of water in the gas and liquid states, *J Chem Phys* 44:4852, 1966.
8. De Poorter J, and others: The proton-resonance-frequency shift method compared with molecular diffusion for quantitative measurement of two-dimensional time-dependent distribution in a phantom, *J Magn Reson Imaging* 103:234, 1994.
9. De Poorter J: Noninvasive MRI thermometry with the proton resonance frequency method: study of susceptibility effects, *Magn Reson Med* 34:359, 1995.
10. De Poorter J, and others: Noninvasive MRI thermometry with the proton resonance frequency (PRF) method: *in vivo* results in human muscle, *Magn Reson Med* 33:74, 1995.
11. Cady EB, and others: The estimation of local brain temperature by *in vivo* ^{1}H magnetic resonance spectroscopy, *Magn Reson Med* 33:862, 1995.
12. Mason RP, Shukla H, Antich PP: *In vivo* oxygen tension and temperature: simultaneous determination using ^{19}F NMR spectroscopy of perflurocarbon, *Magn Reson Med* 29:296, 1993.
13. Young IR, and others: Modelling and observation of temperature changes *in vivo* using MRI, *Magn Reson Med* 32:358, 1994.
14. Young IR, and others: An evaluation of the effects of susceptibility changes on the water chemical shift method of temperature measurement in human peripheral muscle, *Magn Reson Med* 36:366, 1996.
15. International Collaborative Hyperthermia Group: Radiotherapy with or without hyperthermia in the treatment of superficial localized breast cancer: results from five randomized controlled trials, *Int J Radiat Oncol Biol Phys* 35:731, 1996.
16. Edwards AD: Protection against hypoxic-ischaemic cerebral injury in the developing brain, *Perfusion* 8:97, 1993.
17. Cline HE, and others: *A clinical MR guided focused ultrasound surgery system: proceedings of the 2nd Meeting of the Society of Magnetic Resonance*, San Francisco, 1994, Society of Magnetic Resonance.
18. Young IR, and others: Further observations on the measurement of tissue T_1 to monitor temperature *in vivo* by MRI, *Magn Reson Med* 31:342, 1994.
19. Jolesz FA, and others: MR imaging of laser-tissue interactions, *Radiology* 168:249, 1988.
20. Stepanow B, Brix G, Lorenz WJ: *3D temperature mapping: proceedings of the 4th scientific meeting of International Society for Magnetic Resonance in Medicine*, New York, 1996, ISMRM.
21. Matsumoto R, and others: Tissue temperature monitoring for thermal interventional therapy: comparison of T1-weighted MR sequences, *J Magn Reson Imaging* 4:65, 1994.
22. Young IR, Bydder GM, Bryant DJ: Problems with achieving saturation using methods based on bursts of RF pulses with spoilers in magnetic resonance imaging, *Magn Reson Med* 11:127, 1989.
23. Wolff SD, Balaban RS: Magnetization transfer contrast (MTC) and tissue water proton relaxation *in vivo*, *Magn Reson Med* 10:135, 1989.
24. Hajnal JV, and others: Design and implementation of magnetization transfer pulse sequences for clinical use, *J Comput Assist Tomogr* 16:7, 1992.
25. Forsen S, Hoffman RA: Study of moderately rapid chemical exchange reactions by means of nuclear magnetic double resonance, *J Chem Physics* 39:2892, 1963.
26. Mansfield P: Multi-planar image formation using NMR spin echoes, *J Phys C Solid State Phys* 10:L55, 1977.
27. Stejskal EO, Tanner JE: Spin diffusion measurements: Spin-echoes in the presence of a time-dependent field gradient, *J Chem Phys* 42:288, 1965.
28. Le Bihan D, and others: MR imaging of intravoxel incoherent motions: application to diffusion and perfusion in neurological disorders, *Radiology* 161:401, 1986.
29. Moseley ME, and others: Anisotropy in diffusion-weighted MR, *Magn Reson Med* 19:321, 1991.
30. Hajnal JV, and others: Magnetic resonance imaging of anisotropically restricted diffusion of water in the nervous system: technical, anatomic, and pathologic considerations, *J Comput Assist Tomogr* 15:1, 1991.
31. Howe FA, and others: Magnetic resonance neurography, *Magn Reson Med* 28:328, 1992.
32. Mori S, van Zijl PCM: Diffusion weighting by the trace of the diffusion tensor within a single scan, *Magn Reson Med* 33:141, 1995.
33. Arús G, Chang Y-C, Bárány M: N-acetylaspartate as an intrinsic thermometer for ^{1}H NMR of brain slices, *J Magn Reson* 63:396, 1985.
34. Lutz NW, Kuesel AC, Hull WE: A ^{1}H-NMR method for determining temperature in cell culture perfusion systems, *Magn Reson Med* 29:113, 1993.

35. Bottomley PA: Spatial localization in NMR spectroscopy *in vivo, Ann NY Acad Sci* 508:333, 1987.
36. Corbett RJT, Laptook AR, Weatherall P: *Noninvasive measurement of brain temperature in human subjects using volume localized H-1 magnetic resonance spectroscopy: proceedings of the 5th Scientific Meeting of International Society for Magnetic Resonance in Medicine,* Vancouver, BC, 1997, ISMRM.
37. Young IR, and others: An evaluation of the stability of the proton chemical shifts of some metabolites other than water during thermal cycling of normal human muscle tissue, *J Magn Reson Imaging* 1998 (in press).
38. Saeed N, Young IR: *Region of interest tracking in sets of magnetic resonance images with subtle variations in shape: proceedings of the 12th annual meetings of the Society of Magnetic Resonance Medicine,* New York, 1993, Society of Magnetic Resonance Medicine.
39. deSouza NM, and others: Endoscopic laser ablation of the prostate: MR appearances during and after treatment and their relation to clinical outcome, *Am J Roentgenol* 164:1429, 1995.
40. deSouza NM, and others: Laser ablation of the endometrium: MR approaches during and after treatment and the relation of MR appearance to clinical outcome, *Am J Roentgenol* 167:1121, 1996.
41. Saeed N, and others: Regions of interest tracking in temporal scans based on statistical analysis of grey scale and edge properties and registration of images, *J Magn Reson Imaging* 1998 (in press).
42. Hajnal JV, and others: Detection of subtle brain changes using subvoxel registration and subtraction of serial MR images, *J Comput Assist Tomogr* 19:677, 1995.

Chapter 13

FAST IMAGING TECHNIQUES FOR INTERVENTIONAL MRI

Usha Sinha, Shantanu Sinha, Thomas Oshiro

This chapter reviews magnetic resonance (MR) pulse sequences tailored for the specific requirements of MR-guided interventional procedures. The introduction of open-access MR systems has moved MR-guided interventional procedures from the research arena to the clinical realm. MR-guided interventions need to be monitored on real-time or near real-time scales, including fast MR acquisition of dynamic information and real-time image reconstruction and display of data. Furthermore, because the interventional procedure will be performed within the scanner room, appropriate hardware should be available for the display of data near the MR scanner. This chapter discusses the requirements of MR interventional procedures, pulse sequences used in these procedures, general scan methodologies for reducing scan times, and real-time reconstruction and display technologies.

DEVICE TRACKING METHODS

The first step in MR-guided interventional diagnostic or therapeutic procedures is to develop an MR-guided method for positioning the interventional devices (catheters, biopsy needles, radiofrequency [RF] and laser ablation probes) *in vivo.* Two methods of tracking, passive and active, have been implemented (see Chapter 15 and 16 for a fuller discussion).

Passive tracking

In the passive tracking method, the device is visualized by the signal void it creates and by its susceptibility artifact. The field inhomogeneity–induced artifacts are caused by the susceptibility differences between the needle and surrounding tissue. Ferromagnetic stainless steel needles commonly used in interventional procedures cannot be used in MR-guided methods because of the large magnetic field inhomogeneities created on introduction of these devices. The susceptibility artifacts result in large geometric and signal intensity distortions, preventing accurate location of the needle tip. This problem has been solved by the introduction of needles made from alloys composed primarily of cobalt, nickel, chromium, and iron; these needles have susceptibilities closer to that of tissue.[1–3] The MR-compatible needles introduce only a local signal loss of a linear shape, which allows visualization without entirely obscuring the underlying anatomic structures. The extent of artifact also depends on other factors, including main magnetic field strength B_0, echo type, echo time (TE), relative orientation of the needle axis to the main field, needle material composition, and needle diameter. These effects are important to understand to select the optimal sequence, image plane, and device material for MR-guided intervention. Visualization and localization are aided by the presence of a small artifact, although large artifacts will obscure underlying anatomy (an acceptable artifact is 5 mm in a field of view [FOV] of 250 mm). Several studies have investigated these effects.[4–9] The results can be summarized as follows (Fig. 13-1).

1. For the same sequence and orientation of the probe to the main magnetic field, artifacts increase with main magnetic field strength.
2. Gradient echo sequences cause significantly larger artifacts than comparable spin-echo or fast spin-echoes (Fig. 13-1 *A, B*).
3. The artifacts increase with the TE of the gradient echoes (Fig. 13-1 *C, D*).
4. The artifacts increase with the angle to the main magnetic field; a parallel orientation causes the fewest artifacts, and a perpendicular orientation causes the most artifacts (Fig. 13-1 *E, F*). Furthermore, in spin and fast spin-echo sequences the size of the artifact diminishes when the needle is oriented parallel to the read-out axis.
5. Artifact size depends on alloy composition. Among the MR-compatible needles investigated, needles made from higher nickel content alloys show reduced susceptibility artifacts.[8]

Most interventional devices can thus be visualized on MR images by an appropriate selection of MR sequence parameters, which enable conspicuity while minimizing gross susceptibility artifacts. Schenck[10] provided an excellent and exhaustive review of the magnetic susceptibility of different materials, which should help in various interventional applications, including the development of MR-compatible surgical instruments and assessment of the extent of positional errors in MR-guided stereotactic surgery. However, in certain applications (e.g., visualization of plastic catheters for vascular interventions), a problem arises from the total lack of conspicuity on MR images. Modifications for conspicuous and consistent localization include incorporation of a paramagnetic material, dysprosium oxide, into the catheter walls, either uniformly doped or in three equally spaced doped rings.[11]

In passive tracking, the location of the needle is updated at a frequency limited by the time required for image acquisition, reconstruction, and display. Image acquisition times are usually reduced by using two-dimensional Fourier transform (2D FT) spoiled gradient echo or 2D FT steady-state gradient echo sequences. Figure 13-2 shows images acquired every 2 sec using a typical fast low angle shot (FLASH) sequence during a biopsy procedure performed under MR guidance in a 0.2-T open magnet system. The progress of the biopsy needle toward the lesion can be easily seen. In these images, a rectangular FOV was used to reduce the acquisition time. However, gradient echo sequences may produce unacceptably large artifacts at high-field strengths. Fast spin-echoes (TE, 11 sec; repetition time [TR], 120 sec, 4 echo train length; matrix, 256 × 128; scan time, 4 sec); which are less susceptible to artifacts from field inhomogeneities, have been used for breast lesion localization at 1.5 T.[12] A rapid gradient echo sequence with an acquisition time of 800 msec and an interleaved gradient echoplanar sequence with an acquisition time of 350 to 400 msec have been investigated as ultrafast sequences for guidewire placement for vascular interventions under MRI visualization.[7] The studies conducted at 1.5 T showed that with a proper catheter design excellent visualization is possible with the interleaved gradient echoplanar sequence. However, although echoplanar acquisition has adequate temporal resolution, it requires special hardware not usually available on open access MR scanners. The

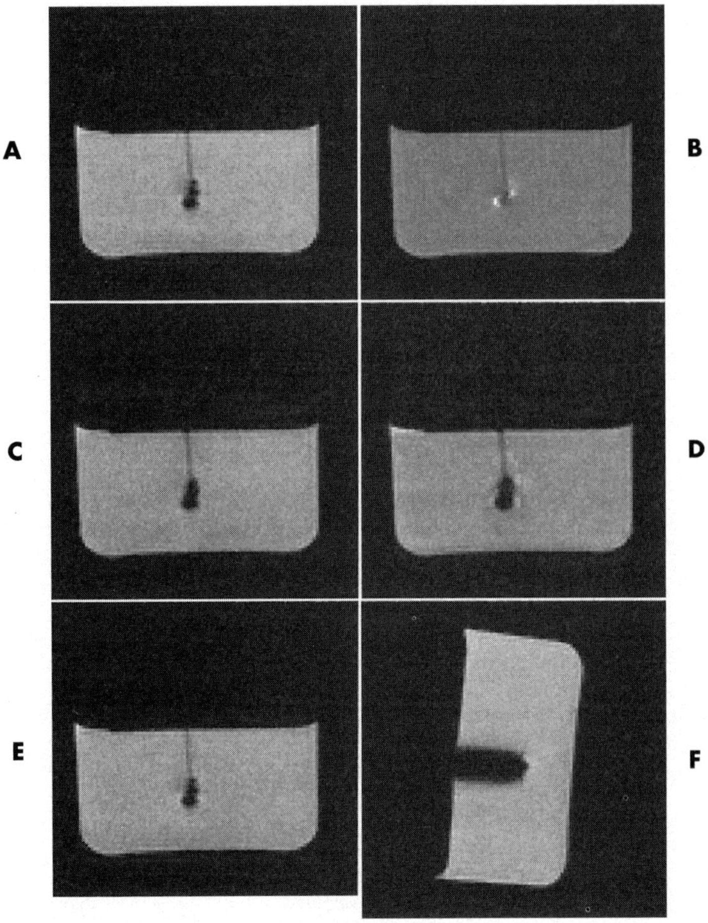

Fig. 13-1. Images of the 18-G needle at 0.2 T acquired under various conditions illustrate the effects of sequence parameters on the magnitude of the susceptibility-induced artifacts. Images were acquired using **A,** a gradient echo sequence (echo time, 15 sec; repetition time, 200 sec; flip angle, 40°; matrix, 256 × 256; slice thickness, 4 mm; field of view, 240 mm) and **B** spin-echo sequence (echo time, 15 sec; repetition time, 300 sec; matrix, 256 × 256; slice thickness, 4 mm; field of view, 240 mm). The susceptibility-induced artifacts at the needle tip are considerably reduced in the spin-echo image compared with the gradient echo image. **C,** An image was acquired using a gradient echo sequence at echo times of 20 msec and 30 msec. All other sequence parameters were maintained as for the image in **A. D,** The increased artifact at the needle tip at the higher echo time is clearly seen. In images acquired with the sequence parameters used in Figure 13-2, *A*, the needle is oriented **E,** parallel to the main magnetic field and **F,** perpendicular to the main field. The increase in artifact size for a perpendicular orientation of the needle can be readily appreciated.

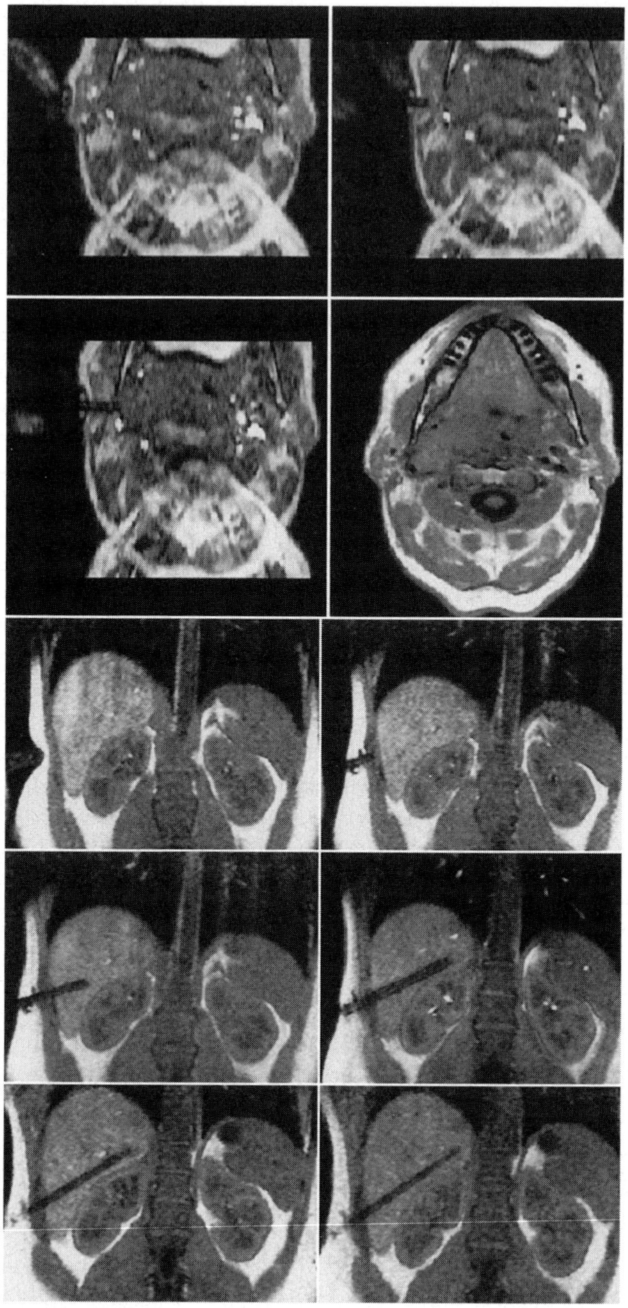

Fig. 13-2. A 57-year-old male with history of squamous cell carcinoma presents after radiotherapy and chemotherapy with a new mass in the lower right parapharyngeal space. Near real-time low-resolution FISP images (echo time, 7 msec; repetition time, 19 msec; matrix, 64 × 256; field of view, 25 cm; slice thickness, 5 mm) using a large flexible coil were sequentially acquired for magnetic resonance imaging–guided fine-needle aspiration. **A,** The radiologist's finger serves as an initial localizer, pointing to the target lesion and gently indenting the retromandibular region. **B** and **C,** A 22-G magnetic resonance–compatible biopsy needle was introduced into the lesion. **D,** High-resolution T1-weighted spin-echo image (echo time, 15 msec; repetition time, 450 msec; matrix, 192 × 256; field of view, 23 cm; slice thickness, 5 mm) confirms needle placement. Necrotizing squamous cell carcinoma was found on cytology. **E** to **J,** Sequential coronal T1 fast low angle shot images were obtained during magnetic resonance imaging–guided biopsy of a hepatic abnormality, which is slightly hypointense to the hepatic parenchyma. The patient had undergone prior left hepatectomy for hepatocellular carcinoma, with recurrence. Percutaneous needle biopsy was performed under magnetic resonance imaging guidance with coaxial technique. After successful needle placement and biopsy, 12 ml of ethanol (corresponding to the volume of the lesion) was infused for ablation without complications.

temporal resolution of the scans should thus be increased by alternate means; several methods have been proposed to improve acquisition efficiency over conventional phase encoding. Some of these acquisition methods and a practical real-time reconstruction system are discussed in Sections III and IV, respectively.

Active tracking

In the passive technique, the device position is updated only as fast as new images are acquired and reconstructed. In active tracking, real-time tracking with the position of the device tip updated 20 times per second is possible. In this technique, a small RF coil, consisting of an untuned single loop less than 1 mm in diameter, is attached to the tip of the interventional device (see Chapter 16).[13] Such a coil is insensitive to signals coming from more than 1 or 2 mm away. The body coil is used to excite all spins within the FOV. Gradient-recalled echoes are generated along three orthogonal axes to frequency encode the 3D position of the coil. The modulation scheme uses a Hadamard encoding method in which all three gradients are applied on each of four excitations with the gradient polarities cycled (Fig. 13-3). The gradient polarities are cycled to minimize the errors in the positional coordinates caused by resonance offset conditions, main magnetic field and local susceptibility-induced field inhomogeneities. The x, y, and z coordinates of the RF coil are found by appropriate combinations of the positions calculated from each excitation.[13] Because only four excitations with a short repetition time (12 to 20 msec) are

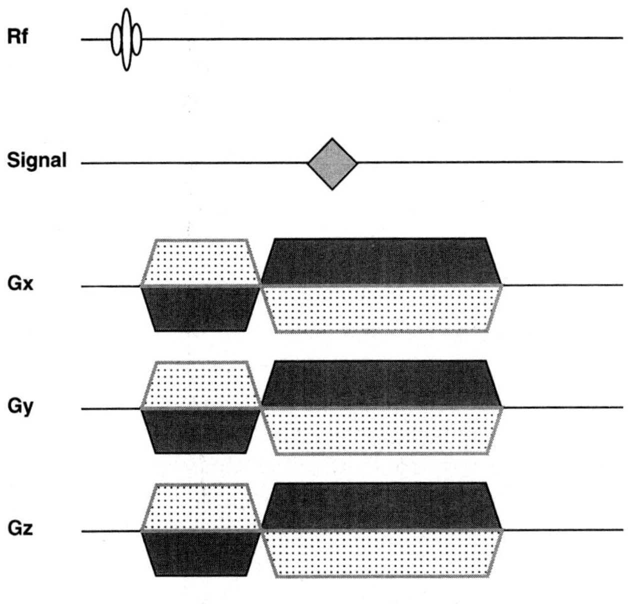

Fig. 13-3. A pulse sequence, based on the Hadamard multiplexing scheme, locates the three-dimensional coordinates of the radiofrequency tracking coil. The gradients are applied along the three orthogonal axes, X, Y, and Z; their polarities (positive or negative) switched in four excitations as (−, −, +), (+, +, −), (+, −, +), and (−, +, +). The *minus* (−) and *plus* (+) signs refer to the direction of the gradient, with *plus* referring to the cross-hatched gradients bounded by the solid lines and *minus* referring to the solid gradients bounded by the dashed lines.

required to update the position of the coil, temporal resolutions of 20 frames per second can be easily achieved. The positional accuracy of the RF coil can be found at a resolution of less than 1 mm, which is typically the in-plane resolution of MR images. The position of the coil, updated 20 times per second, is displayed superposed on a previously acquired MR image. This technique has been verified *in vitro* and *in vivo* when used with intravascular catheters.[14] A modification for tracking on two imaging planes for biopsy and therapy devices has also been verified for positional accuracy.[15] Another modification introduced for the active tracking of biopsy needles is incorporation of an internal MR signal source for a consistent signal from the RF coil.[16] This modification prevents loss of signal when the biopsy needle is passing through tissue areas of low signal.

FAST TEMPERATURE-SENSITIVE SEQUENCES FOR THERMAL MONITORING

This chapter discusses only fast sequences for MR thermometry. A high temporal resolution is required to monitor RF and high-intensity focused ultrasound ablation procedures, whereas the requirements for laser-induced thermotherapy and hyperthermia applications are more relaxed. The temperature dependency of three MR tissue parameters has been used for MR thermometry: spin-lattice relaxation (T1), the diffusion coefficient, and the proton resonance frequency. Each of these parameters has merits and drawbacks when used for MR thermometry. The temperature sensitivity of the diffusion coefficient is 2.4%/°C, which is higher than the temperature sensitivities of T1 (0.8% to 2%/°C) and proton resonance frequency (−0.0107 ppm/°C for pure water, −0.007 to −0.009 ppm/°C for *in vitro* muscle and other organ tissues).[17–19] The T1 dependence on temperature varies in different tissues, and tissue physiologic and metabolic changes during thermal therapy cause deviations from linear behavior. The temperature sensitivity of the diffusion coefficient is high, but diffusion imaging requires large applied magnetic field gradients for rapid imaging. Recent trends in investigations at high field strengths have established that the proton resonance frequency method is more suitable for MR thermometry than is the measurement of diffusion and T1.

Temperature from a measurement of T1 or from T1-weighted sequences

The spin lattice relaxation time T1 for tissues exhibits a linear dependence that can be expressed by the relationship:

$$T1_T = T1_{ref} + S\,(T - T_{ref}) \tag{1}$$

where $T1_T$ is T1 relaxation time at temperature T, $T1_{ref}$ is the spin lattice relaxation time at reference temperature T_{ref}, and S is the temperature sensitivity of T1. T1-weighted images using fast 2D spoiled GRASS or 2D fast spin-echo sequences have been used to monitor temperature changes at 1.5 T during ultrasonic heating.[20] The temporal resolution of these scans was 4 sec for the spoiled GRASS sequence and 5 to 16 sec for the fast spin-echo sequences. A linear variation of the signal intensity of the T1-weighted images with temperature was verified for porcine liver samples and gel phantoms (temperature change, 36° to 66° C). However, these measurements were confined to correlating signal intensity changes to temperature changes and did not involve an explicit calculation of T1 values. Thus, separate calibration will be required for each type of tissue and imaging sequence. However, a recent investigation revealed nonlinear signal intensity variations with temperature using a T1-weighted fast spin-echo for thermometry during interstitial laser photocoagulation *in vivo* in rabbit livers.[21] This latter study showed that changes in the tissue altered the MRI signal intensity, which confounded the intensity changes caused by temperature.

Changes in signal intensity of a T1-weighted image may arise from sources other than temperature alone. A more accurate method of T1-based MR thermometry would be to calculate T1 at each temperature point rather than to use the signal intensities of T1-weighted images. MR temperature mapping has been performed during focused ultrasound surgery using T1 values calculated from an optimized fast spoiled GRASS sequences using the following signal intensity relationship:[2]

$$S_T \propto M_0 \, \frac{(1 - \exp(-TR/T1_T))\sin(\theta)}{(1 - \cos(\theta)\exp(-TR/T1_T))} \tag{2}$$

where S_T is the signal intensity at a temperature T, M_0 is the equilibrium magnetization, and θ is the flip angle. Independent calibration was used to estimate the temperature coefficients.[17] In this and earlier studies, the T1 value at each temperature was calculated using the signal intensity of a reference image at ambient temperature.[17,22] However, the equilibrium magnetization, M_0, is also inversely dependent on the absolute temperature. The effect of M_0 may be significant, as shown in a hyperthermia investigation on the calves of humans. This study confirmed the need for two point measurements at each temperature to preclude the effects of proton density variations to obtain accurate values of T1.[23]

Two point measurements involve acquisition of two sequences at each temperature point, which decreases the temporal resolution. However, high temporal resolutions can be maintained using an inversion-prepared turbo FLASH sequence. Images with two or more values of TI can be acquired at the rate of one image per second, so temporal resolutions of 2 sec can be easily achieved. T1 values can be calculated by a linear fit to the following signal intensity relationship for images acquired with different values of TI (TR and flip angle remain fixed):

(3)

$$S_T \propto (1 - 2 \exp (TI/T1_T))$$

where TI is the effective time of inversion. The linear relationship between T1 and temperature was verified in a gel phantom using a single-shot sequentially ordered inversion-prepared turbo FLASH sequence at 1.5 T using five values of TI at each temperature (Fig. 13-4).[24] Similar measurements in an open configuration system at 0.2 T also confirmed the linear relationship, but problems relating to the lower signal-to-noise ratio at 0.2 T (leading to high standard deviations) have to be addressed before *in vivo* implementation.[25]

Apparent diffusion coefficient

The temperature dependence of the diffusion coefficient is given by the relationship:

(4)

$$(1/T) = (1/T_0) - k/E_a{}^* \ 1n \ (D/D_0)$$

where k is Boltzman's constant, E_a (0.18 eV) is the activation energy for translational molecular diffusion, D_0 is the diffusion coefficient at room temperature, T_0 (in ° K) and D is the diffusion coefficient at temperature T (in ° K). The diffusion coefficient D can be calculated from a two point measurement at each temperature using the relationship:

(5)

$$1n\left(\frac{Sg}{S_0}\right) = D\,(b_g - b_0)$$

where S_g is the signal intensity for an applied gradient g with b value b_g (the b value is proportional to the square of the applied diffusion gradient strength, g, and to the cube of the separation of the diffusion lobes). The accuracy of the temperature measurements can be improved by a linear fit to signal intensities at more than two values of the diffusion gradients, but this calculation would result in increased scan times for each temperature measurement. Measurement of the diffusion coefficient, especially with a high temporal resolution, is difficult. The long acquisition times and the motion sensitivity preclude use of spin-

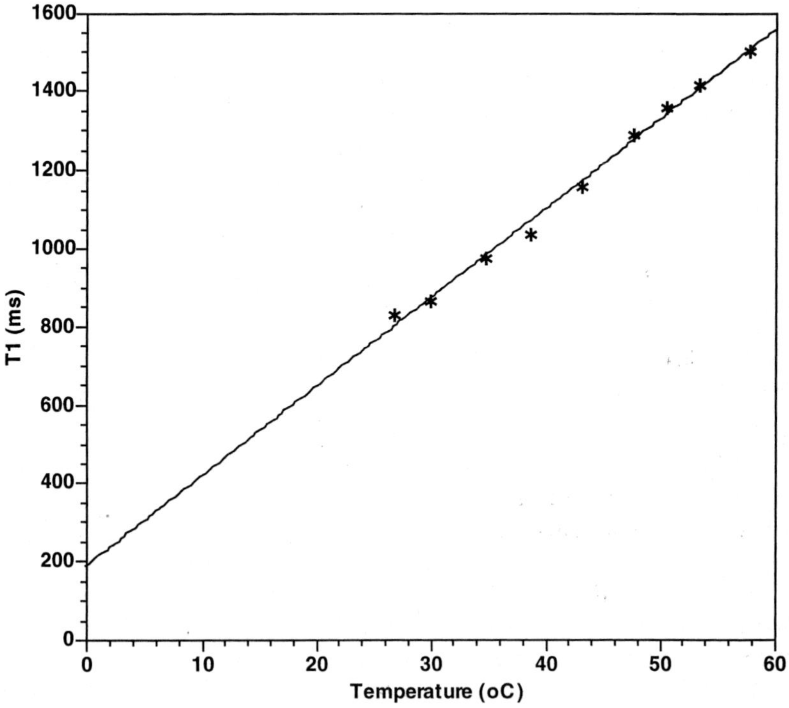

Fig. 13-4. Variation of T1, with temperature measured in a gel phantom at 1.5 T. T1 was calculated by a least squares fit to a signal intensity variation calculated from $S_T \propto (1–2 \exp (TI_{eff}/T1_T))$ where TI_{eff} is the effective time of inversion when the low-order k-space lines were collected (five values of TI_{eff} at 676, 876, 1076, 1476, and 1776 msec were used). A sequentially reordered turbo–fast low angle shot sequence (echo time, 3.9 sec; repetition time, 8.9 sec; flip angle, 12°) was used to acquire images every 1.15 sec. A linear temperature dependence of T1 with a sensitivity of 1.5%/°C was estimated in the temperature range 27°C to 58°C.

echo diffusion-weighted sequences in *in vivo* temperature monitoring. Single-shot diffusion-weighted echoplanar sequences have been used to measure temperature and to monitor hyperthermia procedures.[26] 0.5° C changes can be determined in 1 cm^3 volumes in less than 10 sec using the diffusion-weighted echoplanar imaging sequence. However, this technique has been implemented at 1.5 T in a closed configuration system, and echoplanar upgrades are not available on any commercial open systems. An alternate single-shot diffusion-prepared turbo FLASH sequence was investigated for MR thermometry (Fig. 13-5). The linear dependence of the diffusion coefficient with temperature in a gel phantom was verified at 1.5 T with this sequence (Fig. 13-6).[27] The temporal resolution of the sequence is 2 sec for each diffusion-weighted image, which is adequate for temperature monitoring. Initial experience at measuring temperature at 0.2 T using a diffusion-prepared turbo FLASH sequence revealed problems arising from lower signal-to-noise and artifacts from residual eddy currents.[28]

Proton resonance frequency from gradient echo phase images

Recent investigations of MR thermometry based on the temperature-dependent proton resonant frequency have proved it to be an accurate method that may prove clinically viable. This technique has been successfully applied to map temperature using phase images of gradient echoes. Most measurements have been performed at high fields (1.5 T or greater) in closed configuration systems.[18,19,29–31] Phase-change images are calculated by subtracting either the phase or complex images acquired at higher (or lower) temperatures from a corresponding image at a reference image.[18,29] Before a temperature map can be generated, phase unwrapping and phase drift correction have to be performed using the relationship:

$$\left(\frac{d\Phi\ (x,y)}{dT\ (x,y)}\right) = C^* \ \gamma \ ^* \ B_{ext} \ ^* \ TE \tag{6}$$

where $d\Phi$ (x,y) is the phase difference induced by a temperature change of dT (x,y) at a pixel location (x,y), γ is the gyromagnetic ratio of proton, C is the constant of proportionality, and B_{ext} is the external magnetic field flux.[29] The sensitivity of phase change with temperature is linearly proportional to the main magnetic field. Thus, to achieve an equivalent sensitivity at low field strengths, the TE of the gradient echo has to be increased, which implies a concomitant increase in TR resulting in longer acquisition times. Temperature changes can be measured with a standard deviation of 1.03° C using a navigator echo–corrected gradient echo sequence with a TE of 60 msec and a TR of 100 msec at 0.2 T (Fig. 13-7).[32] The navigator echoes are used to correct for view-to-view phase variations that may result in high standard deviations of the measured

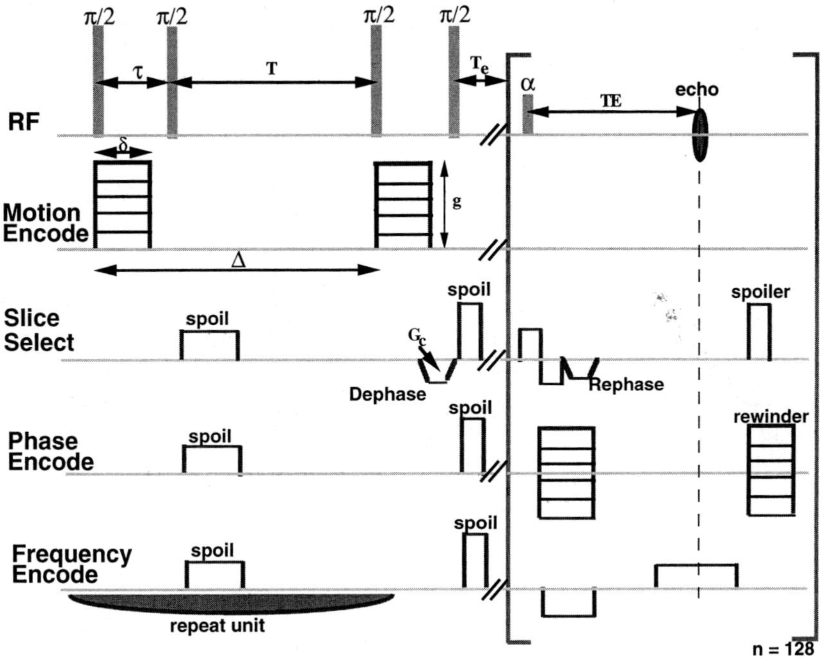

Fig. 13-5. A diffusion-weighted centrally reordered turbo–fast low angle shot sequence is relatively insensitive to the effects of eddy currents. The diffusion gradients are applied during the magnetization preparation period, which has four broadband 90° radiofrequency pulses and two diffusion gradients, g (τ = 24.6 msec, δ = 20 msec, T = 165 msec, Te = 90 msec). The repeat unit of the sequence (in brackets) is applied before any radiofrequency pulse is applied. The crusher gradient (Gc) is applied along the slice-select direction (duration, 1 msec; amplitude, 1 mT/m). Spoiler gradients are applied along all three axes during the two longitudinal evolutions to dephase remnant transverse magnetization.

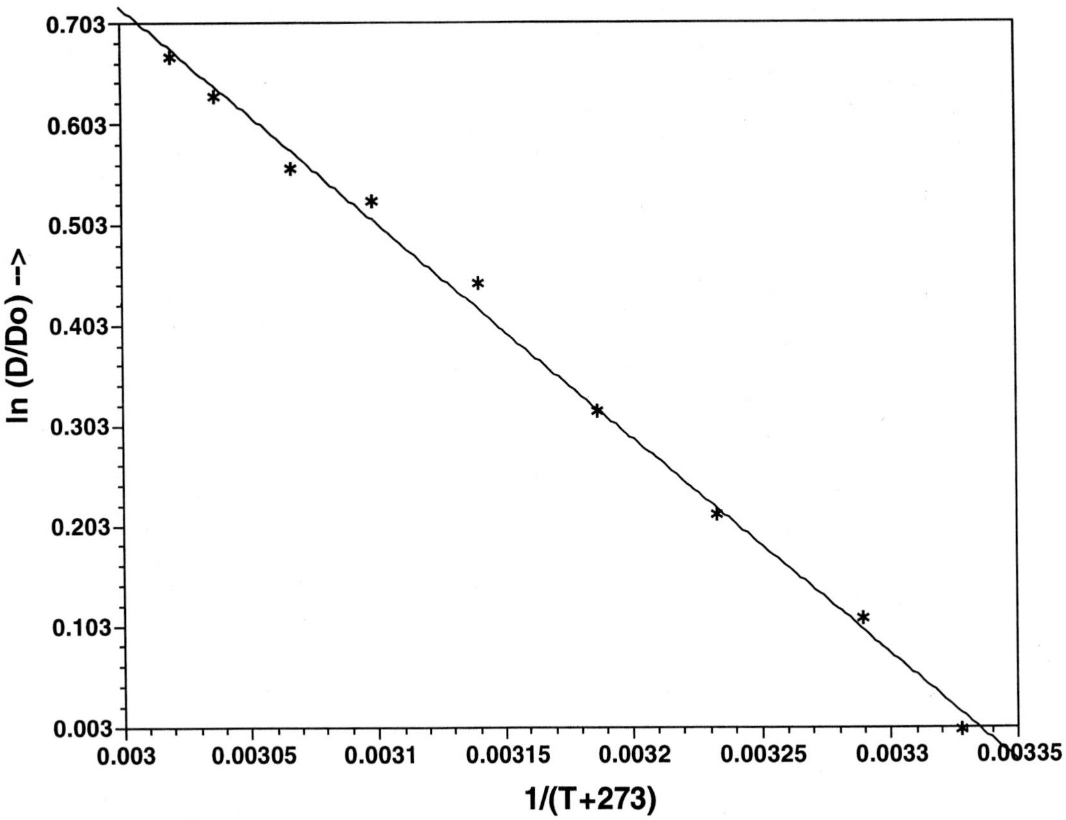

Fig. 13-6. Variation of $\ln(D/D_0)$ with $1/(T + 273)$ in a gel phantom (at 1.5 T) for the sequence in Figure 13-5. Measurements of the diffusion coefficient (D) were made by an exponential fit to the signal intensity variation at three values of the diffusion gradient strength. A temperature sensitivity of 2.9%/°C was obtained for the diffusion coefficient with this sequence.

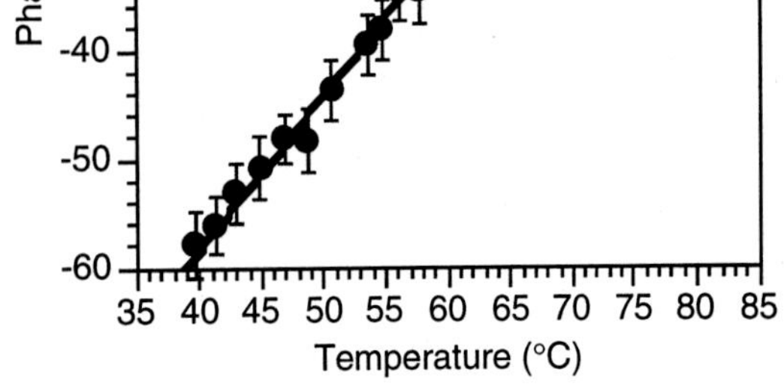

Fig. 13-7. Phase variations with temperature was measured by a navigator echo-based gradient echo sequence at an echo time of 60 msec in a gel phantom at 0.2 T. The other sequence parameters were repetition time, 100 msec; flip angle, 40°; field of view, 200 mm; matrix size, 128 × 128; slice thickness, 7 mm. The temperature sensitivity and temperature uncertainty of the measurement was 2.68 phase degrees/°C and 1.03° C, respectively.

phase. The temporal resolution of these scans (100 msec × 128 = 12.8 sec) is sufficient to monitor RF ablation procedures, which last 1 to 2 min. The authors have successfully implemented a keyholing method, where only the central lines of k-space are collected, thereby reducing scan times by 50%. Simulation experiments showed that contrast and size distortions of a simulated heat lesion were within 10% to 15% for a keyhole size up to 4 (keyhole size is the number of levels in the high-resolution image divided by the number of levels in the keyholed image) (Fig. 13-8). This sequence has been used to monitor the temperature profile of a heat lesion generated by an RF probe in a gel phantom (Fig. 13-9). Some aspects of phase imaging relevant to imaging in an open magnet configuration are the larger phase drifts and higher likelihood of view-to-view phase variations from coupling to external magnetic field perturbations. However, the first problem can be overcome by using a reference phantom maintained at ambient temperature, and the second can be overcome by incorporating navigator echoes.

Echo-shifting methods

The conflicting requirements of long TE for maintaining temperature sensitivity and of high temporal resolution for

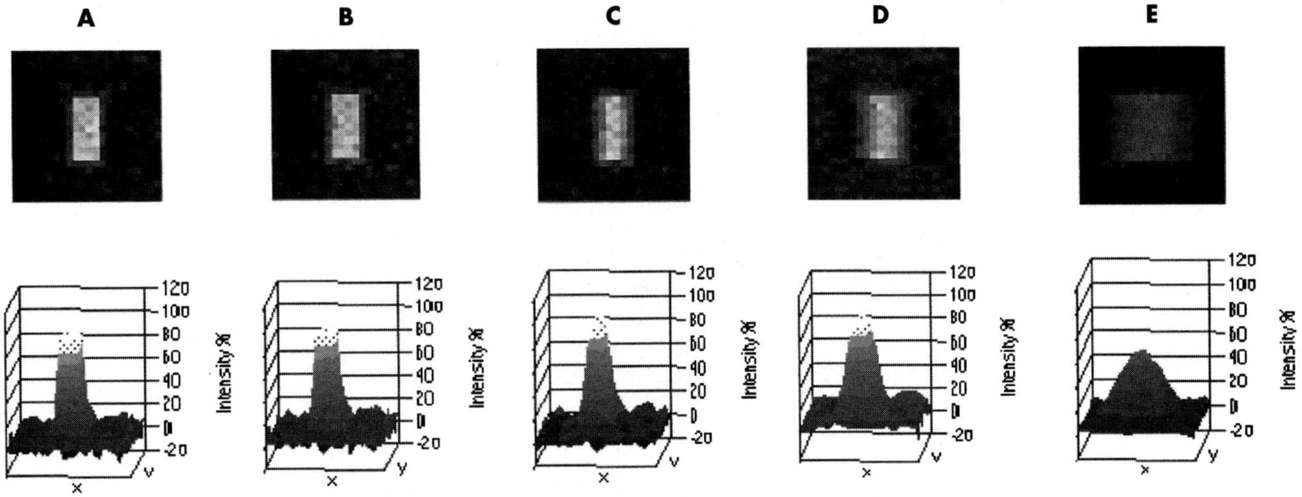

Fig. 13-8. A, Image shows a lesion simulated in a phase image, seen as a rectangular region of hyperintensity. Image shows the lesion reconstructed using **B,** 192; **C,** 128; **D,** 64; and **E,** 32 raw data lines of the image and the remaining high-resolution lines from an image without the simulated lesion. A zoomed region of the phase image centered on the rectangular lesion is shown. Three-dimensional temperature profiles corresponding to the lesions in **A** to **E** are shown in the bottom row.

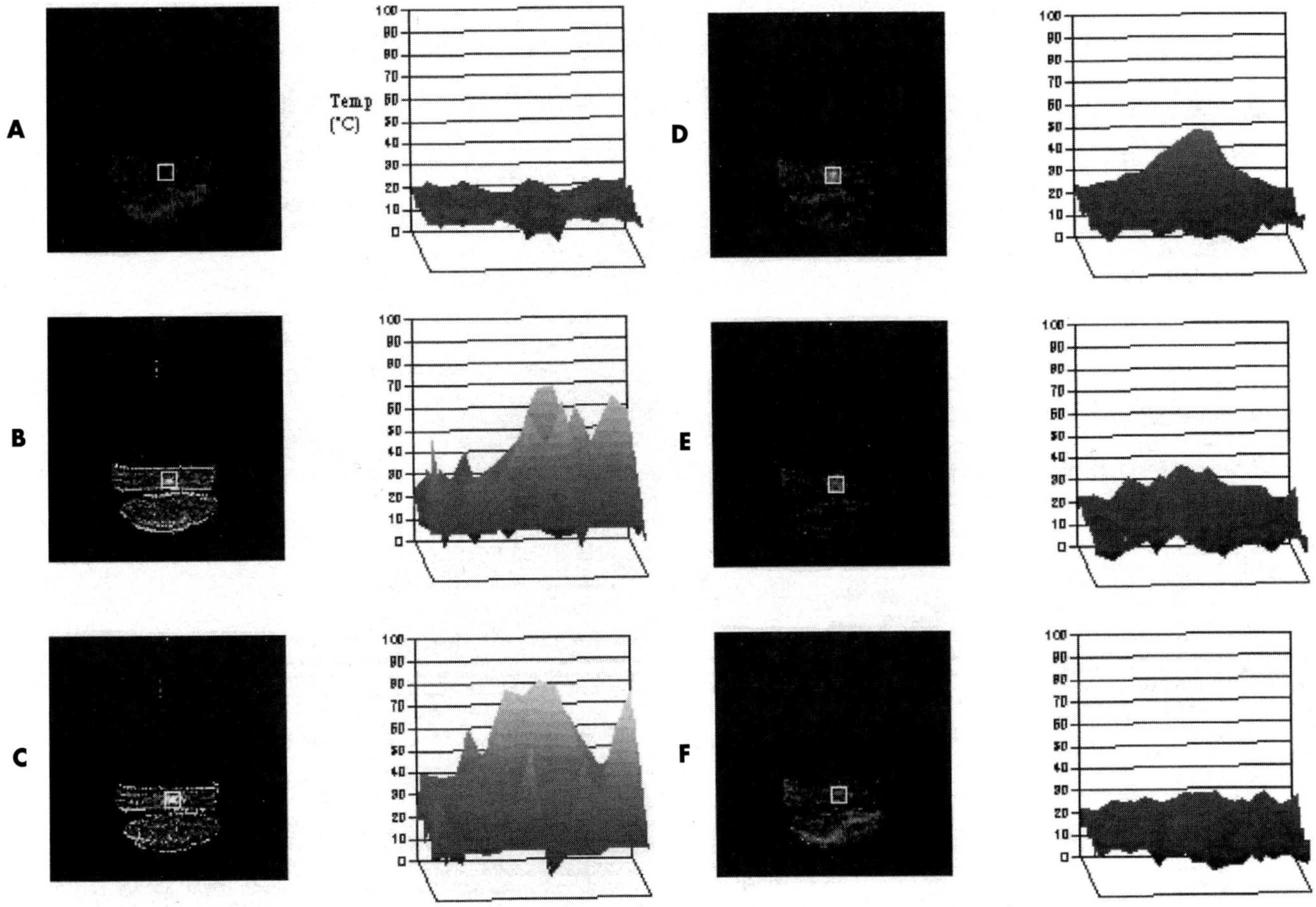

Fig. 13-9. Gel phantom images at different time points of a radiofrequency (RF) ablation procedure have been phase unwrapped and corrected for drifts. Images were acquired **A** to **C,** while the RF power is increased and **D** to **F** after the RF generator is powered down. The three-dimensional temperature profiles are shown (to the right of the image) for the rectangular region of interest (in white) shown superposed on the subtracted phase image.

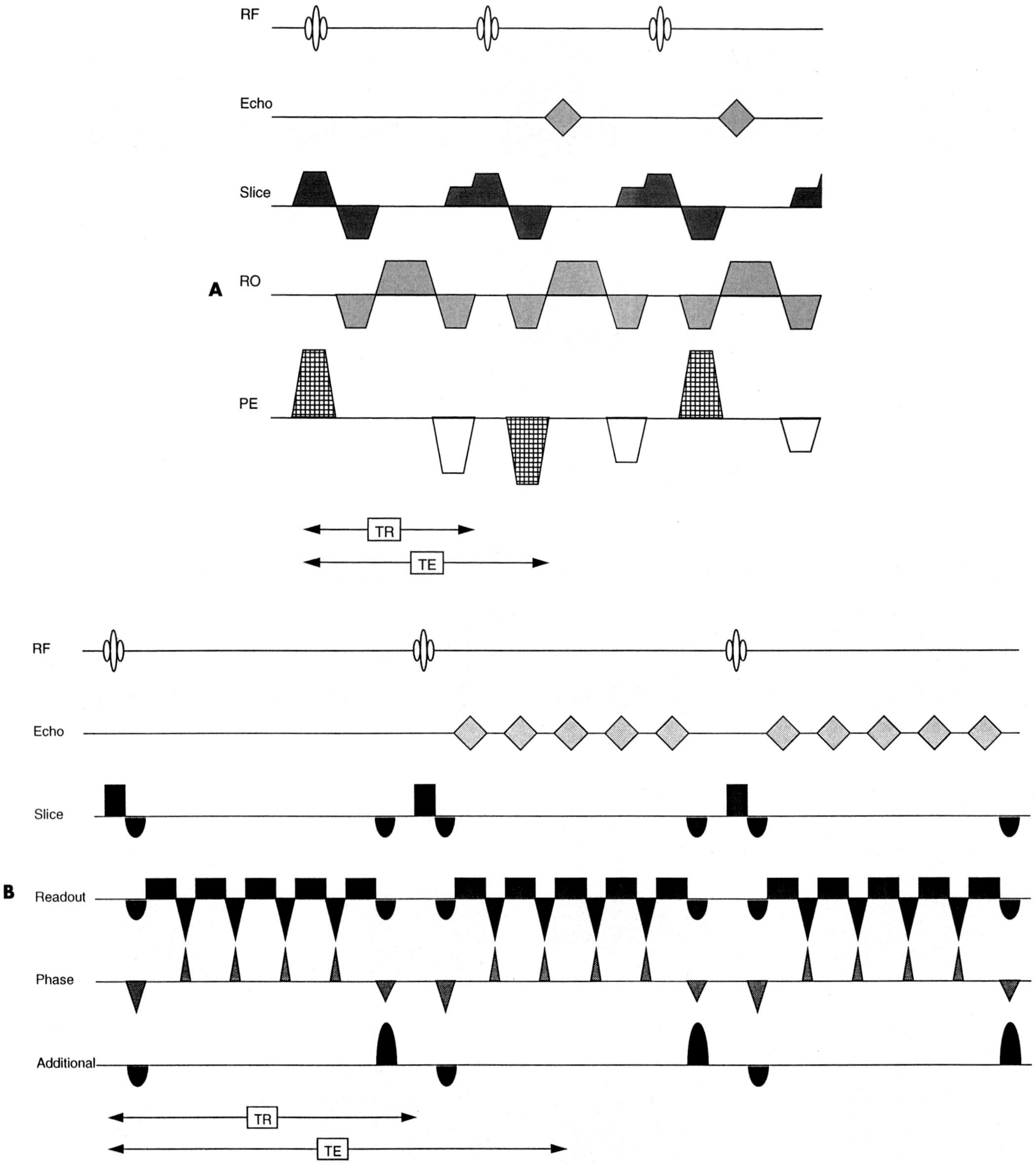

Fig. 13-10. A, Schematic shows the pulse sequence to generate an echo-shifted image. The gradient waveforms are manipulated to cause the spins excited in the (n-1)th repetition time (TR) interval to be focused in the (n)th TR interval. Cross-hatched alternating gradients along the phase direction are crusher gradients. They are shown applied along the phase direction but can be applied along any one of three axes. The first four TR periods show the method by which the spins excited by any radiofrequency pulse are collected in the following TR interval leading to an echo time greater than the TR. **B,** Schematic of the PRESTO pulse sequence, which is a fast version of the echo-shifted sequence. Five echoes are collected at every TR interval, reducing the scan time by a factor of 5 compared with the echo-shifted sequence shown in **A.** The effective echo time is still greater than TR.

monitoring ablation procedures have led to echo-shifted sequences.[33] The idea behind echo shifting is that the TE is greater than the TR accomplished by a special design of the gradient waveforms (Fig. 13-10, *A*). Crusher gradients are included along one of three orthogonal axes, with sufficient strength to dephase any gradient-recalled echo of spins excited in the same TR; however, the phase of the crusher gradient is alternated so that it rephases spins excited by the RF pulse of the previous TR interval. Spins are completely rephased along the read direction within a TR interval, and phase-encode gradients are applied at the end of each TR period. The slice gradient rephases the spins excited by the (n-1)th RF pulse during the nth TR interval (see Fig. 13-10, *A*). Thus, the spins excited by the (n-1)th RF pulse are refocused in the nth TR interval, resulting in a TE greater than TR. An ultrafast version of this sequence, termed *PRESTO*, involves acquisition of multiple gradient echoes per TR, reducing acquisition times to 144 msec for a 64×64 matrix (Fig. 13-10, *B*). The echo-shifted and PRESTO sequences accurately measure temperatures at 4.7 T.[33] However, considerable work remains to be done before either of these sequences is used for thermometry at low fields in open systems.

GENERAL SCHEMES FOR REDUCTION OF SCAN TIMES

Reduction in field of view

The reduction of scan speed by imaging a reduced FOV is applicable to MR therapeutic interventional procedures in which dynamic changes are limited to a small portion of the total FOV. An earlier method was to acquire a base image with the full FOV and acquire subsequent dynamic images with a reduced FOV.[34] This method is accomplished by dense sampling in the phase-encoding direction for the full FOV and sparse sampling for the reduced FOV. The increase in temporal resolution is equal to the ratio of phase lines in the full FOV to those in the reduced FOV. However, the dynamic images cannot be directly Fourier transformed, because this will result in an image with wraparound artifacts from outside the reduced FOV. Difference images formed by the subtraction of corresponding lines of the base and dynamic data can be Fourier transformed without aliasing artifacts. A phase correction has to be applied (for proper positioning) before superposing this dynamic image on the base image. The chief drawback of this system is that changes outside the reduced FOV alias back in the subtracted image resulting in artifacts and, therefore, prior knowledge of the location of the change within the larger FOV is required. This method was successful in tracking the position of moving finger images at 1.5 T and may be clinically applicable. An alternate method of preventing aliasing in the reduced FOV images is to excite a strip rather than the entire slice as proposed in the localized look (LoLo) method.[35] A strip is excited by application of orthogonal gradients during the slice excitation (90°) and slice-focus (180°) RF pulse durations.

A locally focused MR technique has been proposed to image selectively with high resolution in the region of interest.[36] These images require much less scan time than if the entire image was acquired at high resolution. The technique permits user-specified spatial resolution in user-defined portions of the FOV. The user identifies regions of high and low resolution and other regions of no signal intensity in the image. These findings are used to synthesize a set of training images to determine an orthonormal basis set spanning the image reconstruction space. The locally focused images are then reconstructed by using a few acquired phase-encoded signals to calculate image projections onto these basis functions. Greater flexibility is afforded by this method in terms of multiple user-specified regions of high resolution compared with the reduced FOV, but the method is computationally intensive.

Keyhole strategies

Keyhole techniques were initially suggested to improve temporal resolution of dynamic MRI in monitoring contrast agent uptake.[37,38] The simplest keyhole strategy is to acquire a reference image at full resolution and only the central k-space lines for the dynamic images. The dynamic images are then reconstructed after substituting the higher k-space lines from the reference high-resolution image. Simulation of the keyhole technique has shown that spatial and contrast distortions of the dynamic images are less than 10% up to a keyhole factor of 4:1.[39] The temporal resolution is increased compared with that of the reference image because only a subset of the k-space is acquired.

The drawback of conventional keyhole imaging is that the higher spatial frequencies are never updated, which can result in significant blurring and loss of information when attempting to apply keyholing for tracking objects (e.g., a biopsy needle tip) that are spatially small. Several methods have been suggested to ensure that all k-space data are eventually refreshed.[40,41] One technique (termed *CURE*) is based on a random encoding of the phase lines as opposed to the linear update approach of conventional keyholing. In this method, the phase-encode lines are randomly ordered, with the low k-space lines acquired more frequently.[40] An ultrafast gradient echo sequence with a TR of 6.5 msec was used to acquire images using the phase-encode order dictated by the random table. Data were acquired continuously, with the same random phase table used repeatedly. An image at any time point was reconstructed by searching the data outward from that time point until all of the phase line information was available. If two low k-space data were located in the search, the line closer to the desired time point is included. Images of the human heart and a flexed lower leg reconstructed every 90 msec show the feasibility of the technique. This technique could potentially be applied to interventional MR applications if the image reconstruction can be implemented in real-time rather than off-line. An alternate keyhole strategy named *striped k-space scanning* has been proposed in which eight strips are each rotated 22.5° to cover the whole k-space; each dynamic scan acquires one strip. The sequence was implemented on a 0.064-T MR system with open access and shows potential for interventional applications.[42]

A recent simulation study compared the efficacy of different keyhole strategies in tracking a biopsy needle.[43] All of the simulations were performed with 25% of the phase-encode lines acquired every segment and with the needle traversing parallel and perpendicular to the phase-encode axis. The standard keyhole, which repeatedly acquired the central 25% phase lines, was inadequate for needle localization because of lateral blurring of the needle when the phase axis was perpendicular to needle path. When the needle was parallel to the phase-encode axis, no lateral blurring occurred, but the needle tip was poorly defined. The best scheme, based on this simulation study, collected the center 1/8 of phase lines, with the remaining lines ranked and sequentially acquired. Lines were ranked based on the order of maximum to minimum magnitude of the 2D FT of the needle image projected onto the read axis.

Keyhole techniques specifically applied to open-access magnets include conventional keyhole schemes with phase imaging for temperature monitoring during RF ablation studies.[32] A keyhole diffusion weighted spin-echo sequence has also been investigated for low-field (0.064 T) NMR thermometry.[43] A weighted k-space acquisition was implemented in which outer lines were sampled sparsely and inner lines were sampled in the normal way.

Wavelet encoding and singular value decomposition

Various spatial-encoding methods based on separable non-Fourier transformations were recently suggested to increase the speed of acquisitions for interventional and dynamic imaging studies. Considerable work has been done in two areas: wavelet encoding and singular value decomposition (SVD).

Wavelet encoding

Wavelet encoding is an alternative to phase encoding that reduces acquisition times significantly.[44] In wavelet encoding, a distribution of spins is excited by a slice-selective RF pulse along a magnetic field gradient. The spins along the gradient are encoded by changing the excited profile with each RF pulse; the original distribution of spins along the gradient is found with the inverse wavelet transform of the signal. The wavelet transform of a function is the collection of inner products of that function with the wavelet at the proper scales and translations. In wavelet encoding, these inner products are measured by using a selective RF pulse to excite the spin density with a wavelet-shaped profile. The wavelet-based encoding uses the multiresolution characteristics of the wavelet transform to abbreviate data acquisition. Acquisition speeds of 33 sec for a T2-weighted 256 × 256 image are possible using this technique. A modification of this technique which uses 1D Fourier and 1D wavelet-encoding has been implemented on a 0.2-T scanner for dynamic tracking for interventional MRI.[45] Using spatially localized wavelet functions, regions of a spin-echo reference image were updated only where the image was changing (e.g., an advancing biopsy needle). Wavelet encoding reduces scan times by a factor of up to 10 compared with conventional Fourier encoding. A limitation of this method, as with the SVD technique that follows, is that it is based on spatially selective excitations and is thus extremely sensitive to the calculation and excitation of RF profiles.

Singular value decomposition

SVD is based on a matrix decomposition theorem of linear algebra that produces a 2D separable unitary transformation of a matrix.[46,47] This method is implemented, similar to wavelet encoding, by the use of spatially selective RF excitations. The dynamically adaptive MRI based on SVD is specially suited for dynamic or interventional imaging.[48] The spatially selective RF excitation profiles of any dynamic image of a series are determined by the SVD of the image matrix of the previous image in the series. The decomposition algorithm ensures the optimal choice of encoding profiles, which minimizes the number of encoding steps required to update the image. Images with significant detail can be acquired with just 24 encodes. However, a long TR of 1000 msec and low flip angles are required between encodes to ensure that the magnetization recovers between successive pulses. The feasibility of this technique should be further investigated for MR-guided interventional procedures.

REAL-TIME RECONSTRUCTION AND DISPLAY

The first real-time reconstruction system, capable of updating six images per second, was proposed by Wright and others[49] as part of a fluoroscopic MRI system. Recently, a real-time reconstruction system was proposed that enables reconstruction times of 30 frames per second for a 256 × 256 pixel image.[50] The analog data from the MR scanner are input as the first basic functional unit: an analog-to-digital converter capable of digitizing at 0.5 sec for each complex data sample, which is sufficient for the fastest image acquisitions to date (single-shot echoplanar imaging). The data from the analog-to-digital converter are transferred to an interface memory board. The reconstruction system continuously reconstructs the data available in the interface memory at the maximum rate at which it can operate. A dedicated Fourier processor in which 1D Fourier transforms are performed via a direct hardware implementation of the fast Fourier transform algorithm is capable of Fourier transforming at the rate of 122 Hz. The final part of the system is the display processor, which takes the digital image data from the Fourier processor and generates an analog video signal to drive a video monitor. The system is built for data to be stored in a continuous mode; archival is possible on a videotape. A further advantage is that the system can be interfaced to most commercial MR scanners.

REFERENCES

1. Duckwiler G, and others: Head and neck lesions: MR-guided aspiration biopsy, *Radiology* 170:519, 1989.
2. Lufkin R, and others: A technique for MR guided needle biopsy, *Am J Roentgenol* 151:193, 1988.
3. Lufkin R, Teresi L, Hanafee W: New needle for MR guided aspiration cytology of the head and neck, *Am J Roentgenol* 149:380, 1987.
4. Sinha S, and others: Pulse sequence optimization for use with a biopsy needle in MRI, *Magn Reson Imaging* 7:575, 1989.
5. Mueller PR, and others: MR-guided aspiration biopsy: needle design and clinical trials, *Radiology* 161:605, 1986.
6. Farahani K, and others: Effect of field strength on susceptibility artifacts in magnetic resonance imaging, *Comput Med Imaging Graph* 14:409, 1990.

7. Kochli VD, and others: Vascular interventions guided by ultrafast MR imaging: evaluation of different materials, *Magn Reson Med* 31:309, 1994.
8. Frahm C, and others: Visualization of magnetic resonance-compatible needles at 1.5 and 0.2 Tesla, *Cardiovasc Intervent Radiol* 19:335, 1996.
9. Faber SC, Stehling MK, Reiser M: *Artifacts of MR-compatible biopsy needles: optimization of pulse sequences, dependence on MR-parameters, comparison of different products,* New York, 1996, Annual Meeting ISMRM.
10. Schenck JF: The role of magnetic susceptibility in magnetic resonance imaging: MRI magnetic compatibility of the first and second kinds, *Med Phys* 23:815, 1996.
11. Bakker CJ, and others: Visualization of dedicated catheters using fast scanning techniques with potential for MR-guided vascular interventions, *Magn Reson Med* 36:816, 1996.
12. Daniel BL, and others: *Interactive MR-guided breast lesion localization: a phantom study,* New York,1996, 4th Annual Meeting of ISMRM.
13. Dumoulin CL, Souza SP, Darrow RD: Real time monitoring of invasive devices using magnetic resonance, *Magn Reson Med* 29:411, 1993.
14. Leung DA, and others: Intravascular MR tracking catheter: preliminary experimental evaluation, *Am J Roentgenol* 164:1265, 1995.
15. Leung DA, and others: Real-time biplanar needle tracking for interventional MR imaging procedures, *Radiology* 197:485, 1995.
16. Erhart P, and others: Tissue-independent tracking of biopsy needles with an internal signal source, *ISMRM* 3:1740, 1996.
17. Cline HE, and others: MR temperature mapping of focused ultrasound surgery, *Magn Reson Med* 31:628, 1994.
18. Chung AH, and others: Optimization of spoiled gradient-echo phase imaging for in vivo localization of a focused ultrasound beam, *Magn Reson Med* 36:745, 1996.
19. De Poorter J, and others: The proto-resonance-frequency-shift method compared with molecular diffusion for quantitative measurement of two-dimensional time-dependent temperature distribution in a phantom, *J Magn Reson B* 103:234, 1994.
20. Matsumoto R, and others: Tissue temperature monitoring for thermal interventional therapy: comparison of T1-weighted MR sequences, *J Magn Reson Imaging* 4:65, 1994.
21. Fried MP, and others: Dynamic T1-weighted magnetic resonance imaging of interstitial laser photocoagulation in the liver: observations on in-vivo temperature sensitivity, *Lasers Surg Med* 18:410, 1996.
22. Dickinson RJ, and others: Measurement of changes in tissue temperature using magnetic resonance imaging, *J Comput Assist Tomogr* 10:468, 1986.
23. Young IR, and others: Further observations on the measurement of tissue T1 to monitor temperature in vivo by MRI, *Magn Reson Med* 31:342, 1994.
24. Sinha S, Sinha U: *Comparison of MR pulse sequences.* In Black K, Lufkin R, directors: *Interventional MRI,* Marina Del Rey, Calif, 1994 (lecture).
25. Oshiro T, and others: *Comparison of temperature measurements using phase shift and T1 imaging at 0.2 Tesla,* Vancouver, 1997, 5th Annual Meeting ISMRM.
26. MacFall J, and others: Temperature dependence of canine brain tissue diffusion coefficient measured in vivo with magnetic resonance echo-planar imaging, *Int J Hyperthermia* 11:73, 1995.
27. Sinha U, Sinha S: High speed diffusion imaging in the presence of eddy currents, *J Magn Reson Imaging* 6:657, 1996.
28. Sinha S, and others: *Temperature monitoring with single shot diffusion imaging on a 0.2T scanner,* New York, 1996, Proceedings of the ISMRM.
29. De Poorter J, and others: Noninvasive MRI thermometry with the proton resonance frequency (PRF) method: in vivo results in human muscle, *Magn Reson Med* 33:74, 1995.
30. Ishihara Y, and others: A precise and fast temperature mapping using water proton chemical shift, *Magn Reson Med* 34:814, 1995.
31. Vitkin IA, and others: Magnetic resonance imaging of temperature changes during interstitial microwave heating: a phantom study, *Med Phys* 24:269, 1997.
32. Sinha S, and others: Phase imaging on a 0.2 Tesla MR scanner: application to temperature monitoring during ablation procedures, *J Magn Reson Imaging* 7:918, 1997.
33. de Zwart JA, and others: *Ultra fast MRI thermometry,* New York, 1997, Proceedings of the ISMRM.
34. Hu X, Parrish T: Reduction of field of view for dynamic imaging, *Magn Reson Med* 31:691, 1994.
35. van Vaals JJ, van Yperen G, de Boer R: *Real-time MR imaging using the LoLo method for interactive and interventional MRI at 0.5T and 1.5T,* San Francisco, 1994, Proceedings of the SMRM, 2nd Annual Meeting.
36. Cao Y, Levin DN, Yao L: Locally focused MRI, *Magn Reson Med* 34:858, 1995.
37. Van Vaals J, and others: Keyhole method for accelerating imaging of contrast agent uptake, *J Magn Reson Imaging* 3:671, 1993.
38. Jones RA, and others: K-space substitution: a novel dynamic imaging technique, *Magn Reson Med* 29:830, 1993.
39. Spraggins TA: Simulation of spatial and contrast distortions in keyhole imaging, *Magn Reson Med* 31:320, 1994.
40. Parrish T, Hu X: Continuous update with random encoding (CURE): a new strategy for dynamic imaging, *Magn Reson Med* 33:326, 1995.
41. Busch M, and others: *Striped k-space: an extension of the keyhole technique for rapid imaging with high contrast differentiation,* San Francisco, 1994, 2nd Annual Meeting of SMR.
42. Duerk JL, Lewin JS, Wu DH: Application of keyhole imaging to interventional MRI: a simulation study to predict sequence requirements, *J Magn Reson Imaging* 6:918, 1996.
43. Friebe M, Busch M: *Low-field NMR thermometry with diffusion sensitized keyhole and weighted k-space sequencing schemes,* San Francisco, 1994, 2nd Annual Meeting of SMR.
44. Weaver JB, and others: Wavelet-encoded MR imaging, *Magn Reson Med* 24:275, 1992.
45. Wendt M, and others: *Dynamic tracking algorithm for interventional MRI using wavelet-encoding,* Nice, 1995, 3rd Annual Meeting of SMR.
46. Golub GH, Reinsch C: Singular value decomposition and least squares solution, *Numer Math* 14:403, 1970.
47. Dewilde P, Deprettere EF: *Singular value decomposition: an introduction.* In Deprettere EF, editor: *SVD and signal processing,* New York, 1988, North Holland.
48. Zientara GP, Panych LP, Jolesz FA: Dynamically adaptive MRI with encoding by singular value decomposition, *Magn Reson Med* 32:268, 1994.
49. Wright RC, and others: Real-time MR fluoroscopic data acquisition and image reconstruction, *Magn Reson Med* 12:407, 1989.
50. Gmitro AF, and others: A real-time reconstruction system for magnetic resonance imaging, *Magn Reson Med* 35:734, 1996.

Chapter 14

PASSIVE VISUALIZATION STRATEGIES FOR BIOPSY AND NEEDLE PUNCTURE

Christian Frahm, Hans-Björn Gehl

More than 10 years ago, the first activities in the field of interventional magnetic resonance imaging (MRI) started with MR-guided needle punctures of the abdomen and the head and neck.[1–6] At this time, a simple direct depiction of the needle in the MR image was intended, similar to computed tomography (CT)–guided puncture procedure. Therefore, the susceptibility artifact caused by the needle was used to recognize the needle positioned within the tissue. Applying needles made of nonferromagnetic alloys, this idea became feasible. Several years later, this principle was termed *passive visualization* because, unlike active visualization, the interventional device to be visualized does not contribute to the imaging process as a component of the MR system.

Passive visualization was the first principle applied to visualize an interventional device in MRI and is now the most clinically proven; it has been established for MR-guided needle placement. The technical simplicity of this strategy is a considerable advantage because no special hardware or software is necessary. Although passive needle visualization is more complex than needle visualization in CT or fluoroscopy, it is robust and safe if the user is familiar with the main factors influencing the size and visibility of the needle artifact and with the resulting opportunities to visualize an actual needle on the MR scanner.

This chapter discusses the influence of the relevant factors for passive needle visualization and explains the implications for clinical practice.

FACTORS INFLUENCING SIZE AND VISIBILITY OF NEEDLE ARTIFACTS

Susceptibility artifacts occur at interfaces between substances with very different magnetic susceptibilities. The difference in susceptibility results in a local distortion of the magnetic field, which creates spin dephasing and frequency shifts of nearby protons. Therefore, susceptibility artifacts appear in MRI as distortions of signal intensity combined with geometric distortions.[7]

Ferromagnetic stainless steel needles for use under CT, fluoroscopic, or sonographic guidance cannot be applied in MRI because of tremendous susceptibility artifacts and, additionally, the presence of needle deflection caused by magnetic field attraction.[1,8]

MR-compatible needles are made of nonferromagnetic alloys. Such needles cause lower disruption of the local field homogeneity and produce a local, line-shaped susceptibility artifact, which consists only or mostly of a signal loss (Fig. 14-1). However, in some circumstances, a narrow signal rise can be present on the edge of the artifact.

Regarding needle artifact width, the artifact should be clearly visible, so the position of the needle in the body can be checked safely; however, the artifact should not be too broad, so important structures in the region of the puncture path or even in the target region itself are not obscured by the artifact. The size and visibility of the artifact are, however, influenced by many factors (Box 14-1).

Needle orientation to the main magnetic field B_0

The size of the local disruption of B_0 caused by the magnetic polarization of the needle depends on the needle orientation relative to B_0. At a given field strength, the angle of the needle shaft to B_0 is the most important factor influencing the artifact size. A greater angle causes larger artifacts (Figs. 14-1 to 14-5).[1,9–11]

Field strength

At a given needle angle to B_0, needle artifacts are distinctly larger at high field strength than at low field strength.[7,9–11] Field

A

B

C

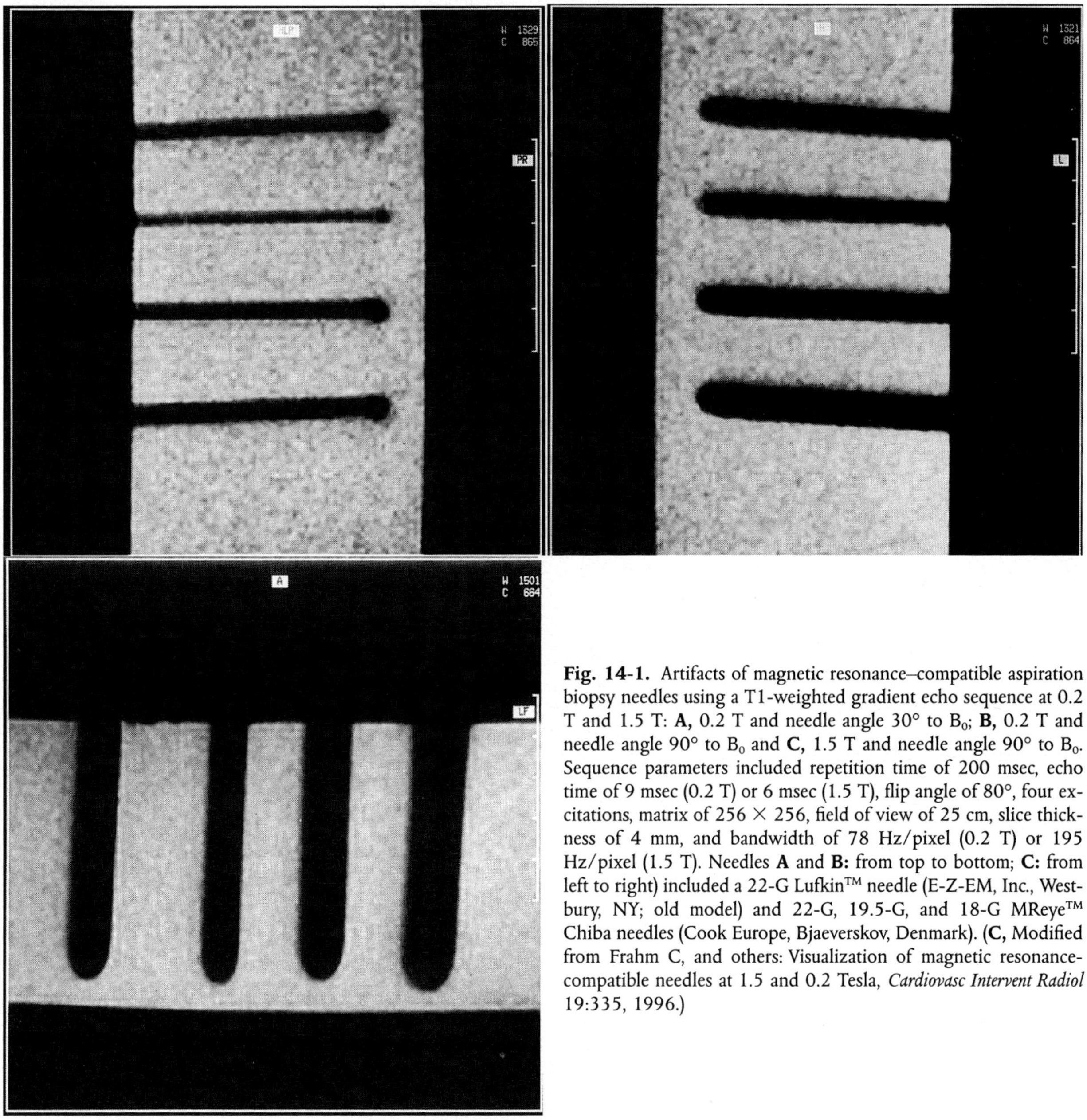

Fig. 14-1. Artifacts of magnetic resonance–compatible aspiration biopsy needles using a T1-weighted gradient echo sequence at 0.2 T and 1.5 T: **A,** 0.2 T and needle angle 30° to B_0; **B,** 0.2 T and needle angle 90° to B_0 and **C,** 1.5 T and needle angle 90° to B_0. Sequence parameters included repetition time of 200 msec, echo time of 9 msec (0.2 T) or 6 msec (1.5 T), flip angle of 80°, four excitations, matrix of 256 × 256, field of view of 25 cm, slice thickness of 4 mm, and bandwidth of 78 Hz/pixel (0.2 T) or 195 Hz/pixel (1.5 T). Needles **A** and **B:** from top to bottom; **C:** from left to right) included a 22-G Lufkin™ needle (E-Z-EM, Inc., Westbury, NY; old model) and 22-G, 19.5-G, and 18-G MReye™ Chiba needles (Cook Europe, Bjaeverskov, Denmark). (**C,** Modified from Frahm C, and others: Visualization of magnetic resonance-compatible needles at 1.5 and 0.2 Tesla, *Cardiovasc Intervent Radiol* 19:335, 1996.)

Box 14-1. Factors influencing size and visibility of needle artifacts

Magnetic resonance

Angle of the needle to the static magnetic field B_0
Field strength of the magnetic resonance imager
Pulse sequence type (e.g., gradient echo or spin- or turbo spin-echo)
Echo time
In case of spin- and turbo spin-echoes, orientation of the frequency-encoding gradient to the needle
Slice thickness
Spatial resolution
Sequence bandwidth or gradient strength

Needle

Alloy
Diameter
Material of the inner stylet within the needle, if present

strength and needle angle to B_0 are the most relevant factors influencing the artifact size of a given needle (see Figs. 14-1 and 14-2).

Pulse sequence type

The 180° refocusing pulses of spin- and turbo spin-echo sequences correct for susceptibility-induced spin dephasing. Generally, using gradient echo sequences causes larger artifacts than using spin- or turbo spin-echo sequences.[2,7,9,10] However, this approach is not accurate in each case and depends on the actual parameters of the pulse sequences to be compared. Thus, pulse sequence type is an important factor but not more important than the relevant sequence parameters, such as echo time and bandwidth (see Fig. 14-3).

Echo time

With use of a gradient echo sequence, the artifact size can be influenced by changing the echo time.[7,9,12] Increasing the echo time allows more time for spin dephasing and results in distinctly increased artifact size (see Fig. 14-3).

Needle orientation to frequency-encoding gradient

With use of spin- or turbo spin-echo sequences and middle or large needle angles to B_0, the artifact width can be considerably diminished or increased by swapping the axes of the phase-encoding and the frequency-encoding gradient. A perpendicular orientation of the frequency-encoding gradient relative to the needle shaft results in a greater artifact width than does a parallel orientation (see Fig. 14-3).[7,9–12] (The geometric distortion and the associated signal attenuation or compression related to susceptibility artifacts are pronounced along the frequency-encoding axis applying echoes refocused by a 180° pulse. When the gradients are swapped, the part of artifact caused by the local nonlinearity of the frequency-encoding gradient remains, but spin dephasing is counteracted by the 180° refocusing pulse. With use of gradient echos, a gradient swap has no provable effect on artifact width.)

Slice thickness

The size of needle artifacts (and susceptibility artifacts in general) can be decreased by the use of thin slices, which reduce dephasing across the slice (see Fig. 14-4).[7]

Spatial resolution

Partial volume averaging is minimized by improving spatial resolution, which improves the visibility of small structures in general and of narrow artifacts in particular. This improvement can be achieved by reducing slice thickness or the field of view (FOV) or by increasing the matrix (see Fig. 14-4). Because the voxel is usually much larger in the direction of slice selection, a reduction of slice thickness generally provides a greater reduction in partial volume averaging than does a reduced FOV.[7]

Bandwidth or strength of frequency-encoding gradient

Needle artifacts (and susceptibility artifacts in general) can be reduced by increasing the strength of the frequency-encoding gradient for a given FOV (see Fig. 14-3).[7,13]

Needle design or alloy

Commercially available MR-compatible needles can be made of one of two alloys: the titanium alloys (used by Daum GmbH, Schwerin, Germany; Somatex GmbH, Berlin, Germany; and C.R. Bard GmbH, Karlsruhe, Germany) and the nonferromagnetic nickel-chromium alloys with high nickel and low iron content (used by E-Z-EM, Inc., Westbury, NY, and Cook Europe, Bjaeverskov, Denmark). If all other factors (e.g., needle diameter) are equal, a titanium needle causes narrower artifacts than a needle of nonferromagnetic nickel-chromium steel (see Fig. 14-5). Furthermore, the artifact width of needles made of nonferromagnetic nickel-chromium alloys may differ depending on the nickel content (see Fig. 14-1).[2,9,10] For a given alloy, the artifact width depends on the needle diameter and on the presence of an inner stylet and its material.

IMPLICATIONS FOR NEEDLE VISUALIZATION IN CLINICAL PRACTICE

Achieving a needle artifact of suitable size is only one aspect of the several considered when an actual MR-guided intervention is performed applying passive visualization. Thus, from the beginning, several important factors influencing artifact size are usually determined or limited in their variability by other important requirements or invariable facts. The actual opportunities to act on artifact size are often less complex than expected in view of the number of influence factors. However, the re-

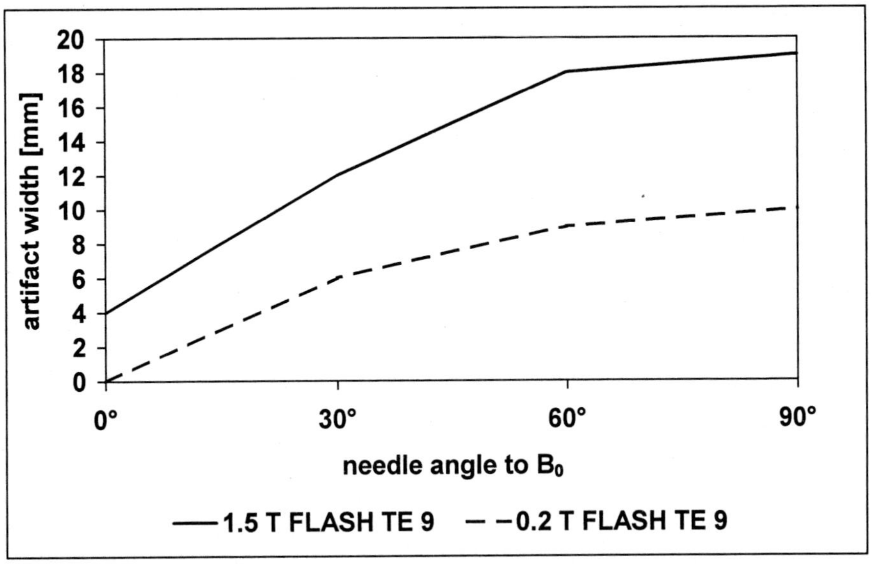

Fig. 14-2. Comparison of artifact sizes for a 14-G core biopsy gun made of a titanium alloy (BiopsyGun™, Daum GmbH, Schwerin, Germany) at 0.2 T and 1.5 T using a T1-weighted gradient echo sequence protocol suitable for abdominal breathhold imaging. Sequence parameters included repetition time of 90 to 120 msec, echo time of 9 msec, flip angle of 80°, one excitation, matrix of 128 × 256, field of view of 35 cm, slice thickness of 8 mm, and bandwidth of 78 Hz/pixel (0.2 T) or 195 Hz/pixel (1.5 T).

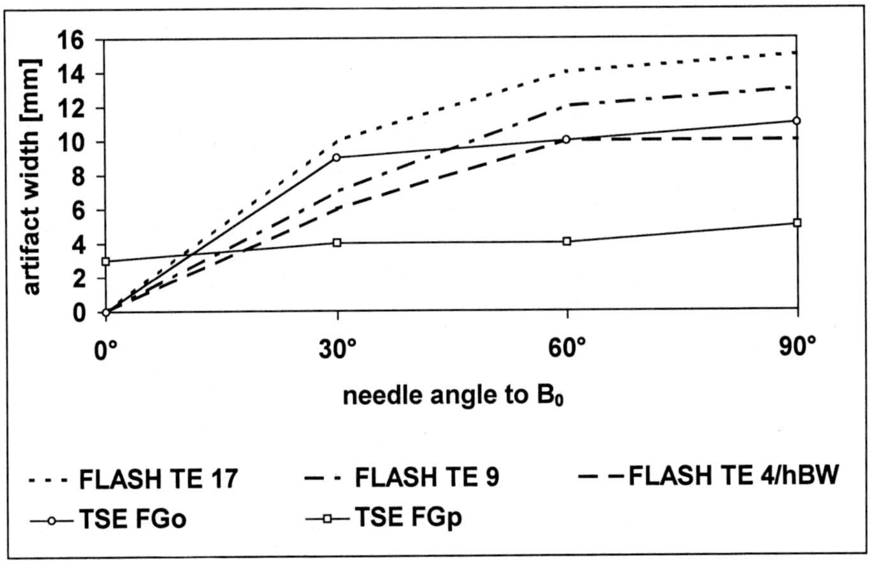

Fig. 14-3. Comparison of artifact sizes applying T1-weighted gradient echo fast low angle shot (FLASH) and turbo spin-echo (TSE) sequence protocols suitable for abdominal breathhold imaging (18 G BiopsyGun™, Daum, Schwerin, Germany) at 1.5 T. General imaging parameters included slice thickness of 8 mm, matrix of 128 × 256, field of view of 35 cm, and one excitation. For FLASH TE 17 and FLASH TE 9, parameters included repetition time of 120 msec echo time of 17 or 9 msec, flip angle of 80°, and bandwidth of 195 Hz/pixel. For FLASH TE 4 with high bandwidth, parameters included repetition time of 120 msec, echo time of 4 msec, flip angle of 80°, and high bandwidth of 355 Hz/pixel. For TSE with a frequency-encoding gradient orthogonal to the needle and TSE with a frequency-encoding gradient parallel to the needle, parameters included repetition time of 351 msec, echo time of 19 msec, echo train length of four, and bandwidth of 130 Hz/pixel.

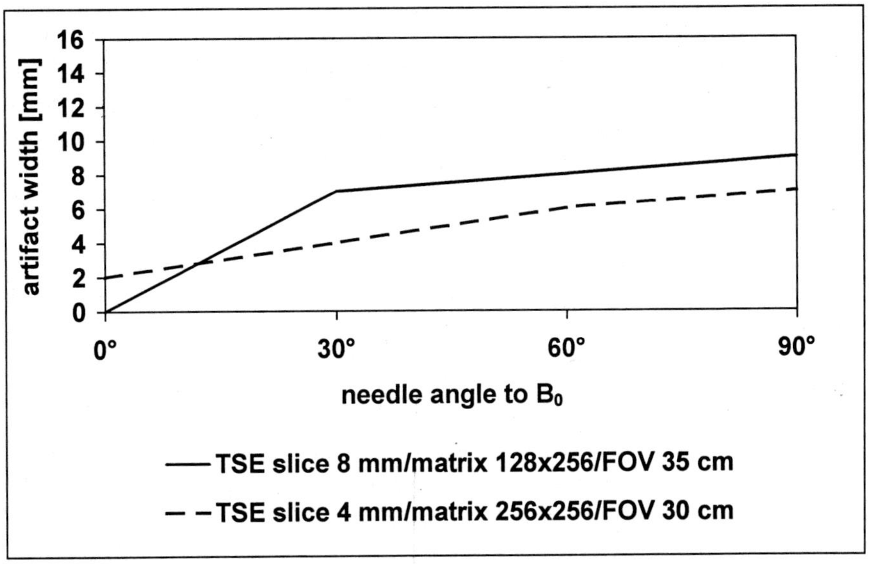

Fig. 14-4. Comparison of artifact sizes for an 18-G puncture needle made of a titanium alloy with a plastic stylet inside (PunctureNeedle™, Daum GmbH, Schwerin, Germany) at 1.5 T using T1-weighted turbo spin-echo sequence protocols with different spatial resolution and slice thickness. Parameters included repetition time of 351 msec, echo time of 19 msec, echo train length of four, one excitation (lower resolution) or three excitations (higher resolution), and bandwidth of 130 Hz/pixel.

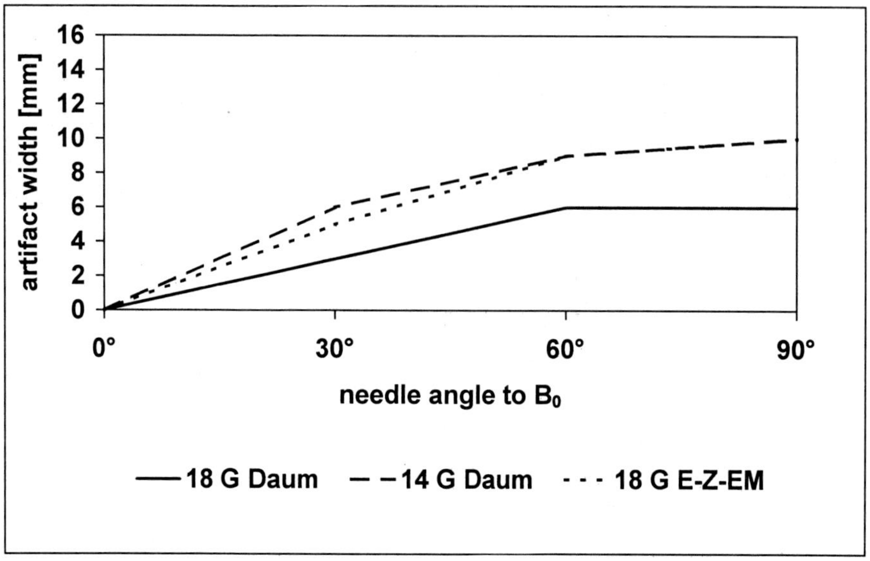

Fig. 14-5. Comparison of artifact sizes for several magnetic resonance–compatible core biopsy devices differing in alloy or needle diameter (0.2-T scanner, T1-weighted gradient echo sequence suitable for abdominal breathhold imaging, repetition time of 90 msec, echo time of 9 msec, flip angle of 80°, one excitation, slice thickness of 8 mm, matrix of 128 × 256, and field of view of 35 cm). For 18-G and 14-G Daum, a BiopsyGun™ (Daum GmbH, Schwerin, Germany) made of a titanium alloy was used. For 18-G E-Z-EM, MRI Biogun™ (E-Z-EM, Inc., Westbury, NY) made of a nonferromagnetic nickel-chromium alloy was used.

maining opportunities to influence needle visualization should be applied consistently.

Of course, only a few users can choose between scanners with different field strengths. Furthermore, the needle angle to B_0 is usually determined by the intended interventional approach (i.e., entry site and puncture path) and the given magnet design. All high-field scanners and most midfield scanners have the conventional tube-shaped magnet design, in which the field axis runs horizontally along the tube (i.e., along the patient's head feet axis). Thus, in most cases of needle punctures on such magnets, the angle of the puncture needle to the static field will be great (approximately 60° to 90°), and the visualization of a puncture needle positioned at a small angle to the static field will not be important. In most low-field imagers, however, the field axis runs vertically through the patient, who is placed in a gap between two horizontal magnetic pole faces. Therefore, the visualization of a puncture needle for any angle of the needle to the static field (0° to 90°) appears practically relevant. However, approaches with a lateral entry site—and thus middle or large angles of the needle to the main magnetic field—are preferred because the physician has greater freedom of movement for manipulations.

Passive visualization in abdominal biopsy and needle puncture

When MR-guided needle punctures are performed in the abdomen, imaging has to be carried out within a very short acquisition time that allows breathhold imaging. Such fast imaging is also necessary for procedures in other regions (e.g., head and neck, musculoskeletal system) when interactive needle guidance is intended. Thus, fast interventional imaging is usually accomplished using gradient echo sequences with short repetition times and only one excitation (as a rule, T1 weighting provides better tissue contrast and is preferred over proton density weighting.) To ensure a sufficient signal-to-noise ratio (SNR) under these conditions, only a relatively low spatial resolution (matrix, approximately 128 × 256; FOV, 24 to 35 cm; slice thickness, 8 to 10 mm) can be used.[14–22] However, although artifact size is generally slightly increased because of thick slices, the visibility of narrow artifacts is reduced because of low resolution and distinct partial volume effect. For this resolution, an artifact width of 5 to 8 mm appears optimal (if possible, not greater than 10 mm), because visibility may be already critical or insufficient if artifact width is less than 4 mm. In this setting, the target lesion should have a diameter of at least 1.5 cm to ensure a safe and successful procedure.

Using a 0.2-T scanner, T1-weighted breathhold gradient echoes with an echo time of about 7 to 9 msec are recommended for image-guided abdominal needle punctures, but a needle angle of 0° to B_0 should be avoided because of critical or insufficient visibility of needle artifact (see Figs. 14-2 and 14-5). With use of thin titanium needles or titanium needles without a metallic stylet, visibility may become critical at a needle angle of approximately 30° to B_0. In this case, the echo time should be increased to 15 to 17 msec.

With use of a high-field scanner and a large needle angle relative to B_0 (as is typical in high-field magnets), reduction of the needle artifact is commonly necessary to obtain a tolerable size. This reduction may be accomplished by applying a gradient echo sequence with a very short echo time and a high bandwidth. For example, with use of titanium needles having a diameter of 20 to 18 G at 1.5 T and large angles to B_0, a T1-weighted gradient echo sequence using an echo time of 4 msec and a high bandwidth of approximately 355 Hz/pixel is recommended (see Fig. 14-3). Alternatively, a T1-weighted turbo (fast) spin-echo sequence with one or two excitations may be used for interventional breathhold imaging (see Fig. 14-3). (T1-weighted turbo spin-echoes are not widely used in diagnostic imaging because only a few slices can be obtained using a short repetition time. For control of needle placement, only a few slices are needed.) The turbo spin-echo allows further reduction of artifact size by arranging a parallel or somewhat parallel orientation of the frequency-encoding gradient to the needle. This approach is recommended when using a 14-G core biopsy needle of a titanium alloy (see Fig. 14-3) or an 18-G biopsy needle of a nickel-chromium alloy on a 1.5-T magnet at large needle angles of 60° to 90° to B_0 (alternatively, the inner stylet of the needle can be removed during imaging, if possible). However, this gradient orientation to the needle will demand gradient swapping in many cases and, therefore, may result in aliasing (wraparound) artifacts. In the case of aliasing, phase oversampling may be used (if possible), or a larger FOV should be chosen. Overall, a 0.2-T scanner is more appropriate than a high-field system for passive needle visualization in large-core biopsies in general and in abdominal core biopsies in particular.

Passive visualization in needle localization or biopsy of breast lesions

If MR-guided needle puncture of breast lesions for localization or biopsy is performed, imaging requirements change distinctly. This procedure should use high-field imagers supplied with dedicated surface coils. Considerably higher spatial resolution (especially lower slice thickness) is necessary, but the time involved for imaging is much less important because no breathhold imaging is required. Thus, an adequate number of excitations or three-dimensional (gradient echo) imaging can be chosen to ensure a good SNR, so imaging protocols with a spatial resolution similar to diagnostic breast imaging (matrix, 256×256 or 256×512; slice thickness, ≤ 4 mm) can be used.[23–26] Decreasing slice thickness and increasing spatial resolution are favorable for passive needle visualization (provided that a sufficient SNR is obtained). The slight reduction of artifact size (resulting from lower slice thickness and, possibly, promoted by applying a three-dimensional technique) is favorable in cases of large artifacts; nevertheless, the visibility of small artifacts is increased because of the higher resolution and the reduced partial volume effect (see Fig. 14-4). For this resolution, therefore, an artifact width of 2 to 5 mm appears optimal (if possible, not greater than 8 mm). With use of a matrix of 256×256, a FOV of 25 to 30 cm, and 4-mm slices, the visibility becomes critical or insufficient at an artifact width less than 2 mm.)

However, achieving similar narrow artifacts of the desirable size may be difficult on a high-field scanner, because high field strength will be combined with a large needle angle to B_0 of 90°, as a rule. Therefore, titanium needles of 18 to 20 G or thin nonferromagnetic steel needles of 20 to 22 G are preferred. If applying a gradient echo, a very short echo time and high bandwidth should be chosen. Alternatively, T1-weighted spin- or turbo spin-echo sequences can be used (see Fig. 14-4). Nevertheless, an artifact width larger than desirable is to be expected in many cases, so it may often be problematic to hit breast lesions smaller than 1 cm in diameter. With use of spin- or turbo spin-echo sequences, the artifact width can be drastically reduced by arranging the orientation of the frequency-encoding gradient parallel to the needle; however, the visibility of needle artifact may become critical or insufficient.

Generally, in most cases, the position of the needle tip does not exactly correspond with the tip position of the needle artifact in MRI. The tip of the needle artifact may be depicted a few millimeters deeper within the tissue than the actual position of the needle tip depending on field strength, needle diameter, alloy, and imaging protocol.[10]

In conclusion, passive needle visualization for puncture and biopsy is predominantly relevant for low-field imagers. Although passive visualization strategies are also practical for high-field magnets, the opportunities to control artifact size appear more favorable for low-field magnets, especially in cases of large-core biopsies. Moreover, considering the advantageous access to the patient in open low-field magnets and the relatively low costs, passive needle visualization is valuable because no further expensive equipment is required. Thus, for image-guided needle puncture and biopsy, passive visualization on low-field magnets has become a practical alternative to other modes of image guidance.

REFERENCES

1. Mueller PR, and others: MR-guided aspiration biopsy: needle design and clinical trials, *Radiology* 161:605, 1986.
2. Lufkin R, Teresi L, Hanafee W: New needle for MR-guided aspiration cytology of the head and neck, *Am J Roentgenol* 149:380, 1987.
3. Lufkin R, and others: A technique for MR-guided needle placement, *Am J Roentgenol* 151:193, 1988.
4. Lufkin R, Layfield L: Coaxial needle system of MR- and CT-guided aspiration cytology, *J Comput Assist Tomogr* 13:1105, 1989.
5. van Sonnenberg E, and others: A wire-sheath system for MR-guided biopsy and drainage: laboratory studies and experience in 10 patients, *Am J Roentgenol* 151:815, 1987.
6. Duckwiler G, and others: Head and neck lesions: MR-guided aspiration biopsy, *Radiology* 170:519, 1989.
7. Wesbey G, Edelman RR, Harris R: *Artifacts in MR-imaging: description, causes, and solutions.* In Edelman RR, Hesselink JR, editors: *Clinical magnetic resonance imaging,* Philadelphia, 1990, WB Saunders.
8. Moscatel MA, Shellock FG, Morisoli SM: Biopsy needles and devices: assessment of ferromagnetism and artifacts during exposure to a 1.5-T MR system, *J Magn Reson Imaging* 5:369, 1995.
9. Frahm C, and others: Visualization of magnetic resonance-compatible needles at 1.5 and 0.2 Tesla, *Cardiovasc Intervent Radiol* 19:335, 1996.
10. Lewin JS, and others: Needle localization in MR-guided biopsy and aspiration: effects of field strength, sequence design, and magnetic field orientation, *Am J Roentgenol* 166:1337, 1996.
11. Ladd ME, and others: Biopsy needle susceptibility artifacts, *Magn Reson Med* 36:646, 1996.
12. Schenck JF: The role of magnetic susceptibility in magnetic resonance imaging: MRI magnetic compatibility of the first and second kinds, *Med Phys* 23:815, 1996.
13. Lüdeke KM, Röschmann P, Tischler R: Susceptibility artifacts in NMR imaging, *Magn Reson Med* 3:329, 1985.
14. Silverman SG, and others: Interactive MR-guided biopsy in an open-configuration MR imaging system, *Radiology* 197:175, 1995.

15. Frahm C, Gehl HB, Weiss HD: *MR-guided drainage and biopsy of upper abdominal lesions: first experiences using an open low-field scanner.* In *Book of abstracts,* Nice, 1995, Proceedings of the Society of Magnetic Resonance, 3rd Scientific Meeting and Exhibition.
16. Frahm C, and others: Technik der MRT-gesteuerten Stanzbiopsie im Abdomen an einem offenen Niederfeldgerät: Durchführbarkeit und erste klinische Ergebnisse, *Rofo Fortschr Geb Rontgenstr Neuen Bildgeb Verfahr* 164:62, 1996.
17. Frahm C, Gehl HB, Weiss HD: *MR-guided core biopsy of upper abdominal and pelvic lesions: results in 18 patients.* In *Book of abstracts,* New York, 1996, Proceedings of the International Society for Magnetic Resonance in Medicine, 4th Scientific Meeting and Exhibition.
18. Gehl HB, and others: Technik der MRT-gesteuerten abdominellen Drainage an einem offenen Niederfeldmagneten: Durchführbarkeit und erste ergebnisse, *Rofo Forstschr Geb Rontgenstr Neuen Bildgeb Verfahr* 165:70, 1996.
19. Lewin JS, and others: *Interactive MRI for procedure guidance on a clinical c-arm system: a pilot biopsy study.* In *Book of abstracts,* New York, 1996, Proceedings of the International Society for Magnetic Resonance in Medicine, 4th Scientific Meeting and Exhibition.
20. Steiner P, and others: Interaktive stereotaktische Interventionen im supraleitenden, offenen 0,5-Tesla-MR-Tomographen, *Rofo Fortschr Geb Rontgenstr Neuen Bildgeb Verfahr* 165:276, 1996.
21. Steiner P, and others: Active biplanar MR tracking for biopsies in humans, *Am J Roentgenol* 169:735, 1997.
22. Lu DSK, and others: Biopsy of hepatic dome lesions: semi-real-time coronal MR guidance technique, *Am J Roentgenol* 168:737, 1997.
23. Heywang-Köbrunner SH, and others: Prototype breast coil for MR-guided needle localization, *J Comput Assist Tomogr* 18:876, 1994.
24. Fischer U, and others: MR-guided biopsy of suspect breast lesions with a simple stereotaxic add-on device for surface coils, *Radiology* 192:272, 1994.
25. Orel SG, and others: MR imaging-guided localization and biopsy of breast lesions: initial experience, *Radiology* 193:97, 1994.
26. Döler W, and others: Stereotaxic add-on device for MR-guided biopsy of breast lesions, *Radiology* 200:863, 1996.

Chapter 15

PASSIVE ENDOLUMINAL TRACKING APPROACHES FOR ENDOVASCULAR INTERVENTIONAL MRI

Henk F.M. Smits, Chris J.G. Bakker

Magnetic resonance imaging (MRI) has several features that make it attractive for guiding endovascular interventions. Compared with conventional x-ray fluoroscopy, MRI offers superior soft-tissue contrast and free selection of scan planes without the need to reposition the patient. It displays vessels without administration of contrast agents and does not use ionizing radiation or other harmful agents. MRI is, therefore, safer than x-ray imaging techniques for the patient and medical staff. In addition, MRI provides anatomic information and can provide functional and metabolic information.

Exploitation of the capabilities of MR with regard to endovascular interventions requires appropriate visualization of devices. Three strategies have been advocated far this task: viz active tracking,[1–3] locally induced field inhomogeneities,[4–6] and passive tracking by visualizing a device on the basis of its associated susceptibility artifacts.[7,8] This chapter discusses the development of suitable devices, scan techniques, and processing and display facilities for passive tracking.

The chapter provides a brief summary of susceptibility and radiofrequency (RF) phenomena pertinent to passive visualization, followed by an overview of current developments with regard to MR-dedicated endoluminal devices. Scan techniques and processing tools for providing near real-time positional feedback of interventional instruments are discussed. Some results obtained with passive tracking are reported, and future developments and perspectives are discussed.

SUSCEPTIBILITY AND RADIOFREQUENCY ARTIFACTS IN MAGNETIC RESONANCE

Definitions

Soon after the introduction of MRI in clinical practice, alien objects were recognized to cause susceptibility artifacts. Magnetic susceptibility is a quantitative measure of a material's tendency to interact with and distort an applied magnetic field.[9] The presence of paramagnetic or ferromagnetic particles in the main magnetic field causes a local magnetic field around these particles, disturbing the homogeneity of the main magnetic field. Because MRI is based on the fact that the NMR resonant frequency is proportional to the magnetic field intensity, any perturbation of the assumed field distribution will cause mismapping of the signals in the frequency-encoding direction and will lead to geometrically distorted images. In addition, local field gradients induce signal losses as a result of intravoxel dephasing.

Findings in the literature

Several publications have investigated the visibility of guidewires and catheters in MRI.[10,11] The observed artifacts depend on multiple imaging parameters and on the orientation of the device with respect to the main magnetic field. With regard to endovascular applications, standard guidewires and catheters,[11–13] balloon catheters,[14] cava filters,[15] and endovascular stents[16–18] have been evaluated as to their disturbance of and visibility in MRIs and angiograms and as to their compatibility with and safety in the MR environment. Some materials pose certain risks because of MRI's hostility for metallic devices.[19] Some metallic devices were heated in the MR scanner because of the rapidly changing RF field,[20] and severe skin burns have been reported. Most standard guidewires have a stainless steel core and are forcefully drawn into the magnet (Fig. 15-1). They also produce large susceptibility artifacts (Fig. 15-2).[15,21,22] Most catheters are braided with thin stainless steel wires for strength and torque control. Because of this braiding, these catheters also give large artifacts. Plastic nonbraided catheters however, cause no artifacts at all, and, because they have such a small cross section, cannot be seen with ultrafast MRI sequences.[12] Some nonbraided balloon catheters are clearly visible because of a local susceptibility artifact caused by tantalum balloon markers.[23] Some cava filters are nonferromagnetic and can theoretically be placed under MR guidance, but they give such a strong susceptibility artifact that the exact position of the stent cannot be determined. Other materials, such as nickel titanium alloy (nitinol), produce no or hardly any susceptibility artifacts and are thus barely visible.[15] However, they cause RF artifacts,[24] visible as noise on the image (Fig. 15-3), and gross intensity distortions. Endovascular stents have been imaged in the deployed mode. The have a very diverse and inconstant appearance (Fig. 15-4).[18]

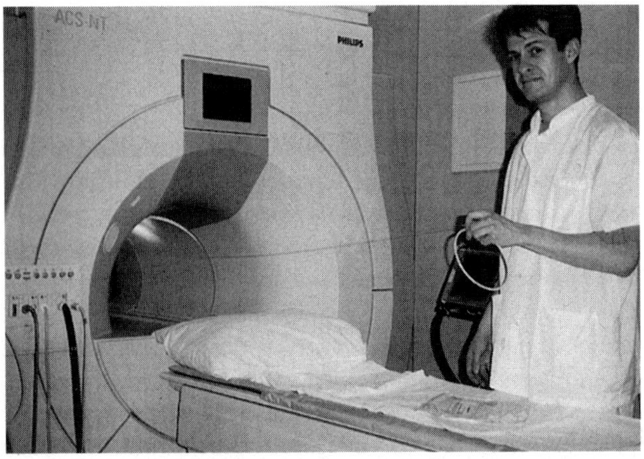

Fig. 15-1. A standard 0.035-inch stainless steel core guidewire is held by its end and forcefully drawn into the scanner. Its use would present a safety risk to the patient. (Courtesy of R. Springorum; with permission.)

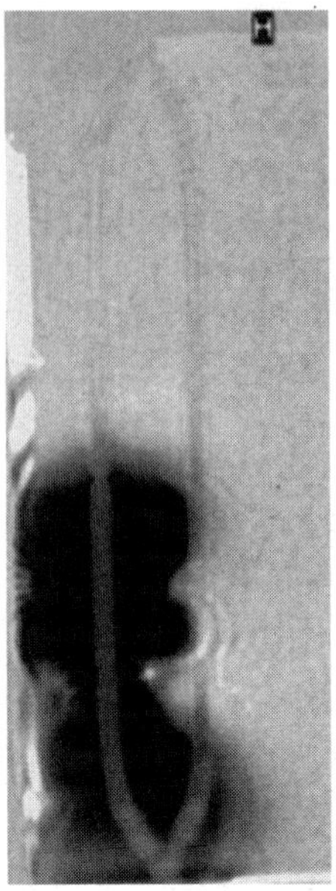

Fig. 15-2. Large susceptibility artifact of a standard 0.035-inch stainless steel core guidewire.

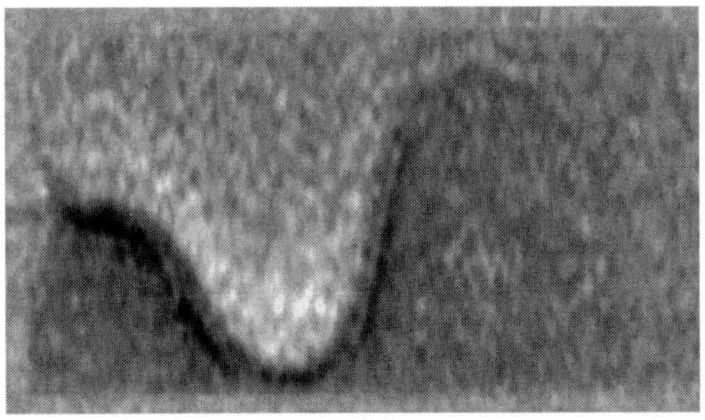

Fig. 15-3. Radiofrequency artifact caused by a standard 0.035-inch nickel titanium alloy guidewire.

A

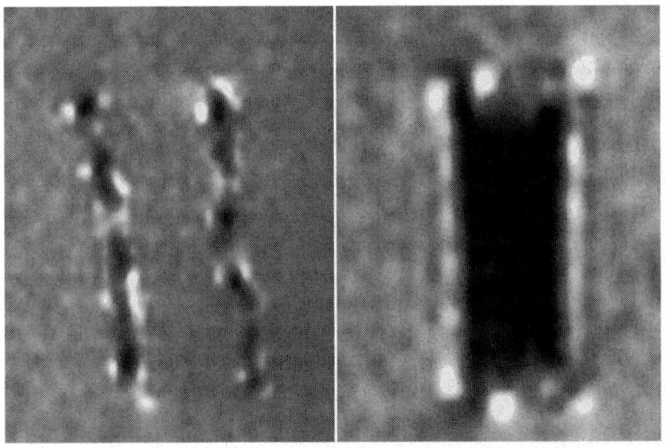

B

Fig. 15-4. **A**, Nickel titanium alloy stent oriented along B_0 reveals mild susceptibility artifacts. **B**, A stent made of a different alloy of nickel titanium oriented along B_0 reveals mild susceptibility artifacts; however, signal void is present inside the stent because of radiofrequency shielding.

Parameters affecting the appearance of susceptibility artifacts

The appearance of susceptibility artifacts depends on the magnetic properties of the object, on the object's orientation within the magnetic field, and on the imaging technique used.[9,25–27] Usually, the artifact is visible as a dark area of signal void on the MR image. Susceptibility artifacts increase with higher field strength and tend to be more severe for gradient echo than for spin-echo sequences. The artifacts also increase with longer echo times and smaller receiver bandwidths. Typically, the severity of susceptibility artifacts strongly depends on the orientation of the paramagnetic substance to B_o. Aligned with B_o, the artifact is minimal. When perpendicular to B_o, the artifact becomes maximal. This orientational dependency of susceptibility artifacts is shown in Figure 15-5. In contrast, the susceptibility artifact of a small dot of paramagnetic substance does not depend on its orientation to B_o (Fig. 15-6). The field of a paramagnetic material appears as a horizontally oriented biconcave linear structure with two teardrops perpendicular to its center (Fig. 15-7).

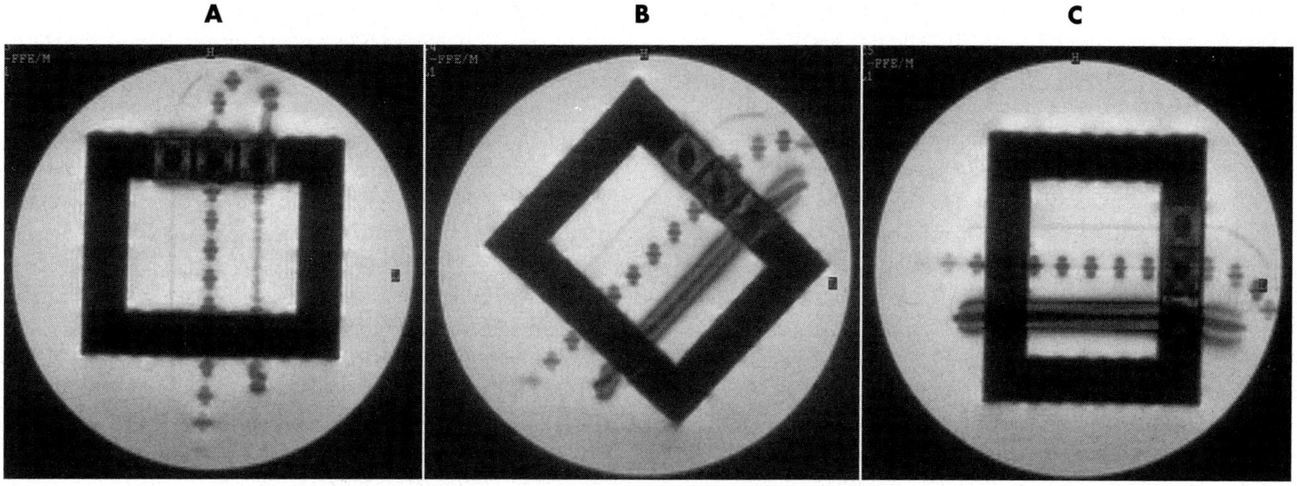

Fig. 15-5. Three catheters in water at various rotations: **A,** parallel to B_o; **B,** 45° to B_o; and **C,** 90° to B_o. A plain catheter, a catheter with ring markers, and a catheter uniformly doped with a paramagnetic substance; B_o is along the Z (vertical) axis. Aligned with B_o, the uniformly doped catheter is barely visible, but the susceptibility artifact becomes large perpendicular to B_o. The ring markers are consistent.

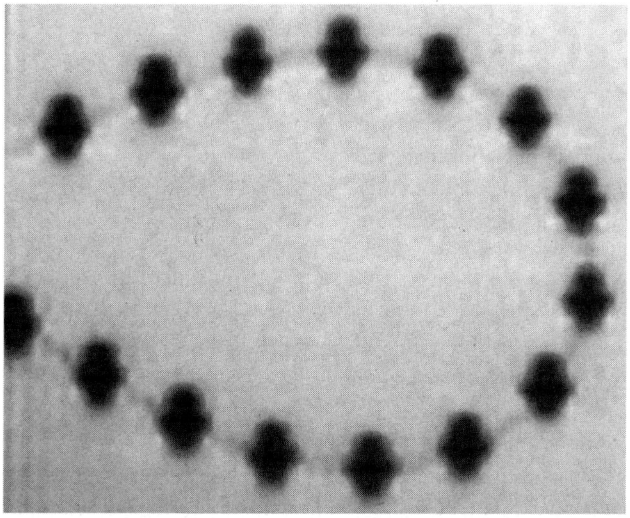

Fig. 15-6. A fiberoptic guidewire is prepared with dysprosium marker rings. The orientation of the main magnetic field is vertical. The presentation of the artifact is independent of the orientation to B_o.

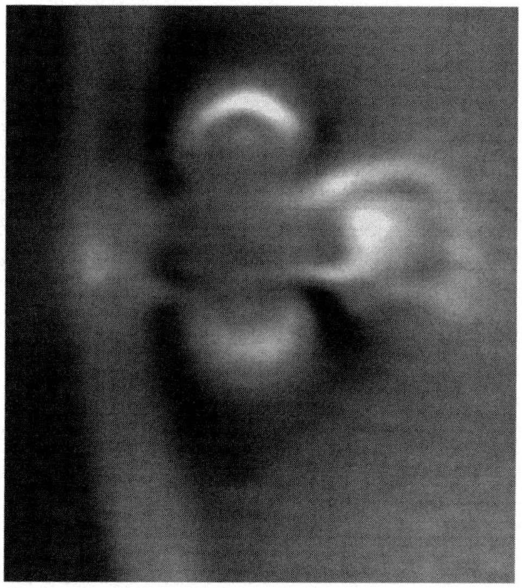

Fig. 15-7. Gradient echo image shows the typical shape of the artifact of a dot-shaped amount of paramagnetic substance in an external static field B_o.

MAGNETIC RESONANCE–DEDICATED DEVICES

Recently, testing of standard devices was determined to be an ineffective way to develop appropriate devices for MR-guided endovascular interventions. Dedicated MR devices had to be developed that were safe and consistently well-visualized with consistent visualization. Moreover, it was realized that susceptibility artifacts not only produce image degradation but also constitute a source of information. These realizations led to the conscious application of paramagnetic substances to achieve visualization of MR devices.

Definitions

When undergoing an MR-guided procedure, the patient should be excluded from any dangers or harm, especially in reference to devices. According to the United States Food and Drug Administration, the term *MR safe* indicates that the device, when used in the MR environment, presents no additional risk to the patient; however, it may affect the quality of the diagnostic information. The term *MR compatible* refers to a device that, when used in the MR environment, is MR safe and has been shown to neither significantly affect the quality of the diagnostic information nor be affected by the MR device. A device can be MR compatible with one scanner but not with another scanner.[28] To be defined as *MR dedicated*, a device must be MR safe, may not provoke image degradation (MR compatible), and should be well-seen in MRIs with consistent appearance. These issues govern the choice of materials for developing MR-dedicated devices.

Materials for magnetic resonance–dedicated devices

Guidewires

The MR environment is very hostile toward ferromagnetic materials, which should thus be avoided. This drawback is problematic for the development of guidewires, which usually have a stainless steel core to assure robustness and torque control. Simple plastic wires are too floppy and have unsatisfactory torque control. They have unsatisfactory pushability and too much whip (the tendency to rotate 360° after a certain amount of torque, caused by the accumulation of energy in the material itself). Fiber optics may be an alternative for the core of a guidewire.[17] Construction of a fiberoptic guidewire with excellent torque and without the risks associated with the introduction of conductive materials is possible.[29] For passive visualization, incorporation of paramagnetic markers seems to be promising. Dysprosium oxide, similar to gadolinium, has high magnetic susceptibility and can readily be incorporated in the plastic shaft of catheters or wires. A dysprosium oxide concentration of 10% (by weight), a ring length of 1 mm, and an interspacing of 10 to 20 mm gave satisfactory results in phantom experiments[7] and preliminary volunteer work.[8]

Catheters

Development of MR-dedicated balloon catheters is not difficult. Most standard balloon catheters are nonbraided and are simply adapted to the needs of susceptibility-based visualization by placing paramagnetic markers in the wall of the balloon catheter. The position of the markers is preferably just outside the balloon to avoid camouflage of the balloon lumen by the signal void of the markers. For optimal visualization, a balloon is inflated with gadolinium-doped water. Before determining the optimal concentration for inflation of the balloon, one should identify the circumstances in which the balloon will be deployed. With a subtraction technique, the contrast between the contents of the vessel and the balloon should be maximal, not the contrast between the vessel environment and the contents of balloon. For direct visualization of the balloon, a concentration of 2% to 5% gadolinium in water gives the highest signal intensities in the inflated balloon. To get a dark balloon, it should be inflated with more concentrated gadolinium.

Standard introducer sheaths can be provided with a distal MR marker to immediately recognize dislocation of the sheath as long as the tip is within the field of view (FOV). For interventional MR procedures, the patient is typically situated in the bore of the magnet. Depending on the region of interest, the patient is more or less covered by the magnet. A sheath extension device, which covers the distance between the standard sheath and the position of the radiologist outside the bore, can be helpful.

In addition to MR-dedicated devices, many small surgical tools and additional equipment should be MR safe. Most indeflators contain few screws or coils that are ferromagnetic. The Encore indeflator (Boston Scientific, Boston, Mass) is completely inert to the strong magnetic field.

DEDICATED SCAN TECHNIQUES FOR PASSIVE TRACKING

The pulse sequence of choice should image the susceptibility artifact well. Gradient echo techniques are well-known for their sensitivity to susceptibility artifacts. To enable a paramagnetic marker to produce a signal void, the chosen pulse sequence should produce high signal intensities inside the vessel lumen and in the direct surroundings of the vessel. The latter is necessary because the susceptibility artifact can measure up to 7 mm, giving a void partially outside of the vessel lumen. The relative signal intensity can be influenced by the chosen flip angle.

In passive tracking, a new image is required each time new information about the actual position of the device is requested, so acquisition time should be short. Three-dimensional (3D) angiographic sequences are too time-consuming and should be made before the introduction of the devices. The angiogram serves as a road map. The endovascular intervention can be guided by dynamic 2D gradient echo techniques.[29] The endovascular position of devices can be monitored by on-line subtraction and overlay techniques. Measures to increase tracking speed include a reduced FOV[30,31] and keyhole imaging.[32] Use of subtraction allows reduction of the FOV to a greater extent because artifacts caused by aliasing are subtracted. Moving structures outside the FOV but within the area of image wraparound are not subtracted and should be avoided (e.g., bowel movement), which can be achieved with a deliberate choice of image plane. To track the device through tortuous vessels, a relatively thick slice is preferred. With a standard gradient capability of 15 mT/m, a field strength of 1.5 T, a reconstruction time of 0.1 sec per 256 × 256 image, a repetition time of 15 msec, an echo time of 9 msec, an FOV of 128 × 256 mm, a matrix of 128 × 256, a flip angle of 10°, and first-order flow compensation, imaging times of 0.5 sec are possible.[29]

POSTPROCESSING AND DISPLAY

For MR-guided interventions, images should be displayed in the MR suite with minimal delay time (i.e., the time between end of acquisition and display in the scanning room).

The delay time should be added to the scan time, resulting in MR fluoroscopy with a refresh rate of one frame per 1 to 2 sec (assuming a delay time of 0.5 sec). Thus, the guidewires can be negotiated through created stenoses in phantoms and balloon catheters can be positioned properly.[29] For most clinical indications, however, a tracking speed of 1 frame per second is probably insufficient, and faster scan techniques should be developed. Fast scan techniques, such as radial scanning and spiral scanning, are promising, but their use for interventional MR should be evaluated. With the subtraction technique, the markers of the device are very well visualized; however, the vessel contour and the

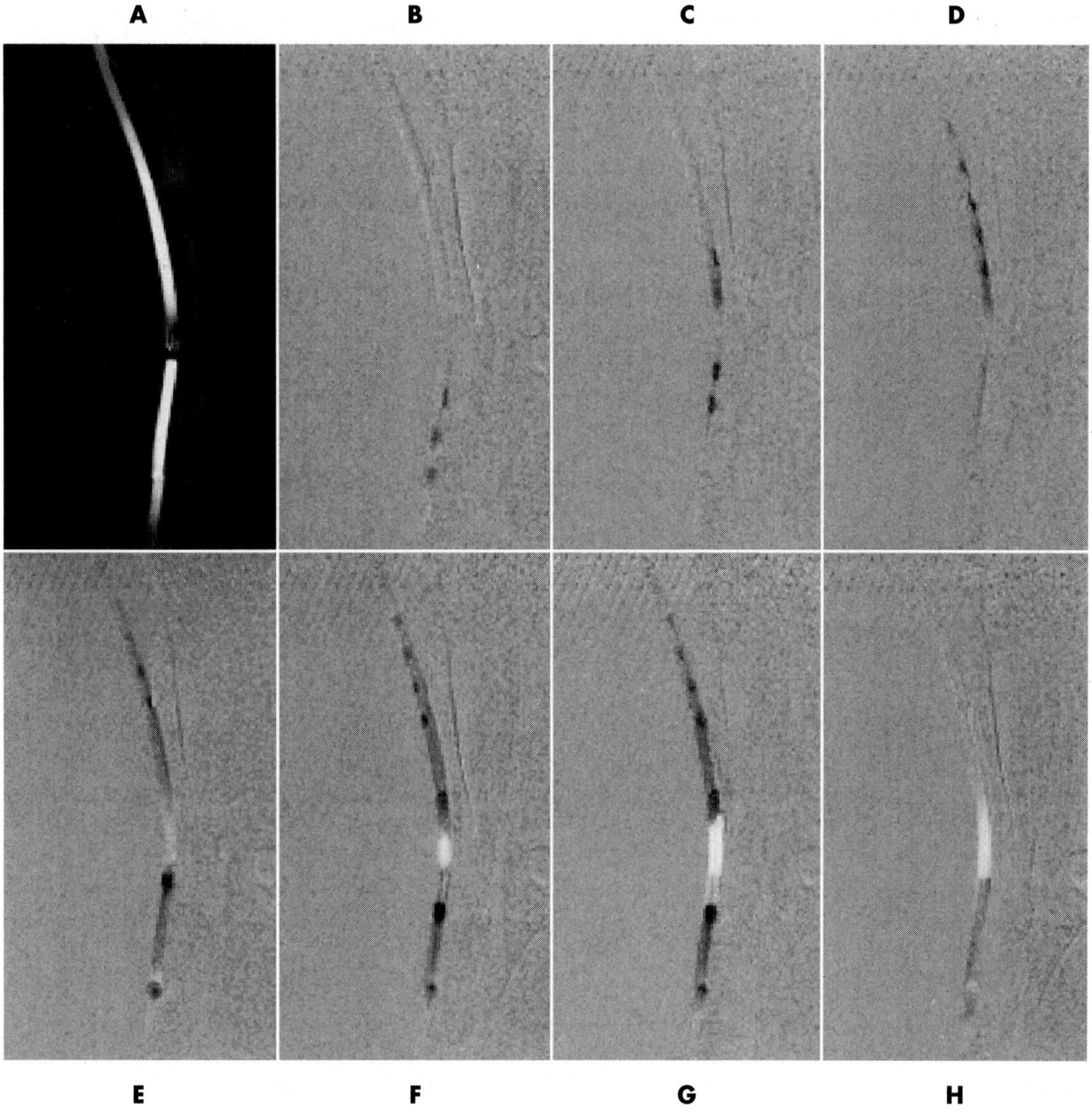

Fig. 15-8. Eight selected frames from a balloon angioplasty procedure in a flow phantom with a dilatable stenosis: **A**, A two-dimensional phase contrast angiogram shows the signal void caused by the stenosis. **B** to **D**, The fiberoptic guidewire (five dysprosium rings 30% by weight, interspacing 16 mm, near the tip 8 mm) is negotiated through the stenosis. A balloon catheter (6 mm, 4 cm) is **E**, introduced and **F**, positioned over the stenosis. **G**, The balloon is inflated with gadolinium-doped water; the stenosis is dilated and the devices are withdrawn. **H**, The disappearance of the void causes a bright spot.

location of the stenoses are subtracted. Projection of the markers onto a previously acquired angiogram results in a tool equal to the road map in the angiosuite. This overlay technique indicates the position of the markers of the device with respect to the vasculature.

To display the dynamic images with subtraction and overlay techniques in the MR suite, fast and powerful computers and sophisticated software are necessary. For display in the MR suite, data should be transported via fiberoptics into the suite, where they can be displayed on liquid crystal display screens. The time consumed by these postprocessing tools should be added to the latency.

DISCUSSION AND FUTURE PROSPECTS

With recent evolution of MR technology, MR fluoroscopy has become reality. MR-guided endovascular interventions are a topic of research focusing on visualization of MR-dedicated devices. With susceptibility-based passive tracking, consistent visualization of MR-dedicated fiberoptic guidewires and polyethylene catheters in near real-time 2D gradient echo images is feasible. The paramagnetic markers clearly show up in dynamic subtraction images. Visualization of the markers with respect to the vessels of interest is readily achieved with overlay techniques by mapping these subtraction images onto a previously acquired angiogram. In this manner, the entire interventional procedure—from the introduction and placement of a guidewire to the positioning of a catheter across the stenosis—the inflation of the balloon, and the dilation of the stenotic region can be performed under MR guidance (Fig. 15-8). One advantage of doing this procedure under MR guidance is that the intervention's effects can be assessed immediately by MR angiography and MR flow measurements.

Results reported so far are restricted to phantom experiments and animal studies. Before MR-guided vascular interventions can be introduced in clinical practice, some items need further attention. A complete armamentarium of MR-dedicated interventional devices should be developed. The steerability of fiberoptic guidewires should be improved to make them appropriate and safe for clinical application. Development of MR-dedicated stents and delivery systems should be initiated, with attention to safety aspects. Performing complex procedures in the MR suite introduces persons, materials, and equipment in the MR suite, which can be dangerous for the patient. Staff members should be well-trained, and equipment should be thoroughly tested before use in the MR environment. Current MR equipment that has been designed for optimal image quality should be transformed into a system with sufficient image quality but maximum flexibility. Flexibility can be enhanced with interactive scan parameter modification during scanning and intermittent execution of MR fluoroscopy, angiography, or flow measurements.[33] Manufacturers should create a silent scanner: what is the use of avoiding radiation risks if it is traded for the risk of hearing loss? Another issue is the development of faster scan techniques and faster reconstruction algorithms providing shorter latency times. With stronger gradient capabilities, repetition times of 5 msec are possible, resulting in a substantial reduction of acquisition time. Postprocessing should include motion compensation techniques to reduce gross motion artifacts; with computed marker detection, determination of the spatial position of the device may be possible, which can steer image acquisition. Interventional MR will benefit from further maturation of functional tests. The evolution of functional MR will help determine the clinical applications of vascular interventional MR.

For some clinical applications, passive tracking seems to offer a feasible solution that can be performed on a standard modern MR scanner with few restrictions concerning safety issues.

REFERENCES

1. Ackerman JL, and others: *Rapid 3D tracking of small RF coils.* In *Book of abstracts,* Montreal, 1986, Society of Magnetic Resonance in Medicine, 5th Annual Meeting.
2. Dumoulin CL, Souza SP, Darrow RD: Real-time position monitoring of invasive devices using magnetic resonance, *Magn Reson Med* 29:411, 1993.
3. Leung DA, and others: Intravascular MR tracking catheter: preliminary experimental evaluation, *Am J Roentgenol* 164:1265, 1995.
4. Frahm C, and others: *Passive visualization: a suitable approach for MR-guided vascular interventions in low-field systems? In vivo evaluation of a new guide wire.* In *Book of abstracts,* Vancouver, 1997, International Society for Magnetic Resonance in Medicine, 5th Scientific Meeting and Exhibition.
5. Glowinski A, and others: Catheter visualization using locally induced, actively controlled field inhomogeneities, *Magn Reson Med* 38:253, 1997.
6. Sonderegger M, Dohi T: *MagTip: a catheter visible in the MRI, CAR.* In Lemke HU, and others, editors: *Proceedings of the International Symposium on Computer and Communication Systems for Image Guided Diagnosis and Therapy,* Paris, 1996, Elsevier Science.
7. Bakker CJG, and others: Visualization of dedicated catheters using fast scanning techniques with potential for MR-guided vascular interventions, *Magn Reson Med* 36:816, 1996.
8. Bakker CJG, and others: MR-guided endovascular interventions: susceptibility-based catheter and near-real-time imaging technique, *Radiology* 202:273, 1997.
9. Schenck JF: The role of magnetic susceptibility in magnetic resonance imaging: MRI magnetic compatibility of the first and second kinds, *Med Phys* 23:815, 1996.
10. McKinnon GC, and others: *Towards visible guide wire antennas for interventional MRI.* In *Book of abstracts,* San Francisco, 1994, International Society of Magnetic Resonance in Medicine, 2nd Annual Meeting.
11. Koechli VD, and others: Vascular interventions guided by ultrafast imaging: evaluation of different materials, *Magn Reson Med* 31:309, 1994.
12. Rubin DL, Ratner AV, Young SW: Magnetic susceptibility effects and their application in the development of new ferromagnetic catheters for magnetic resonance imaging, *Invest Radiol* 25:1325, 1990.
13. Lenz G, Drobnitzky M, Dewey DH: *MR-visible catheters for intra-vascular interventional MRI procedures.* In *Book of abstracts,* New York, 1996, International Society of Magnetic Resonance in Medicine, 4th Scientific Meeting and Exhibition.
14. Gmitro AF, Ehsani AR, Yee DC: *Real-time MRI guided balloon angioplasty.* In *Book of abstracts,* Vancouver, 1997, International Society of Magnetic Resonance in Medicine, 5th Scientific Meeting and Exhibition.
15. Teitelbaum GP, Bradley WG, Klein BD: MR imaging artifacts, ferromagnetism, and magnetic torque of intravascular filters, stents, and coils, *Radiology* 166:657, 1988.
16. Matsumoto AH, and others: Tantalum vascular stents: in vivo evaluation with MR imaging, *Radiology* 170:753, 1989.
17. Stroman PW, and others: Will it be feasible to insert endoprostheses under interventional MRI? *J Endovasc Surg* 3:396, 1996.

18. Olree M, and others: MRI of endovascular stents: in vitro analysis of imaging artifacts, *Cardiovasc Intervent Radiol* 20:60, 1997.
19. Lufkin R, and others: Interventional magnetic resonance imaging in the head and neck, *Top Magn Reson Imaging* 2:76, 1990.
20. Shellock FG, Slimp G: Severe burns of the finger caused by using a pulse oximeter during MRI, *Am J Roentgenol* 153:1105, 1989.
21. Girard MJ, and others: Wallstent metallic biliary endoprosthesis: MR imaging characteristics, *Radiology* 184:874, 1992.
22. Moscatel MA, Shellock FG, Morisoli SM: Biopsy needles and devices: assessment of ferromagnetism and artifacts during exposure to a 1.5-T MR system, *J Magn Reson Imaging* 5:369, 1995.
23. Yee DC, Roach DJ, Gmitro AF: Real-time MR imaging for vascular interventions, Radiological Society of Northern America, 82nd Scientific Assembly and Annual Meeting, Chicago, *Radiology* 210:376, 1996.
24. Camacho CR, Plewes DB, Henkelman RM: Nonsusceptibility artifacts due to metallic objects in MR imaging, *J Magn Reson Imaging* 5:75, 1995.
25. Bakker CJG, and others: Simulation of susceptibility artifacts in 2D and 3D Fourier transform spin-echo and gradient-echo magnetic resonance imaging, *Magn Reson Imaging* 12:767, 1994.
26. Bakker CJG, and others: Parameters affecting the appearance of susceptibility artifacts in magnetic resonance imaging, 9th European Congress of Radiology, Vienna, *Eur J Radiol* 5:399, 1995.
27. Farahani K, and others: Effect of field strength on susceptibility artifacts in magnetic resonance imaging, *Comput Med Imaging Graph* 6:409, 1990.
28. Silverman SG, and others: Design and implementation of an interventional MR imaging suite, *Am J Roentgenol* 168:1465, 1997.
29. Bakker CJG, and others: MR-guided balloon angioplasty: in vitro demonstration of the potential of MRI for guiding, monitoring and evaluating endovascular interventions, *J Magn Reson Imaging* 8:245, 1998.
30. Fredrickson JO, Pelc NJ: Temporal resolution improvement in dynamic imaging, *Magn Reson Med* 35:621, 1996.
31. Hu X, Parrish T: Reduction of field of view for dynamic imaging, *Magn Reson Med* 31:691, 1994.
32. Van Vaals JJ, and others: `Keyhole' method for accelerating imaging of contrast agent uptake, *J Magn Reson Imaging* 3:671, 1993.
33. Holsinger AE, and others: Real-time interactive magnetic resonance imaging, *Magn Reson Med* 14:547, 1990.

Chapter 16

ACTIVE TRACKING OF INTERVENTIONAL DEVICES

Charles L. Dumoulin

Although magnetic resonance imaging (MRI) is a well-established diagnostic method, use during therapeutic procedures is only beginning.[1–6] If MR is to become a viable interventional modality, several issues will have to be addressed and overcome, including patient access, patient monitoring, MR compatibility of therapeutic devices, and the need for real-time visualization of interventional devices.

Passive and active methods have been proposed for following the location of invasive devices (e.g., catheters, biopsy needles, endoscopes) in an MR scanner. Passive methods use MRI for visualizing a device within the patient and can usually be performed without additional scanner hardware.[7–9] Active visualization methods, on the other hand, require the creation of a signal, which is emitted or detected by the device. One method of active visualization uses light as the locating signal.[10] However, because the body is not transparent, optical methods can be applied only outside the body; devices inside the body should be fixed to external optical markers.

Active tracking of devices using radiofrequency (RF) signals has also been described.[11,12] RF tracking is not restricted to rigid devices because an RF signal can be easily carried over a flexible cable in the device. Although optical and RF tracking methods can be used in an MR scanner, both techniques require calibrated mapping of tracking coordinates into MRI coordinates because geometric distortions in an MRI scan are unrelated to the geometric distortion in optical or RF tracking coordinate space.

Active visualization methods using MR signals are being used for clinical interventions at a few sites. With MR-based methods, MR signals are collected and used to determine device locations. Signals can be detected along the length of the device[13] or with small receiver coils built into the device.[14,15] MR-based tracking uses the same instrumentation and physical phenomena as MRI and thus can be well registered with an MRI scan. Unlike most MRI, however, MR tracking can be performed at rates as high as 20 frames per second over the entire three-dimensional (3D) volume of the patient.

OPTICAL TRACKING OF INTERVENTIONAL DEVICES

Several device tracking systems using optical emitters and sensors are commercially available, and at least one has been

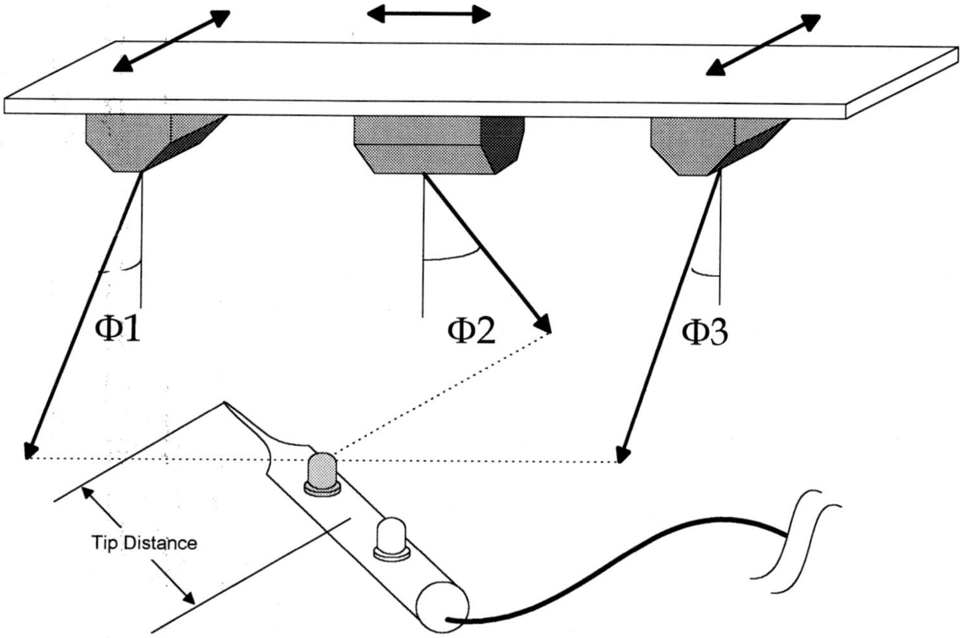

Fig. 16-1. An optical tracking system uses three linear detectors spaced apart on a bar suspended over the work area. Infrared light-emitting diodes (LEDs) on a probe sequentially light up and are detected by the sensors. The three measured angles Φ1, Φ2, and Φ3 are sufficient to locate the LED in three-dimensional space. When the location of the second LED is measured, the orientation of the probe can be determined and the location of the probe tip calculated.

used extensively with an MRI system.[10] Active optical tracking systems use one or more light-emitting diodes (LEDs), which typically operate in the infrared spectrum. These LEDs are tracked with an array of sensors near the working volume of the procedure. Typically, the optical tracking system controller activates one LED at a time. While the LED is illuminated, the sensors determine its location within their field of view (FOV). Locations from multiple sensors are triangulated to obtain the 3D location of the activated LED. In one implementation (Fig. 16-1), three linear arrays placed on a rigid bar over the working region are used to determine three deflection angles (as viewed from three locations). In a different implementation, two or more infrared-sensitive cameras simultaneously measure two deflection angles each.

Because an infrared-emitting diode is a point source, an optical tracking system can determine only the position of a device having a single emitter, not the device's orientation. However, full position and orientation information can be determined if three LEDs are arranged on the device in a triangular fashion.

Optical tracking systems operating in an MR scanner are fully functional at all times, even during MRI acquisition. They can also track devices over relatively large volumes, potentially covering regions inside and outside the MR scanner. A major limitation of optical tracking, however, is that a clear visual path must be maintained between the sensor and the LEDs. Consequently, the tracked device must be carefully positioned and manipulated so that neither the operator nor the patient obscures the LEDs. Because of the need to maintain a line-of-sight path between each LED and the sensor array, optical tracking of a device internal to the patient can occur only if a rigid geometric relationship exists between the LEDs and the portions of the device inside the body. Optical tracking of biopsy needles is one application in which such a geometric constraint can sometimes be assumed, but deflection of the needle should always be considered as a possible source of positional error.

TRACKING USING ELECTROMAGNETIC FIELDS

Tracking interventional devices using RF electromagnetic fields has several attractive aspects. Variations of this technology have been used to follow 3D pointers[16] and, more recently, to place catheters in the ventricles of the heart.[17] Although RF tracking shows great promise, it has not yet been shown in clinical applications on MR scanners.

RF tracking uses low-frequency electromagnetic fields broadcast from a set of transmitter coils and detected by one or more receiver coils. The RF fields used for tracking are independent of the RF fields used for MRI, and the coils built into the interventional device can act as the transmitter or receiver. In principle, measurement of the strength of the detected magnetic field helps determine the location and orientation of the receiver coils if the position of the transmitter coils is known. Conversely, the position of the transmitter coils can be determined if the position and orientation of the receiver coils are known.

RF tracking systems use very low-frequency signals (typically less than 10 kHz or, in some cases, a pulsed direct current

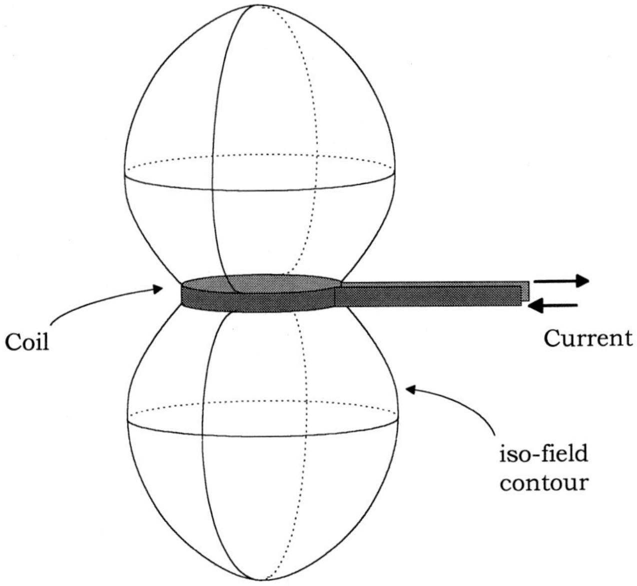

Fig. 16-2. An isofield contour is generated by passing electrical current through a circular coil.

(DC) field). At these frequencies, the wavelength is so long that only near-field effects need be considered. Although many geometric system designs are possible, a simple system might use three transmitting RF coils at known locations, which broadcast their signals one at a time. The magnetic fields created by these transmitting coils are detected by a set of receiving coils embedded in the interventional device.

As current flows in each transmitting coil, a magnetic field is generated. This magnetic field has a dipole geometry (Fig. 16-2). A tracked probe can detect the magnetic field generated by each transmitting coil by measuring the amount of current induced in a pick-up coil as the magnetic field changes. Static magnetic fields, such as those created by an MRI system, do not induce current in the receiving coil.

The sensitivity of a pick-up coil depends on how the coil is oriented to the detected magnetic field. Maximum sensitivity will occur when the axis of the pick-up coil is parallel to the magnetic field, and minimum sensitivity occurs when the axis of the pick-up coil is perpendicular to the field. Consequently, one pick-up coil cannot be used to quantify the magnetic field at a given point in space. This limitation is easily overcome, however, by using three pick-up coils, each oriented perpendicular to one another. By simultaneously detecting the induced currents in three mutually orthogonal coils, the vector (i.e., the direction and magnitude) of the magnetic field at the location of the probe can be determined.

Given the strength of the magnetic field detected by the probe and the strength of the magnetic field dipole created by the transmitting coil, the isofield contour that the pick-up coils experience can easily be determined. However, knowing the isofield contour experienced by a probe is not sufficient to locate that probe. Enough information to locate the probe can be obtained by measuring the magnitude of the isofield contour created by a second and third transmitting coil.

Knowledge of one isofield contour restricts all possible locations of the probe to a surface within the tracked volume. Knowledge of a second isofield contour restricts possible locations of the probe to the intersection of two surfaces (i.e., the probe can be located anywhere along a curve) (Fig. 16-3). Knowledge of a third isofield contour restricts possible locations to the intersection of the three surfaces (i.e., a point). This approach is similar to the way that the Global Positioning System (GPS) operates (although GPS relies on time delays in signals rather than on the strength of the detected signal). Mathematically, this process is carried out by solving three equations with three unknown variables.

When metallic structures, such as an MRI magnet, are located near transmitting RF coils, the magnetic field sensed by the pick-up coils can be disturbed, in turn creating an error in the computed position and orientation of the pick-up coil. Two mechanisms are possible: first, if the metallic structure is nonferromagnetic but conducts electricity, eddy currents are created in the structure. These eddy currents create an image field that partially cancels the field at the pick-up coil. Larger structures, particularly those that permit eddy currents to flow in large loops, are more prone to creating eddy currents. In addition, eddy currents tend to build up and decay with time constants, which are determined by the content and geometry of the eddy current–inducing structures. Thus, eddy currents make detection of the signal time dependent. The second mechanism in which metallic structures interact with the receiving or transmitting coils occurs when ferromagnetic material is brought near the coils. Ferromagnetic material placed near a coil can change its inductance and can thereby change the efficiency with which the coil makes or detects the magnetic field.

In addition to overcoming the artifacts arising from nearby metallic structures, successful use of RF tracking of interventional devices within MR scanners requires the development of

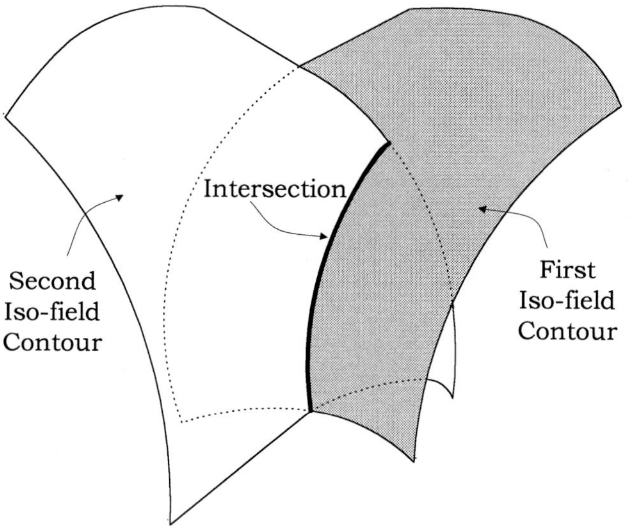

Fig. 16-3. The intersection of two isofield contours. With electromagnetic tracking, isofield contours generated by several sources are measured. The intersection of these contours is then used to identify the location of the device. The intersection of two isofield contours defines a curve in space. The intersection of a third isofield contour with this curve defines a point.

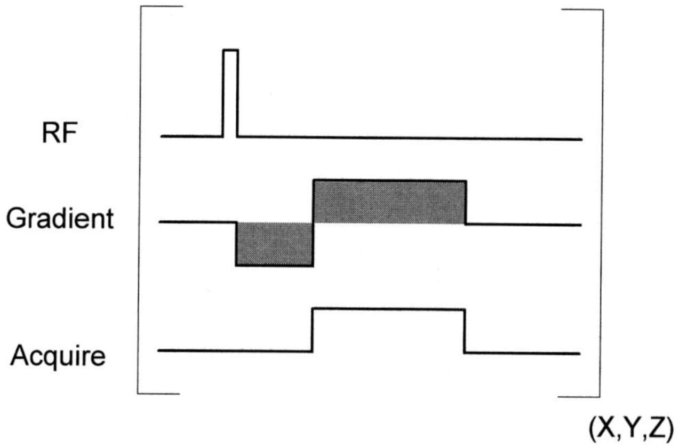

Fig. 16-4. A simple pulse sequence for locating a small coil. A spatially nonselective radiofrequency pulse is used to excite all nuclear spins in the excitation coil. Data are then acquired in the presence of a magnetic field gradient. The pulse sequence is repeated for the orthogonal axes to obtain three-dimensional data.

small receiver coils suitable for inclusion in interventional devices. Other issues, such as the interaction between the changing electromagnetic fields of the scanner and the RF tracking system, should also be addressed. However, the most significant hurdle may be that the MRI space, with its distortions, must be mapped into the RF tracking space, with its distortions. Although this feat may be possible with a calibration procedure, whether it can be reliably accomplished is unknown.

MAGNETIC RESONANCE TRACKING

Principles

A fundamental principle of MR is that the resonant frequency of a nuclear spin is directly proportional to the magnetic field that the spin experiences. In MRI, this relationship is used to determine positional information by subjecting nuclear spins to a magnetic field gradient, which causes the resonant frequency of each spin to have a spatial dependency. Images are then reconstructed using frequency analysis methods, such as the Fourier transform.

Location of a device using active MR tracking relies on the same fundamental principle. In the presence of a field gradient, the Larmor frequency of each spin in the patient varies along the axis of the gradient. Unlike conventional MRI, however, the MR signal in an MR tracking procedure is detected by a small coil embedded in the device, which is capable of receiving signals from only a limited volume. Consequently, when the detected MR signal is subjected to frequency analysis, one sharp peak is observed in the power spectrum. The frequency of this peak indicates the location of the coil within the sample.

Several localization pulse sequences suitable for tracking an interventional device have been described.[14,15] The simplest pulse sequence (Fig. 16-4) creates transverse spin magnetization over the entire volume of the transmitting RF coil using a spatially nonselective RF pulse. A gradient-recalled echo is then generated with a frequency-encoding gradient pulse applied on one axis. Frequency analysis of the MR signal detected in the presence of this magnetic field gradient is performed to determine the location of the coil along the axis of the applied gradient (Fig. 16-5). The full 3D coordinates of the device can be determined by repeating the entire process using orthogonal magnetic field gradient pulses.

The peak in the power spectrum is easily located by identifying the point having the greatest signal intensity. This method is insensitive to the phase of the peak and works well even when the signal-to-noise ratio is relatively low. Alternative methods in which the data are fit to a parametric model of the expected shape of the peak are also possible.

With the pulse sequence shown in Figure 16-4, any phenomena that change the local magnetic field (and hence the resonance frequency of the spins) will create an offset in the detected location of the coil. These field errors can arise from inhomogeneities in the main magnetic field and from local inhomogeneities of the magnetic field created by magnetic susceptibility differences of materials within the sensitive volume of the coil. Magnetic susceptibility can be of particular concern for tracking procedures because interventional devices may not have a magnetic susceptibility that exactly matches the surrounding tissue.

Resonance frequency offset errors can be removed during MR tracking by modulating the magnetic field gradient pulses. For example, the pulse sequence described above can be applied twice, each application having opposite polarity of the frequency-encoding gradient. Frequency offset errors can then be separated

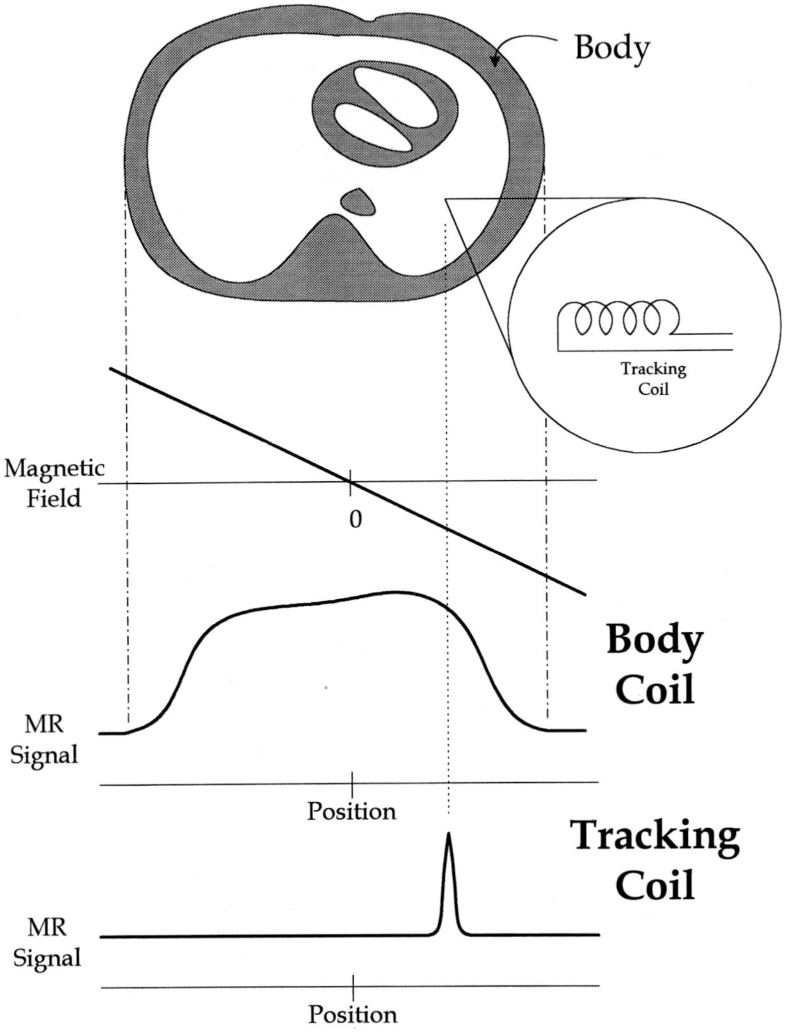

Fig. 16-5. Magnetic resonance signals detected by a small coil are Fourier transformed to give a frequency spectrum. Because the data are acquired in the presence of a magnetic field gradient, the frequency of the signal is proportional to the position of the coil along the gradient.

and removed from the coil position by computing the average coil location in the two acquisitions. Although effective, this technique requires six excitations to be performed for each localization.

Resonance offset errors can also be removed by using various multiplexing schemes (Fig. 16-6). In one scheme, the first excitation is performed without a frequency-encoding gradient to provide a reference. The subsequent excitations provide positional information for the three orthogonal directions. The X, Y, and Z coordinates of the coil are computed by removing the offset determined in the first acquisition from the locations found with subsequent acquisitions.

A second modulation scheme uses Hadamard multiplexing, in which three orthogonal localizing gradient pulses are simultaneously applied for each of four excitations. The polarity of each gradient pulse varies with each excitation. With the Hadamard multiplexing method, the true X, Y, and Z locations are computed by taking linear combinations of the positions determined in each acquisition:

$$X = -P(\text{ex } 1) + P(\text{ex } 2) + P(\text{ex } 3) - P(\text{ex } 4) \quad (1)$$
$$Y = -P(\text{ex } 1) + P(\text{ex } 2) - P(\text{ex } 3) + P(\text{ex } 4) \quad (2)$$
$$Z = -P(\text{ex } 1) - P(\text{ex } 2) + P(\text{ex } 3) + P(\text{ex } 4) \quad (3)$$

where P(ex 1), P(ex 2), P(ex 3), and P(ex 4) are the coil positions determined in the first, second, third, and fourth excitations, respectively.

Uses

An MR tracking system using the pulse sequences described above creates a continuous stream of 3D coordinates from the MR tracking coil. The speed of this stream of numbers is limited by the repetition time TR of the pulse sequence. Tracking rates as fast as 20 frames per second are easily achieved with modern scanning equipment.

The coordinates generated by an MR tracking system can be used in several ways and for many applications.[18–21] For example, the coordinate stream can provide a real-time representation of a device's location. This representation can be a numeric output or a graphic symbol (i.e., an icon) superimposed on a reference image. The image can be a conventional MRI scan, an MR angiogram, a computed tomography image, or even a live video image of the patient.

An alternative use of an MR tracking system combines the imaging and tracking functions of the MR scanner. With this

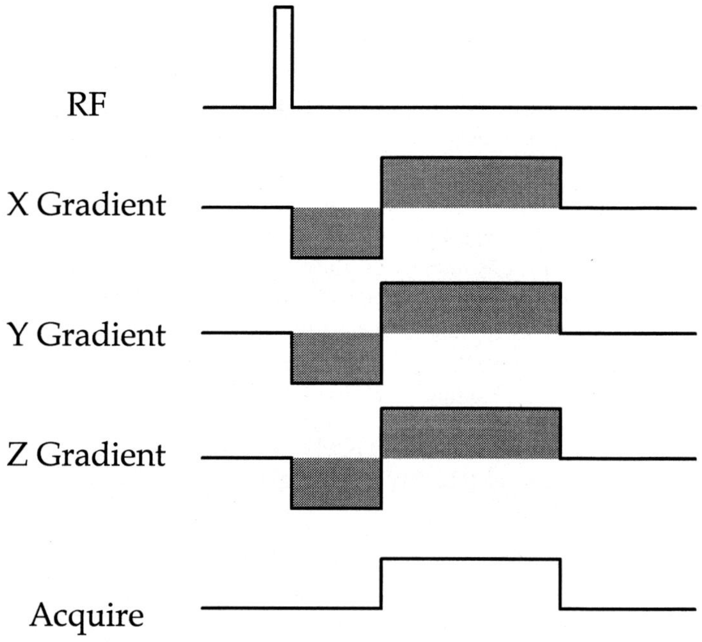

Encoding Schemes

Zero-Reference

excitation	X	Y	Z
1	0	0	0
2	1	0	0
3	0	1	0
4	0	0	1

Hadamard

excitation	X	Y	Z
1	-	-	-
2	+	+	-
3	+	-	+
4	-	+	+

Fig. 16-6. A multiplexed pulse sequence is used to locate a small coil. As with the simple pulse sequence (see Fig. 16-4), a spatially nonselective radiofrequency pulse is used. During data acquisition, however, magnetic field gradients are applied on all axes. The polarity (or amplitude) of these gradients is varied in each acquisition. With the appropriate modulation scheme, resonance offset artifacts can be removed from the positional data.

approach, the MR tracking system is used to locate a coil and then "steer" the MR scanner. The process can be repeated indefinitely; thus, as the tracked coil is moved in the body, MRI scans of the patient at the device location are continuously obtained. This guided scan mode of operation can be used for biopsy needle placement and for imaging of moving joints.[22]

Biplane and three-dimensional display

MR tracking data can use any image as a reference. Furthermore, because any image plane can be acquired with MR and combined with the 3D tracking coordinates, superimposing the tracking icon on two independent images is relatively straightforward. Because MR tracking demands relatively modest computation resources, a tracking icon can be superimposed on as many image planes as desired, even if the images are oblique to one another. Biplane formats similar to those used in x-ray fluoroscopy are particularly useful, especially during vascular procedures in which orthogonal maximum pixel projection images from 3D MR angiograms are used as reference images.[19]

Tracking multiple devices

With MR tracking, MR signals are generated from the entire patient but are detected by a small tracking coil. Because the tracked coil can be anywhere in the excitation coil and because small RF coils do not interact unless very close to each other, simultaneous tracking of multiple coils is possible. Multiple coil tracking can be used to monitor multiple positions in one device or to monitor the location of multiple devices. Multiple coil tracking can also be used to determine the orientation and location of a device. If such a multiple coil device is used for guided scan operations, image obliqueness and location can be controlled by the device.

Characteristics

The design and construction of an invasive device are important. For example, the materials used in the construction of the device should be chosen carefully. These materials must be biocompatible and strong enough to prevent breakage during normal use. They must also withstand the rigors of sterilization.

MR tracking devices have attributes beyond those normally considered for the construction of an invasive device. To operate properly, an MR tracking device should have all of the components that permit tracking and should be compatible with MRI.

Magnetic resonance compatibility

An invasive MRI device cannot be ferromagnetic. Ferromagnetic devices will exhibit an attraction to the static magnetic field of the MRI system. This attraction can occur with substantial force and can result in serious injury to the patient.

Ferromagnetism, however, is not the only magnetic property of concern to a device designer.[23] Devices constructed with nonferromagnetic materials but having a magnetic susceptibility different from that of human tissue can create large signal voids in MRI scans. The effect is more severe in higher field MR systems and is made worse with longer echo times, particularly for gradient-recalled imaging sequences.

The geometry of the invasive device should also be considered by the invasive device designer. Devices containing one or more electrical conducting loops may couple with the RF excitation coil of the MR scanner. This coupling can result in a localized change in signal intensity in the image or, in some cases, a focusing of RF power into a small region in the patient and corresponding generation of heat. An electrical conducting loop need not be entirely composed of the device because biologic tissue is itself conducting.

It is prudent to choose nonmetallic materials for device construction whenever possible. Many plastic and ceramic materials are suitable for use in an MR scanner. Even nonmetallic materials, however, can have a magnetic susceptibility that does not match that of human tissue. Because the severity of a susceptibility-induced artifact is determined by the strength of the magnetic field and by the size and shape of the material, a new material for device construction should be evaluated carefully.

Magnetic resonance tracking compatibility

An MR tracking device has several unique attributes. It should have one or more receiving coils to detect MR signals. Most invasive devices, however, are by necessity small, and tuning and matching elements are difficult to incorporate into the device. The lack of these elements can reduce the impedance match between the coil and the MR system's preamplifier, which in turn degrades the signal-to-noise ratio of the device. Simple coils constructed without tuning and matching elements typically have sufficient sensitivity for MR tracking.

The signals detected by an invasive device's receiving coils should be propagated to the MRI system. Consequently, the device should incorporate wires or cables. With the MR tracking techniques described in this chapter, detection of MR signals from parts of the device other than the coil may disturb tracking. For example, MR signals present along the length of a twisted-pair cable may be unintentionally received and sent to the preamplifier. If these signals are stronger than the signal detected by the tracking coil, then the MR tracking system will follow the location of the cable not the coil. Coaxial cables provide greater shielding than twisted-pair cables and typically perform much better for MR tracking. Nonferromagnetic miniature coaxial cables having little susceptibility-induced artifacts are readily available.

Multiple coils

Frequently, it is useful to incorporate multiple tracking coils in one invasive device. Multiple coils permit the orientation and the location of the device to be determined. Alternatively, multiple coils placed at several locations along a flexible device (e.g., a catheter or guidewire) permit the curvature of the device to be visualized.

The designer of a multiple coil device might be tempted to place the coils in series so that one receiver channel can be used. Although this placement may facilitate construction of the device and reduce the cost of the tracking system, it creates major challenges for safe use. Signals acquired from multiple coils but detected with one receiver cannot always be separated by the tracking software. For example, a two-coil device attached to one receiver will give a tracking power spectrum with two peaks. However, when the tracking magnetic field gradient is orthogonal to the line formed by the two coils, the two peaks will overlap, causing identification of each peak to be ambiguous. Consequently, multiple coil tracking is most safely performed with multiple receivers.

SAFETY CONSIDERATIONS FOR TRACKED DEVICES IN INTERVENTIONAL MAGNETIC RESONANCE IMAGING

The design and use of any interventional device should minimize danger the patient. Although safety issues concerning active device tracking are not unique, the use of invasive devices with an MR scanner is novel enough that a full safety analysis should be performed before any device is used in patients. Safety issues related to interventional device tracking in an MR scanner include the accuracy and precision of tracking, electrical patient isolation, and heating of the patient (see Chapter 10).

Registration of tracking data with a magnetic resonance image

Because the same physical process and instrumentation are used for imaging and tracking, MR tracking provides excellent registration of tracking data with the MRI scan. However, care is required when using MR tracking in regions of the body where local geometric distortions caused by susceptibility differences in tissue (e.g., near the petrous bone) occur. The MR tracking method described in the preceding text compensates for these local susceptibility differences, whereas the imaging procedure may not.

Registration of tracking data with an MRI scan is more problematic for optical and electromagnetic tracking methods because they provide a coordinate space determined by parameters independent of the MRI formation process. Calibration procedures for optical and electromagnetic tracking are necessary but not always adequate.

Although interventional device tracking in an MR scanner serves the same purpose as an x-ray fluoroscope, x-ray fluoroscopes provide real-time images of the patient and the invasive device, whereas devices tracked in MR scanners do not provide simultaneous tracking and imaging. With currently available tracking systems, interventional MR procedures are performed with a "road map" image rather than with one reflecting the immediate condition of the patient. Use of a "road map" image is not a serious limitation for most clinical applications. Interventional vascular procedures using "road map" images have been routinely used in x-ray fluoroscopy for years. Nevertheless, patient motion should be minimized during the procedure to maintain registration of the tracking and image data. Navigator echoes[24] may be useful for maintaining registration of images and tracking data in regions of anatomy subjected to breathing motion. Registration of tracking data in the heart may be possible with the acquisition of a dynamic "road map" image synchronized to the patient's heartbeat during device tracking.

Electrical isolation of the patient

Electrical isolation of the patient from surrounding equipment is an important safety consideration. A prudent design is robust and provides full isolation, even in the presence of two or more simultaneous failures. For example, a properly designed isolation circuit will prevent harm to a patient, even if an exposed conductor is located in a coronary artery and an electrical failure has placed full-line voltage on the nonisolated side of the circuit.

As a safety precaution in a properly designed isolation circuit, the maximum current and voltage a patient can be exposed to in the event of a system failure are limited. The most stringent and widely used safety criterion applies to electrical exposure to the heart. Although several regulatory agencies have established various criteria, any isolation circuit that can protect the patient from at least 4000 V and limits the maximum leakage current to 10 μA will meet these criteria.

Figure 16-7 illustrates one way in which an isolation circuit can be designed. The circuit consists of an air-core transformer and DC-blocking capacitors. Ferrite core transformers are not used because they would become saturated in the presence of the MR scanner's magnetic field. Capacitors limit the band pass of the circuit, thereby increasing the isolation.

Heating

A patient in an MR scanner is subjected to rapidly changing magnetic and electric fields. If a conducting structure (e.g., a guidewire or a cable) is placed in the patient, transfer of energy into the structure and generation of heat is possible. Significant heating in patients caused by a scanner's magnetic field gradient pulses has not been observed. However, heating induced by RF pulses has been observed and should be fully considered before an interventional device is used in an MR scanner.

RF pulses in an MR scanner create rapidly changing magnetic and electric fields in the patient. However, human tissue is not perfectly transparent to the RF energy, and some energy in the RF pulse is converted to heat. The most commonly used measure for heat deposition with an MR scanner is the specific absorption rate (SAR), which is measured in watts per kilogram of tissue.

Although the deposition of heat in the human body during an MR scan has been extensively studied, relatively little is known about the generation of heat in and near interventional devices. Nevertheless, experiments have been performed[25,26] that suggest that the RF pulses of an MR scanner can induce heating in tissue surrounding a conducting structure (e.g., a wire or cable). This heat appears to be created by high electric fields at the tip of the conducting structure.

In one set of experiments, heating in the tip of a copper wire placed in saline solution was intentionally maximized. Body coil excitation was performed in a 1.5-T scanner with a maximum transmitter amplifier gain. A very aggressive fast spin-echo pulse sequence was used to maximize the number of RF pulses. Temperature rises in the saline solution were monitored with a fiberoptic temperature probe and found to be highly localized at the tip of the device. Different locations and orientations of the copper wire were investigated, and the configuration yielding the greatest amount of heat was used in subsequent measurements.

In one representative experiment, significant heating was observed, and a SAR of 6048 W/kg was calculated. However, the heating was highly localized and appeared to be deposited in a region approximately 1 mm^3 in volume. Thus, only approximately 1 mg of saline was heated. Consequently, the SAR of the 1 g of saline containing this hot spot was approximately 6 W/kg, which was well below the International Electrotechnical Commission specification of 8 W/kg in any gram of tissue. Although the observed heating was within the regulatory SAR limit, in this experiment some saline was excessively heated. Clearly, the traditional guidelines for SAR are inappropriate when the source of heating is highly localized; a guideline based on local temperature rise may be more appropriate.

In these experiments, worst case conditions were used. In lower field scanners, heating would be much less, even for equivalent worst case procedures, because the power of an RF pulse needed to achieve a specific flip angle in MRI is proportional to the square of the magnetic field. Consequently, an imaging procedure will generate $\frac{1}{9}$ the heat in a 0.5-T scanner as it does in an identical 1.5-T scanner. Furthermore, the

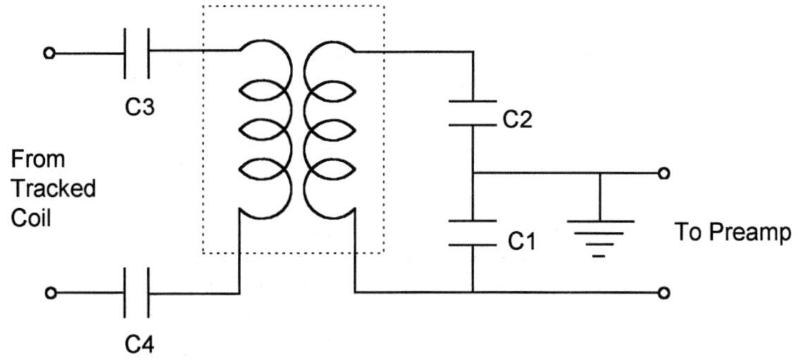

Fig. 16-7. An isolation circuit protects the patient from accidental exposure to electrical current, including ground loops.

wavelength of the Larmor frequency at 0.5 T is three times longer than it is at 1.5 T. Thus, devices appear to be shorter from an electrical point-of-view at lower fields, resulting in less efficient coupling to the excitation coil. The experimental results indicate that RF-induced heating of interventional devices is of concern only at higher field strengths.

The heating observed in these experiments is a consequence of applying RF pulses in the presence of a long conducting structure and is unrelated to the ability to track a device. Tissue heating should be a concern whenever any conducting structure (e.g., guidewire, electrocardiography lead, endoscope) is placed in a patient in higher field magnets.

COMPARISON OF ACTIVE AND PASSIVE VISUALIZATION TECHNIQUES

Temporal resolution

Active visualization of invasive devices during interventional MR procedures has advantages and disadvantages with respect to passive methods. For example, optical, electromagnetic, and MR tracking methods can follow devices at rates as fast as human perception (approximately 20 frames per second) and with little latency. However, the temporal resolution of passive methods is limited to the temporal resolution of the MRI pulse sequence. Very fast imaging methods (e.g., spiral scanning, echoplanar imaging) may achieve acceptable rates, but low-latency reconstruction and display of these 2D images remain challenging.

Although active tracking methods provide the location of one or more points in a device, passive visualization methods provide an image of a large portion of the device. However, for temporal resolution to be acceptable, passive visualization methods are limited to 2D image acquisition, and the invasive device should be manipulated within the confines of the imaging slice.

Spatial resolution

The in-plane spatial resolution of a passively visualized device is limited by the spatial resolution of the imaging scheme. Likewise, the through-plane resolution is limited by the image slice thickness. If the device cannot be constrained to lie in the image plane, multiple planes will need to be acquired (at the expense of temporal resolution) or a relatively thick image slice should be used (at the expense of through-plane resolution). If a thick slice is used, imaging characteristics of the device may need to be changed for greater visibility. This goal can be accomplished by doping the device with a substance having a magnetic susceptibility different from that of human tissue. Unfortunately, the size of a susceptibility-induced void in an image varies with the orientation of the device and the direction of the imaging gradient pulses. In general, the dependency on voids decreases the accuracy of device localization while degrading the visualization of the tissue surrounding the device.

However, with active tracking, the limit of spatial resolution is determined by the attributes of the method. Optical methods will be limited by the size of the LED and the resolution of the detector. MR and electromagnetic tracking resolution will be limited somewhat by the size of the RF coils. In general, the spatial resolution limit of a tracked coil is approximately equal to the coil size. In the case of MR tracking, the tracked coil can incorporate its own MR signal source.[27] If the detected MR signal is made to be stronger than the signal arising from the tissue surrounding the coil, then the spatial accuracy limit is determined by the sample size not the coil size.

CONCLUSIONS

Visualization of a device using active tracking methods is being evaluated at several institutions. Optical tracking and MR tracking have been used to follow rigid biopsy needles and external anatomic markers. MR tracking has also been used to track flexible devices (e.g., catheters).

Although active tracking methods require more device modification than typical passive visualization methods, they can provide real-time 3D information with minimal latency. An unmodified device (e.g., a biopsy needle) can be used with active tracking methods if the device is used with a tracked holder and assumed to be rigid. With the MR and electromagnetic tracking methods, even flexible devices (e.g., catheters) can be tracked by incorporating suitable receiving coils.

With active tracking methods, the location of the device can be represented in real-time as a graphic symbol, or icon, superimposed on one or more reference images. Alternatively, the numeric coordinates generated by the tracking system can be used to control the imaging plane of the scanner.

The ultimate role of MR and active device tracking in interventional radiology remains to be determined. Nevertheless, the use of MRI systems for interventional procedures offers unique possibilities, and the role of interventional MRI will grow with time.

REFERENCES

1. Jolesz FA, and others: MR imaging of laser-tissue interactions, *Radiology* 168:249, 1988.
2. Bleier AR, and others: Real-time magnetic resonance imaging of laser heat deposition in tissue, *Magn Reson Med* 21:132, 1991.
3. Darkazanli A, and others: *MRI guided ultrasonic surgery*, Berlin, 1992. Proceedings of the 11th Annual Meeting of the Society of Magnetic Resonance in Medicine.
4. Kahn T, and others: *MR guided laser interventions in cerebral gliomas*, Berlin, 1992, Proceedings of the 11th Annual Meeting of the Society of Magnetic Resonance in Medicine.
5. Gewiese B, and others: *MRI-controlled laser-induced interstitial thermotherapy (MR-LITT)*, Berlin, 1992, Proceedings of the 11th Annual Meeting of the Society of Magnetic Resonance in Medicine.
6. Matsumoto R, and others: *Real-time MR monitoring of cryoablation in the liver: predictability of the histological outcome*, Berlin, 1992, Proceedings of the 11th Annual Meeting of the Society of Magnetic Resonance in Medicine.
7. Lufkin RB, Teresi L, Hanafee WN: New needle for MR-guided aspiration cytology of the head and neck, *Am J Radiology* 149:380, 1987.
8. Koechli VD, and others: Vascular interventions guided by ultrafast MR imaging: evaluation of different materials, *Magn Reson Med* 31:309, 1994.
9. Bakker CJ, and others: Visualization of dedicated catheters using fast scanning techniques with potential for MR-guided vascular interventions, *Magn Reson Med* 36:816, 1996.

10. Schenck JF, and others: Superconducting open-configuration MR imaging system for image guided therapy, *Radiology* 195:805, 1995.
11. Dumoulin CL, and others: *Tracking system to follow the position and orientation of a device with radiofrequency field gradients,* 1993, US patent 5,211,165.
12. Dumoulin CL, and others: *Tracking system to follow the position and orientation of a device with radiofrequency fields,* 1995, US patent 5,377,678.
13. McKinnon GC, and others: *Towards visible guide wire antennas for interventional MRI,* San Francisco 1994, Proceedings of the 2nd Annual Meeting of the Society of Magnetic Resonance.
14. Ackerman JL, and others: *Rapid 3D tracking of small RF coils,* Montreal, 1986, Proceedings of the 5th Annual Meeting of the Society of Magnetic Resonance in Medicine.
15. Dumoulin CL, Souza SP, Darrow RD: Real-time position monitoring of invasive devices using magnetic resonance, *Magn Reson Med* 29:411, 1993.
16. Polhemus Inc., P.O. Box 560, Colchester, Vt (USA).
17. Non-fluoroscopic in-vivo navigation and mapping technology, *Nature–Medicine* 2:1393, 1996.
18. Leung DA, and others: Real-time biplanar needle tracking for interventional MR imaging procedures, *Radiology* 197:485, 1995.
19. Leung DA, and others: Active visualization of intravascular catheters with MRI: in-vitro and in-vivo evaluation, *Am J Radiology* 164:1265, 1995.
20. Wildermuth S, and others: MR-guided percutaneous intravascular interventions: evaluation of preliminary catheter design, *Radiology* 202:578, 1997.
21. Steiner P, and others: Active biplanar tracking for biopsies in humans, *Am J Radiology* 169:735, 1997.
22. Daniel BL, and others: *Active scan plane registration during dynamic musculoskeletal MR imaging using an external MR-tracking coil,* Vancouver, 1997, Proceedings of the 5th Annual Meeting of the Society of Magnetic Resonance.
23. Schenck JF: The role of magnetic susceptibility in magnetic resonance imaging: MRI magnetic compatibility of the first and second kinds, *Med Phys* 23:815, 1996.
24. Ehman RL, Felmlee JP: Adaptive technique for high-definition MR imaging of moving structures, *Radiology* 173:255, 1989.
25. Maier SE, and others: *Safety of MR tracking catheters,* Nice, 1995 Proceedings of the 3rd Annual Meeting of the Society of Magnetic Resonance.
26. Wildermuth S, and others: MR-guided percutaneous angioplasty: assessment of tracking safety, catheter handling and functionality, *CVIR* (in press).
27. Erhart P, and others: Tissue-independent MR tracking of invasive devices with an internal signal source, New York, 1996, Proceedings of the 4th Annual Meeting of the Society of Magnetic Resonance.

Chapter 17

FEASIBILITY OF MR–GUIDED NEUROENDOSCOPY

Andreas Melzer, Martin Scholz, Rainer M.M. Seibel

In complex neurosurgical procedures, it may be difficult to differentiate the anatomic relationships of tumors and critical structures while dissecting and removing pathologic tissue (i.e., in the region of the internal capsule, thalamus, and basal ganglia).[1] Although the microscope makes it possible to distinguish the borders of a tumor, keeping a three-dimensional (3D) orientation within the operative field is difficult, particularly when the ventricle is collapsed.[2,3]

Neuroendoscopic visualization provides detailed information of the surfaces of the operative field with decreased invasiveness of the procedure.[4] However, the colored video image is generated only from the light reflected from the surfaces of tissue. The limited field of view restricts assessment of areas outside of the optical field. The small access and the remote nature of tissue handling lead to further restrictions. Nevertheless, several neuroendoscopic diagnostic and surgical procedures have been developed in recent years.[5–8] In endoscopic surgery, only indirect manipulation is achieved via a direct eye-hand coordination axis because the surgeon has to watch the video monitor.[9] The surgical procedures have to be carried out with lack of tactile feedback and reduced kinematic response. Structures cannot be palpated. Evaluation of local anatomy and pathology is achieved via visual inspection only.

In open neurosurgery, the experienced operator has mentally stored information of the patient's anatomy below and behind the surfaces within the operative field. The operator can plan the correct surgical access to avoid critical structures. Orientation and tissue assessment are achieved through tactile feedback and kinematic response. The purpose is to merge magnetic resonance imaging (MRI) with neuroendoscopic technique to add information on structures that cannot be distinguished nor seen underneath the surface because of the limited access.

The surfaces of the operative field in conjunction with the organs and the underlying structures represent the volume of interest. This tissue volume can be more or less visualized with various imaging systems. However, which imaging technology best serves as an additional intraoperative imaging system? Because of excellent soft-tissue contrast, temperature and flow sensitivity, and arbitrary slice orientation, some physicians choose MRI as the imaging technology for endoscope and instrument guidance. In 1994, a project was started on the development of MR-compatible endoscopes, ancillary equipment, and techniques for MR guidance. This chapter presents the results of a preliminary feasibility cadaver study of MR-guided neuroendoscopy.

PREREQUISITES FOR MAGNETIC RESONANCE–GUIDED ENDOSCOPY

Video endoscopes provide an excellent image of the surfaces of the operative field in real-time and on-line. Two types of endoscopes have been evaluated *in vitro* and *ex vivo:* flexible fiberscopes and rigid rod lens endoscopes.

Endoscopes and equipment were tested in three open magnets: 0.067-T ACCESS (Toshiba Inc., San Francisco, Calif),[10] 0.2-T Magnetom OPEN (Siemens, Erlangen, Germany),[11] and 0.23-T Outlook (Picker, Cleveland, Ohio). The newly developed endoscopes, instruments, and ancillary equipment were evaluated with the Magnetom OPEN. Fast gradient echoes (fast low-angle shot [FLASH], fast imaging with steady-state precision [FISP]) with repetition times (TR) between 30 and 120 msec and echotimes (TE) between 9 and 14 msec were used as sequences.

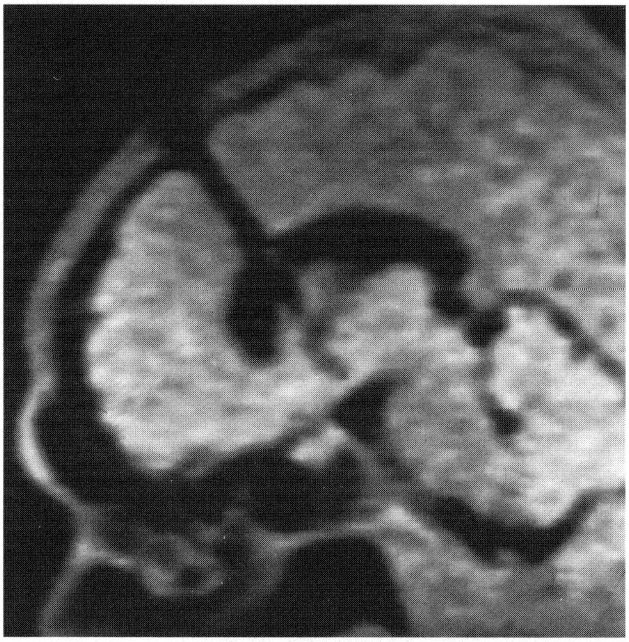

Fig. 17-1. Magnetic resonance image of an endoscope within the right ventricle of a cadaver (spin-echo, 0.067-T magnet).

Flexible endoscopes

Flexible fiberscopes can be produced in small sizes to an outer diameter of 0.3 mm. The flexible endoscopes were 0.5, 0.7, and 0.9 mm in diameter. Image resolution and color accuracy of fiberscopes are generally less than those of rigid rod lens scopes. Most flexible microscopes are equipped with stainless steel object lens housing and are thus not fully MR compatible. In the ultra-low field of the ACCESS magnet, this problem was not major, but the MRI quality was insufficient (Fig. 17-1). Tests in the 0.2-T Magnetom OPEN revealed incompatibility for imaging purposes. Recently improved fiber technology provides 10,000 fibers in an 0.97-mm endoscope, and synthetic material for the front lens housing allows acceptable image characteristics and MR compatibility (Fig. 17-2). For surgical purposes, however, higher image quality is required.

Rigid endoscopes

Rod lens endoscopes with an outer diameter of 4 mm provide acceptable image quality and illumination of the neurosurgical operative field. Standard rigid reusable endoscopes and laparoscopes have been evaluated, but none featured adequate MR compatibility (not even in the 0.067-T open system). Different alloys suitable for endoscopic lens construction were evaluated. New lenses were further tested because the materials can frequently cause significant artifacts. Lens housings and ocular and other parts of the rod lens system underwent extensive testing as well. A low artifact endoscope was developed (1:1 artifact size; instrument:diameter ratio) (Fig. 17-3). Endoscopes with different sizes (4, 5, and 10 mm; 0° and 30° viewing angle) are available. These endoscopes will undergo premarket approval for neuroendoscopy.

Video endoscopes

Video endoscopy comprises the following devices that require approval for MRI applications (Fig. 17-4):

- Camera
- Light transmission cable
- In-room monitor

A

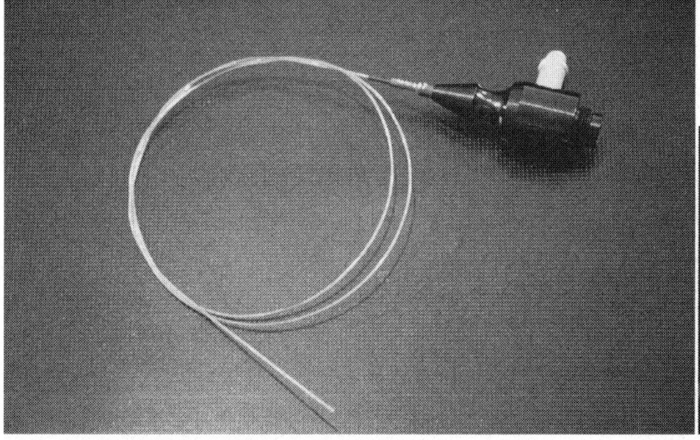

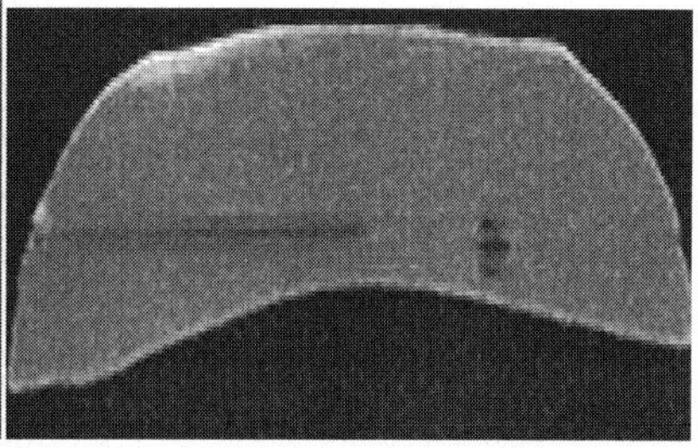

B

Fig. 17-2. A 0.97-mm flexible magnetic resonance (MR)–compatible endoscope. **A,** External view; **B,** MR image of endoscope within a phantom.

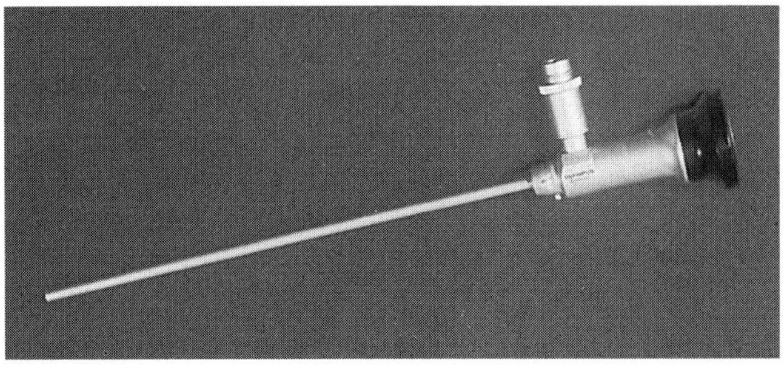

Fig. 17-3. A 4-mm rigid magnetic resonance–compatible endoscope (Olympus Winter & Ibe, Hamburg, Germany).

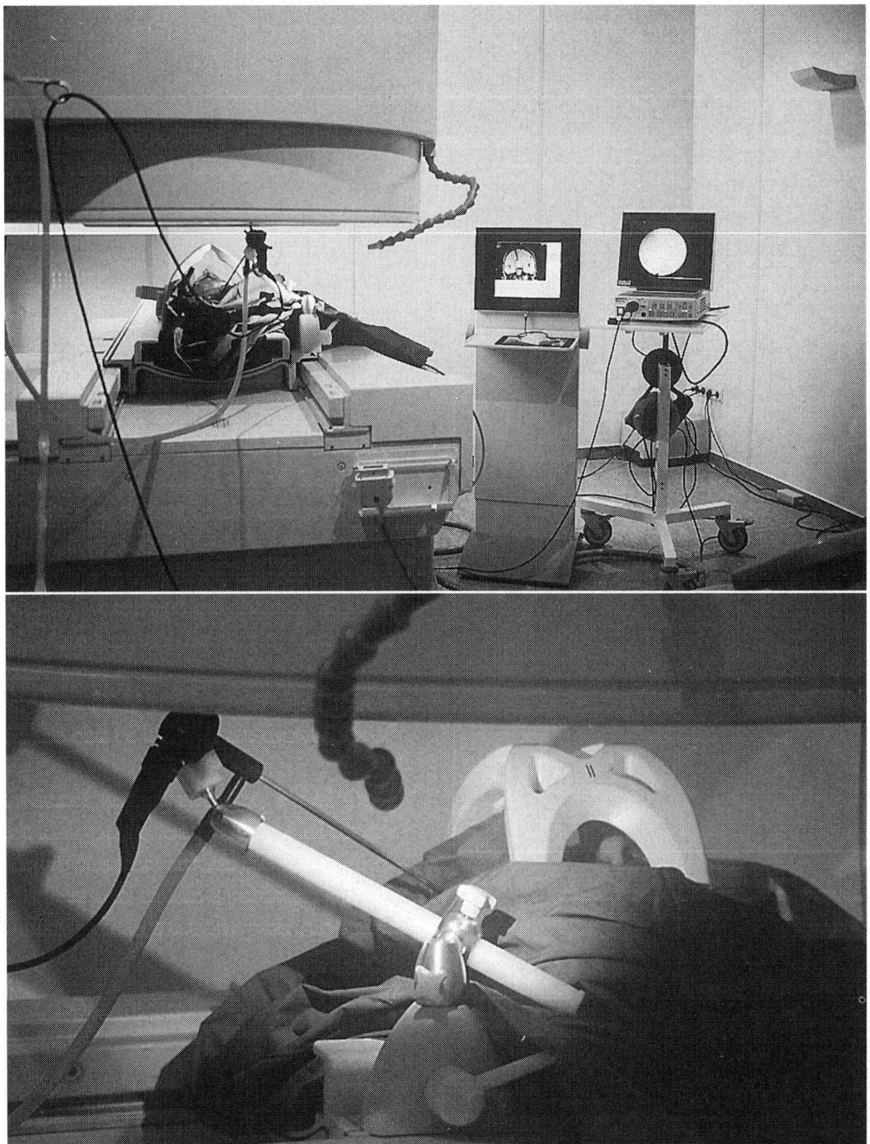

Fig. 17-4. The system set up for magnetic resonance–guided endoscopy, including the light source and cable, video camera, and thin-film technology matrix screen.

The light source and video recorder can be placed outside of the radiofrequency (RF) cabin of the magnet.

Neuroendoscopy requires high-resolution color monitors, but those containing cathode ray tubes cannot be used close to the magnet because of image distortion. Particularly, if fluoroscopic-like sequences are used to control the endoscopic approach, immediate observation of the intraoperatively gathered MRI scans and endoscopic images is mandatory. A second in-room monitor with standard video quality is required. Technologic realization of an MR-compatible color screen with high-quality display is difficult. The magnetic field leads to image distortion of tube monitors, and most liquid crystal display (LCD) monitors do not feature adequate resolution and color grades. A thin-film technology (TFT)–active matrix monitor with analog control of each pixel provides excellent MRI scans and can be equipped with a specially developed color processor (Pritzel Electronic, Prutting, Germany). A 14-inch display with 1024 × 768 lines was chosen for the in-room console. Electric shielding with an ultrathin metal net in front of the screen is required to eliminate high-frequency interference with the MRI scan, and specially developed electric circuits are necessary to provide resistance of the display to the magnetic field. The first prototype has been tested during various endoscopic and neuroendoscopic procedures (Fig. 17-5). Further development and improved displays led to an excellent image that fulfills the diagnostic requirements for endoscopy. In one test, a Sony black matrix monitor was compared with a 14-inch TFT and a digital LCD using a 10-mm laparoscope adapted to an Olympus (Tokyo, Japan) 5 MR-compatible camera. According to tests with standard-resolution charts and color charts during endoscopic procedures, the TFT flat screen displayed superior resolution to the tube monitor.

Light sources and light cables

New low-power light sources with no interference with the imaging system are available. This type of light source can be used only for the magnet illumination. Endoscopy requires higher power, the better color temperature of xenon light, and connection to light cables.

For endoscopic procedures, high-power light sources with daylight quality are necessary. The light source (CLV 20 Olympus, Tokyo, Japan) can be used in the MR suite. If placed on the floor near the magnet, the light source does not cause significant artifacts. However, this position is unacceptable in terms of safety because the light cable may interfere with the surgeons' legs and with the chair. For this drawback to be avoided, a 10-m light cable with full MR compatibility was developed (Fig. 17-6), thereby any light source can be placed outside the RF cabin and does not interfere with imaging or the procedure. The light cable can be used throughout the procedure; even when located within the image plane, the cable does not cause artifacts. Two types are available: 3.5- and 5-mm light transmission.

Light intensity is adjusted through the camera control unit, which can be connected to the light source via a coaxial cable. The placement of the camera unit outside of the magnet is preferable because RF emissions could not be eliminated completely. However, the line between the chip camera and the control unit should not exceed 5 m to allow optimal image quality. Longer cables increase the signal-to-noise ratio (SNR) of the video image.

TECHNIQUE OF MAGNETIC RESONANCE–GUIDED ENDOSCOPY

In cadaver studies, a right and left frontoparietal approach to the ventricular system, including the foramen of Monro and the

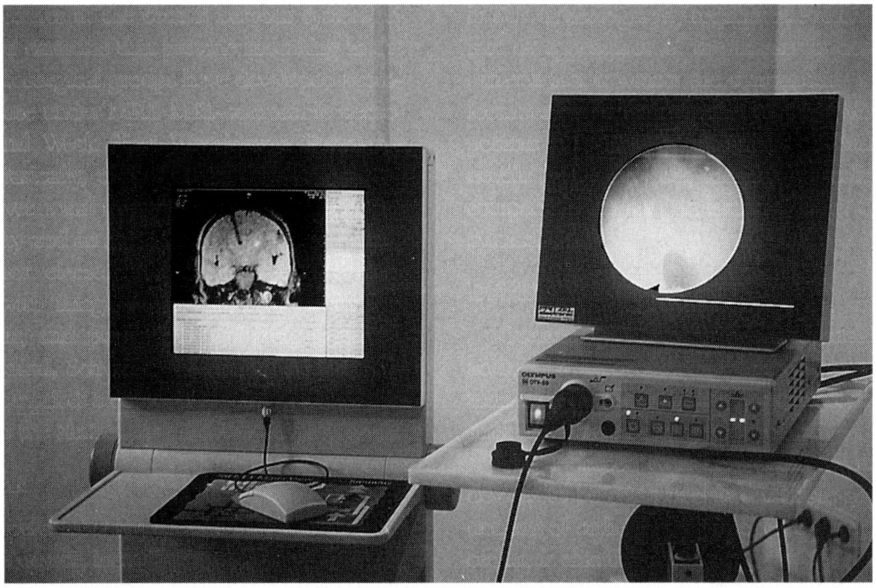

Fig. 17-5. Prototype of a magnetic resonance (MR)–compatible analog thin-film technology matrix flat screen for MR-guided endoscopy (Pritzel, Prutting, Germany).

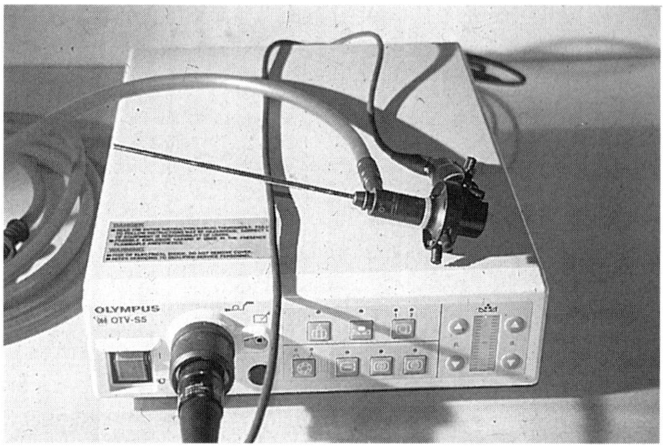

Fig. 17-6. Magnetic resonance–compatible endoscope and 10-m light transmission cable (Olympus Winter & Ibe, Hamburg, Germany).

third ventricle, has been evaluated.[4] For this purpose, two anatomic preparations of a male and a female head were placed in a foam bed to provide stable position. A multipurpose large and standard head coil were used. The following test protocol aspects were assessed: endoscope and instrument handling, sterile conditions, free access to the head, and convenience to the surgeon.

Magnetic resonance endoscopic guidance technique

Subsequent to initial T1 spin-echo imaging, the burr hole was visualized. For the correct trajectory to be determined, a gadolinum contrast–filled syringe or an MR Grid (Daum Medical, Schwerin, Germany) was used. For correlation of the access trajectory with the endoscope, a Wasculap laser pointer (Daum, Schwerin, Germany) was adjusted according to the preoperative planning. The endoscope was then aligned with the laser beam during insertion. Direct optic visualization can be achieved to increase the safety of access to the ventricular system. The insertion pathway was MR controlled by FISP 2D and FLASH 2D gradient echoes. Because the head is prepared, most of the cerebrospinal fluid (CSF) disappears because the head is leaking from the cut at cervical level 3. The ventricles were partly air filled, which impedes visualization of the endoscope. Thus, artificial CSF with the same signal characteristics as natural CSF was evaluated. Gelifundol, saline, and 5% glucose/saline solutions were examined by FLASH 2D, FISP 2D, spin-echo, and turbo spin-echo. For this purpose, a 6-F urinary catheter (Cook, Bjaeverskov, Denmark) was introduced through the preformed burr hole into the right ventricle, and the ventricular system was then filled with 150-ml Gelifundol (Biotest Pharma, Dreieich, Germany) under MR control. For leakage of the artificial CSF to be avoided, the neck was sealed by a polyamide film, which was firmly attached with rubber bands.

RESULTS

The head coil turned out to be preferable because of image quality. A further advantage of the head coil is its optimal and stable position.

Artificial CSF Gelifundol revealed the best signal characteristics. Although this substance has light yellow color, it is used for refilling the CSF compartments.

Under liquid-filled conditions, MR-guided endoscopy was feasible. The endoscope could be detected in all tested sequences. For initial guidance, the fluoro-like FISP 2D sequence is appropriate (Fig. 17-7). For final assessment of the endoscope position, FLASH 2D with a full 256×256 matrix and a 26-sec acquisition time is appropriate. Surrounding anatomy and CSF can be detected by using T1-weighted spin-echo, 3D gradient echo, and T2-weighted turbo spin-echo. For this purpose, the endoscope should be fixed (see Fig. 17-4, *B*) to have optimal image quality. The current coil holder was modified to provide attachment of the endoscope. The precision of endoscope placement was approximately 2 mm.

DISCUSSION

It is possible to achieve localization and guidance of endoscopes for neuroendoscopic procedures. Instruments can be localized with an accuracy of approximately 2 mm. MRI provides excellent soft-tissue contrast, arbitrary slice-orientation, temperature, and flow sensitivity. Application of FLASH and FISP gradient-recalled echo enables breathhold and fluoroscopy-like imaging with acceptable contrast, SNR, and resolution. Commercially available equipment with adequate surgical function was not fully MR compatible. However, instruments are difficult to display, and the manufacturing of MR-compatible instrumentation is costly and time-intensive.

Conventional x-ray fluoroscopy provides poor soft-tissue contrast; only a biplanar system provides limited 3D information. Display of vascular structures and the ventricular systems is poor and requires administration of contrast media. Preoperative access trajectory planning and instrument tracking are impossible and are thus not applicable for most neuroendoscopic guidance.

Although ultrasound provides sectional images of real-time and 3D information and Doppler function displays venous and arterial blood flow, the ultrasound image is operator dependent,

A

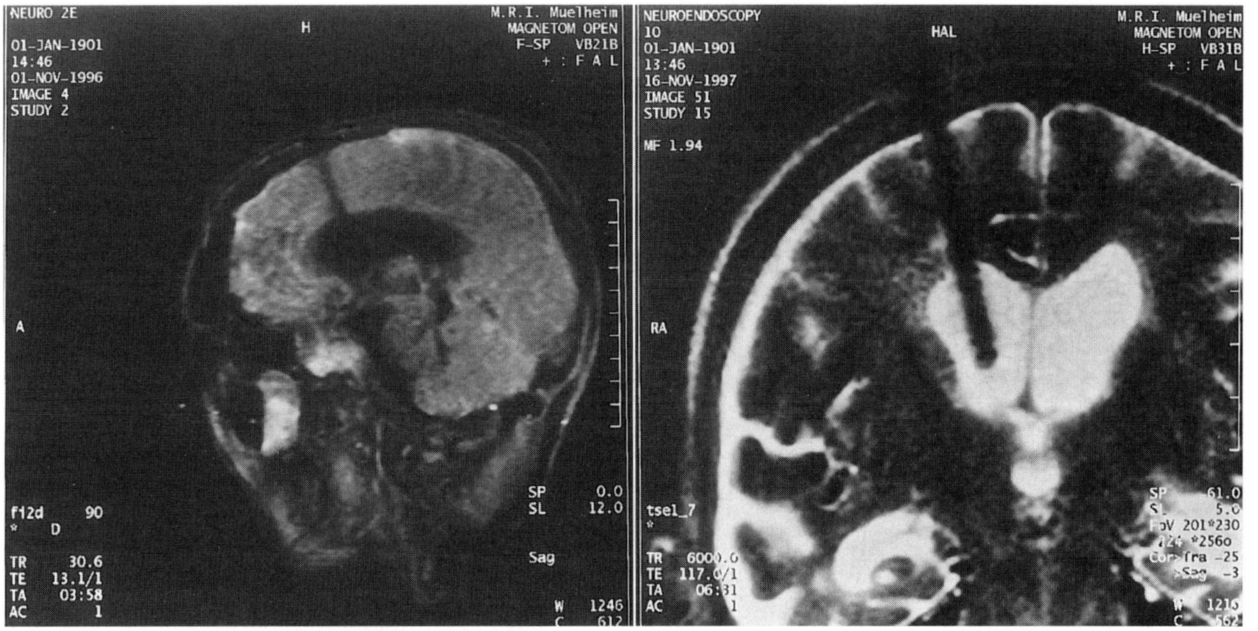

B

Fig. 17-7. **A,** Fluoroscopic-like magnetic resonance guidance of a 5-mm rigid endoscope to the lateral ventricle (gradient-recalled echo; fast imaging with steady-state precision; two-dimensional; repetition time, 30.6 msec; echo time, 13.1 msec; acquisition time, 4 sec). **B,** T2-weighted control image (turbospin-echo, repetition time, 6000 msec; echo time, 117 msec).

requires an ultrasonic window, and does not permit a complete view behind structures. Bone or air-filled compartments create a sound shadow, and penetration is poor. The obligatory sound coupling with gels or water as interface between scanner and tissue surface confines the intraoperative use, particularly for endoscope guidance. Because current systems are not stationary, interactive instrument guidance requires manual control or adaptation of the tool to the scanning probe. Instruments are only displayed if their surfaces provide sound scattering and reflection; usually, only the tip of an instrument can be visualized. Preoperative access trajectory evaluation is difficult, and the reproducibility is user dependent.

Computed tomography (CT) has become an excellent tool for interventional procedures, such as those pioneered by Seibel and others.[12] CT provides reproducible high-resolution images with superior details of bone structures and is useful for preoperative planning and stereotactic guidance.[13] Differentiation of soft tissue and critical structures with the brain is, however, limited. The contrast of instruments during CT-guided procedures is less than that during MR. Although material selection for CT instrumentation is less critical than for MRI, metallic objects larger than 3 mm create significant artifacts and, in the longitudinal direction distally to the tip, impede orientation and accuracy of localization. In addition, x-ray exposure and monoplanar imaging in axial and paraxial directions limit the 3D information. Excellent bone structure representation and high resolution can be used to overlay information on MRI scans, thereby closing the gap of information.[14]

Instruments in neurosurgery can be guided by stereotactic navigation methods.[15] The concept of stereotactic guidance was taken further with implementation of optoelectronic tracking of the instrument and 3D localization within a preoperatively reconstructed set of CT or MRI scans. Small light-emitting diodes are attached to the instrument's handle and traced by linear cameras. The controlling workstation continuously obtains information on the instrument's position and orientation. A virtual instrument is displayed in the respective image of the patient, and thus maneuvering of the probe can be controlled in space.[16] However, changes and anatomic shift in the operative volume during surgery are not detected. Thus, update imaging or an additional on-line imaging system is required.

Further studies on MR guidance of neuroendoscopic procedures will implement the use of navigation systems to guide the endoscope and instruments. Active systems with light-emitting diodes and passive systems with light-reflecting elements will be examined. The interventional tool should be aligned completely with the orientation of the image planes. The current situation requires a predetermined slice orientation according to a certain access trajectory. Change of orientation of the endoscope leads to loss of the artifact in the image. If slice orientation and position are changed, the instrument position path can be changed. This process is time consuming and awkward because the sequence needs to be reloaded for each step of the localization process.

MRI acquisition parameters of the slice orientation can be externally gathered and processed by the MR computer, enabling an interactive slice orientation to the moved instrument accordingly. The principle of optoelectronic frameless instrument navigation can be implemented in the control system of an MRI unit, whereby the tracking of a tool within the

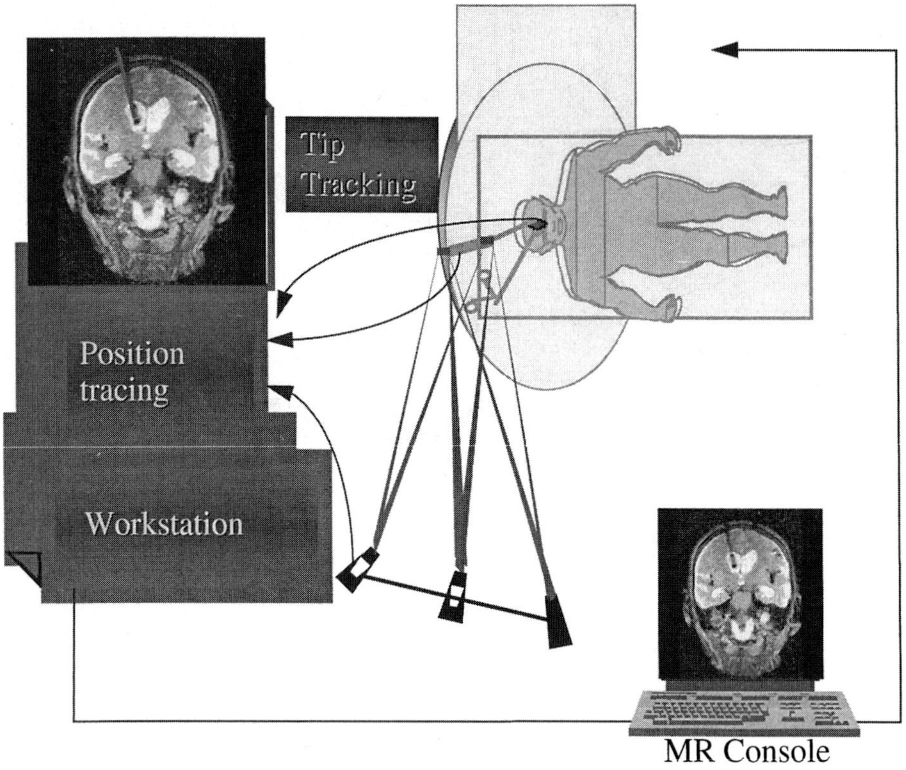

Fig. 17-8. The principle of optoelectronic instrument guidance and tip tracking for neuroendoscopy.

magnetic field can be directly transferred to the slice orientation of the respective sequence. Although the sequence needs to be loaded, images can be acquired automatically according to the position in alignment with the instrument or perpendicular to the distal tip of the instrument. The image plane orientation can be changed and redefined without moving the instrument. This ability ensures constant control of the endoscope and instrument during movement. Unattended curvature or bending of the instrument may distort the position of the instrument tip.[17] Tip tracking allows direct display of the instrument tip signal in a complete set of MRI scans, whereby interactive slice orientation in axial or perpendicular position in accordance to the instrument can be obtained (Fig. 17-8).[18] This technique is based on active tip tracking that uses a small RF antenna coil[19,20] located at the distal tip of the endoscope. The position of this tip coil can be traced and used for slice positioning and orientation. In combination with interactive slice orientation, MR guidance will be significantly improved.

REFERENCES

1. Greenwood J Jr: Radical surgery of tumors of the thalamus, hypothalamus and third ventricle area, *Surg Neurol* 1:29, 1973.
2. Ehni G: Interhemispheric and percalosal approach to the cingulate gyri: interventricular shunt tubes and certain deeply placed brain lesions, *Neurosurgery* 144:99, 1984.
3. Sugita K: *Microneurosurgical atlas,* Berlin, 1985, Springer-Verlag.
4. Perneczky A, Tschabitscher M, Resch K: *Endoscopic anatomy for neurosurgery,* Stuttgart, 1993, Thieme.
5. Bauer BL, Hellwig D: Minimally invasive endoscopic neurosurgery: a survey, *Acta Neurochir (Wein)* 61 (suppl) 1:12, 1994.
6. Oka K, and others: An observation of the third ventricle under flexible fiberoptic ventriculoscope: normal structure, *Surg Neurol* 40:273, 1993.
7. Camaert J, Abdullah J: Diagnostic and therapeutic stereotactic cerebral endoscopy, *Acta Neurochir (Wein)* 124:11, 1993.
8. Harris LW: Endoscopic techniques in neurosurgery, *Microsurgery* 15:541, 1994.
9. Cuschieri A: *General principles of laparoscopic surgery: operative manual of endoscopic surgery,* Heidelberg, 1992, Springer-Verlag.
10. Scholz M, and others: MRI-guided endoscopy in the brain: a feasibility study, *Min Neurosurg* 39:33, 1996.
11. Melzer A, and others: Technology and principles of image-guided interventions and surgery, *Surg Endosc* 11:946, 1997.
12. Seibel R, and others: CT and MRI guided microtherapy, *Seminars in Laparoscopic Surgery* 4:167, 1997.
13. Apuzzo MLJ, Sabshin JK: Computed tomographic guidance stereotaxis in the management of intracranial mass leasons, *Neurosurgery* 12:277, 1983.
14. Hill DLG, and others: Feasibility study of magnetic resonance imaging guided intranasal flexible microendoscopy, *Computer Aided Surgery* 2:264, 1997.
15. Scholz M, and others: Endoskopische Neuronavigation. Eine praklinische Srudie mit dem Easy Guide Neuro System, *Endoskopie heute* 3:299, 1997.
16. Melzer A: *Instruments for laparo-endoscopic surgery: conventional and intelligent endosurgery,* New York, 1996, Churchill-Livingstone.
17. Silverman SG, and others: Interactive MR-guided biopsy in an open configuration MR imaging system, *Radiology* 197:175, 1995.
18. Busch M, and others: Active tip tracking as a control method for the positioning of medical instruments during MR-guided interventional procedures, *Proc Int Soc Magn Reson Med,* 1922, 1997.
19. Davis CP, and others: Ultra-high-speed MR imaging, *European Radiology* 6:297, 1996.
20. Leung DA, and others: Real-time biplanar needle tracking for interventional MR imaging procedures, *Radiology* 197:485, 1995.

Chapter 18

MR–COMPATIBLE POSITRON EMISSION TOMOGRAPHY

Keyvan Farahani, Randal B. Slates, Yiping Shao, Masao Sugita, Simon Cherry

For any device to be used in an interventional magnetic resonance (MR) procedure, it should first satisfy the conditions of MR compatibility. Namely, the device should be nonferromagnetic, and its presence and operation in the magnetic field environment of MR should not produce susceptibility or electromagnetic interference artifacts on MRI. Furthermore, operation of the device should not be affected by MRI and should not harm the patient. Positron emission tomography (PET) is no exception. But why MR-compatible PET? And what is the relationship with interventional MRI?

PET is an imaging technique that uses positron-emitting tracers to provide images of biochemical activity in the organ of interest.[1] Over the past 2 decades, PET has been used extensively to perform functional studies of the brain. More recently, PET has been shown to be highly sensitive in detecting brain tumors.[2,3] PET also can detect head and neck squamous cancers not seen on MRI.[4] Although PET images provide quantitative information, they lack the fine spatial resolution (<1 mm) achievable with MRI. Therefore, many studies of brain function rely on coregistration of PET and MRI to match the patient's functional and structural anatomies. MR-compatible PET would allow the acquisition of PET and MRI pairs that are intrinsically coregistered and spatially and temporally correlative. It would also allow simultaneous acquisition of PET and MR studies of physiologic nature, such as functional, spectroscopic, or angiographic MRI.

By the same token, it is conceivable to imagine interventional MRI studies that are aided by the information provided by MR-compatible PET technology. In research applications, when PET is performed simultaneously with MR-guided ablations of soft tissue, it can provide information on functional activity surrounding a treated region. In clinical applications, this technique is powerful for minimally invasive treatments in the brain, where sparing of healthy and functional tissue is essential. Furthermore, because of its high specificity for the detection of brain tumors, MR-compatible PET can help the interventionalist by guiding in management of residual or recurring tumors.

POSITRON EMISSION TOMOGRAPHY OVERVIEW

PET is a functional imaging method for scanning the human body. Physicians and scientists use PET to study the function of various organs and tissues. The functional imaging technique of PET provides different information than anatomic imaging techniques, such as computed tomography (CT) or MRI. Function of the body is studied by using a radioactive tracer that is injected into a vein. An image is then acquired by a PET scanner, and the tracer's location in the body can be determined. Tracer tissue uptake can be studied to determine the function of a particular organ or tissue of interest.

Positron-emitting isotopes (e.g., ^{11}C, ^{18}F, ^{13}N, ^{15}O) can be chemically attached to many types of molecules and used as functional probes. The positron emitter, now attached to a molecule, emits a positron that travels a short distance, colliding into atoms and losing energy along the way, and eventually interacts with an electron. Two 511-keV photons are then created from the annihilation of the electron-positron pair. These two photons are emitted in opposite directions (180°) and are detected in coincidence by photon detectors within the PET camera. The photon detectors are typically arranged in a circular ring geometry within the PET camera and are comprised of scintillation crystals coupled to a photomultiplier device. The scintillation crystals (i.e., bismuth germanate, lutetium oxyorthosilicate) convert the high-energy 511-keV photons into lower-energy photons in the visible light range. The photomultiplier devices, typically photomultiplier tubes, convert the visible light photons into electrons, which are multiplied and sent as an electronic signal to acquisition electronics. The acquisition electronics process the data, which are sent to a computer for reconstruction (by filtered backprojection) to form an image. The image, a cross-section of the patient, is defined by the plane of the detector ring and represents the activity distribution of the radioactive probe. Volumetric images can be obtained if several detector rings are placed next to each other, acquiring coincidence photons between detectors in the same ring and in different rings.

PET can also be used in dynamic studies by acquiring the distribution of the radioactive probe over time. Information about the change in distribution over time and the regional distribution of the probe in the body can be obtained by collecting repeated images over time; therefore, kinetic processes can be studied. PET can also provide quantitative information about the function of organs or tissues in the body.

This chapter describes a prototype of MR-compatible PET developed at the University of California, Los Angeles (UCLA).

DESIGN OF THE MAGNETIC RESONANCE-COMPATIBLE POSITRON EMISSION TOMOGRAPHY SYSTEM

Two prototype MR-compatible PET systems have been developed at UCLA.[5,6] McPET I system, a small benchtop system, shows proof of principle. McPET II system, a single-slice PET scanner with a detector ring diameter of 54 mm, consists of 72 lutetium oxyorthosilicate scintillator crystals. Each crystal measures 2 × 2 × 5 mm^3, and the array of crystals is held in a lucite ring holder. The slice thickness is about 1 mm at full-width half maximum. The system has a reconstruction resolution of 2.1 mm, a coincidence time resolution of 26 nsec, and an energy resolution of 45%.[7]

The lutetium oxyorthosilicate crystals are optically coupled with three multichannel photomultiplier tubes via a 4-m long bundle of optical fibers. The photomultiplier tubes and associated electronics are electromagnetically shielded in an aluminum enclosure. During operation in the MRI suite, the photomultiplier tube assembly and the counting electronics are placed more than 3 m away from the center of the magnet.

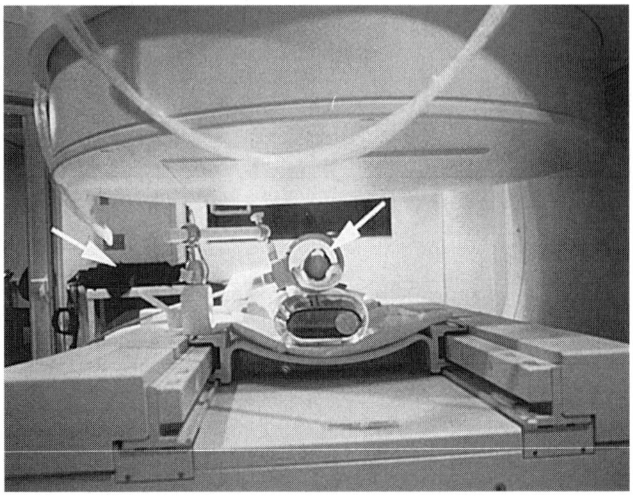

Fig. 18-1. Set up of the prototype magnetic resonance (MR)–compatible positron emission tomography (PET) inside an open MRI system. The PET detector array is placed inside an MR surface oil (*right arrow*). The photomultiplier tubes and electronics are shielded and placed 3 m away from the magnet (*left arrow*).

SIMULTANEOUS POSITRON EMISSION TOMOGRAPHY AND MAGNETIC RESONANCE IMAGING AND ARTIFACT ASSESSMENT

MRI scans have been acquired simultaneously with PET on a conventional 1.5-T superconducting unit (Siemens Magnetom Vision, Islein, NJ) and on an open-configuration interventional 0.2-T resistive system (Siemens Magnetom Open, Erlangen, Germany). Image quality and artifacts have been assessed using phantoms and biologic tissues.[8,9]

A rod phantom was filled with a solution of ^{18}F, a positron emitter, and $NiSO_4$ to provide the MR signal. Each phantom was held inside the PET detector ring using a lucite holder. The PET detector in turn was centered and held in place inside the MR coil (Fig. 18-1). Figure 18-2 shows a pair of PET and MRI scans acquired simultaneously from the phantom. The phantom source activity was about 25 mCi. The PET image data were obtained from approximately 21,000 events collected, and the image was reconstructed using a standard filtered backprojection algorithm with a Shepp-Logan filter rolled off at the Nyquist frequency. The MRI scan was obtained using a small surface coil and a gradient echo sequence with an echo time of 9 msec, a repetition time of 66 msec, a field of view of 10 cm, and a slice thickness of 7 mm.

Assessment of artifacts has included determination of counting artifacts (false-positives) on the PET data and MRI artifacts. MRI artifacts were assessed with the PET electronics on and off. Image subtractions to determine image artifacts showed no signs of artifacts on standard clinical spin-echo and gradient echo MRI.[8,9]

A 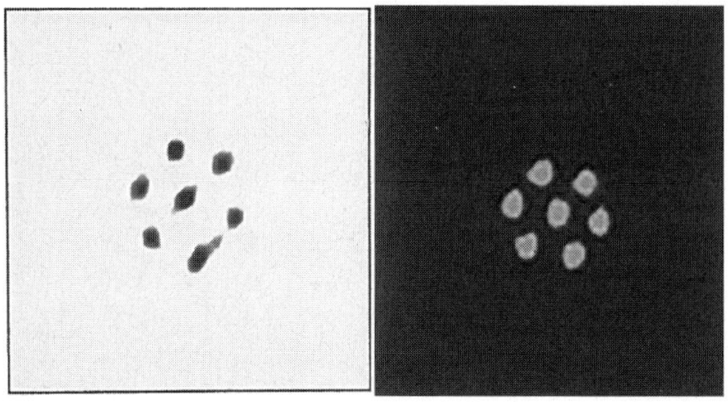 B

Fig. 18-2. Contemporaneous **A,** positron emission tomography scan and **B,** magnetic resonance image obtained from a 15-mm diameter rod phantom. Each rod is 1 mm in diameter.

A 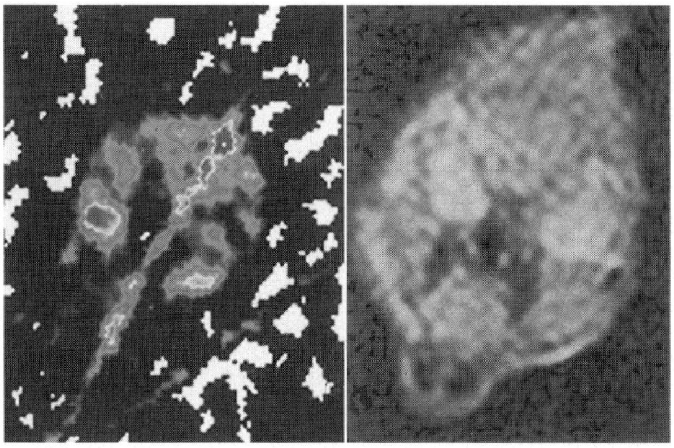 B

Fig. 18-3. Contemporaneous **A,** positron emission tomography scan and **B,** magnetic resonance image acquired from a rat's brain *in vivo.* See Color Plate 4.

SUMMARY

MR-compatible PET is feasible. Although interventional MRI and MRI-compatible PET technologies are in their infancy, there is potential for MRI-guided interventions aided by PET. Future investigations will focus on designing large-diameter MR-compatible PET systems, suitable for humans.[10] Figure 18-3 shows the first pair of simultaneous PET and MRI scans acquired *in vivo.*

REFERENCES

1. Phelps ME, Mazziotta JC, Schelbert HR, editors: *Positron emission tomography and autoradiography,* New York, 1986, Raven Press.
2. Di Chiro G: Positron emission tomography using [18F]fluorodeoxyglucose in brain tumors: a powerful diagnostic and prognostic tool, *Invest Radiol* 22:360, 1987.
3. Alavi JB, and others: Positron emission tomography in patients with gliomas: a predictor of prognosis, *Cancer* 62:1074, 1988.
4. Jabour BA, and others: Extracranial head and neck: PET imaging with 2-[F-18]fluoro-2-deoxy-D-glucose and MR imaging correlation, *Radiology* 186:27, 1993.
5. Shao Y, and others: Development of a PET detector system compatible with MRI/MRS systems, *IEEE Trans Nuc Sci* 44:1167, 1997.
6. Shao Y, and others: Simultaneous PET and MR imaging, *Phys Med Biol* 42:1965, 1997.
7. Shao Y, and others: Development of a PET detector system compatible with MRI/NMR systems, *IEEE Trans Nuc Sci* 44:1167, 1997.
8. Farahani K, and others: Contemporaneous positron emission tomography and MR imaging at 1.5 T, *J Magn Reson Imag* (in press).
9. Slates R, and others: *Assessment of artifacts in simultaneous PET and MR imaging,* 1997, Proceedings of the IEEE Transactions on Medical Imaging.
10. Shao Y, and others: *The road to simultaneous PET/MR images of the brain.* In Carson RE, Daube-Witherspoon ME, Herscovitch P, editors: *Quantitative functional brain imaging with positron emission tomography* (in press).

Chapter 19

THERAPY PLANNING FOR INTERVENTIONAL MRI

Shantanu Sinha, Usha Sinha, Thomas Oshiro

Interventional magnetic resonance imaging (MRI) is a growing application of MRI that combines minimally invasive therapeutic techniques with diagnostic imaging. Interventional MR refers to MR-guided therapy techniques, which include thermal ablation procedures (hyperthermia, high-intensity focused ultrasound [HIFU], laser-induced interstitial thermotherapy [LITT], radiofrequency [RF], microwave, and cryoablation), ethanol ablations, endoscopic sinus surgery, bone biopsies, and sympathectomy.[1–6] Therapy planning for interventional MRI will vary depending on the accessibility to the patient in the scanner. The conventional closed MR scanner configuration provides limited accessibility to the patient, but recently, several dedicated interventional open scanners with wide-angle accessibility have become commercially available. However, because the closed configuration is more widely installed, this chapter discusses strategies for therapy planning in conjunction with closed- and open-configuration MR scanners. Planning an interventional MR procedure includes target definition, trajectory selection, dosage calculation, guidance of the interventional probe, and monitoring during and after the procedure. Planning is largely determined by accessibility of the magnet and by MR compatibility of the therapeutic devices. If the therapeutic device is not MR compatible, real-time MR monitoring during intervention cannot be included as part of the therapy plan. Alternate methods of monitoring have to be used to control the interventional procedure. This chapter provides a brief discussion of MR-compatible equipment to emphasize the effects on therapy planning.

SPECIAL TOOLS FOR MAGNETIC RESONANCE–GUIDED THERAPEUTIC INTERVENTIONS

Conventional surgical tools are made of stainless steel, which cannot be readily used in the MR scanner. These ferromagnetic objects are subject to significant magnetic forces, and the resultant torque is a source of potential hazard to patients and personnel. Even alloys that experience insignificant torque near the scanner may produce considerable susceptibility-induced image distortions that preclude use of these alloys for MR-guided intervention. Several MR-compatible biopsy and aspiration needles made from high-nickel content needles are commercially available.[7] One important advantage with the open-access magnet system is that MR monitoring during the interventional procedure allows real-time visualization and feedback of the therapeutic procedures. However, monitoring should be coupled with the development of MR-compatible therapeutic devices and fast-pulse sequences with sufficient sensitivity to detect changes caused by intervention. MR-compatible devices for cryoablation, ethanol infusion, HIFU ablation, and LITT have been developed. The advantage of an interventional procedure using LITT is that the entire laser power supply can be situated outside the scanner room while the laser fiberoptic cable is brought into the scanner room via electrically shielded conduits. This shielding minimizes interference from the laser electronics and permits MR acquisition during laser ablation. However, the technical challenge to develop an MR-compatible RF ablation device is considerably greater. This device should include a nonmagnetic RF probe to reduce susceptibility-induced artifacts in MRI and an RF generator, which introduces minimal electronic noise into the MR signal. A combination hardware and software filter was recently developed, which reduces the electronic noise from the RF generator to a level that MR phase images for temperature mapping can be acquired during RF ablation (Fig. 19-1).

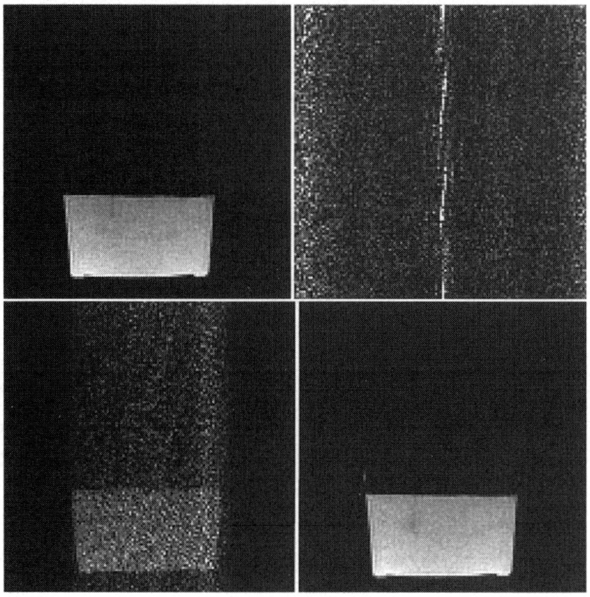

Fig. 19-1. A magnetic resonance (MR)-compatible radiofrequency (RF) generator is critical to the development of real-time MR image monitoring of RF lesions. **A,** An MRI scan shows a gel phantom acquired with the RF generator turned off. **B,** Conventional RF generators cause considerable electronic noise that completely degrades image quality. **C,** Incorporation of a software filter improves image quality but not sufficiently for temperature monitoring. **D,** The cropping of edges of the image can be eliminated by increasing the bandwidth of the filter. Electronic noise is reduced to acceptable levels by including software and hardware filters.

PREPLANNING

Preplanning refers to planning before the interventional procedure. The goals of preplanning are to locate the target, to ascertain the best surgical approach to the target point (i.e., to define the entry and target point on a three-dimensional [3D] dataset acquired before the procedure), and to calculate the dosage. For interventional biopsies, the first two steps of preplanning are sufficient. For thermal or cryoablation procedures, the dosage (e.g., laser, RF, or HIFU power and duration) and number of thermal lesions required to cover the tumor should be calculated based on the tumor size and location.

Localization of the target

Typical imaging sequences acquired before MR intervention for brain lesions are 2D T1- and T2-weighted images and 3D T1-weighted images acquired before and after administration of the contrast agent Gd-DTPA.[3,8] These images help establish the location and extent of the enhancing tumor. A similar protocol is also followed for liver lesions. MR angiograms can be obtained to map the relative location of the tumor with respect to major blood vessels, which is important for two reasons: (1) to plan the trajectory to the target, which avoids major blood vessels, and (2) to plan the dosage required in thermal ablation procedures. For example, in RF ablation procedures, a large blood vessel or cerebrospinal fluid (CSF) spaces near the electrode tip will act as a heat sink, preventing a full lesion from developing or making the lesion asymmetric.[9,10] Because many interventional MR scanners are operated at low fields (0.064 to 0.5 T), acquisition of high-resolution 3D time of flight MR angiograms in a high-field system (1.5 T) may be necessary. T1- and T2-weighted images acquired on the low-field interventional units can then be registered to the MR angiograms from the high-field scanners. Furthermore, multimodality image registration, such as MR–positron emission tomography (PET) or MR-magnetencephalography (MEG), may be necessary when PET or MEG images are used in the presurgical evaluation of brain function.[11] Registration can be readily accomplished when a stereotactic frame is included. In a frameless procedure, registration can be performed using fixed markers attached to the patient or surface-matching algorithms.[12] Fast, completely automated registration algorithms are preferred if real-time registration is required.[13] *Real-time* refers to registration of images acquired during the interventional procedure with images acquired at a previous examination or in a different scanner. Real-time registration introduces additional complications because the data set acquired during the procedure is often, because of temporal considerations, of poor image quality, is of poor resolution, and is restricted to a couple of slices.

Trajectory selection

The second step of preplanning is to optimize the surgical trajectory. 3D images acquired in the previous step are normally downloaded to a 3D workstation. The ideal 3D workstation for preplanning should have several features: image visualization in 2D and 3D, multimodality image registration and fusion, and tools for simulating trajectories from the entry point to the target. Workstations with these functions are described in the literature.[14,15] The surgeon can align multimodality images and subsequently display the registered images in 2D and 3D format. Simulated trajectories of the interventional probe are then viewed superimposed on these images, with the option of displaying in 3D format also. However, preplanning to optimize the surgical trajectory is not as important when intraoperative MR guidance is available. This step may be optional if intraoperative guiding techniques (described in the section on guidance of the interventional probe) are available. The details of preplanning will depend largely on the guidance technique used: frame-based stereotaxy, frameless stereotaxy, or MR-guided target tracking.

Dosage calculation

Calculation of dose should be adapted to the physical requirements of the therapy, the anatomic region involved, the type of ablation (tumor ablation, functional ablation), and location of the target region (proximity to blood vessels or ventricles). The term *dose calculation* is loosely used and does not strictly refer to dose as much as to optimization of the different parameters for delivering the appropriate therapy to the target region. For instance, in an RF ablation procedure of a tumor, in addition to the thermal power and duration of the RF, the length of the exposed electrode tip and the diameter of the electrode tip may need to be optimized according to the size of the tumor. Similar to the determination of the optimal trajectory to the target, accurate power and duration calculations as part of preplanning are optional with the availability of MRI techniques to monitor the progress of the ablation procedure. However, real-time MR monitoring techniques are recent developments that should be validated. Some preliminary studies have investigated the validity of MR monitoring techniques by correlation to pathologic findings.[16] Because MR monitoring techniques are at an infancy stage, dose calculations should be based on pretherapy images. Some guidelines based on experimental and theoretic considerations exist for planning different interventional procedures; they are given below:

Radiofrequency ablation

RF ablation for management of certain brain pathology was established at least 30 years before the advent of MR interventional techniques. However, MR-guided RF ablation provides, for the first time, the ability to guide the probe and monitor the thermal ablation and postablation effects. The established technique for managing brain tumors is to create an RF lesion by increasing the temperature to 80° C and maintaining it for 1 min.[3] The size and shape of the thermal lesion are determined by various physical and tissue factors. At the University of California, Los Angeles (UCLA) patients with brain tumors underwent RF thermal therapy using a 5- or 10-mm exposed tip straight electrode or a side-advanced spring that describes a 10-mm diameter semicircle from the tip of the electrode to create a 3D treatment volume.[3] Extensive literature exists on physical parameters (e.g., electrode diameter, exposed tip length, wattage, duration) to create lesions of a desired size in different target areas.[17,18] Saline-cooled RF electrodes can generate larger lesions than can noncooled RF electrodes for a given diameter of the RF electrode.[19] For MR monitoring, a small-diameter needle is desirable for optimal visualization of tissue, free from susceptibility artifacts. Thus, a small-diameter saline-cooled RF probe may be preferred over a noncooled probe when larger thermal lesions (2 to 3 cm) are desired. The parameters in the literature provide a good starting point for therapy planning, which, coupled with real-time MR monitoring, should provide accurate control of the lesion size.

In addition to the data available from experimental studies, several thermodynamic models have been proposed for tissue heating.[20,21] Direct tissue volume heating during RF ablation is less than 1 mm, so all deeper tissue heating, which is most of the thermal lesion volume, results from passive heat conduction from this small region of heating. Thus, conductive heating from an RF source can be analyzed in terms of tissue heating from a pure thermal source. At steady-state conditions, the heat generated by the RF current equals heat loss by conduction (heat diffusion) and convection (via microcirculation). A simplified model, in which the effects of metabolic heat production and microvascular perfusion based connective cooling are ignored, leads to the following relationship (when a constant temperature source is maintained):

$$d/d_i = (t_o - T)/(t - T)$$

where d is the distance from the center of the thermal source, d_i is the radius of the heat source (slightly larger the electrode radius), t_o is the temperature at the electrode-tissue interface, T is the ambient tissue temperature, and t is the temperature at radius d.[18] This model predicts that at steady state, the lesion size should be proportional to the electrode-tissue interface temperature and the electrode radius. Although *in vitro* determinations of lesion size correlate well with temperature at the electrode-tissue interface, *in vivo* correlations are poorer, possibly because of variability in the amount of RF catheter contact pressure and different amounts of convective heat loss based on the tissue perfusion status.[22] Fast temperature-sensitive MR sequences provide an unique opportunity to map, in real-time, the spatial temperature distribution during the ablation process. MR temperature mapping techniques can provide better control over lesion size than afforded by pretherapy calculations based on thermodynamic models alone. Correlation of thermal maps obtained during RF ablation in gels and *in vitro* tissue to the thermodynamic model is being attempted.

Laser-induced interstitial thermotherapy

Kahn and others[8] used a neodymium:yttrium-aluminum garnet (Nd:YAG) laser source for brain lesions and established typical power and time of irradiation to be 4 to 5 W and 10 to 20 min, respectively (see Chapter 29). In this study, MR temperature sequences (see below) were used to monitor the size of the thermal lesion, and the ablation was terminated when the diameter of the laser-induced peripheral zone was similar to the diameter of the tumor. The diameter of the tumors ranged from 18 to 35 mm. The duration of irradiation was determined by the feedback obtained from the MR-generated thermal maps, obviating the need for accurate dosage calculation in the preplanning stage.

A low-powered Nd:YAG laser has also been used for LITT of breast tumors. In this study, a precharred 400-μ diameter laser probe at 2 W was applied for 9 min to create 1- to 2-cm lesions. Real-time MR monitoring was not used in this study; however, MRI scans were acquired after therapy to confirm the size and location of the thermal lesion. LITT has also been applied successfully to the management of prostate cancer and bladder outlet obstruction, with MR used to monitor postablative changes.[24,25] Recently, preliminary attempts have been made toward planning therapy based on computer simulation. The model initially calculates the expected light distribution in the irradiated areas. This is followed by a calculation of the heat and damage distribution through the targeted tissue structures. The model accounts for the specific geometry of the applicator, the changes of the optical and thermal properties of the tissue during coagulation, blood perfusion, and thermal exchange between the tissue, the applicator, and the ambient medium.[26] These simulation studies can be used to design new types of laser diffuser tips to obtain larger or asymmetric thermal lesions.

High intensity focused ultrasound

The acoustic intensity pattern and temperature distribution created by a diffraction-limited spherical transducer have been analyzed for HIFU ablations conducted in gel phantoms and bovine muscle.[27] The intensity created at a point (r,z) depends on the acoustic waves generated at the surface. The relative intensity pattern near the focus can be approximated by an elliptic gaussian with characteristic radii r_o and z_o that corresponds to 60% of the maximum intensity. The half-intensity radii estimated from the intensity analysis were used to calculate the temperature profiles. The ultrasound spot radius measured from the temperature profile measured in gel phantoms using T1-weighted sequences agreed with acoustic intensity calculations. However, the agreement is not as good in muscle, in which the focal spot spreads to almost twice the theoretic estimation. This discrepancy based on focal spot spreading was possibly caused by fat in the muscle or microbubbles in the aging bovine meat. These studies emphasize the need for a real-time MR temperature monitoring because theoretical models do not always provide accurate estimates.

GUIDANCE OF THE INTERVENTIONAL PROBE

Frame-based stereotaxy

Frame-based stereotactic MRI has been implemented for guiding biopsies, tumor resections, tumor ablations, deep electroencephalogram electrode placement, and functional target localization for functional ablation.[28,29] Several stereotactic systems with localizer frames designed for MRI localization are commercially available: Cosman Robert-Wells (Radionics, Burlington, Mass), Leksell (Elekta Instruments, Atlanta, Ga), and Laitinen (Sandstorm Trade & Technology, Welland, Ontario, Canada). In addition to helping localize the coordinates of the target area, the stereotactic frame also serves as a fixation device during imaging and as a probe carrier during surgery. The 3D workstation is used in conjunction with the preoperative images to determine the optimum trajectory from which the settings of the stereotactic arc are calculated automatically. In an open-access scanner, images are not necessarily acquired preoperatively because the patient with the frame can be positioned during the entire procedure within the scanner without needing to be removed from the gantry, as in the case of closed systems. The accuracy of stereotactic MRI guidance is limited by various factors: susceptibility artifacts at interventional probe-tissue, frame fiducial–air, or tissue-air interfaces; the linearity and calibration of magnetic field gradients; and eddy currents of the pulsed gradients excited in the cryoshield. It is important to maintain a rigorous quality control program that periodically assesses gradient performances and eddy current effects.[30] Assessing these errors in positioning is essential for high accuracy of target location. Correction algorithms to improve the accuracy of the spatial coordinates have been suggested.[31] The final localization of the probe should be confirmed by imaging with the probe in position at the target.

Frameless stereotaxy

Frame-based stereotactic systems are accurate and well-proven but require the fixation of the frame to the patient. Frameless stereotactic localization further reduces patient discomfort and makes the therapeutic procedure more minimally invasive. Furthermore, stereotactic frames can be used only when rigidity and immobility of the organ with respect to the frame have been accomplished. These prerequisites are satisfied only for brain and bone surgery; they are not satisfied for most organs or soft tissue.[32]

Interactive operating arm

The advent of the open magnet configuration combined with real-time imaging capabilities enables successful targeting even in regions that are flexible and mobile. One such system is composed of an MR-compatible arm (referred to as the *digitizer*); a 3D workstation; and a liquid crystal display screen, which permits viewing inside the scanner. The potential of open interventional MR scanners is increased in conjunction with mechanical arm–based frameless stereotaxy. In this technique, no preoperative images are required because the computer is calibrated to the scanner's internal coordinate system. A digitizer can supply information about its location and orientation, and this information is relayed to the 3D workstation. Researchers at UCLA have used a mechanical digitizer, whereas researchers at other sites have implemented an optical digitizer with an open interventional MR system.[15] The digitizer is calibrated with respect to the interventional magnet coordinate system by touching the digitizer to three or more points on the magnet. This calibration permits the 3D workstation to locate the position of the digitizer as it moves in the magnet bore. The MR scanner host system and the 3D workstation are linked, so the physician can specify scan planes by moving the digitizer to the desired locations. Near real-time images can be acquired directly in the plane of the digitizer location and orientation. The therapeutic probe (RF, laser, cryotip, or alcohol needle) is attached to the mechanical arm, so the probe's location is known from the digitizer's position. The 3D workstation provides multiple viewing capabilities to facilitate the surgeon, including a 3D view with the probe overlaid, an image in the plane of the probe, and a view perpendicular to the probe. Because the physician controls the arm's 3D location, this technique accurately guides the probe to the target area with real-time feedback.

Magnetic resonance–guided target tracking

The scanner itself can be used to update images rapidly as the interventional device approaches the target or update the position of an RF coil (attached to the probe tip) on a 3D image dataset acquired just before insertion of the probe.

Passive tracking

In the passive tracking method, the device is visualized by the signal void it creates and by its susceptibility artifact (see Chapter 15). In this technique, the location of the needle is updated at a frequency limited by the time required for image acquisition, reconstruction, and display. Image acquisition times are usually reduced by using 2D Fourier transformed spoiled gradient echo (spoiled gradient recalled echo in steady state or fast low-angle shot) or 2D Fourier transformed steady-state gradient echo (steady state free precession or fast imaging with steady-state precision) sequences. However, gradient echo sequences may produce unacceptably large artifacts at high-field strengths. Fast spin-echoes (echo time, 11 msec; repetition time, 120 msec; echo train length, 4; matrix 256 × 28; scan time, 4 sec), which are less susceptible to artifacts from field inhomogeneities, have been used for breast lesion localization at 1.5 T.[33] A rapid gradient echo sequence with an acquisition time of 800 msec and an interleaved gradient echoplanar sequence with an acquisition time of 350 to 400 msec have been investigated as ultrafast sequences for guidewire placement for vascular interventions under MRI visualization.[7]

Active tracking

Active tracking, a method of internal tracking first suggested by Dumoulin, Souza, and Darrow,[34] has been implemented successfully in an interventional MR scanner for guiding a laser probe for vascular interventions (see Chapter 16). In active tracking, real-time tracking with the position of the device tip updated 20 times per sec is possible. In this technique, a small RF coil, consisting of an untuned single loop less than 1 mm in diameter, is attached to the tip of the interventional device. Such a coil is insensitive to signals coming from more than 1 mm away. The body coil is used to excite all spins within the field of view. Gradient-recalled echoes are generated along three orthogonal axes to frequency encode the 3D position of the coil. The positional accuracy of the RF coil can be found to a resolution of less than 1 mm, which is typically the in-plane resolution of MRI. The position of the coil, updated 20 times per sec, is displayed superimposed on a previously acquired MRI scan. This technique and variants thereof have been verified *in vitro* and *in vivo*.[35,36] This technique is ideally suited for an open scanner configuration because the device location is tracked by MRI. A 3D dataset in the region of interest may be acquired before intervention, and the surgeon can view the trajectory as the position of the device tip is shown superposed on the 3D volume. As in the case of passive tracking, images are displayed inside the scanner room on a liquid crystal display screen to provide real-time feedback to the physician.

MAGNETIC RESONANCE MONITORING OF THE THERAPEUTIC PROCEDURE

Once the probe is located in the desired target volume, therapy is initiated. MRI is excellent for monitoring, controlling, and assessing the therapy procedure. The choice of the imaging sequence depends on the type and the temporal demands of the therapeutic procedure. MRI is unique in its ability to noninvasively measure spatial temperature distributions through the effect of temperature on MR parameters (T1, diffusion, and proton chemical shift). The demands on temporal resolution are high but do not necessarily require real-time frame rates as in tracking. The ablations typically are in the range of 20 to 40 sec for HIFU, 1 to 2 min for RF, and 10 to 20 min for LITT. For temperature to be monitored with sufficient temporal resolution in HIFU and RF ablations, it is necessary to be able to acquire temperature maps at least every 5 to 10 sec. Of the three MR parameters sensitive to temperature, phase imaging appears most promising (see Chapter 12).

Phase imaging to monitor temperature changes during ablation

Recent investigations of MR thermometry based on the temperature-dependent proton resonant frequency have proved that this method is accurate and may be clinically viable. This technique has been applied successfully to map temperature using phase images of gradient echoes. Most measurements have been performed at high fields (1.5 T) in closed-configuration systems.[37,38] Phase imaging has been used to monitor temperature changes during RF, LITT, and HIFU procedures. Phase change images are calculated by subtracting the phase or complex images acquired at higher (or lower) temperatures from a corresponding reference image.[39] Phase unwrapping and phase drift correction should be performed before a temperature map can be generated. At UCLA, an off-line system has been developed in which phase images are automatically transferred from the host scanner system to the external computer and processed (phase unwrapped, drift corrected, and subtracted) to obtain the temperature maps.[40] These maps are color coded and displayed superimposed on the original images (Fig. 19-2). The therapy is terminated when the lesion size (as determined from the temperature maps) matches the size of the tumor. The termination

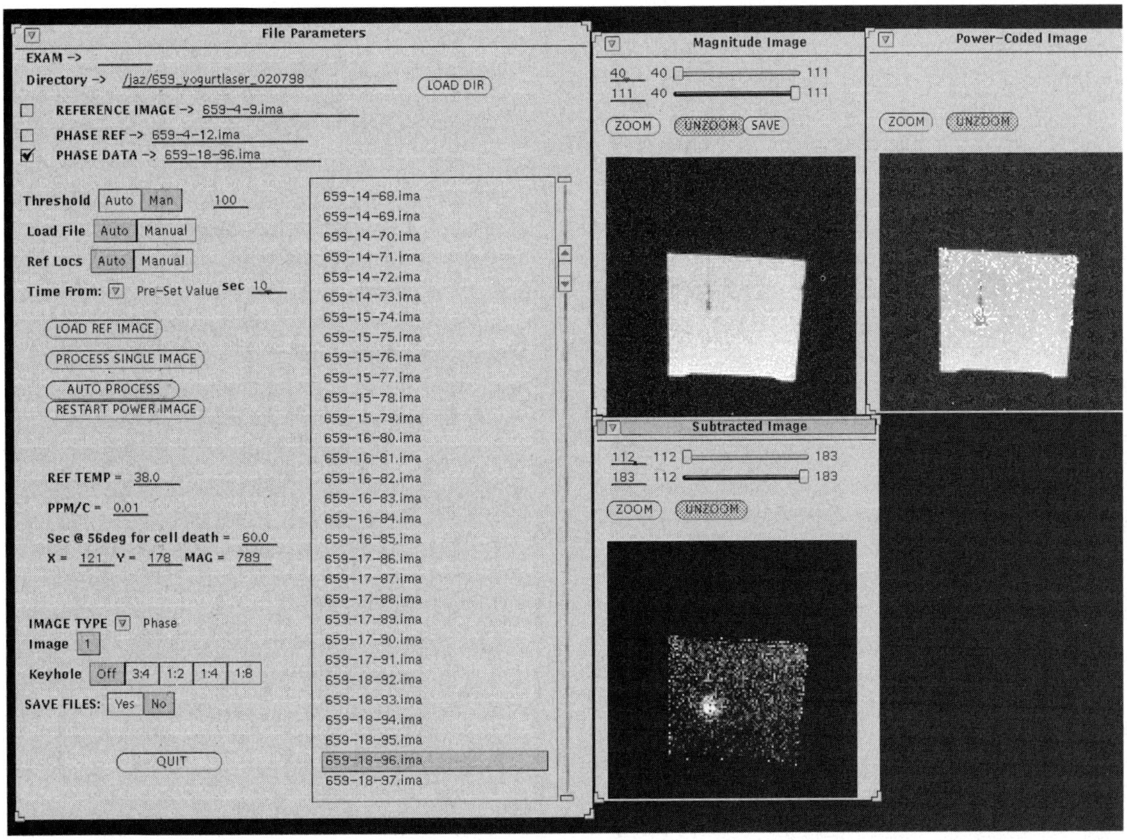

Fig. 19-2. This computer display package allows real-time visualization of heat lesions. Temperature maps are generated from phase images and displayed in color for ease of visualization. User interaction is minimal and involves only identification of the reference image before the dynamic ablation procedure. In addition to the temperature maps, the integral under the temperature-time curve is also displayed because this parameter is an indicator of cell death. The map of this integral is also displayed in color superposed on the original images. See Color Plate 5.

criterion can be based on isocontours of temperature or on an integral of temperature and time. This latter criterion is used because the dose required for cell death has been estimated (based on hyperthermia experience) to be 43° C for 240 min.[41] As the temperature increases, the required time is reduced by half for every 1° increase in temperature.

Cryoablation

Freezing has been investigated as a means of ablating deep pathology (see Chapter 22). MR-guided cryoablation has recently become possible only with the development of MR-compatible freezing devices.[42] It is important to monitor the temperature inside the frozen region induced by cryoablation. However, the MR signal from the solid tissue is too weak to use MR thermal sequences for monitoring temperature. A technique combining MRI data with a finite difference formulation of the energy equation has been developed to map the temperature profile of the frozen region.[43]

Alcohol ablation

Injection of ethanol into tissues in sufficiently high concentration results in local dehydration necrosis. Ethanol infusion can be readily monitored using T2-weighted imaging sequences.[4] The lesion signal intensity decreases on T2-weighted images during the time course of the ethanol injection. Low spatial resolution, rectangular field of view, T2-weighted fast spin-echo sequences are used to obtain images with a temporal resolution of 1 min, which is adequate to monitor the ethanol ablation of tissues (approximately 3 to 4 min to completion).

CONCLUSIONS

MR-guided therapy has remarkable potential, although it is in a stage of infancy. Further developments in scanners with better patient access and MR-compatible therapeutic devices will help establish MR-guided therapy as a viable surgical option. Concurrently, other areas to be investigated are ultrafast MR sequences for guiding and monitoring of the procedure. These developments and improved image viewing and scan control options from within the scanner room will provide the surgeon or radiologist with real-time information that was previously not available during surgical intervention. The combined advancement in these areas may establish the MR scanner as an integral part of the operating room.

REFERENCES

1. Hathout G, and others: MR-guided aspiration cytology in the head and neck at high field strength, *J Magn Reson Imaging* 2:93, 1992.
2. Hynynen K, and others: MRI-guided noninvasive ultrasound surgery, *Med Phys* 20:7, 1993.
3. Lufkin RB, and others: *MR guided radio-frequency ablation of brain tumors.* In De Salles A, Lufkin R, editors: *Minimally invasive therapy of the brain,* New York, 1997, Thieme.
4. Lu DS, and others: MR-guided percutaneous ethanol ablation of liver tissue in a 2-T open MR system: preliminary study in porcine model, *J Magn Reson Imaging* 7:303, 1997.
5. Castro D, Saxton RE, Lufkin R: Interstitial photoablative laser therapy guided by magnetic resonance imaging for the treatment of deep tumors, *Semin Surg Oncol* 8:233, 1992.
6. Huang AY, and others: *Interventional MRI for neurosurgery.* In Hadley MN, editor: *Perspectives in neurological surgery,* St Louis, Mosby, 1995.
7. Kochli VD, and others: Vascular interventions guided by ultrafast MR imaging: evaluation of different materials, *Magn Reson Med* 31:309, 1994.
8. Kahn T, and others: *Clinical applications of laser-induced interstitial thermotherapy in the brain.* In De Salles A, Lufkin R, editors: *Minimally invasive therapy of the brain,* New York, 1997, Thieme.
9. Cosman ER, Cosman BJ: *Methods of making nervous system lesions.* In Wilkins RH, Rengachar SS, editors: *Neurosurgery,* vol 3, New York, 1985, McGraw-Hill.
10. Hriz MI: *Image-guided functional ablation of the brain.* In De Salles A, Lufkin R, editors: *Minimally invasive therapy of the brain,* New York, 1997, Thieme.
11. Witte OW: Magnet encephalography as a tool for presurgical evaluation of brain function, *Eur Radiology* 7:1158, 1997.
12. Sinha S, and others: Structure-function correlation in gated cardiac MR and PET studies, *Am J Roentgenol* 164:301, 1995.
13. Jyrkinen L, and others: A method for patient movement registration during MRI intervention, *Eur Radiology* 7:1150, 1997.
14. Smith KR, Frank KJ, Bucholz RD: The Neuro Station: a highly accurate, minimally invasive solution to frameless stereotactic neurosurgery, *Comput Med Imaging Graph* 18:247, 1994.
15. Williams ML: *Graphics workstations for therapy of the brain.* In De Salles A, Lufkin R, editors: *Minimally invasive therapy of the brain,* New York, 1997, Thieme.
16. Kahn T, and others: Correlation of neuropathological findings and phase-based MRI-temperature maps in experimental laser interstitial thermotherapy (LITT), *Eur Radiology* 7:1147, 1997.
17. Organ LW: Electrophysiologic principles of radiofrequency lesion making, *Int Symp Radiofrequency Lesion Making Procedures* 39:69, 1976.
18. Cosman ER, Rittman WJ: *Physical aspects of radiofrequency energy applications.* In Huang SKS, editor: *Radiofrequency catheter ablation of cardiac arrhythmias: basic concepts and clinical applications,* Mount Kisco, 1994, Futura.
19. Boaz TL, and others: MR guidance and monitoring of radiofrequency thermal ablation performed in rabbit liver utilizing saline cooled and non-cooled radiofrequency electrodes, *Eur Radiol* 9:1157, 1997.
20. Haines DE, Watson DD: Tissue heating during radiofrequency catheter ablation: a thermodynamic model and observations in isolated perfused and superfused canine right ventricular free wall, *PACE Pacing Clin Electrophysiol* 12:962, 1989.
21. Haines DE, Watson DD, Verow AF: Electrode radius predicts lesion radius during radiofrequency energy heating: validation of a proposed thermodynamic model, *Circ Res* 67:124, 1990.
22. Haines DE: *Temperature monitoring in radiofrequency catheter ablation.* In Huang SKS, editor: *Radiofrequency catheter ablation of cardiac arrhythmias: basic concepts and clinical applications,* Mount Kisco, 1994, Futura.
23. Mumtaz H, and others: Laser therapy for breast cancer: MR imaging and histopathologic correlation, *Radiology* 200:651, 1996.
24. Bomni RA, and others: Laser ablation-induced changes in the prostate: findings at endorectal MR imaging with histologic correlation, *Radiology* 202:232, 1997.
25. Flynn RJ, and others: Endoscopic laser ablation of the prostate (ELAP): changes in magnetic resonance imaging and clinical outcome at 1 year, *Br J Urol* 78:747, 1996.
26. Schwarzmaier HJ, and others: Laser-induced interstitial thermotherapy (LITT): applicators and therapy planning, *Eur Radiology* 7:1154, 1997.
27. Cline HE, and others: MR temperature mapping of focused ultrasound surgery, *Magn Reson Med* 31:628, 1994.
28. Kondziolka D, and others: A comparison between magnetic resonance imaging and computed tomography for stereotactic coordinate determination, *Neurosurgery* 30:402, 1992.
29. Maciunas R, and others: A universal system for interactive image-directed neurosurgery, *Stereotact Funct Neurosurg* 58:108, 1992.
30. Alexander E III, and others: Magnetic resonance image-directed stereotactic neurosurgery: use of image fusion with computerized tomography to enhance spatial accuracy, *Neurosurg* 83:271, 1995.
31. Fitzpatrick J, and others: *A technique for improving accuracy in position and intensity within images acquired in the presence of field inhomogeneity.* In *Book of abstracts,* New York, 1990, 9th Annual Meeting of the Society of Magnetic Resonance in Medicine.
32. Gybels J, Suetens P: Image-guided surgery, *Verh K Acad Geneeskd Belg* 59:35, 1997.
33. Daniel BL, and others: *Interactive MR-guided breast lesion localization-a phantom study,* New York, 1996, 4th Annual Meeting of ISMRM.
34. Dumoulin CL, Souza SP, Darrow RD: Real time monitoring of invasive devices using magnetic resonance, *Magn Reson Med* 29:411, 1993.
35. Leung DA, and others: Intravascular MR tracking catheter: preliminary experimental evaluation, *Am J Roentgenol* 164:1265, 1995.
36. Gohde SC, and others: MR-guided cholecystostomy: assessment of biplanar, real-time needle tracking in three pigs, *Cardiovasc Intervent Radiol* 20:295, 1997.
37. De Poorter J, and others: The proto-resonance-frequency-shift method compared with molecular diffusion for quantitative measurement of two-dimensional time-dependent temperature distribution in a phantom, *J Magn Reson Imaging,* 103:234, 1994.
38. De Poorter J, and others: Noninvasive MRI thermometry with the proton resonance frequency (PRF) method: in vivo results in human muscle, *Magn Reson Med* 33:74, 1995.
39. Sinha S, and others: Phase imaging on a 0.2 T MR scanner: application to temperature monitoring during ablation procedures, *J Magn Reson Imaging* 7:918, 1997.
40. Oshiro T, and others: Design of a computer interface system for MR image guided monitoring of heat lesions in vivo, *Radiology,* 205:176, 1997.
41. Damianou C, Hynynen K: The effect of various physical parameters on the size and shape of necrosed tissue volume during ultrasound surgery, *J Acoust Soc Am* 95:1641, 1994.
42. Hong JS, and others: MR imaging assisted temperature calculations during cryosurgery, *Magn Reson Imaging* 12:1021, 1994.
43. Richardson ML, and others: MR appearance of skeletal neoplasms following cryotherapy, *Skeletal Radiology* 23:121, 1994.

Chapter 20

IMAGE PROCESSING STRATEGIES FOR INTERVENTIONAL MRI

Ferenc A. Jolesz, Joachim Kettenbach, Nobuhiko Hata, Ron Kikinis

Rapid progress in imaging techniques and advances in computer technology in the past decade have had a profound effect on radiology and related clinical fields. The role of imaging in diagnosis and therapy has become accepted, and neuroradiology has been boosted by technologic advances. Image-based spatially localized descriptions of the brain have forwarded the understanding and diagnosis of numerous neurologic and neurosurgical conditions. Although no method is optimally sensitive or specific for the assessment of central nervous system disorders, several imaging methods carry independent and complementary information. Although magnetic resonance imaging (MRI) has substantial advantages over other modalities to depict the brain, integration and quantification of image-based information obtained with multiple imaging methods, such as MRI, functional MRI, MR angiography, x-ray computed tomography (CT), and single photon emission tomography (SPECT), are necessary to obtain enough information for neurosurgical guidance.

From the point-of-view of technology, achieving the goal of image-guided therapy considers two steps: image acquisition and image postprocessing. The choice of the image acquisition will determine the tissue specificity of the images. Postprocessing techniques for tissue segmentation extract quantitative volumetric information for tissue classes in the brain: white matter, grey matter, cerebrospinal fluid (CSF), white matter abnormalities, and other pathologies (e.g., brain tumors). Although tissue specificity mostly depends on tissue characterization with a given physical system (i.e., CT, MRI), anatomic specificity is primarily determined by postprocessing techniques.

Neurosurgery and radiology are important in the development and implementation of intraoperative imaging. One major goal of intraoperative image guidance is reduced surgical morbidity. While working toward this goal, surgeons have assessed their performances and have discovered the weaknesses of conventional surgical techniques.

LIMITATION OF SURGICAL VISUALIZATION

Visualization during neurosurgery is incomplete; the surgeon cannot see the anatomy beyond the exposed surfaces. For example, conventional craniotomy is markedly constrained by the relatively small area of exposed brain surface, which lacks spatial clues that surgeons need to comprehend all of the relevant anatomy. Such limitations of direct surgical visualization have several consequences: (1) Cortical localization is not accurate, and it is even more compromised within the brain parenchyma. (2) The definition of exact trajectories for targeting is impossible without stereotactic guidance. (3) If the anatomic and pathologic boundaries are unclear (and, thus, accurate tumor localization is impossible), healthy tissue should be removed to ensure complete resection.

Full integration of advanced imaging in neurosurgery will result in fundamental changes in therapeutic strategies and approaches. Advances in technology have resulted in sweeping changes in diagnostic radiology, and more widespread use of modern therapeutic devices, computers, and advanced imaging technologies will have a far-reaching effect on neurosurgery.

COMPUTER-BASED IMAGE GUIDANCE

Image guidance, in general, can reduce the inherent invasiveness of surgery and improve localization and targeting by intraoperative imaging via ultrasound or, more recently, MRI. Alternatively, intraoperative image guidance can be based on previously acquired images using reference frames attached to the patient (frame-based stereotaxy), or images that have been registered to the patient (frameless stereotaxy). In the latter case, computers can navigate the operator through three-dimensional (3D)-coordinates and thus fulfill the need for enhanced visibility during interventional radiologic and minimally invasive surgical procedures.

Image-derived information for management can be applied to every stage of therapy. The increasing demand for refinement of imaging and image representation for neurosurgery requires unique methods for data acquisition, processing, and display and full understanding of the process of imaging and its applications to therapy. Image-based modeling requires computerized image-processing methods (segmentation, registration, and display) and image integration techniques, replacing the mental process of generating 3D representations of patient anatomy. Although advanced imaging modalities and information processing or display methods are widely used in planning, monitoring, and guiding various therapies, these imaging techniques can be integrated into interventional and surgical procedures.

SURGICAL PLANNING AND SIMULATION

For full comprehension of image-based information, neurosurgeons prefer appropriately rendered and interactively displayed 3D data, which resemble the visual information seen during surgical exploration. Adequate use of volumetric data for preoperative planning is formidable, particularly for surgeons who have little understanding of image-based modeling and computer sciences. Depending on the particular application, preoperative planning implies image reconstruction and integration of various display, image manipulation, and visualization tools that help simulate and plan an intervention.

The role of surgical planning in tumor surgery is to define the safest possible approach with the least possible damage to healthy tissue. In this trajectory optimization process, alternative navigational paths and movements through the physical space are tested and analyzed using a preoperative model. In craniofacial and orthopedic surgical applications, the role of surgical planning is the optimal execution of preoperative plans.[1–6] Further expansion of surgical planning and simulation techniques into other surgical fields requires more complex methods (e.g., elastic warping) and more information about shape, position, and orientation, which may correct or account for unavoidable tissue deformation and organ shifts during surgery.[7] Establishing a simulated procedural environment is critical for creating image-based virtual reality, which allows the user to actively enter the 3D environment and perform simulated procedures.

INTRAOPERATIVE IMAGE GUIDANCE

Useful image-guided surgery needs solutions to three key problems: segmentation of MRI or other scans into relevant anatomic structures, registration of graphic models to the patient, and tracking of surgical instruments relative to the patient and the registered scans. Finally, tools for visualizing the segmented models and the scans in concert with the tracked instruments are needed to provide direct feedback to the surgeon. The segmentation stage converts the standard medical imaging data into a set of labeled structures defined by the coordinate system attached to the scanner. These labeled structures highlight key anatomy for the surgeon (e.g., the position of a tumor relative to vessels or critical cortical areas). However, this detailed model patient needs to be directly related to the position of the patient. A coordinate frame transformation should map the structures of the reconstructed model to a coordinate frame centered on the patient. Thus, the optimal means of registering or aligning the geometric information of the segmented model with the geometry of the patient requires a mathematical solution. After these two coordinate frames have been connected, the next stage relates the coordinates of a trackable probe to these two frames. Thus, the position of the probe relative to the segmented structures and the original scan is presented, thereby providing the surgeon with an enhanced view of the surgical field relative to the entire anatomic model of the patient.

As noted, to support minimally invasive surgical procedures, the surgeon must be presented with a rich set of image information. The goal is to support surgical interventions with minimal opening and disruption of tissue, while at the same time giving the surgeon a working experience equivalent to that of proceeding with no concern for collateral tissue damage. Thus, the surgeon should be provided with a detailed reconstruction of the patient's anatomy, although the direct field of view (FOV) may be very limited.

For accurate models of anatomy to be obtained, the raw imagery (e.g., MRI) should be converted by first labeling individual volume elements (voxels) by their associated tissue type, followed by connection or adjacent voxels of similar type into higher-level models of anatomic structures. A detailed approach to this segmentation problem is beyond the scope of this chapter, which reviews the main issues involved in segmenting MRI (or related imagery) into useful structures. The major components of this system are based on the following concepts: 3D models of a patient's internal anatomy; registration or alignment of these models with the position of the patient for enhanced reality visualization and planning; and the tracking through surgery of changes in patient position, position of key surgical instruments, and changes in anatomy caused by surgical procedures.

A skillfully prepared, geometrically correct preoperative plan and a well-developed simulation of the procedure are components of an executional operational model that can be implemented in the operating room. Intraoperative image guidance is based on functional integration of the previously acquired and processed 3D information and the corresponding anatomy of the patient within the same frame of reference. During neurosurgery, an interactive real-time display can show the otherwise hidden anatomic information generated by a single modality or composed from multimodal volumetric images.[7–13] Trajectories from the preoperatively prepared executional plans and models can also be exhibited.

Patient-specific anatomic models

A detailed model of patient anatomy should be created by analyzing medical imagery (e.g., MRI). This analysis includes classifying each voxel in the image into bit-map files for different tissue types (e.g., skin, fat, bone, grey matter, white matter, CSF, tumor, and blood vessels) in the case of neuroscans. Although perfect automatic systems are not available, considerable prior effort[14–25] has resulted in reliable semiautomatic methods. These segmented models should be in direct relationship with the patient, so the surgeon can easily relate what is seen in the model to what is seen in the patient. This approach supports visualization (in which the surgeon can see aligned views of the patient and internal model structures [Fig. 20-1]) and navigation (in which the surgeon can specify points within the patient—e.g., by touching a point—and can see the full context of the corresponding point within the MRI scan [Fig. 20-2]).

Registration

For registration of the 3D model to the patient to be achieved, the following should be specified: the characteristics of the model data set to be used in matching (e.g., skin surface, natural landmarks or artificial fiducials); the characteristics of the second data set, taken from the patient on the operating table (e.g., preattached artificial fiducials, features from dense surface scans, sparse surface scans, video images); and the class of transformations over which a registration solution is sought (e.g., rigid 3D, affine 3D, or flexible or elastic deformations).[26–38]

Intraoperative guidance requires matching of the two frames of reference. The coordinates within which the models exist should be mapped or registered into the physical space of the patient. Links between these two components are realized by combining image-to-patient registration and by tracking instruments within the operational field. These ingredients are key for frameless stereotactic targeting methods, which capitalize on interactive control of image planes and exploit the full information content of perceived 3D space.

Patient-to-model registration is substantially different from multimodality coregistration. Image fusion requires matching all image-based geometric data in a unique coordinate system. The matched data coexist within a single virtual database but, for image-guided procedures, should also be registered into the physical space of the patient. In addition, these data should be overlaid or projected onto the patient's exposed surface if surgical guidance is necessary. Various methods are available for patient-to-model registration. In the original, frame-based stereotactic method, 3D points (of the physical frame) are matched with 2D points (seen on the images). Alternatively, surface points are matched with selected anatomic landmarks or external fiducial markers visible on the images and the patient. In these methods, registration requires pointers attached to position-sensing devices, which establish the relationship between the reference frame of the patient and the images. Other registration techniques match visible anatomic objects, features, or shapes represented on the patient and the reconstructed images.

Video camera–based methods detect visible features on the patient (ear, nose, eyes) appearing on the reconstructed surfaces and the video images.[39] Skin surface–based registrations can be

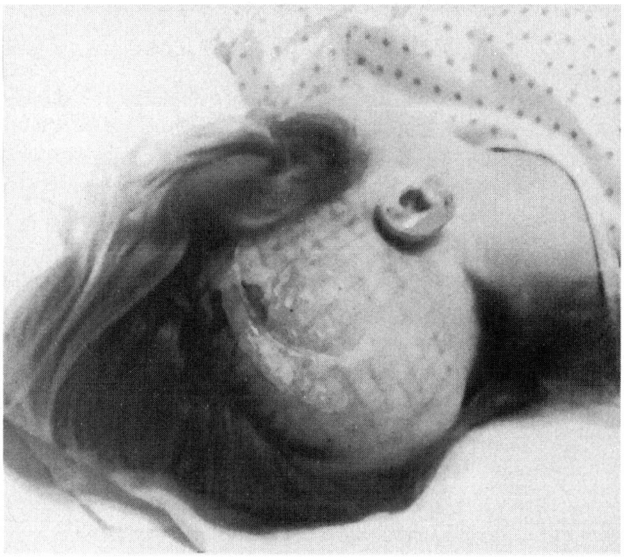

Fig. 20-1. Magnetic resonance imaging reconstruction with the patient on the operating table shows a brain tumor and the ventricles overlaid onto a live video view of the patient. See Color Plate 6. (From Grimson, and others: An automated registration method for frameless stereotaxy, *Image Guided Surgery and Enhanced Reality Visualization,* April 1996.)

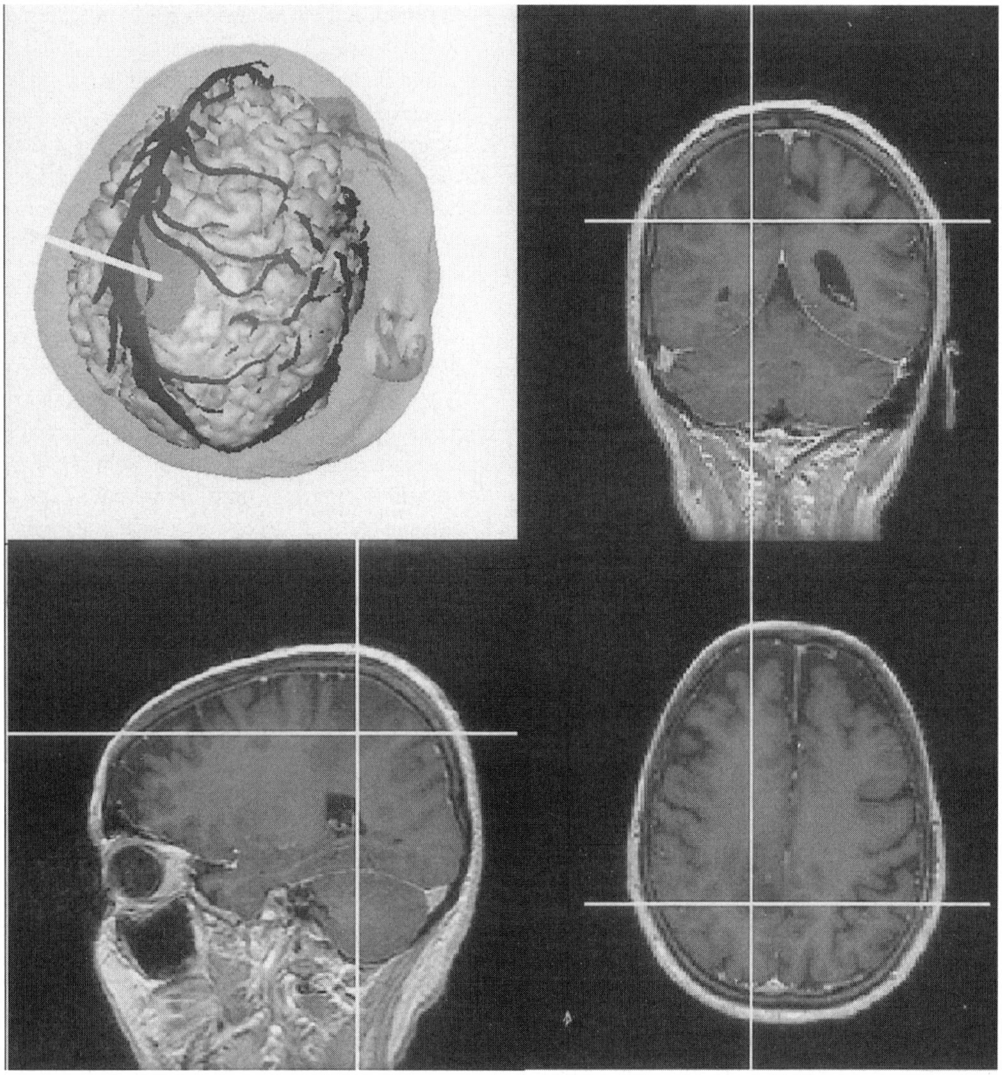

Fig. 20-2. Tracking of a surgical probe. A three-dimensional graphic reconstruction of the patient's head displays the position of the probe and three cross-sectional slices of the patient's magnetic resonance data. *Crosshairs* denote the probe's tip. See Color Plate 7. (From Jolesz FA, Kettenbach J, Kikinis R: *Image-guided neurosurgery with intraoperative MRI.* In Debatin JF, Adam G, editors: *Interventional magnetic resonance imaging,* Heidelberg, 1998, Springer-Verlag.)

refined by readjusting them to inner surfaces of the organs as they become exposed during surgery. For example video registration can be improved by matching cortical vessels, visible on the surface of the exposed brain and on 3D reconstructions based on MR angiograms.[40] Currently, laser scanning is used to obtain digitized surfaces and later match 3D curves with those obtained with automated methods.[41]

In a current system, 3D data from the patient's position on the operating table are obtained by scanning the skin surface of the patient with a laser ranging device. This scanner operates by passing a low-power laser beam through a cylindrical lens to create a plane of light. This plane is directed onto the patient and is observed in a video camera oriented at a fixed angle offset to the laser plane. As a result, points at different depths relative to the baseline separating the camera and laser appear at different positions or offsets in the camera. The camera's position relative to the laser is carefully calibrated to relate the position of the observed laser points in the image to the 3D position of the reflecting point in the world. The laser is mounted on a stepper motor, and the laser plane is swept across a range of positions, thus scanning depth positions over a volume of space. Typically, only 15 to 20 lines of data are scanned, allowing for rapid acquisition of data, albeit only at a sparse set of lines. As a consequence, there is no guarantee that the lines intersect distinctive features (e.g., tip of the nose, corner of the eye). Instead, a set of 3D points, measured relative to a coordinate frame attached to the laser ranger, lie on a small set of planes because of the nature of the laser data-acquisition process. Hence, registration methods are required that do not rely on a small set of distinctive features or fiducial landmarks,

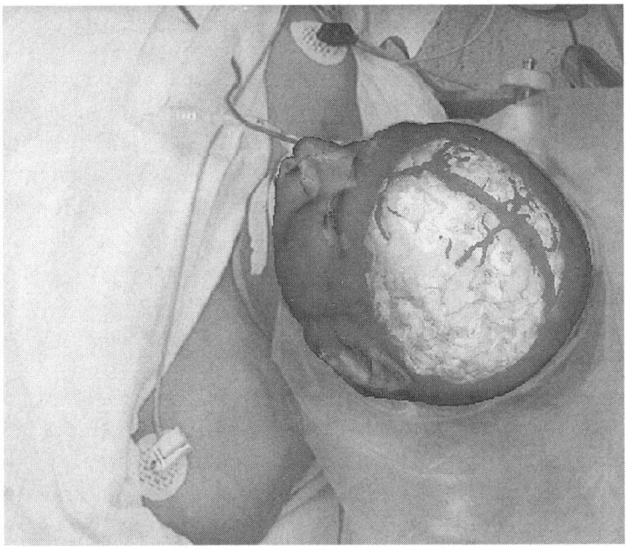

Fig. 20-3. Magnetic resonance imaging reconstruction with the patient on the operating table shows an overlay of the skin, skull, and internal structures onto a live view of the patient. See Color Plate 8.

but rather can align sets of data features based on goodness of surface fit. Thus, the problem is to align two data sets: a dense surface representation (the skin surface from the MRI reconstruction), and a set of points (the sampled laser points).

The model information can thus be brought into the coordinate frame of the laser. Once the position and orientation of a video camera relative to the laser are solved, images of the internal structures of the model can be rendered through the associated camera model, providing a synthetic view of what internal structures look like with no intervening material. These views are combined with live shots from the camera to create enhanced reality visualizations (Fig. 20-3), allowing guided surgical procedures to be planned. This registration allows the surgeon to visualize the patient's internal anatomy. Ideally, however, the surgeon can query the system about points within the patient. Thus, for example, the surgeon should be able to take a probe, touch a point on or in the patient, and see the location of this point in the full original or segmented MRI scans.

In a current system, this capability is accomplished by an optical digitizer (Flashpoint 5000, Image Guided Technologies, Inc., Boulder, Colo), which tracks a set of several light-emitting diodes (LEDs) and uses triangulation by three high-resolution cameras (charged-coupled-device [CCD]) to determine the LED's positions relative to a coordinate frame attached to the camera system. Thus, by attaching a set of LEDs to the probe, the position and orientation of the probe in the Flashpoint's coordinate frame can be determined. The position of the Flashpoint's probe is calibrated with respect to the laser system to connect all these coordinate frames together, allowing probe points to be related to the laser coordinate frame and hence to the MRI scans (see Fig. 20-3). This patient-to-model registration assumes that the patient has not been moved since the original registration. LEDs are attached directly to the patient and any changes in position are tracked to account for changes in patient position.

The Flashpoint system can be used as an acquisition device. If the probe is traced along the skin surface of the patient and the position of the probe tip is recorded, additional data points can be included with the laser data as part of the registration process.

For accuracy to be improved various registration methods can be combined. By merging the view of the surgical field with a surface representation of 3D images and, in some cases, with the correlated maps of functional cortical physiology (obtained from preoperative transcalvarial stimulation, intraoperative electrode recordings, and functional MRI), sufficient control of neurosurgical procedures can be provided even in high-risk areas.[42] Multimodality data from MRI, MR angiography, SPECT, or positron-emission tomography (PET) scans and spatially recorded functional physiologic and preoperative surgical plans can be registered to the patient to intraoperatively integrate all available information.[10,11]

Tracking

Reliable and completely automated registration methods can integrate the image-based information with the patient's anatomy. Nevertheless, intraoperative 3D position sensing and tracking are essential to account for the inevitable movements of the patient and the path of the surgical instruments. If the position of surgical instruments, anatomic landmarks, and image-derived 3D anatomy do not correspond, geometric accuracy is impossible, and precise plans cannot be executed consistently. After initial registration, patient motion can be tracked by reregistration of the updated images if real-time imaging is available. Tracking is the process by which objects are dynamically localized in the patient's coordinate system. Of particular interest is the tracking of medical instruments and the patient's head. Common methods of tracking include articulated arms, optical tracking, passive systems, sonic digitizers, and electromagnetic localizers. In computer-assisted surgery in which only previously acquired images are used, so-called navigational systems establish the relationship between the surgeon's movements and the image-based information within the physical space of the patient.[43-50] Intraoperative 2D and 3D displays—virtual or enhanced (augmented) reality representation—allow navigation within the patient's body to be guided by direct visibility and by the images themselves.

To follow the movements of the surgeon's hand or instruments, encoders continuously detect the position and orientation of passive mechanical arms at the articulations.[51] Alternatively, various 3D positional sensors can be mounted on the patient or standard surgical tools.[52-54] These noncontact devices can be used for tracking patient or physician movements or the path of rigid surgical instruments. Optical and ultrasound digitizers cannot transmit through the tissues; therefore, to detect positions deep in the body, the digitizers should be placed on the proximal end of rigid instruments. Conventional electromagnetic sensors can be detected through the body but cannot fit within needles or endoscopes unless the sensors are miniaturized. Smaller electromagnetic sensors have become available; they can be attached to the tip of flexible catheters and inserted into the working channel of endoscopes.[55] Tracking technology with single or multiple sensors permits the use of instruments as pointers or tracing tools and enables the physician to outline regions or define trajectories. The most important aspect of sensor technology and tracking is interactivity. Conventional stereotactic frames impede freedom of motion and use calculations instead of displays to define positions. In interactive frameless stereotaxy, the computer displays the position and the motion of the instruments accurately and immediately with respect to image-defined anatomic boundaries. Repetitive display of target, trajectory, and volume information allows interaction with the surgical plan and monitoring of the progress of the procedure.

Most navigational systems developed in the past decade are relevant only for interactive image-guided neurosurgery and endoscopic sinus surgery. The use of preoperative images for intraoperative image guidance is limited by potential intraoperative changes in anatomy. If navigation is based solely on preoperative images, intraoperative tissue distortions, shifts, and displacements (caused by retraction of tissues, removal of tumor masses, loss of CSF, hemorrhage, or edema) cause substantial errors. Modeling of elastic deformations and correction of the images are possible but only within a limited range; beyond this range, intraoperative imaging becomes necessary.

Standard application of the existing system in neurosurgical cases proceeds as follows:

1. The patient is prepared for surgery as usual up until head sterilization. The head is visible.
2. The system registers MRI segmentation to the patient. This step is achieved by scanning the patient's head using a laser triangulation device to acquire 3D information about the patient's scalp. At the same time, additional data points can be acquired using the Flashpoint tracking system and a nonsterile probe. All of these points are registered to the skin surface of the MRI segmentation, thereby aligning the full MRI reconstruction with the position of the patient on the operating table.
3. Simultaneously, the position of the head clamp or marked skin points on the patient are acquired using an optical tracking system.
4. The patient is sterilized and draped. At this stage, the surgeon is presented with augmented reality visualizations, in which all internal structures of the MRI segmentation are overlaid in exact alignment with a live video view of the patient, taken from the perspective of the surgeon (usually with a camera looking over the shoulder).
5. Throughout surgery, the system can track sterile surgical probes and display the position of the probes in the 3D volume of MRI data, with segmented structures overlaid (see Fig. 20-2). This step enables the surgeon to visualize surgical position relative to other nearby structures at any point in the procedure.

Intraoperative magnetic resonance imaging

Near real-time imaging during interventional and surgical procedures provides updates about the patient anatomy or the changing position of movable organs, depicts the position of instruments, and, without registration, establishes the necessary relationship between the patient and the images. Advances in imaging technology, particularly in 3D ultrasound, high-speed CT, and MRI with high performance computing, permit the combination and integration of near real-time, high-contrast, and spatial resolution volumetric images with frameless stereotactic, interactive localization methods during image-guided therapy.[56-58]

MRI, because of its high tissue contrast and spatial resolution and its multiplanar and functional imaging capabilities, has the most appeal for monitoring and controlling therapy. Open-configuration magnets, which permit full access to the patient and are equipped with instrument tracking systems, provide an interactive environment in which biopsies, percutaneous or endoscopic procedures, and minimally invasive interventions or open surgeries can be performed. In addition, various thermal ablations with image-based control of energy deposition can be performed to exploit the intrinsic sensitivity of MRI to temperature and tissue integrity.

Nevertheless, several obstacles hindered the evolution of MRI-guided interventions. MRI's value for guiding biopsies of tumors best detectable by MRI was apparent, but the closed magnets conventional at the time made it cumbersome to perform. The incompatibility with the electromagnetic environment, the inaccessibility of patients within the magnets, and the expense of MRI impeded its widespread acceptance for percutaneous procedures. Advances in low-field open-configuration magnet design and recognition of MRI's potential for monitoring and controlling thermal ablations and other percutaneous therapies initiated this new direction in interventional radiology. Because of the lack of direct visualization of thermal ablations, a 3D imaging technique is used to monitor these processes. Use of temperature-sensitive MRI sequences during therapy allows heat deposition and the resulting tissue alterations to be observed.[59]

This unique potential of MRI provided the impetus for a midfield open-configuration MR system. The goal was to develop a new generation of imaging systems that provided relatively unlimited access to the patient, near real-time monitoring, localization, targeting, interactive scanning, MR-compatible instruments, and equipment necessary for an MR-based interventional suite or operating room. MRI coupled with direct visualization can realize many interventional and surgical procedures better than either technique alone. Such a combination of MRI and invasive procedures meets the present trends toward safe and accurate image-guided minimally invasive therapies.

The configuration of magnet determines the scope and the ease with which interventional or intraoperative imaging can be performed. Most percutaneous procedures and open surgeries, however, require freehand techniques based on hand-eye coordination and close and direct contact with the patient's exposed anatomy. The horizontal gap configuration does not permit open surgeries and makes more complicated percutaneous procedures difficult to perform. Only the vertical gap allows the physician to enter between the two components of the magnet and directly manipulate the patient's anatomy. This configuration allows the use of endoscopes, laparoscopes, and operating microscopes.

The vision of interventional MRI[59] initiated research and development. As a result, a 0.5-T interventional MRI system, SIGNA SP, was developed by General Electric Medical Systems (Milwaukee, Wis) in collaboration with the Brigham & Women's Hospital.[60] This system has a unique open configuration, which allows the surgeon to perform procedures on patients placed within it. Images are acquired using optical tracking of surgical instruments to establish accurate intraoperative correlation between instrument position and anatomic structures.[61] The images can be viewed on monitors located conveniently within the vertical gap of the magnet. The neurosurgeon is thereby equipped with a near real-time, interactive navigational method.[62–64]

The constantly updated images help eliminate errors that can arise during framed and frameless stereotactic surgery, whereby anatomic structures, which can alter their position because of shifting or displacement of brain parenchyma, are correlated with images obtained preoperatively. Interventional MRI allows anatomic structures and lesions to be precisely localized and targeted, and the progress and extent of a procedure can be evaluated continuously. This on-line guidance helps determine tumor margins, optimize surgical approaches, achieve complete resection of intracerebral lesions, and monitor potential intraoperative complications.

SIGNA SP and the interventional surgical suite in which it resides (Fig. 20-4) combine key enabling technologies: a superconductive MR system, flexible transmitter or receiver coils, computer workstations, position sensors, intraoperative display, and audio and video equipment.[60,61,65–67] The facility is equipped with MR-compatible anesthesia delivery and monitoring devices and instruments for biopsies, thermal ablations, endoscopies, and open surgical procedures. It incorporates and integrates functions related to imaging, image guidance, and therapy. The high technology environment and its components represent cross-fertilization among interventional radiology, minimally invasive therapy, and image-guided computer-assisted surgery. The system was installed at the Brigham & Women's Hospital in 1994. Although the initial application domain included primarily percutaneous biopsy, the capability ultimately became applicable in many interventional and surgical applications, which consolidated direct imaging and real-time image guidance.[68–70]

The most salient characteristic of interventional MRI is the ability to interactively use imaging to localize, target, and monitor the procedure. Instead of covering an image volume with preplanned serial cross-sections, the operator can define scan planes and their location as needed. This capability is similar to what can be done using ultrasonography. Navigational systems used in neurosurgery and endoscopic sinus surgery also have interactive selection of scan planes for localization or targeting but use previously acquired images. Without real-time monitoring or

A

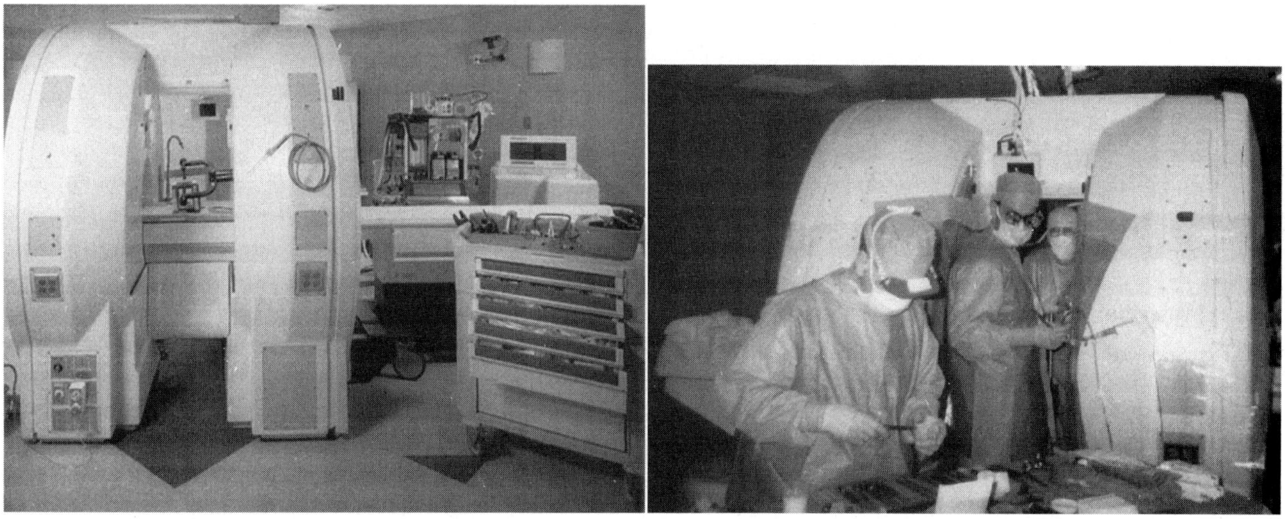

B

Fig. 20-4. Interventional magnetic resonance: **A,** The open-magnet system provides an opening between two superconducting magnetic coils to permit access to the patient during imaging. Depending on the procedure, the patient's table may be positioned along or perpendicular to the axis of the image. **B,** A neurosurgical procedure is performed in the General Electric (Milwaukee, Wis) interventional magnetic resonance system. (From Jolesz, and others: Image-guided procedures and the operating room of the future, *Radiology* 204:601, 1997.)

frequent image updating, these methods cannot adopt intraoperative changes.

The interactive image plane selection and definition implemented in General Electric's interventional MRI system (Flashpoint Scan Plane Pointer) use an optical tracking system (LEDs localized by infrared sensitive video equipment). This method shares some aspects with frameless stereotactic or navigational systems. In particular, it provides direct control of scan plane location, orientation, and angulation with enough flexibility and convenience for freehand procedures and enough accuracy for stereotactic biopsies.[59–61] The system can capture images along interactively defined coordinates to obtain geometrically correct information about patient's anatomy and location of instruments. This system has provided localization and targeting of brain biopsies even in extremely high-risk areas (hypothalamus, pineal region, brainstem). Application of interactive MRI scan plane selection for performing biopsies of abdominal organs and other body parts also introduced frameless stereotaxy into the field of cross-sectional interventional radiology.[62–64]

Interactive image guidance within the interventional MRI system using optical or other tracking systems can be applied to many interventional and surgical procedures (Fig. 20-5). In all imaging modes, information is acquired according to the position and orientation of the sensors and three orthogonal planes generated within a moving frame of reference. The most straightforward mode is interactive scanning, in which the operator intuitively moves the device to obtain a comprehensive view of the scanned 3D volume. This mode resembles ultrasonography, except that the three orthogonal planes can be displayed without changing the position of the probe. In the localizing mode, the probe is used as a virtual pointer with a computer-displayed icon that can point to or outline an anatomic object within the body. This mode can also be used to trace contours of organs or margins of lesions or to obtain points or surfaces from inside the body for registration.

In the targeting mode, the tip or the shaft of a virtual needle is displayed on three orthogonal planes, showing the expected path of the needle as an annotation. If the predicted position of the tip and the planned trajectory are acceptable, the real needle or probe can be advanced into the target. In the tracking mode, the trail of instruments or the motion of body parts can be followed and displayed on the images.[62]

For interactive image guidance, images should be generated and displayed quickly enough to be used without disrupting or slowing the procedure and before considerable changes occur within the operational field. The definition of real-time imaging or dynamic image update is relative and contingent on the time constants of the procedures or the processes being imaged. Imaging of needle placement may require an update of multiple slices or planes. Monitoring thermal ablation of a tumor should incorporate a volume (several slices). Most localization, targeting, tracking, and monitoring requirements can be satisfied by the commonly available fast imaging techniques (fast spin-echo, gradient echo). Several novel imaging techniques offer improved temporal resolution, achieved by less redundant spatial encoding, without considerably affecting spatial resolution and signal-to-noise. MR fluoroscopy and other dynamic imaging approaches use preexisting information for adaptive encoding of changing image data.[71–76]

Application of the open magnetic resonance system for neurosurgery

Combination of direct vision and beyond-the-surface imaging was possible in a environment that incorporates the operat-

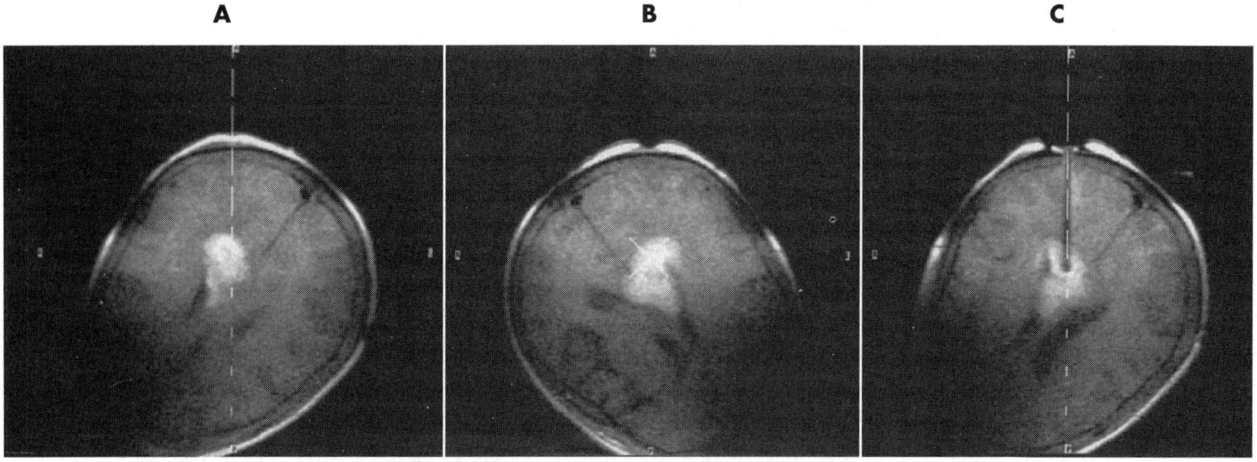

Fig. 20-5. Interactive image guidance, frameless stereotactic targeting, and brain biopsy using optical tracking of the needle holder. These orthogonal views were acquired with a T1-weighted fast spin-echo sequence (repetition time, 400 msec; echo time, 170 msec) obtained after intravenous contrast administration. **A,** The virtual needle (predicted needle path) is displayed as a segmented line. **B,** The virtual needle tip is perpendicular to the predicted needle path *(crosshatch)*. **C,** The biopsy needle is seen as a metallic artifact behind the segmented line and introduced along the predicted path. (From Jolesz, and others: Image-guided procedures and the operating room of the future, *Radiology* 204:601, 1997.)

ing room and an MRI scanner. This integrated system allowed more accurate localization and targeting during surgery. Definition of histopathologically correct tumor margins, comprehension of the full extent of disease processes, and accurate definition of anatomic landmarks improved surgical efficiency and decreased invasiveness. Complete resection of tumors, decreased vulnerability of surrounding tissues, and avoidance of critical structures should improve clinical outcome and reduce complication rates. When MRI was merged with frameless stereotaxy, navigational tools, and multimodality image fusion, combination of all available spatial information with real-time image update became possible. Use of this composite information during open surgeries may revolutionize minimally invasive therapy, leading to the development of new surgical strategies and approaches.[77]

The interventional MR scanner has two separate superconducting magnetic coils with an outer diameter or 1840 mm. A 560-mm gap is located between the coils, allowing the surgeon to access the interventional field by placing the operative bed in the gantry. The main magnet field strength is 0.5 T, and homogeneity is 12.3 ppm over 300 mm or 1.6 ppm over 200 mm.

Interventional MRI has two modes called *standard scan* and *interactive scan:* the former is similar to that available in a conventional diagnostic scanner, and the latter is the interactive oblique mode in which surgeons and radiologists can interactively select the position and orientation of the scanning plane. For this interactive mode, the system is equipped with an optical scan plane locator and its detector (Flashpoint 5000). The locator has two to three LEDs that are tracked by 3 CCD cameras attached on the rail above the interventional filed. The locator can be mounted on surgical devices, such as a biopsy needle holder, a suction tube, or a sinus endoscope. The scan plane locator is calibrated to the imager; thus, its spatial relationship is known.

Early neurosurgical experience based on more than 150 cases illustrates most of the anticipated benefits of intraoperative MRI.[64,77] Interactive localization and targeting provided on-line planning of optimal trajectories for biopsies and real-time image feedback during needle advancement and tissue sampling. Using this method, lesions in deep and high-risk regions (e.g., hypothalamus, pineal region, brainstem) have been biopsied.[62,77] Unavoidable hemorrhagic complications were immediately recognized, localized, and managed surgically by open craniotomy within the magnet. Intraventricular, relatively mobile, and unstable targets have been reached safely, and cystic structures in various locations have been drained under continuous image control (Fig. 20-6).

The potential advantages of precise localization and optimized access route have been shown by combining an operative microscope with MRI-guided resection of deep-seated small tumors and cavernous hemangiomas. Surgical removal of extra-axial tumors may benefit from the delineation of surrounding, directly invisible anatomy. In addition, intraoperative MRI-guided laminectomies in the lumbar and cervical

A

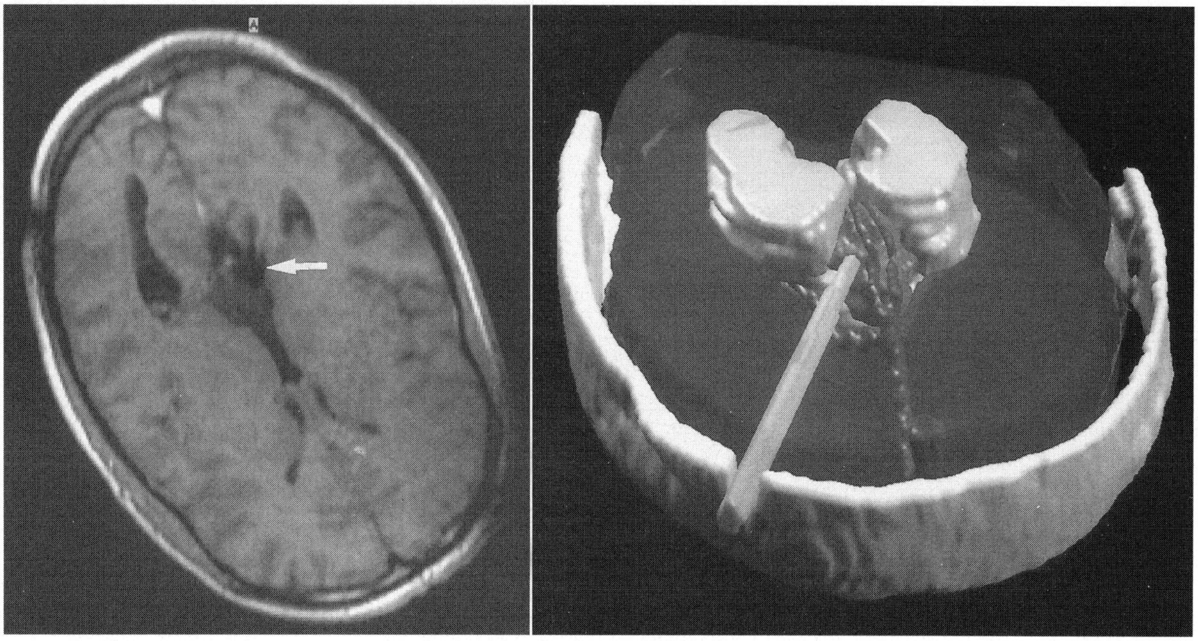

B

Fig. 20-6. Image-guided drainage of a pineal cyst using magnetic resonance imaging guidance. **A,** The tip of a biopsy needle is guided into the pineal cyst (*arrow* shows the needle artifact). **B,** For better visualization, three-dimensional rendering from the volumetric dataset shows the cyst, thalami, and surrounding veins. For hemorrhage to be avoided, the needle was introduced between the internal cerebral vein and the vein of Rosenthal. See Color Plate 9. (From Jolesz, and others: Image-guided procedures and the operating room of the future, *Radiology* 204:601, 1997.)

A 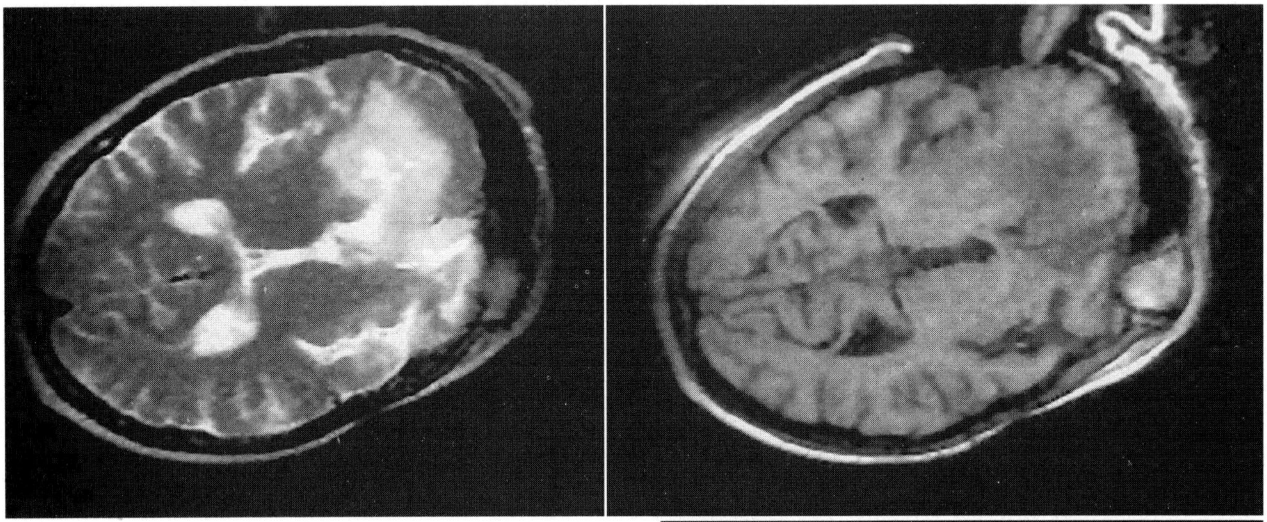 B

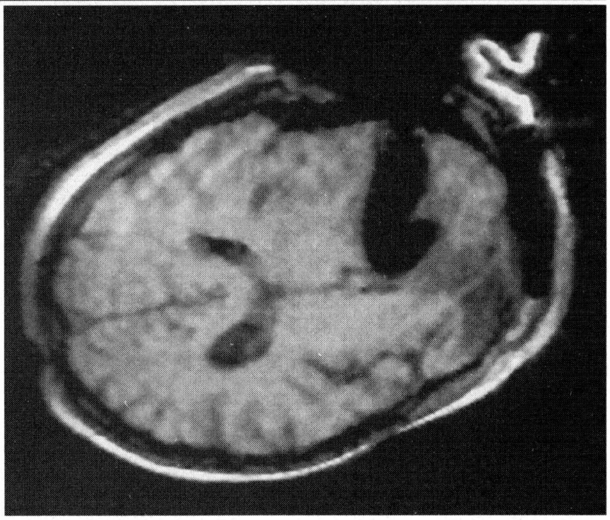 C

Fig. 20-7. Intraoperative image guidance. **A,** Brain tumor (malignant glioma) on T2-weighted images (fast spin-echo: repetition time, 2100 msec; echo time, 100 msec) were acquired within the open magnet preoperatively. Localization for the best entry site for craniotomy was accomplished by the surgeon's finger. **B,** This T1-weighted image (fast spin-echo: repetition time, 400 msec; echo time, 17 msec) was taken after the craniotomy. Localization was accomplished by the surgeon's fingertip on the brain surface before tumor resection. **C,** T1-weighted intraoperative image shows tumor resection. (From Jolesz, and others: Image-guided procedures and the operating room of the future, *Radiology* 204:601, 1997.)

spine may represent a new minimally invasive approach to this high-risk area.

The most exciting and potentially rewarding neurosurgical application of interventional MRI guidance is resection of malignant intra-axial tumors (Fig. 20-7).

When viewing the exposed brain surface without imaging, the neurosurgeon cannot define the spatial extent of the tumor; even after the neurosurgeon surgically enters the brain tissue, the tumor is indistinguishable from healthy cerebral tissue in most patients. Preoperative image data may help show the extent of the tumor in some instances. During resection of large, deep tumors, however, brain structures may move and become deformed, negating the value of preoperative images. Using intraoperative optical tracking and refreshing the volumetric images, surgeons can locate the tumor margins and completely resect the tumor while preserving the integrity of surrounding healthy brain tissue. Similar methods can be applied to resection of other intraparenchymal tumors, such as breast cancer or soft-tissue sarcoma, in which the margins are difficult to define with the naked eye.

NEW DEVELOPMENTS AND APPLICATIONS

Interventional magnetic resonance imaging front-end workstation and network settings

Most interventional MRI system-specific functions are controlled by the front-end workstation (SPARC station 20, model 612MP, Sun Microsystems, Mountain View, Calif). The functions include the real-time imaging control, temperature monitoring to prevent overheating of the magnets, and an audio and video switcher (Fig. 20-8).

In addition to these functions, implemented as a default clinical setting, a server software can send and receive the locator and imaging data to and from another workstation. If a client process running on the research workstation requests locator information, the server software accesses the locator device and transfers the position and orientation of the tracking device. If

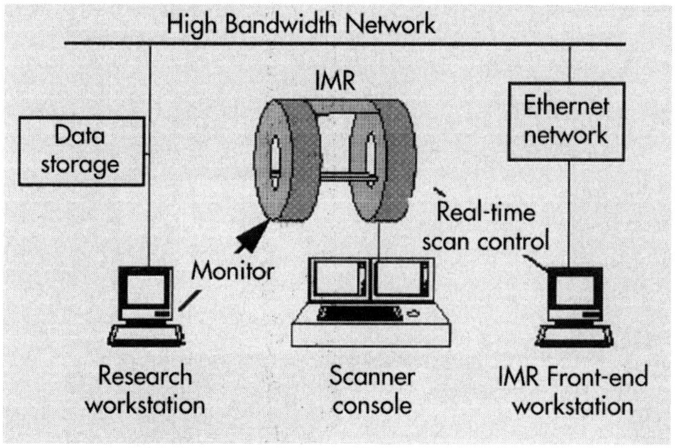

Fig. 20-8. Configuration of the interventional magnetic resonance imaging (MRI) system. The interventional MRI system is connected to two major computers: an interventional MRI front-end workstation dedicated for scan control and a research workstation with high-performance graphics capability. Each workstation and scanner is connected to an Ethernet network that operates nominally at 10 megabits/sec.

the client process requests the image data, the server software returns the latest data stored in the interventional MRI memory buffer, which is updated by an interactive scan in the default clinical package. Because the front-end workstation is dedicated for imaging control, the running server process must not damage its performance or affect any of its associated resources. Thus, the server software will not allocate its own image buffer but will access the shareable buffer offered by the imaging control. In terms of computational power, the server software restricts its functionality to sending and receiving the data and excludes image processes that would otherwise consume the front-end computer's computational resources. One preliminary study showed that the server software consumes about 1% of memory and central processing unit power for primary scan control tasks.

Research workstation

Because registration, thermal monitoring, or other client processes require high-performance 3D graphics manipulation, fast network communication with other machines, and vast memory or disk storage, a research workstation is specifically designed and dedicated to meet these purposes. Therefore, a research workstation (Ultra 1, Sun Microsystems, Mountain View, Calif) with a graphics card (Creator 3D, Sun Microsystems) was dedicated for image registration and a visual interactive interface.

Enhanced graphics interface within a real-time interventional magnetic resonance imaging system

A method to fuse multimodality (pre- and intraoperative) images for interventional MRI-guided surgery has been developed. The preliminary work included engineering of a setting for high-performance computing, use of the hospital network, and integration of the interactive guidance system into the open-configuration MRI scanner.[59,61,78–80]

Multimodality representation of morphology can be integrated from previous CT or MRI, along with functional physiologic data (transcranial magnetic stimulation, MR angiography, functional MRI) and metabolic information (SPECT). These combined data can then be coregistered with intraoperative real-time MRI data. The resulting composite provides the surgeon with the most comprehensive view of the operative field and helps the surgeon plan and execute the procedure. Coregistration of CT, MR angiography, and MRI is especially helpful in skull base surgery. The combination of functional MRI with cortical physiology is invaluable for executing surgical resection without sacrificing critical brain functions. SPECT registration to intraoperative MRI differentiates metabolically active tumor parts from necrotic areas.

The interventional MRI environment requires information from multiple pre- and intraoperative sources integrated into a single database. From this resource, enhanced visibility or virtual reality representation can be achieved using various 3D interactive display systems. Navigational and other human interface tools can be used for localization, targeting, and correlation of anatomic models and surgical procedures within the physical space of the patient. Real-time updating of the image database will be required to follow the progress of the procedures and to find exact tumor margins within deformable soft-tissue structures.

The Image Guided Therapy Program of Brigham & Women's Hospital represents a concentrated effort of radiologists, surgeons, and computer scientists to introduce advanced imaging, image processing, and image-controlled therapy techniques into interventional radiology and surgery. Already implemented image-guided procedures provide a glimpse to the future and show that enabling technologies are available. Using these advances, interventional radiologists have developed new procedures and techniques. Diagnostic radiologists have also been involved in the therapeutic process; their relationship with their surgical colleagues has extended beyond the constraints of the traditional consultation. By entering together into the "operating room of the future," they have developed a closer interaction. This association has resulted in a greater understanding of the interplay between diagnosis and management and in greater appreciation of each other's role in patient care.

Highly accurate and complex surgical procedures are possible using an interactive 3D graphics display (Fig. 20-9) in which multiple modalities (MRI [T1, T2, MR angiography], CT, SPECT, and intraoperative MRI data) are integrated. Using this method, surgeons and interventional radiologists can localize a trajectory path that is minimally invasive to critical anatomic structures, such as vessels and critical cortical functional areas. This approach attempts to use multimodality guidance in combination with intraoperative MRI to perform biopsies and surgeries of brain tumors (Fig. 20-10).

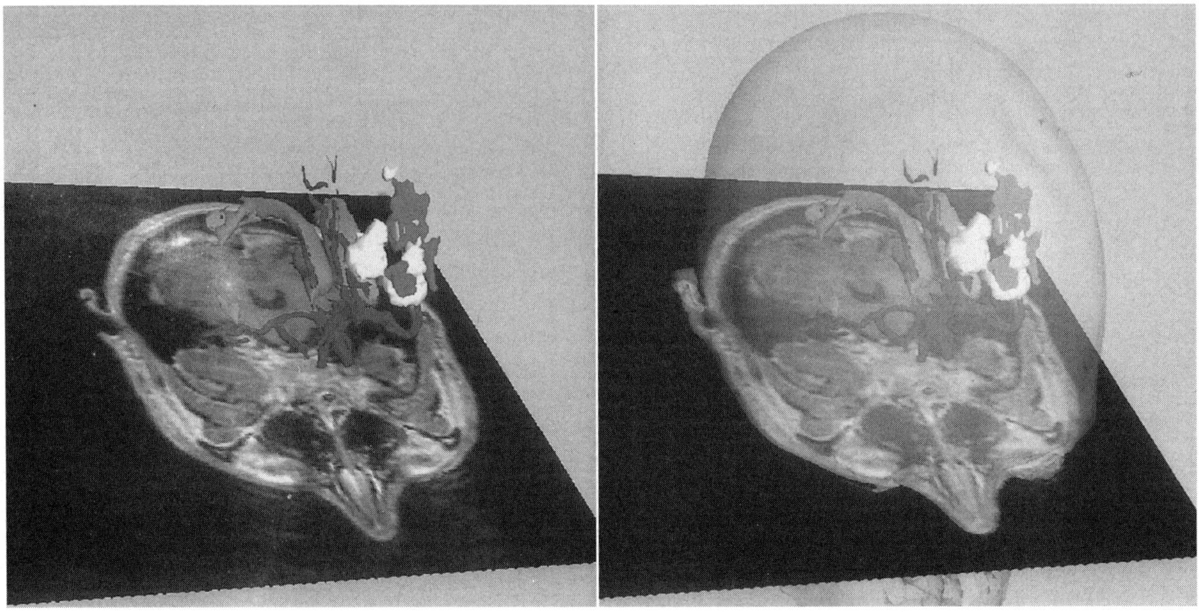

A B

Fig. 20-9. Multimodality images in three-dimensional graphics display. **A,** An axial magnetic resonance image (MRI) spoiled gradient-recalled echo sequence (SPGR) with a vessel model extracted from MR angiography and a tumor model from gadolinium-enhanced SPGR. **B,** The same axial MRI (SPGR) and a skin model extracted from MRI (SPGR). See Color Plate 10.

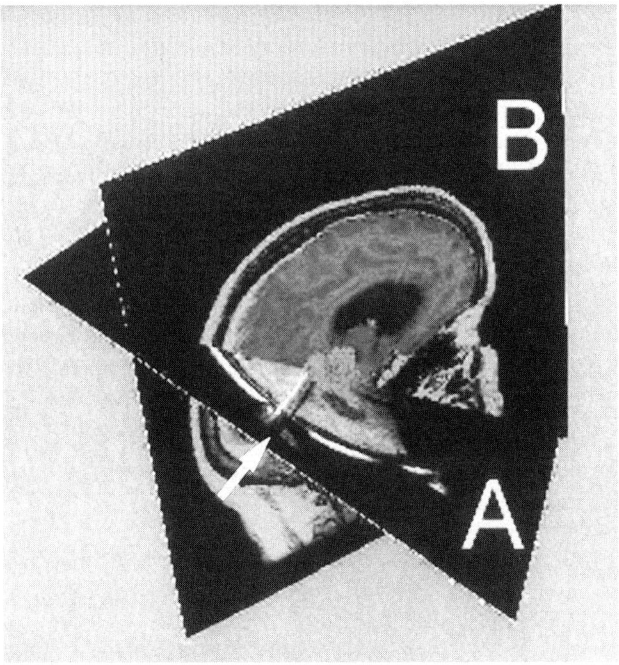

Fig. 20-10. Three-dimensional graphics interface for better spatial recognition and access to registered preoperative magnetic resonance imaging (MRI). **A,** Intraoperative MRI with biopsy needle *(arrow)* and **B,** preoperative MRI are fused and displayed together. See Color Plate 11. (From Hata N, and others: Registration of pre-operative and intraoperative images for MR-guided therapy, *SPIE* [in press].)

Monitoring and control of magnetic resonance–guided ablation therapy with interventional magnetic resonance imaging

The greatest potential of MRI is in monitoring and in delivery of various energies by means of thermal probes. This application is particularly important because achieving the full potential of these techniques requires good localization and targeting and quantitative spatiotemporal control of energy deposition, which requires monitoring of the thermal changes and the resulting tissue alterations.

Computer-assisted temperature-sensitive MRI for interstitial laser therapy has been developed.[71–75, 81–83] Clinical applications involving tumor ablation in the brain and liver have been initiated (Fig. 20-11). The interventional MRI system was used to guide and monitor the accurate placement of the laser source (needle with optical fiber) at the targeted lesion. T1-weighted fast spin-echo and spoiled gradient-recalled echo sequences with phase mapping of the water proton chemical shift images, transferred to a research workstation from the MR scanner, were used to reconstruct temperature mapping for monitoring the effect of laser ablation. Newly developed software in the imaging system and the research workstation enabled rapid (27 to 221 msec) and on-line temperature image reconstruction. In the case of a highlighted brain tumor, subtraction images from T1-weighted scans and proton chemical shift images clearly showed the signal intensity peak at the tip of the laser guide. The preliminary study indicated that the presented system de-

A 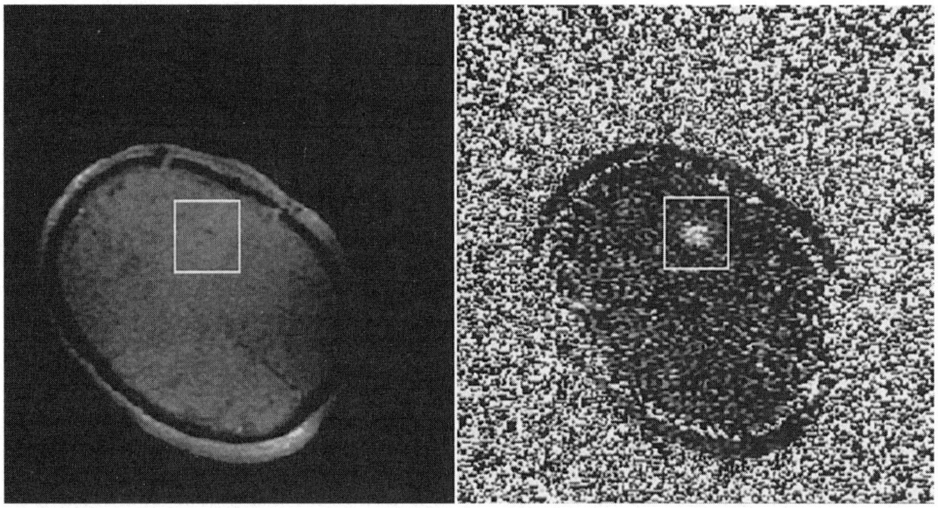 B

Fig. 20-11. Thermal monitoring of interstitial laser therapy with temperature mapping of the water proton chemical shift. **A,** Two-dimensional spoiled gradient-recalled echo phase mapping of the water proton chemical shift. **B,** The reconstructed temperature map. The high-intensity area inside the *square box* indicates the high-temperature lesion in the tumor.

A B C

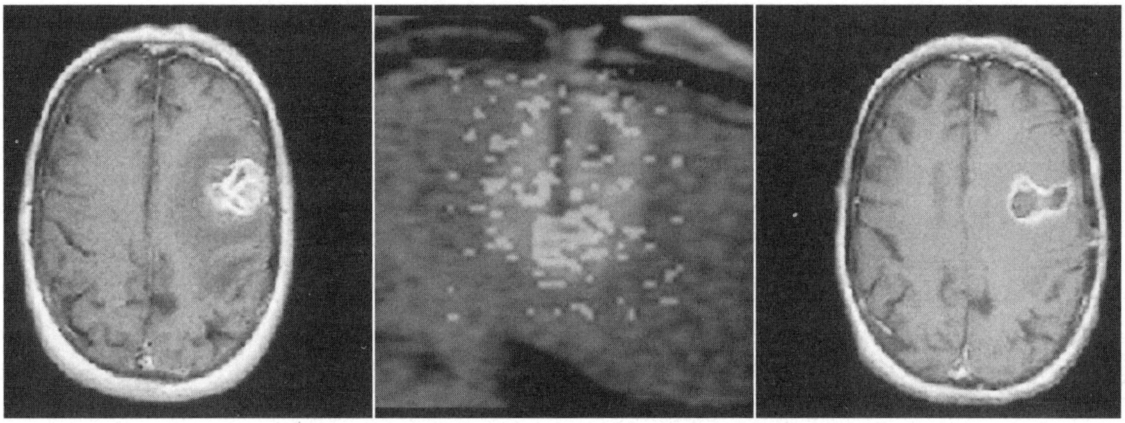

Fig. 20-12. Interstitial laser therapy of brain tumor. **A,** T1-weighted (repetition time [TR], 500 msec; echo time [TE], 20 msec) contrast-enhanced image acquired with a 1.5-T scanner before the procedure showed the enhancing brain tumor. **B,** Thermal monitoring of interstitial neodymium:yttrium-aluminum-garnet laser therapy with pixel subtraction of T1-weighted fast spin-echo images (TR, 400 msec; TE, 17 msec) acquired within the open magnet during a 4-W power deposition. Changes in signal intensity around the laser fiber were color-encoded in red. **C,** T1-weighted (TR, 500 msec; TE, 20 msec) contrast-enhanced image at 1.5-T 24 hours after laser management. Note the lack of enhancement within the tumor. The ring enhancement around the coagulated tumor is consistent with the breakdown of the blood-brain barrier. See Color Plate 12. (**A, C,** From Joachim Kettenbach, and others: MRI paper #976243, Monitoring and visualization techniques for MR-guided laser ablations in open MR-system.)

sign is feasible for real-time and on-line monitoring of interstitial laser therapy (Fig. 20-12).

DISCUSSION

The role of image processing

Significant challenges exist in the technical aspects of converting conventional MRI scan information into a 3D data set. However, from the standpoint of neurosurgery, the potential benefit from an advanced 3D imaging program to enhance surgical visualization will depend heavily on the presentation of enough information in a form that allows safe and effective attainment of surgical goals but simplifies the visual presentation to avoid visual information overload on the surgeon during various facets of the procedure.

In addition to the data provided by MRI scans, valuable information can be obtained from functional mapping of anatomic data sets, which can then be incorporated directly into the 3D MRI reconstruction. Modalities include thallium-201 and technetium-99m-hexylmethylpropylene amineoxine dual-isotope SPECT 3D imaging or fluorine-18-labeled deoxyglucose or methionine PET. Other modalities might offer significant enhancement of the available preoperative information to help in guiding neurosurgical procedures. Various motor, speech, or visual areas might be mapped using SPECT or transcranial magnetic stimulation. Other modalities might be incorporated into the enhancement of 3D and functional data. Electrocorticography with 3D definition of epileptiform activity is also possible.

All of these data can be merged into a unified model for presentation to the surgeon. The final stage is to use enhanced high-speed computer graphics to support guidance of neurosurgical and other surgical procedures. Most surgical specialties have other anatomic cues to identify various structures as the surgeon proceeds through a surgical endeavor. The neurosurgeon has a significant knowledge base about neuroanatomy, which can be significantly distorted by the local pathology to a point at which the functional anatomy of motor, sensory, or cranial nerves or other pathways cannot be determined from standard or magnified operative visualization alone. The tremendous benefit gained by bringing stereotactically linked MR, CT, SPECT, and functional mapping data into the active field of perception of the neurosurgeon during a neurosurgical operation is tremendous. The efforts of the Surgical Planning Laboratory at Brigham & Women's Hospital, especially as they apply in the intraoperative MR project, are actively addressing these challenges at multiple levels. The benefit to the neurosurgeon and patient has been increasingly clear to the neurosurgical community worldwide.[84]

THE FUTURE OF IMAGE-GUIDED NEUROSURGERY

As the computer becomes more integral in the surgical process, the need to provide information to the surgeon in a convenient and intuitive way becomes greater. This relationship is most significant in the interventional MRI system, in which image information acquired by MRI and augmented and annotated by computer data is a powerful tool for intraoperative planning and guidance.

Thus, the goals are to extend existing work in segmentation, registration, visualization, and tracking to provide useful tools to the neurosurgeon. The hope is that such tools will serve as an enhancing mechanism, enabling the surgeon to execute surgeries in a minimally invasive manner, while proceeding as if the entire surgical field were available. Such image-guided surgical systems should enable the surgeon to perform more accurate surgeries, with less invasion of neighboring tissue; perform these surgeries in less time; and plan and execute safer paths to desired targeted tissue. Initial neurosurgical experience is illustrated by more than 250 neurosurgical cases with excellent results. Researchers intend to build on the experience with this system to build the next generation of image-guided neurosurgical systems.[77]

For the next generation of image-guided neurosurgical systems, three fronts need to be addressed: (1) The solution of various scientific and technical issues would significantly enhance the range of capabilities of image-guided systems. (2) A range of issues concerning the development and use of the system should be addressed to fully leverage the usefulness of these systems in supporting more effective surgical practice. (3) The utility and practicality of such systems should be evaluated through detailed interaction with neurosurgeons using these systems in a range of procedures.

CONCLUSIONS

The concept of image guidance demands a strategic shift in the focus of medical imaging from diagnosis to management. Continuous commitment from imaging experts, interventionalists, and surgeons is necessary to expedite development of technology in a rapidly changing healthcare environment. Image-guided therapy offers the possibility of improving safety, efficacy, and cost-effectiveness of existing procedures, and it may result in new procedures that cannot be conceived outside of this environment.

As the computer becomes more integral in the surgical process, the need to provide information to the surgeon in a convenient and intuitive way becomes greater. This relationship is most important in the interventional MRI system, in which image information acquired by MRI and augmented and annotated by computer data is a powerful tool for intraoperative planning and guidance.

REFERENCES

1. Vannier MW, Marsh JL, Warren JO: Three dimensional CT reconstruction images for craniofacial surgical planning and evaluation, *Radiology* 1:179, 1984.
2. Cutting C, and others: Three-dimensional computer assisted design of craniofacial surgical procedures: optimization and interaction with cephalometric and CT-based models, *Plast Reconstr Surg* 77:877, 1986.
3. Altobelli DE, and others: Computer-assisted three-dimensional planning in craniofacial surgery, *Plast Reconstr Surg* 92:576, 1993.
4. Jolesz FA, Kikinis R, Cline HE, Lorensen WE: *The use of computerized imaging and image processing for neurosurgical planning.* In Black PMcL, Lampson LA, editors: *Astrocytomas,* Cambridge, Mass 1993, Blackwell Scientific.
5. Vogl TJ, Assal J, Bergman C: Three-dimensional MR reconstruction images of skull base tumors, *J Magn Reson Imaging* 3:357, 1993.
6. Hu XP, Tan KK, Levin DN: Three-dimensional magnetic resonance images of the brain: application to neurosurgical planning, *J Neurosurg* 72:433, 1990.
7. Chernoff DM, and others: Three-dimensional imaging and display of renal tumors using spiral CT: a potential aid to partial nephrectomy, *Urology* 43:125, 1994.
8. Jolesz FA: Image-guided procedures and the operating room of the future, *Radiology* 204:601, 1997.
9. Zhang J, and others: Multimodality imaging of brain structures for stereotactic surgery, *Radiology* 175:435, 1990.
10. Holman BL, and others: Computer-assisted superimposition of magnetic resonance and high-resolution technetium-99m HMPAO and thallium-201 SPECT images of the brain, *J Nucl Med* 32:1478, 1991.
11. Levin D, and others: The brain: integrated three-dimensional display of MR and PET images, *Radiology* 172:783, 1989.
12. Wells WM, and others: Multi-modal volume registration by maximization of mutual information, *Medical Image Analysis* 1:35, 1996.

13. Kall BA, and others: Methodology and clinical experience with computed tomography and a computer-resident stereotactic atlas, *Neurosurgery* 17: 400, 1985.
14. Axel L, Costantini J, Listerud J: Intensity correction in surface-coil MR imaging, *Am J Roentgenol* 148:418, 1987.
15. Cline HE, and others: Three-dimensional segmentation of MR images of the head using probability and connectivity, *J Comput Assist Tomogr* 14:1037, 1990.
16. Gerig G, Kubler O, Jolesz FA: Nonlinear anisotropic filtering of MRI data, *IEEE Trans Med Imaging* 11:221, 1992.
17. Gerig G, and others: *Medical imaging and computer vision: an integrated approach for diagnosis and planning,* Hamburg, 1989, Proceedings of the 11th DAGM Symposium.
18. Hohne KH, Hanson W: Interactive 3D segmentation of MRI and CT volumes using morphological operations, *J Comput Assist Tomogr* 16:285, 1992.
19. Hohne KH, and others: New kinds of three-dimensional atlases of the anatomy and function of the human body, *Z Arztl Fortbild (Jena)* 89:430, 1995.
20. Kikinis R, and others: Computer-assisted interactive three-dimensional planning for neurological procedures, *Neurosurgery* 38:640, 1996.
21. Kikinis R, and others: Routine quantitative analysis of brain and cerebrospinal fluid spaces with MR imaging, *J Magn Reson Imaging,* 2:619, 1992.
22. Lim KO, Pfefferbaum A: Segmentation of MR brain images into cerebrospinal fluid spaces, white and gray matter, *J Comput Assist Tomogr* 13:588, 1989.
23. Sandor S, Leahy R: Surface-based labeling of cortical anatomy using a deformable altlas, *IEEE Trans Med Imaging* 16:41, 1997. *A 3D morphological algorithm for automated labelling of the cortex in magnetic resonance brain images,* Palo Alto, Calif, 1994, AAAI Spring Symposium Applications of Computer Vision in Medical Image Processing.
24. Wells W, and others: *Statistical intensity correction and segmentation of magnetic resonance image data,* In Rochester, Minn, 1994, Proceedings of the 3rd Conference on Visualization in Biomedical Computing.
25. Wells W, and others: Adaptive segmentation of MRI data, *IEEE Trans Med Imaging* 15:429, 1996.
26. Adams L, and others: An optical navigator for brain surgery, *IEEE Computer* 29:48, 1996.
27. Barnett GH, and others: Use of a frameless, armless stereotactic wand for brain tumor localization with two-dimensional and three-dimensional neuroimaging, *Neurosurgery* 33:674, 1993.
28. Henderson JM, Smith KR, Bucholz RD: An accurate and ergonomic method of registration for image-guided neurosurgery, *Comput Med Imaging Graph* 18:273, 1994.
29. Cinquin P, and others: Medical imaging and computer-assisted interventions, *Rev Prat (France)* 46:319, 1996.
30. Colchester ACF, and others: Development and preliminary evaluation of VISLAN: a surgical planning and guidance system using intra-operative video imaging, *Medical Image Analysis* 1:73, 1996.
31. Galloway RL Jr, Maciunas RJ, Edwards CA II: Interactive image guided neurosurgery, *IEEE Trans Biomed Eng* 39:1226, 1992.
32. Maciunas RJ, Galloway RL Jr, Latimer JW: The application accuracy of sterotactic frames, *Neurosurgery* 35:682, 1994.
33. Heilbrun MP, and others: Stereotactic localization and guidance using a machine vision technique, *Stereotact Funct Neurosurg* 58:94, 1992.
34. Maciunas RJ, and others: A universal system for interactive image-directed neurosurgery, *Stereotact Funct Neurosurg* 58:108, 1992.
35. Peters T, and others: Three-dimensional multimodal image-guidance for neurosurgery, *IEEE Trans Med Imaging* 15:121, 1996.
36. Ryan MJ, and others: Frameless stereotaxy with real-time tracking of patient head movement and retrospective patient-image registration, *J Neurosurg* 85:287, 1996.
37. Sipos EP, and others: In vivo accuracy testing and clinical experiences with the ISG viewing wand, *Neurosurgery* 39:194, 1996.
38. Watanabe E, and others: Open surgery assisted by the neuronavigator, a stereotactic, articulated, sensitive arm, *Neurosurgery* 28:792, 1991.
39. Gleason PL, and others: Video registration virtual reality for nonlinkage stereotactic surgery, *Stereotact Funct Neurosurg* 63:139, 1994.
40. Nakajima S, and others: Use of cortical surface vessel registration for image-guided neurosurgery, *Neurosurgery* 41:403, 1997.
41. Grimson WEL, and others: An automatic registration method for frameless stereotaxy, image-guided surgery, and enhanced reality visualization, *IEEE Trans Med Imaging* 15:129, 1996.
42. Ettinger GJ, and others: *Non-invasive functional brain mapping using registered transcranial magnetic stimulation,* San Francisco, Calif, 1996, IEEE Workshop on Mathematical Methods in Biomedical Image Analysis.
43. Kosugi Y, and others: An articulated neurosurgical navigation system using MRI and CT images, *IEEE Trans Biomed Eng* 35:147, 1988.
44. Kato A, and others: A frameless navigational system for computer-assisted neurosurgery, *J Neurosurg* 74:845, 1991.
45. Roberts DW, and others: A frameless stereotaxic integration of computerized tomographic imaging and the operating microscope, *J Neurosurg* 65:545, 1986.
46. Koivukangas J, and others: Ultrasound-controlled neuronavigator-guided brain surgery, *J Neurosurg* 79:36, 1993.
47. Kall BA, Kelly PJ, Goerss SJ: The computer as a stereotactic surgical instrument, *Neurol Res* 8:201, 1986.
48. Apuzzo ML, Sabshin JK: Computed tomographic guidance stereotaxis in the management of intracranial mass lesions, *Neurosurgery* 12:277, 1983.
49. Zamorano L, Jiang Z, Kadi AM: Computer-assisted neurosurgery system: Wayne State University hardware and software configuration, *Comput Med Imaging Graph* 18:257, 1994.
50. Iosifescu DV, and others: Evaluation of an automated registration algorithm for the volumetric measurement of MRI brain structures, *Neuroimage* 6:13, 1997.
51. Zinreich SJ, Tebo SA, Long DM: Frameless stereotaxic integration of CT imaging data: accuracy and initial applications, *Radiology* 188:35, 1993.
52. Korves B, and others: Image- and model-based surgical planning in otolaryngology, *J Otolaryngol* 24:265, 1995.
53. Fried MP, and others: Image-guided endoscopic surgery: results of accuracy and performance in a multicenter clinical study using an electromagnetic tracking system, *Laryngoscope* 107:594, 1997.
54. Fried MP, and others: Image-guided surgery in a new magnetic resonance suite: preclinical considerations, *Laryngoscope* 106:411, 1996.
55. Acker DE, Jimenez DF: *Miniature position sensor for image-guided surgery,* Montreal, Canada, 1996, Abstract in 4th Congress of Neurosurgical Surgeons.
56. Lufkin R, and others: MR body stereotaxis: an aid for MR guided biopsies, *J Comput Assist Tomogr* 12:1088, 1988.
57. Lufkin R, and others: A technique for MR-guided needle placement, *Am J Roentgen* 146:351, 1986.
58. Silverman SG, and others: Interactive MR-guided biopsy in an open-configuration MR imaging system, *Radiology* 197:175, 1995.
59. Jolesz FA, Shtern F: The operating room of the future: report of the National Cancer Institute workshop, "imaging guided stereotactic tumor diagnosis and treatment," *Invest Radiol* 27:326, 1992.
60. Schenck JF, and others: Superconducting open configuration MRI system for image-guided therapy, *Radiology* 195:805, 1995.
61. Silverman SG, and others: Interactive MR-guided biopsy in an open-configuration MR imaging system, *Radiology* 197:175, 1995.
62. Moriarty TM, and others: *Magnetic resonance imaging therapy: intraoperative MR imaging.* In *Neurosurgery Clinics of North America: Clinical frontiers of interactive image guided neurosurgery,* Philadelphia, 1996, WB Saunders.
63. Alexander E, Kikinis R, Jolesz F: *Intraoperative magnetic resonance imaging therapy.* In Barnett GH, Roberts D, Guthrie B, editors: *Image-guided neurosurgery: clinical applications of interactive surgical navigation quality medical publisher,* St. Louis, (in press).
64. Alexander E, and others: Innovations in minimalism: intraoperative MR, *Clin Neurosurg* 43:338, 1996.

65. Silverman SG, and others: Design and implementation of an interventional MR imaging suite, *Am J Roentgenol* 168:1465, 1997.
66. Jolesz FA, and others: Interactive image-guided interventions in an open configuration MR imaging system, *Radiology* 197:175, 1995.
67. Jolesz FA, Kahn T, Lufkin R: Genesis of interventional MRI, *J Magn Reson Imag* 8:2, 1998.
68. Hsu L, Fried MP, Jolesz FA: Interactive MR-guided sinus endoscopy, *Radiology* 197:237, 1995.
69. Fielding JR, and others: MR-imaging of the female pelvic floor in the supine and upright positions, *J Magn Reson Imaging* 6:961, 1996.
70. Winalski CS, and others: Functional musculoskeletal imaging with a vertically open MR-imager, *Radiology* 193:404, 1994.
71. Matsumoto R, Oshio K, Jolesz FA: Monitoring of laser and freezing-induced ablation in the liver with T1-weighted MR imaging, *J Magn Reson Imaging* 2:555, 1992.
72. Matsumoto R, and others: Tissue temperature monitoring for thermal interventional therapy: comparison of T1-weighted MR sequences, *J Magn Reson Imaging* 4:65, 1994.
73. Bleier AR, and others: Real-time magnetic resonance imaging of laser heat deposition in tissue, *Magn Reson Med* 21:132, 1991.
74. Matsumoto R, and others: Interstitial Nd:YAG laser ablation in normal rabbit liver: trial to maximize the size of laser-induced lesions, *Lasers Surg Med* 12:650, 1992.
75. Cline HE, and others: Focused US system for MR imaging-guided tumor ablation, *Radiology* 194:731, 1994.
76. Duckwiler G, and others: Head and neck lesions: MR-guided aspiration biopsy, *Radiology* 170:519, 1989.
77. Black PM, and others: Development and implementation of intraoperative MRI and its neurosurgical applications, *Neurosurgery* 41:831, 1997.
78. Fried MP, and others: Image-guided surgery in a new magnetic resonance suite: preclinical considerations, *Laryngoscope* 106:411, 1996.
79. Fried MP, Jolesz FA, Morrison PR: Image guidance with laser applications, *Otolaryngol Clin North Am* 29:63, 1996.
80. Jolesz FA, Blumenfeld SM: Interventional use of magnetic resonance imaging, *Magn Reson Q* 10:85, 1994.
81. Cline HE, and others: MR temperature mapping of focused ultrasound surgery, *Magn Reson Med* 31:628, 1994.
82. Kuroda Y, and others: Temperature mapping using water proton chemical shift obtained with 3D-MRSI: feasibility in vivo, *Magn Reson Med* 35:20, 1996.
83. Kettenbach J, and others: Monitoring and visualization techniques for MR-guided laser ablations in an open MR-system, *J Magn Reson Imaging* 8, 1998.
84. Kettenbach J, and others: *Surgical planning laboratory: a new frontier of radiology?* Vienna, 1997, European Congress of Radiology.

Chapter 21

DATABASES FOR INTERVENTIONAL MRI

Ricky K. Taira, Alfonso F. Cardenas

Magnetic resonance (MR)–guided interventional treatment methods are highly complex and require the clinician to make various incremental decisions during the procedure. Many clinical variables should be considered in deciding the best treatment strategies for a patient. For example, radiofrequency (RF)-ablation for a brain tumor requires information acquired over many clinical events, including (1) initial consultation (e.g., age, sex, neurologic status, family history, laboratory test results); (2) pre-treatment diagnostic imaging examinations (e.g., description of tumor appearance and location); and (3) the interventional procedure itself (e.g., number, size, localized placement of RF electrodes, neurologic symptoms and findings). Each physician on the team performing the interventional procedure needs timely access and intelligent presentation of these data to make informed decisions. Post-treatment assessment of the intervention introduces even more variables to manage and correlate.

Given this multitude of patient data, a comprehensive database management system is needed for the interventional physician to function optimally. An intelligent database management system can help physicians make more objective decisions by providing a support system for quickly accessing, organizing, summarizing, and presenting technical and patient data accumulated over many encounters. Several important data management issues should be addressed, including:

1. How can data measured during the interventional operation be included as part of the electronic procedural record?
2. How can the complete patient record be integrated and accessed from a single easy-to-use interface? The fragmentation of the patient record among heterogeneous distributed databases (e.g., hospital information systems, radiology information systems, picture archiving and communication systems [PACS]) limits its practical availability.
3. How can database, analysis, and visualization software interoperate? These software programs are independent and require the user to deal with incompatibilities in data file formats, unit values, storage structures, and

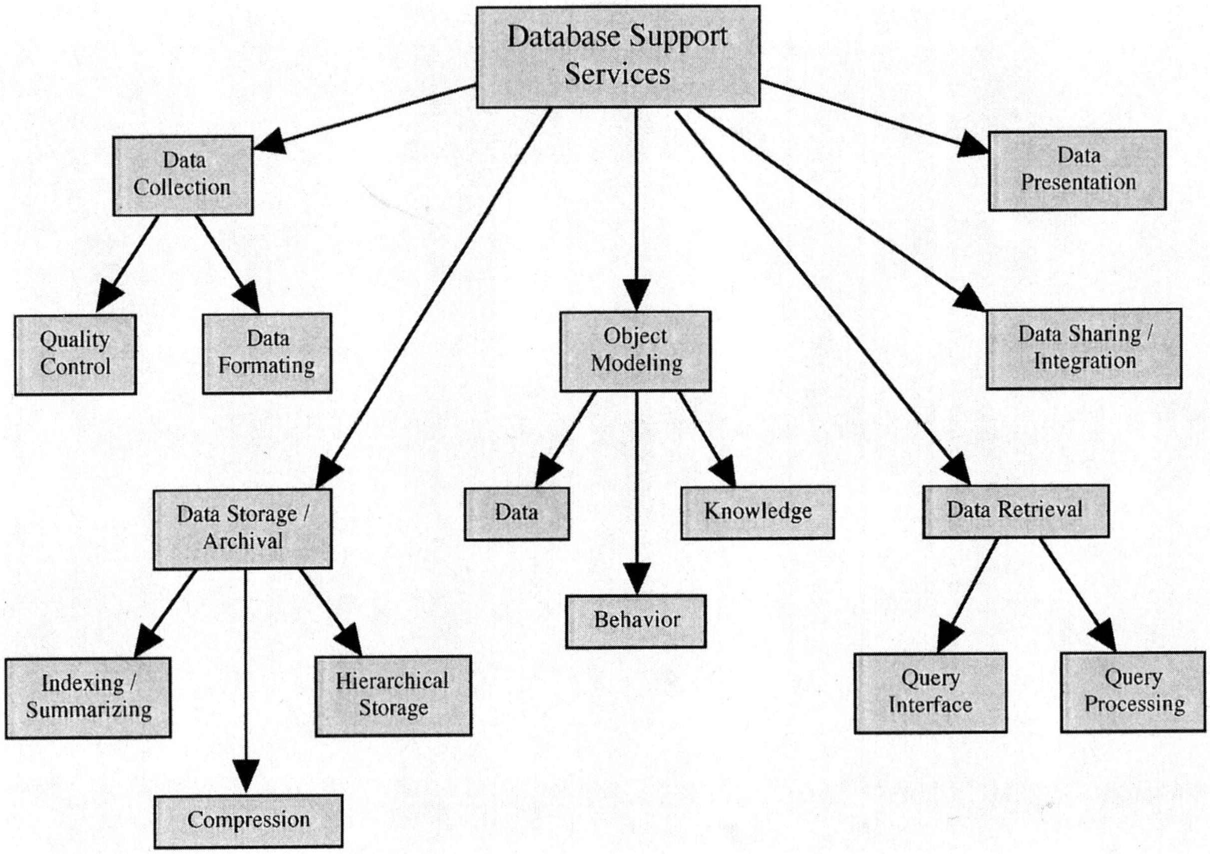

Fig. 21-1. Generic database services are provided by state-of-the-art information management systems.

internal machine representations (e.g., byte ordering, byte boundaries).

4. How can a busy clinician efficiently navigate through the many data available for a patient? One patient may undergo multimodality management over months or years, which includes evaluation with sequential imaging and laboratory and other tests.
5. How can archived cases be retrieved based on patient demographics, presented pathology, and radiographic findings?

The answers to these questions and others are being addressed by several research groups. Important research areas include object-oriented analysis and design,[1–4] active databases,[5,6] intelligent agents,[7,8] multimedia visual query languages,[9,10] distributed database management,[11,12] and cooperative query answering systems.[13] These information management advances will be necessary for interventional methods to optimize patient care, research, and teaching. This chapter describes how these important database management advances can be applied to the management of interventional data. Data management issues include data collection, data storage, object modeling, information retrieval, and multimedia presentation. Figure 21-1 summarizes these basic database services provided by state-of-the-art information management systems. Specific examples from interventional neuroradiology will be used in describing some of the problems and solutions associated with providing these services.

DATA COLLECTION

Medical data are often highly variable, incomplete, imprecise, and inaccurate. They often do not meet the quality standards of other scientific disciplines.[14] All efforts should be made to use a disciplined, meticulous approach to data collection to ensure data availability and quality for patient management and procedure evaluation studies. Proper data collection requires that the data be fully characterized (i.e., so results are reproducible) and be recorded and available for retrieval, processing, distribution, and visualization. Two aspects of data collection should be addressed: (1) What information needs to be collected? (2) How do data get into an appropriate general computing environment?

What data to collect

Ideally, as much detail as possible should be recorded to fully document the clinician's observations, thought processes, and actions during an interventional procedure.[15] The choice of data collection is iterative and involves modeling the entities (e.g., patient, machines, instruments) and processes and later identifying the most important factors that may affect the outcome of the intervention. An explanation of why each parameter is important should be recorded as part of the preintervention analysis. A simple evaluation model can be initially formulated for independent variables that have an effect on the outcome of the intervention (e.g., RF energy delivered) and dependent response variables (e.g., tumor volume). Once sufficient clinical data are available, statistical tests can determine if certain factors are not being considered or if extraneous noise variables are present in the model.

The circumstances under which the data were obtained should be recorded, including schematically diagramming the configuration of the equipment and patient. The temporal relationship of observations and actions may be important to accurately reconstruct a timeline of events, which requires various time stamps be associated with the data.[16,17] "Holes" in the database (i.e., missing data), in which certain data are recorded for some procedures and not for others, lead to inconsistent data sets that can affect analytical results.[18] Data collection forms (i.e., check sheets) help ensure that all necessary data are collected.[19] A quality control person should be designated before the start of an interventional procedure to ensure data completeness and accuracy.

The uncertainty of recorded data should be estimated whenever possible. (A measurement is not very useful without knowing its precision.) Because the structure and application of science depend on measurements, these uncertainties should be evaluated and kept to a minimum. Precision can be especially important in instances in which the same parameter (e.g., blood flow velocity) is measured with different methodologies (e.g., *in vivo* Doppler ultrasound probe versus analytic videodensitometric techniques).

Entering the data into the computing environment

Recorded data are of little use without a means to retrieve, analyze, and visualize them. The data from an interventional procedure can be diverse and include image data (e.g., MR), narrative data describing the procedure and follow-up evaluation, numeric data from various measuring instruments (e.g., thermistor), graphic data (e.g., contours outlining tumor boundaries on MR images), and schematic data that capture the configuration of the patient and instrumentation during the procedure. Often narrative, numeric, schematic, and documentary data are acquired in analog form via audio dictation systems, handwritten notes, or video taping and may need to be filtered, edited, and converted to digital form. Handwritten notes can be recorded digitally using a pen-based "digital notebook" device (e.g., Apple's Newton).[20] Structured data collection templates with computer or paper interfaces can assist in data recording. Data should be entered into these templates by a data recorder or abstract rather than by a physician, who may find the interface too cumbersome. Poor user interfaces have inhibited the clinical acceptance of many computerized data entry systems. Therefore, user interface design is critical.

Some data (e.g., images) have an interface to a computer, but the computer (e.g., a computer that comes with an MRI machine) has limited assess to global system resources (i.e., storage subsystems, distribution services, analysis programs, visualization software, indexing algorithms). In most PACS architectures, image data are sent to a general computing environment using a capture computer, which mediates the transfer between the image acquisition system and the rest of the PACS network.[21] The emergence of various image communication standards in medicine (e.g., Digital Imaging and Communication in Medicine v3.0-DICOM v3.0) will improve image information exchange between heterogeneous medical imaging computers,[22–24] including interoperability among scanners, archives, and display workstations.

DATA STORAGE AND ARCHIVAL

The main storage difficulties in the management of interventional MR data concern images. For example, a typical MR interventional study samples 256 × 256 × 8–bit images at rates of up to several frames per second for 10 sec to several minutes. Several runs during a procedure may be necessary, resulting in several hundred megabytes of data. An image archive can soon exceed several terabytes of data within a few years. A storage management system should have the following features: (1) reliable, long-term, on-line image archival; (2) timely, on-demand image retrieval of current and historic image data; (3) reasonable cost; and (4) scalable architecture to accommodate system growth.

Hierarchical storage strategy

The commonly proposed solution to large-scale image storage involves organizing fast-, medium-, and slow-access storage subsystems into a three-tiered hierarchy (Fig. 21-2). This hierarchy parallels an analog film library that includes short-, medium-, and long-term storage filing.[25] In the analog film library, storage levels are differentiated by their storage capacity, speed of retrieval, and probability of a given request being directed to a particular level.[26] In the digital world, level 1 storage devices consist of fast devices that can support approximately real-time access to 512 × 512 × 8–bit images. These devices are more expensive per megabyte of storage than are level 2 and level 3 devices.

Redundant arrays of inexpensive disks (RAID) are the emerging level 1 storage device of choice in many imaging applications.[27,28] RAID systems arrange multiple independent disks into a logical disk and use redundancy and parallel data transfers to enhance the reliability and bandwidth of the logical disk. Level 2 storage uses medium-priced storage media (about 5 cents per megabyte) that are high capacity, reliable, and moderate in access performance. Optical disk jukeboxes are the current level 2 devices of choice.

Optical disk jukeboxes consist of one or more optical disk drives, a library of optical disk cartridges, and robotics. The robotics are responsible for inserting optical disk platters into the drives, removing platters from drives, and shelving platters into their library storage slots.[29] Optical disk jukeboxes can access data faster than tape systems (random access devices) but slower than magnetic disk systems. Optical jukeboxes can manage a

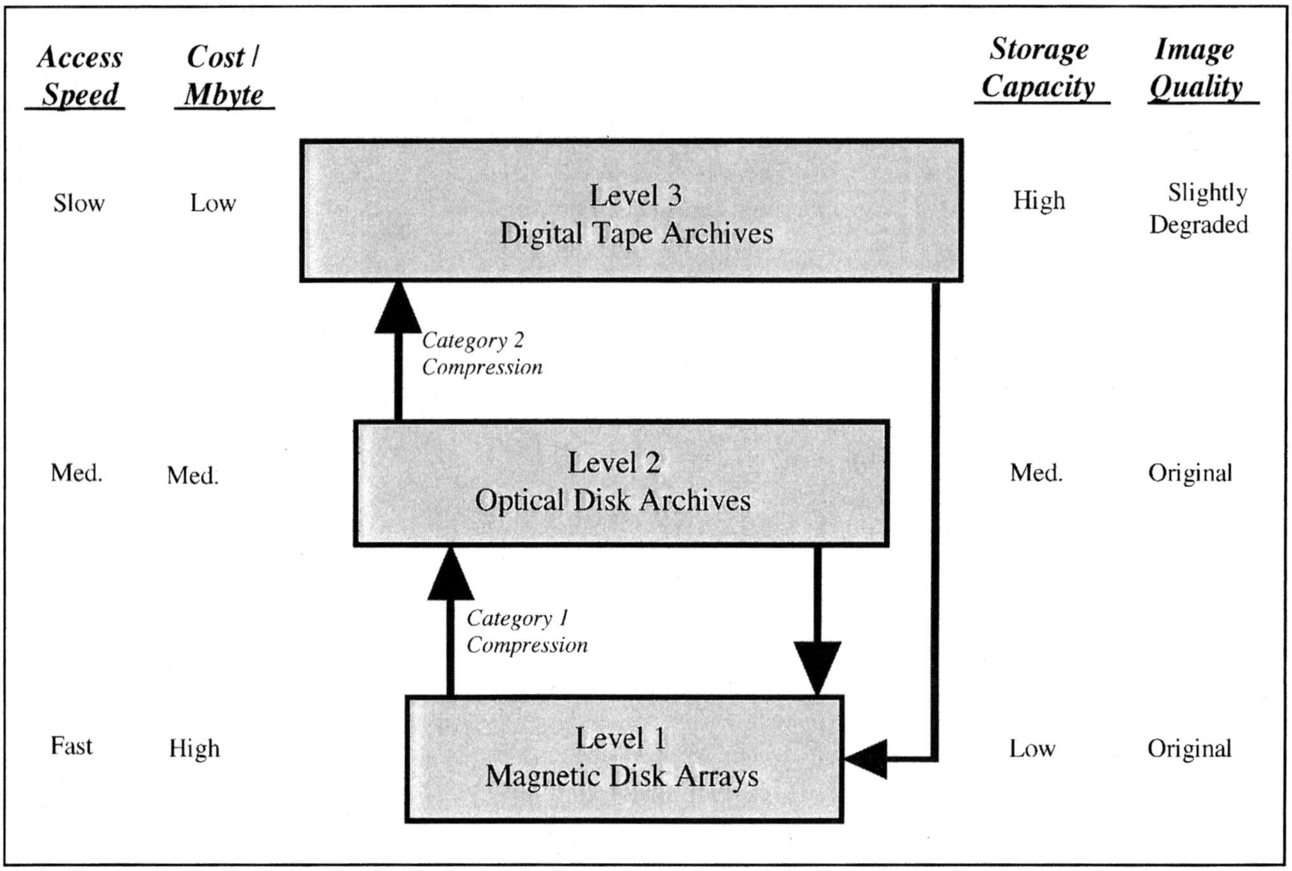

Fig. 21-2. A three-tiered hierarchy is used to store medical images.

few thousand optical disk cartridges. Several optical jukebox systems may exist in a medical network.

Level 3 storage uses slow, high-capacity, inexpensive digital storage media, such as videotapes, digital video disks, 4-mm digital audio tape, 19-mm helical scan tape, or digital linear tape.[30–32] Digital tape storage systems are sequential access systems and therefore slow. Tape jukeboxes support multiple tape drives and can manage a few thousand tapes.

The hierarchical storage architecture relies on calculated placement and movement of files to provide fast access to patient images. Image files can move vertically between levels in the storage hierarchy (e.g., from a slow level 3 tape system to a fast level 1 RAID device) and horizontally between computers within the same level (e.g., from a RAID device connected to an emergency room workstation to a RAID device on a neuroradiology workstation). Movement and access are controlled by a virtual file system, which shields the user from the complication of accessing data from various classes of distributed storage devices.

Newly generated images from an interventional procedure (e.g., MR, digital subtraction angiography) are placed onto a fast-access level 1 storage device. Level 1 storage is allocated only for high-access probability images. To avoid networking and image reconstruction delays, level 1 images should be uncompressed and stored near the display workstation of most probable usage.[33]

The acquisition of new images for a patient should trigger movement of all relevant historic images for this patient from level 2 or level 3 storage to faster level 1 storage. Other clinical events that can trigger this automatic staging of historic images to level 1 storage include patient scheduling and patient arrival. The relevant comparison images (temporal and intermodality) to retrieve are based on how each historic image for a patient correlates with the current study in regards to the organ system, imaging modality, date, and image type (e.g., admission image, discharge image, preoperative image, postoperative image).

The movement of image files from faster level 1 to slower level 2 storage is necessary to allocate level 1 storage space for newer studies (level 1 storage is volatile) and to make permanent copies of images for archival. This movement of image files is typically controlled by how long an image has remained on level 1 storage and its viewing frequency. The images with the lowest access probability are moved to level 2 storage and deleted from level 1 storage. This process is analogous to that in a manual film system, in which patients' folders are moved from short-term to medium-term storage if not viewed for several days (e.g., 10 days). Other image movement strategies are further discussed elsewhere.[34,35]

The horizontal movement of the images between storage nodes in the same level occurs primarily in level 1.[36] Images can migrate to various workstations as their access characteristics change (e.g., when a patient moves from one clinical service to another). Image files may reside on several diagnostic workstations if it is probable that access will occur from many locations. Factors that determine image file placement include radiology service of study, supervising radiologist, clinical service attending the patient, patient status (inpatient, outpatient, emergency patient), the patient's current activity at a particular workstation, and type of examination. New developments arising from the need for distributed digital video servers will soon make the horizontal placement of images less critical.[37] These developments include improved operating systems and faster network interfaces to RAID devices that minimize the network overhead to distributed banks of RAID storage.

Image compression: numeric encoding methods

Image compression methods aim to reduce the storage requirements of imaging studies without significantly affecting their information content. They are particularly of concern in high-volume imaging studies, such as interventional MR. They can extend the image storage capacity of an archive from 2 to 50 times. Reduction in the volume of data for an imaging study also reduces read-time from a storage device and reduces network transmission time. The two categories of numeric data compression methods are reversible (i.e., "lossless" or "error-free") and irreversible (i.e., "lossy"). Reversible methods preserve all information content within the image. That is, the compressed image after reconstruction is numerically identical to the original image. The common reversible compression methods includes Huffman encoding,[38] Ziv-Lempel encoding,[39] and arithmetic coding.[40] Typical compression ratios—ratio of compressed file size to uncompressed file size—are between 2 and 5.

Irreversible methods can attain much higher compression ratios but result in "approximately equivalent" images after reconstruction. A conservative irreversible compression would result in a "visually lossless" image; that is, no differences are perceptible between the original and the reconstructed compressed image as determined by a panel of expert radiologists. This rather subjective definition and the variability of visualizing artifacts and image detail under various viewing conditions make "lossy" image compression methods controversial. Common irreversible methods include Joint Photo Experts Group (JPEG) for still images,[41,42] Moving Pictures Expert Group (MPEG) for timed sequenced images,[43] cosine transform-based methods,[44,45] and wavelet transform-based methods.[46–48] The choice of algorithm depends on the desired image quality, processing speed, and cost. The processing speed depends on the degree to which the algorithm can be parallelled and the ease with which it can be implemented in hardware.

The strategy for applying compression to medical images is unsettled. In general, only reversible image compression methods are acceptable. Whether to apply compression methods on new imaging studies depends on the speed of compression or reconstruction, the speed of the imaging network, the accuracy of image placement within the network, and the speed and capacity of the level 1 storage system. Chao and others[49] proposed that level 2 images be compressed using a reversible compression scheme, such as arithmetic coding. The rationale is to increase the storage capacity of these storage centers, retain original image quality, and improve image transmission speed to distributed workstation sites. Chao and others also proposed that level 3 storage (images that have not been accessed within about 2 years) be irreversibly compressed because: (1) the probability of a clinical request for a study older than 2 years is low;[26] (2) an original copy of the imaging study has been written to a level 2 volume that is permanent but may be off-line; (3) the radiologist's interpretation of the imaging study is available in the form of a text report; (4) irreversible compression methods can attain high compression ratios (>25), thus making an on-line 10-year image archive (tens to hundreds of terabytes large) economically feasible.

Image compression: semantic encoding methods

Additionally, filtering methods based on image content may soon be routine in real-time or spectroscopic imaging studies that generate many images per study. This scheme, often referred to as clinical compression or selective compression, uses information obtained through an image analysis system (computer or human) to decide which parts of the image are important or which frames of an image sequence are important. The important parts of the imaging study are stored using information preserving techniques, whereas less important parts may be more highly compressed or filtered out. Summarization methods can be used to compress important aspects of an imaging sequence. For example, the specific area of the aneurysm with the highest pressure is usually of most interest to the physician.

Noncritical areas could be represented by summary information (e.g., average, maximum, and minimum temperatures in the region). These summarization techniques are useful for cases (regions) in which, for example, the temperature is relatively stable.

DATA MODELING

Medical data derived from patients undergoing interventional MR procedures can be complex. Intelligent search, sort, association, and presentation methods optimize the retrieval, review, and analysis of these data. These requirements have prompted much interest in the development of comprehensive data models for medicine.[50,51] Data models provide an information management system with knowledge of the types of entities stored within the system, their relationships, their attributes, and their possible values. Such knowledge is necessary for a database system to assist in answering complex questions, such as: How do the shape and volume of a tumor change with regard to time after therapy? What other cases of lesions similar in size, intensity, and growth or shrink rate as the current case are there? Can cases showing a tumor in the posterior fossa adjacent to the dura or next to the 4th ventricle be found? Can cases in which the tumor continued to grow after treatment be found?

Basic modeling constructs

A logical data model for medicine formally describes all patient information. Most data models are based on the entity-relationship model,[52] which describes the basic constructs for formally representing data. These constructs include entities (any object, event, or process that contains information), attributes (descriptors attached to entities that characterize their state), and relationships (correlating verb phrases that describe the interaction among entities). Data models for medical image entities are being defined by Part 3 of the DICOM v3.0[23,24] and other efforts. General data models for medicine have been developed by the National Library of Medicine (Unified Medical Language System Semantic Network for Medicine).[53,54] A partial data model for an MR-guided RF thermal ablation procedure is diagrammed in Figure 21-3.

Modeling extensions

Recent advances in data modeling have extended the descriptive capabilities of the entity-relationship model. These extensions include semantic data models,[55,56] object-oriented data models,[1,4,57,58] temporal data models,[17,59] spatial data models,[60,61] and temporal-evolutionary data models.[62,63]

Generalization or specialization

Generalization or specialization relates a specific object type to a more generic type. Subtypes inherit characteristics of their parent supertype. This modeling construct is useful in describing the type-classification of objects. This hierarchy helps the database system understand the domain of general concepts (e.g., neoplasms, nervous tissue) and the relationship to more specific concepts (e.g., glioblastoma multiforme). Figure 21-4 shows the generalization or specialization inheritance hierarchy for histologic classes of human neoplasms of the nervous system. This knowledge allows a database system to infer that a glioblastoma multiforme tumor is a type of glioma, which is a type of neoplasm originating from nervous tissue.

These advanced modeling constructs often are not yet supported by the native database system storing the data. For example, most current medical database systems do not support object-oriented functionality. In these situations, logical entities are created to reference physical data items. These logical entities give the physical data object-oriented, stream, or spatial modeling capabilities.[64] These logical entities use pointers to allow access to the physical data, which may be distributed among various database sites.

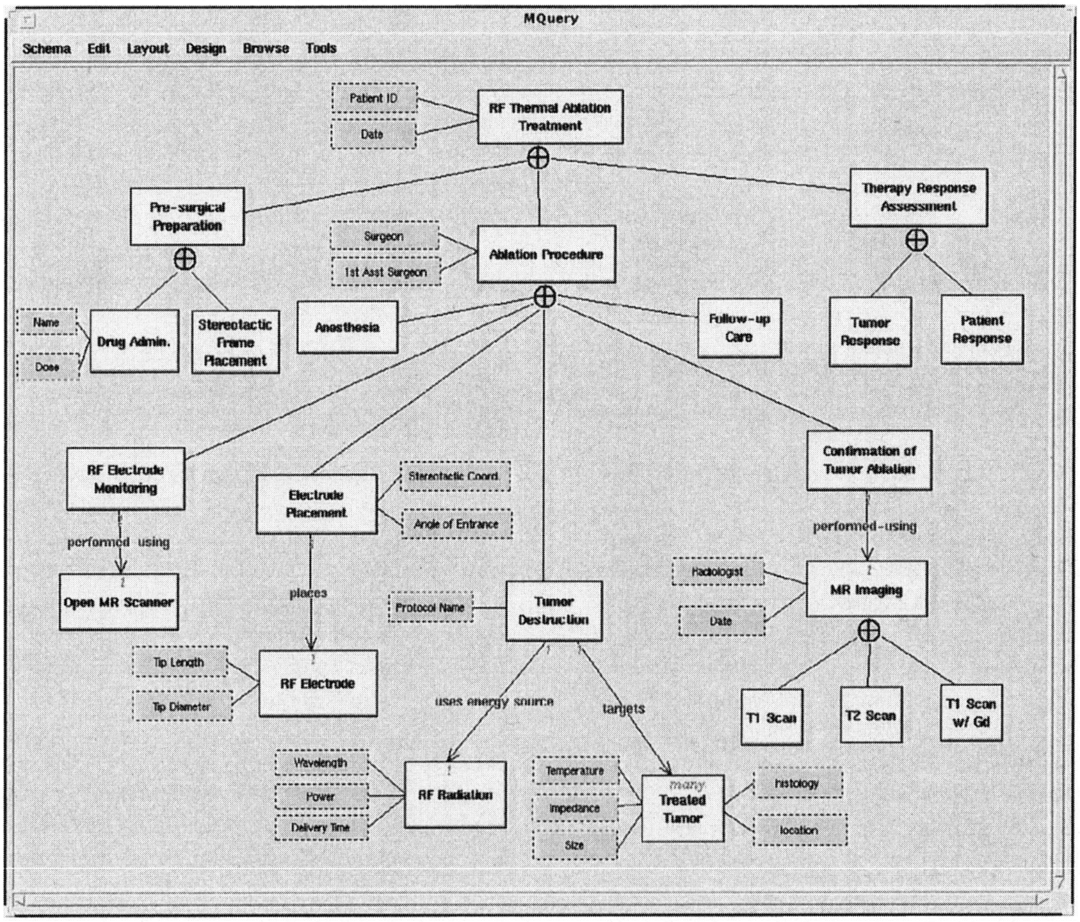

Fig. 21-3. In this partial data model for a magnetic resonance–guided radiofrequency thermal ablation, the *ring-cross* is used to indicate a "consists-of" relationship. *Dotted boxes* represent entity attributes.

Aggregation

Aggregation models the composition of a complex object into its constituent parts. This construct is useful for describing complex objects or procedures consisting of multiple aspects or parts (e.g., the brain consists of several substructures or a lesion's appearance is a function of brightness, uniformity, border characteristics, texture, shape etc.). For example, the aggregation relation describes an RF thermal ablation procedure as consisting of a presurgical preparation step, the ablation procedure, and a therapy response assessment step (see Fig. 21-3). These steps can be further decomposed using the aggregation construct. Figure 21-5 shows the aggregation hierarchy for various components of the brainstem.

Methods

The object-oriented extensions to the entity-relationship model allow methods (i.e., procedures) to be associated with entities. These methods describe behavioral characteristics of the entity. For example, a method that calculates temperature flow from an MR sequence can be associated with the entity brain tumor. This method allows specialized programs to be automatically attached to high-level data entities.

Temporal constructs

Temporal modeling constructs describe how the state (e.g., size, position, shape) of an entity changes. Temporal changes are described in terms of direction (e.g., growing, shrinking) and rate (e.g., fast, stable, slow). Temporal constructs also model the order of events (e.g., noticeable changes were seen 2 weeks after surgery, process A co-occurs with process B). Snodgrass and Ahn[17] provide a taxonomy of time terminology. Interval- and point-based temporal models characterize time-dependent data and relationships.[16,59,65] Streams are specialized entities that represent a sequence of objects related in time.[66] The sequenced objects are often different versions of the same object but with different states. For example, a lesion whose volume is changing because of a therapeutic process is modeled as a type of stream.[67]

Evolutionary constructs

Evolutionary constructs describe the transformation of an object as it goes through an evolutionary change (i.e., high-entropy change). This modeling construct can be used to represent the embryonic development of an organ or the transition of tumors through different gross pathologic classifications (e.g., a

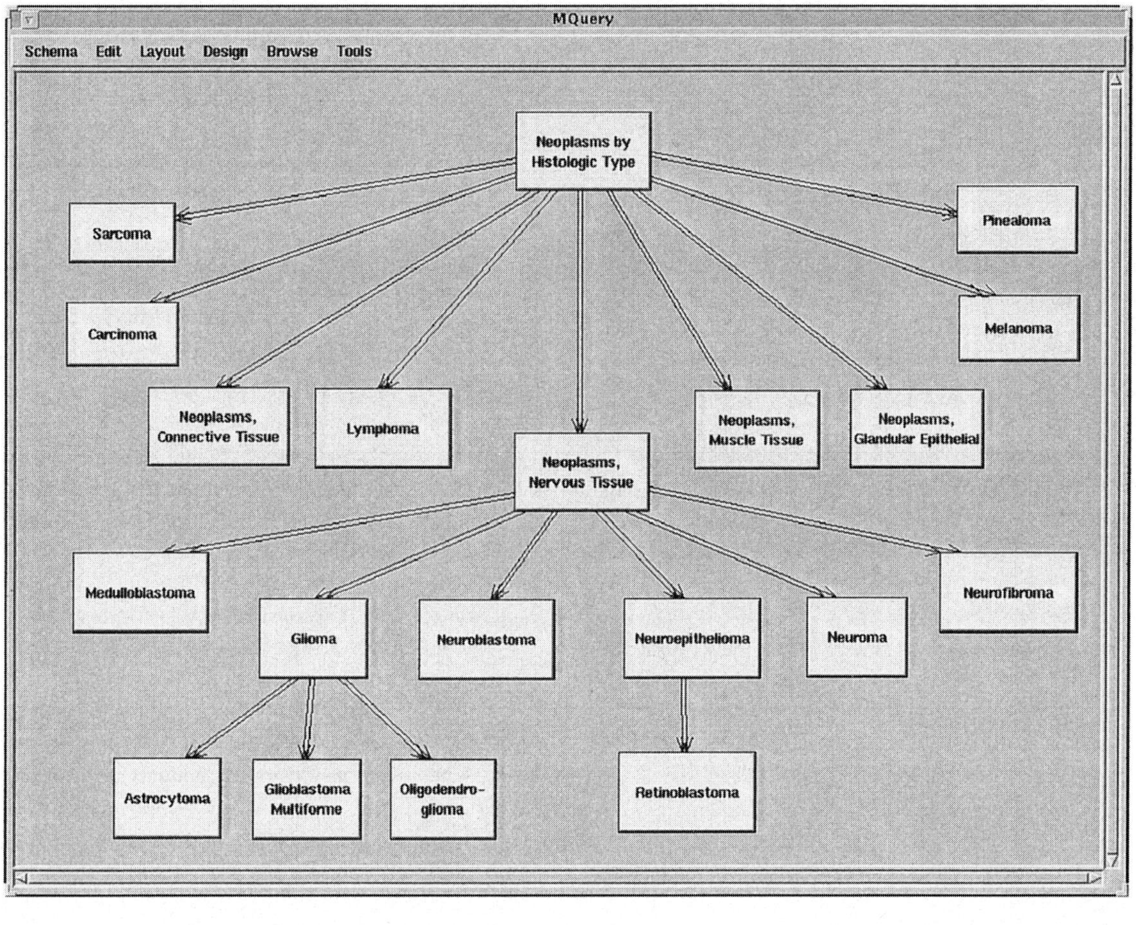

Fig. 21-4. Generalization or specialization inheritance hierarchy shows classes of nervous system tumors. The *double arrow* indicates a specialization relationship.

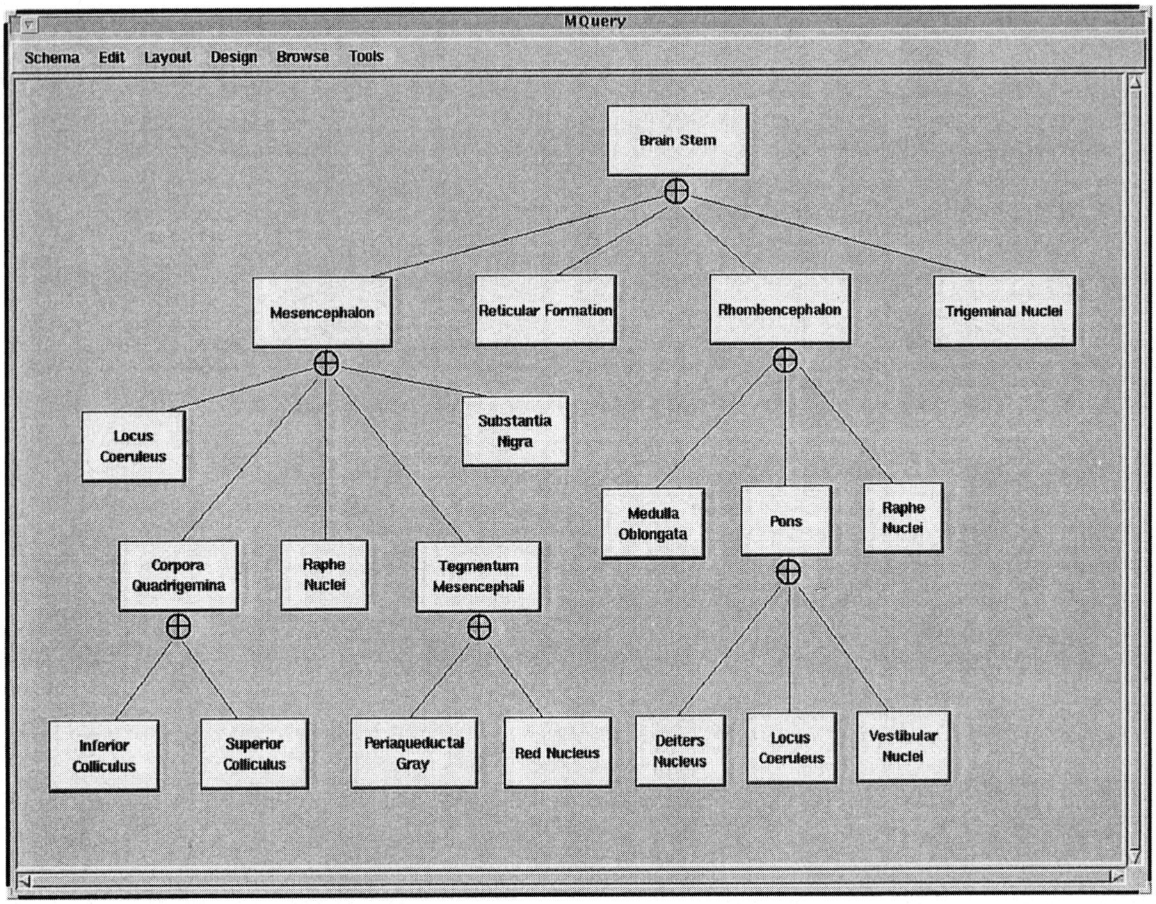

Fig. 21-5. In this aggregation hierarchy for the brainstem, the *ring-cross* is used to indicate a "consists-of" relationship.

micro-adenoma evolves into a macroadenoma). An evolutionary sequence of an object describes the various evolutionary stages with respect to some active entropy-altering phenomenon (development, aging, therapy, disease). These data constructs allow medical entities to be queried as a function of various gross transformations.

Spatial constructs

Spatial constructs relate the spatial extent, confinement, or direction of nearby objects. A more complete discussion can be found in the literature.[56,60] These constructs help to solve queries such as find a tumor near, next to, invading, or contained within the sphenoid sinus?

Other relationships

The *Unified Medical Language System Metathesaurus* developed by the National Library of Medicine specifies approximately 45 relationships between medical terms,[54] including *causes, connected to, degree of, diagnosis, indicates, precedes, process of, manifestation of, functionally related to,* and others.

Model instantiation

Once a logical data model is constructed for an interventional application (see Fig. 21-3), the newly acquired images, reports, and measurements generated by the procedure should be inserted into the data to be intelligently queried. This step is necessary because most imaging studies are referenced by their content (i.e., body location, presence of tumor) or in terms of other entities, relationships, or attributes in the data model. For example, before using a new MR examination for a patient, an investigator should know the following:

1. What imaging technique was used? This question may reference basic acquisition parameters, such as echo and relaxation times; slightly more abstract descriptions, such as T1- or T2-weighted; or high-level descriptions, such as a protocol name.
2. What views and body regions does this examination cover? This question may refer to general body regions or more specific anatomic organs or sites.
3. Why was this examination performed? The clinical history or suspected pathology of the patient should be linked to the imaging study.
4. What were the important findings associated with this examination? Findings may include low-level radiologic findings (e.g., densities) or high-level process descriptions (e.g., tumor).
5. Which image slices best show the important findings?

The data associated with the MR procedure need to be logically organized into a data model to efficiently answer such

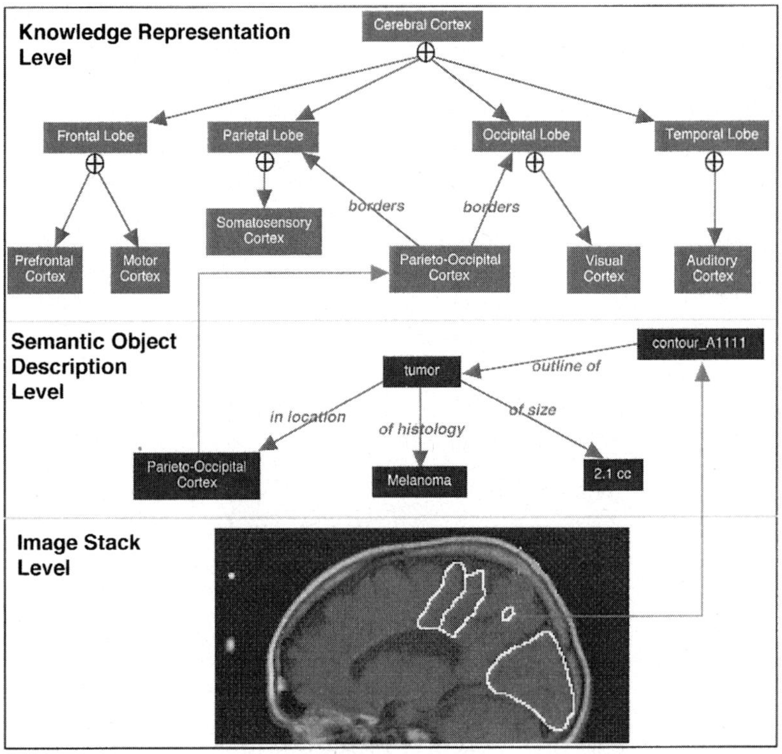

Fig. 21-6. A three-level data model is used to formally characterize the content of medical images and to integrate general domain knowledge.

questions. Data describing an imaging procedure may be obtained from various sources including:

1. The DICOM-defined header fields that accompany radiologic images complying with the American College of Radiology-National Electrical Manufacturer's Association DICOM standard.[23] The DICOM v3.0 standard defines image acquisition description fields that are to accompany medical imaging studies.
2. Abstract descriptive values that are calculated. If not available, abstract values such as "T1-weighted" should be calculated based on low-level parameter values (i.e., echo and repetition times) and scanner specifications. This transformation is necessary because low-level values are often meaningless to nonradiologists.
3. Dictated medical reports. An information-rich text report is associated with each medical procedure. This report includes descriptions of radiologic findings, pathologic processes, and areas of disease involvement. Natural language analysis methods are becoming more successful and are moving toward the goal of formally structuring important concepts dictated within a medical free text report.[68–71]
4. Important findings in an image that are directly annotated using graphic drawing or writing tools. This step helps improve the labeling of observations within the image.
5. Image analysis methods. Segmentation methods and contour analysis routines provide the most precise method for capturing spatial features (e.g., shape, extent, location) and spatial relationships (relative position, containment information, intersections, clustering patterns) of image objects.[72–76] Analytical descriptors (e.g., Fourier coefficients to describe shape) complement semantic terms (e.g., *spherical, triangular, popcorn-shaped*). Both are useful indices to medical image objects.

The complete model for medical image data should include the raw data, high-level semantic or numeric descriptions of the data, and general knowledge about the data. Figure 21-6 shows one method for comprehensive representation of these types of data. It shows the use of a three-level data model.

The lowest level, the **image stack level,** represents raw patient images and contours. It uses a dynamic stacked logical data structure.[77] Stacks are aggregations of related images along a third dimension. This dimension can be space (e.g., image volume), time (image sequence), or energy (spectroscopic images). Image stacks map well to the volumetric nature of cross-sectional images. For example, multiple stacks of pictures can provide additional temporal or spectral information. Stacks may consist of a hierarchy of other stacks.

The middle level, the **semantic object description level,** provides a formalized semantic description of the important characteristics of the images stored in the image stack level. These descriptions are derived from headers, free-text analysis programs applied to the corresponding radiology reports, or mathematical analyses of contoured imaging data (see above). The semantic object description level provides a data model for a particular image. That is, each radiology imaging study results in a data model unique to the findings and characteristics of the image. An object-oriented semantic data model is used to describe these findings.[56,78]

The top layer, the **knowledge representation level,** models medical concepts at the class level (generic level) rather than the instance level. This layer contains data structures that capture domain knowledge.[79] This domain knowledge is needed by a database management system to infer additional information about a concept. For example, an aggregation hierarchy (see Fig. 21-5) is effective for providing a system with the ability to infer that the pons is part of the rhombencephalon, which is part of the brainstem, which is part of the brain. A generalization-specialization hierarchy (see Fig. 21-4) provides a query-processing system with the ability to automatically determine all related concepts to a parent concept (e.g., types of nervous tissue neoplasms include medulloblastoma, glioma, neuroblastoma, neuroepithelioma; types of gliomas include astrocytomas, glioblastoma multiforme, oligodendrogliomas). Nodes in the knowledge representation layer have instance mappings to nodes or relationships in the semantic object description level; thus, object instances within an image can be mapped to the larger general data model. The *Unified Medical Language System Metathesaurus* developed by the National Library of Medicine is an excellent electronic resource that can be applied to this level of the data model.[53,54]

CASE RETRIEVAL

Once the medical data for an interventional procedure have been collected, modeled, and indexed, sophisticated case-retrieval strategies can be applied. A case-retrieval system for medicine can be complex because the data are distributed among multiple data repositories and because of the imprecise or abstract terms used to describe medical objects, events, and procedures. For example, several difficulties are associated with the following medical data:

Retrieve magnetic resonance images and all medical reports of middle-aged patients that demonstrate a malignant spherical mass in the vicinity of the sphenoid sinus that has reduced in size by greater than 70 percent post thermal ablation therapy.

Problems that should be addressed include the following:

- How can this natural language query be translated to a computer? Conventional query languages have limited ability to understand spatial relationships (e.g., "in the vicinity of"), spatial patterns (e.g., shapes), and temporal concepts (e.g., "reduced in size by 70% post thermal ablation therapy").
- What methods are used to match cases in the system to conditions specified in the query? The system should be able to mimic the response of a trained expert in the medical field. It should be knowledgeable about a concept's attributes, relationships (e.g., a malignant mass can be an adenoma or one of several other cancerous growths), and reference variations (e.g., synonyms, lexical variants).
- How does the system retrieve cases similar to the case specified within the query? Exact matches of cases in the database may not exist. For example, the system may need to relax the shape of the mass from spherical to elliptical.
- What is the user's role in performing queries? A flexible user interface allows the user to express the query, refine the query, and navigate through the presented query solutions. The user requires tools to visualize the presented data in a specific format (e.g., pictoral, graphic, tabular).

Various system architectures to support advanced medical information processing needs are emerging.[7,11,51] The KMeD system (Knowledge-Based Multimedia Medical Distributed Database System) is a prototype system that attempts to create a complete application that allows a physician to perform all database, image processing, and study tasks with a consistent intuitive interface.[80] The KMeD system uses several methods to perform the tasks of query formulation and query template matching.

Query formulation

Query formulation is concerned with how to express English-like queries. In the KMeD system, queries can be formulated using generic tabular and iconic interfaces or custom form-based interfaces.

The tabular format, PicQuery^{+},[9] is based on a query-by-example paradigm.[81] It uses a five-column table to describe the query search constraints, including the object attribute name (e.g., lesion size); the relational correlator (e.g., greater than); the attribute value (e.g., 3 cm); the logical operator (e.g., and, or), which allows construction of compound complex predicates; and the predicate group identification number, which is needed to definite clauses (in parentheses) in complex predicates. The tabular format expresses *ad hoc* queries on data that can be constrained using alpha-numeric expressions. Graphical browsing tools for the global data dictionary allow the user to easily review the entities and attributes maintained within the database.[29]

The iconic interface, MQuery,[67] uses icons to visually represent prototypical objects. This interface format is useful for queries that specify spatial relationship constraints that are difficult to describe alpha-numerically. An example spatial query is to find all cases of a tumor in a specific brain location (e.g., frontal lobe) in the database. To specify this query, the user browses a visual dictionary containing iconic representations of visually oriented database entities. Icons representing a brain object and a tumor object are copied from the dictionary into a query window palette, where they can be freely moved and manipulated. The tumor object is overlaid on top of the brain object and positioned over the site of interest (i.e., frontal lobe) to indicate the tumor location in brain tumor cases.

An example of an application-specific query interface is shown in Figure 21-7. A common research query involves combined specifications of patient demographics, disease pathology, and radiologic findings. In the main menu, when the "pathology of interest" icon is selected, a custom pathology format is presented. Figure 21-7 shows the brain tumor specification template. The upper portion of this template provides the user with a hierarchical list corresponding to the histologic

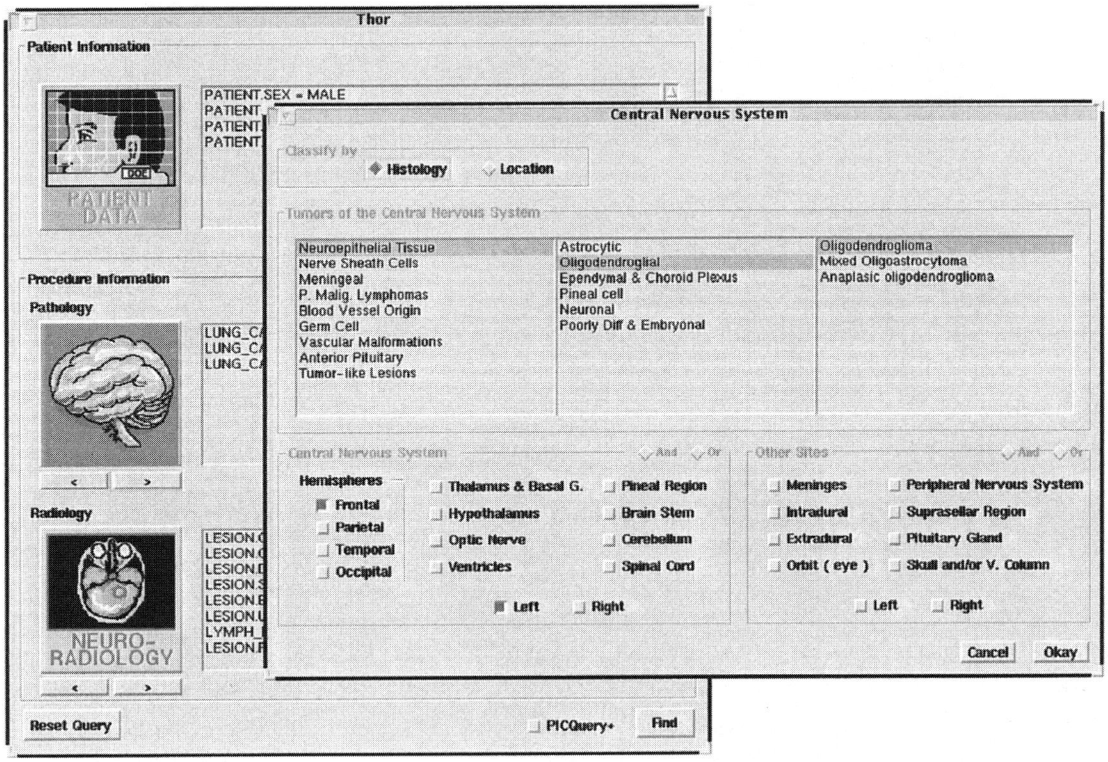

Fig. 21-7. An application-specific query interface specifies patient demographics, disease pathology, and radiologic findings.

classification of brain tumors. The histology class filter allows the investigator to be very specific (e.g., oligodendroglioma) or very general (e.g., tumors originating from neuroepithelial tissue) in qualifying the histology characteristics for the case to be retrieved. Subclasses of general concepts are known via the knowledge representation layer within the data model (see the section on model instantiation). Radio buttons allow the user to specify the location of the tumor. When multiple values for an attribute are allowed (e.g., tumor location), the user should specify whether to perform an "or" or "and" search constraint.

Query answering

In the KMeD system, once the user has specified the patient demographics, disease pathology, and radiology constraints, query processing begins by parsing the query into individual predicates and interpreting the attribute names and values for each predicate. A user-specified query might naturally reference an abstract concept value, which has no direct matches within the database. For example, in the query "Find cases that show central nervous system tumors," the KMeD system recognizes the term *central nervous system tumor* as a conceptual entity, which is a node within the knowledge representation level of the data model (i.e., generalization-specialization hierarchy—see the section on modeling extensions). The data model is used to construct a revised query that includes all the leaf nodes under this concept (i.e., astrocytoma, oligodendroglioma, glioblastoma multiforme, retinoblastoma).

The revised interpreted query is processed by a case-matching module, which uses various indices within the instantiated data model to identify cases that match the query template. References to logical entities (e.g., streams—see the section on modeling extensions) are identified, and the physical location of the data is determined. Once cases and data items are identified, a plan for retrieving the data is constructed. These data may be physically distributed among several federated information systems (e.g., hospital information system [HIS], radiology information system [RIS], PACS). The plan is determined dynamically based on the location of the data, the availability of database server processes, and the availability of network services.

To execute the plan, KMeD makes use of a collection of data access and formatting agents. These agents are software robots that can access the hospital network, make session connections with various database server machines, communicate with remote databases in the appropriate language, read targeted data items, communicate results to a designated workspace, and translate data from a source to target format. Data integration computer-aided software engineering tools are commercially available to assist in the rapid prototyping and debugging of these software agents.[82,83] As a way to improve user performance, distributed data can be staged into a centralized database cache. The staging process can be

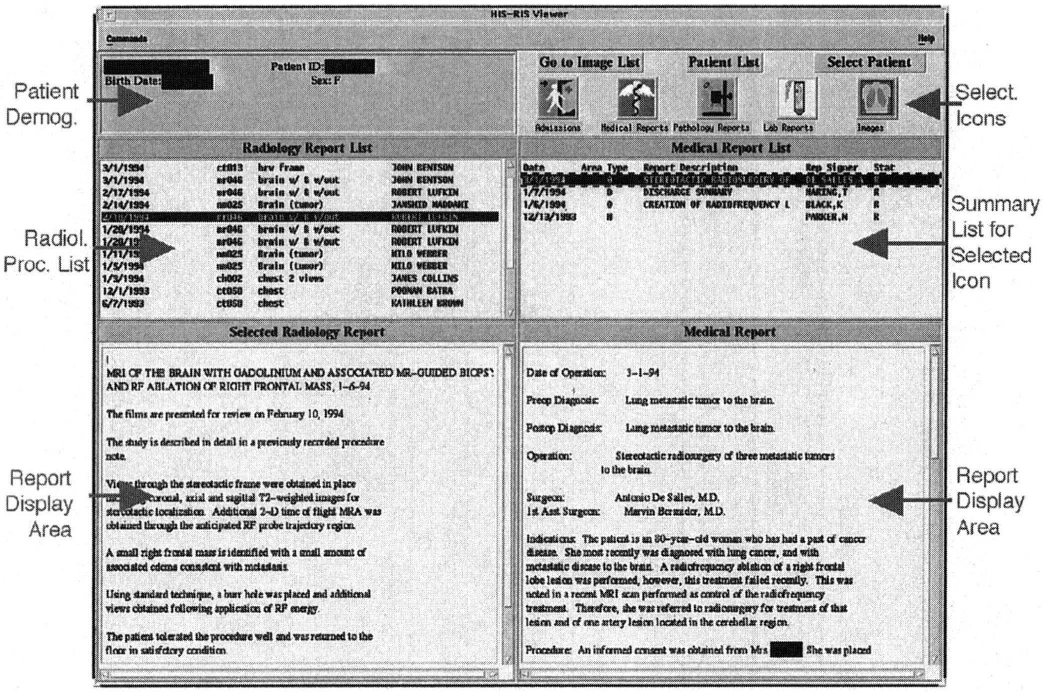

Fig. 21-8. User interface displays hospital information system, radiology information system, and picture archiving and communications system medical records using a file-folder organization paradigm.

triggered by clinical events, such as patient admission or patient scheduling.

DATA PRESENTATION

One of the most challenging tasks in the construction of a medical information system is the design of the user interface for an integrated electronic patient record.[84,85] How to develop mechanisms to allow a user to easily visualize and access voluminous record-oriented data has not been given due priority. A user may be interested in several data items, some of which should be displayed simultaneously with related items, whereas others are disjointed and can be reviewed separately. Interventional physicians increasingly require rapid access to past radiologic reports and other medical record data, such as admission and discharge summaries, pathology reports, operative reports, and clinical laboratory data. If these data are not effectively summarized or organized and have cumbersome interfaces, users will be overloaded with information or become frustrated because of operational difficulties.

The success of any intelligent data presentation system for interventional radiology relies on developing a comprehensive model of the types of data, tasks, interaction paradigms, and queries that the system may potentially encounter. The system's goal is to develop and execute a display strategy that anticipates the expectations and logic processing of the user. This problem is complex given the innumerable combinations of image sequences, pathology conditions, display hardware configurations, user preferences, and supplementary medical and radiologic report information for any case.

File-folder approach

One means of organizing the electronic patient record uses a file-folder approach. In this paradigm, documents are classified according to type and arranged in reverse chronology. Summary lists facilitate document selection. Figure 21-8 shows such a user interface developed at the University of California, Los Angeles (UCLA), for displaying HIS, RIS, and PACS medical records. The left half of the user screen includes patient demographic information, a selectable list summarizing radiology procedures performed on the patient, and an area that shows radiology reports for the selected procedure in full. On the right half of the interface, selectable icons allow the user to specify the type of HIS or PACS information to be displayed in the central listing area. These icons correspond to admissions and discharge information, medical reports, laboratory reports, pathology reports, and PACS images. From the summary listing, the user can select a record, which triggers display of the corresponding full-text report below. A PACS image, if selected, can be viewed directly on a selected monitor.

Timeline approach

In many instances, the sequence of events and object changes are most important to a diagnostician or therapist (e.g., tracking the volume of a treated tumor). In such cases, a patient's history may be more effectively displayed using a visual timeline.[86–88] The timeline may be general, including all documents, or it can be configured by the user to include only documents of interest. For example, a timeline for a patient undergoing an MR-guided RF thermal tumor ablation procedure may

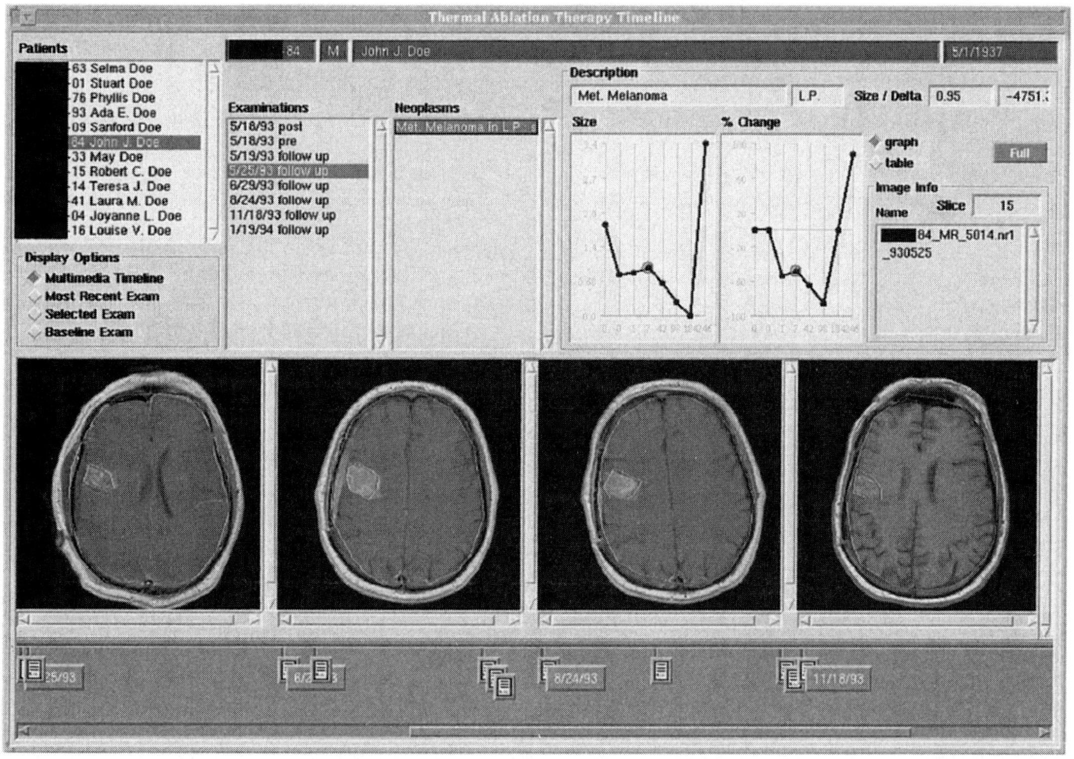

Fig. 21-9. Visual timeline approach presents patient data. The horizontal axis represents time. This image used the UCLA KMeD system developed at the University of California, Los Angeles.

include sequences of select images, giving a visual record of the size of the primary tumor (Fig. 21-9).[88] Appropriate icons are "hung" off the timeline to provide easy review of pathology, radiology, and medical reports generated during the window of time being viewed.

SUMMARY

Interventional MR applications in the brain have placed increased demand for faster data processing, decision support, and near real-time acquisition and display of digital image data in the procedure room. The advancement and quality assurance of interventional procedures depend on a disciplined approach to all aspects of data management. These aspects include improving the recording of fine-grained detail needed for documenting the interventional procedure, designing integrated data models that describe the accumulated characteristics and behavior of the data, and developing intelligent sorting, summarizing, and retrieval techniques for achieved clinical cases.

The long-term goal of a data management system for minimally invasive therapy of the brain is to provide a user-friendly system that can retrieve historic cases based on the combination of patient demographics, clinical history, lesion pathology, therapy description, and radiographic findings. A data management system that can capture the entire inventory of accumulated multimedia data on interventional patients with similar lesions would be a powerful resource for decision support and for outcomes research. The database technologies necessary to provide this type of intelligent case retrieval have only recently been formalized with clinical prototype systems now being developed. Much research remains, however, to achieve the goal of developing flexible, expandable, and intelligent information processing architectures to manage the vast decentralized image and text data repositories prevalent in healthcare environments.

REFERENCES

1. Zdonik S, Maier D: *Readings in object-oriented databases,* Palo Alto, Calif, 1990 Morgan-Kaufmann.
2. Coad P, Yourdon E: *Object-oriented analysis,* ed 2, Englewood Cliffs, NJ, 1991, Prentice-Hall.
3. Atwood TM: The case for object-oriented databases, *IEEE Spectrum,* 1991.
4. Henderson-Sellers B: *A book of object-oriented knowledge: object-oriented analysis, design, and implementation: a new approach to software engineering,* New York, 1992, Prentice-Hall.
5. Miller JA, and others: The active KDL object-oriented database system and its application to simulation support, *Journal of Object-Oriented Programming* 4:30, 1991.
6. Kappel G, and others: TriGS: making a passive object-oriented database system active, *Journal of Object-Oriented Programming* 7:40–51, 1994.
7. Wiederhold G: Mediators in the architecture of future information systems, *IEEE Computer* 25:38, 1992.
8. Waldrop MM: Software agents prepare to sift the riches of cyberspace, *Science* 265:882, 1994.
9. Cardenas AF, and others: The knowledge-based object-oriented PICQUERY + language, *IEEE Transactions on Knowledge and Data Engineering* 5:644, 1993.
10. Del Bimbo AD, Campanai M, Nesi P: A three-dimensional iconic environment for image database querying, *IEEE Transactions on Software Engineering* 19:997, 1993.

11. van Mulligen EM, Timmers T, van Bemmel JH: A new architecture for integration of heterogeneous software components, *Methods Inf Med* 32:292, 1993.
12. Attalur GK, Bradshaw DP, Coburn N: The CORDS multidatabase project, *IBM Systems Journal* 34:39, 1995.
13. Chu WW, Chen Q: A structured approach for cooperative query answering, *IEEE Transactions on Knowledge and Data Engineering* 6:738, 1994.
14. Kamaroff AL: The variability and inaccuracy of medical data, *Proceedings of the IEEE* 67:1196, 1979.
15. Shortcliffe EH, Barnett GO: *Medical data: their acquisition, storage, and use.* In Shortcliff EH, and others, editors: *Medical informatics: computer applications in health care,* 1990, Addison-Wesley.
16. Allen JF: Maintaining knowledge about temporal intervals, *Communications of the Association of Computing Machinery* 26:832, 1983.
17. Snodgrass RT, Ahn I: *A taxonomy of time in databases,* 1985, Proceedings of Association of Computing Machinery SIGMOD International Conference on the Management of Data.
18. Little RJA, Rubin DB: *Statistical analysis with missing data,* New York, 1987, John Wiley & Sons.
19. Parsaye K, Chignell M: *Intelligent quality control.* In Parsaye K, Chignell M: *Intelligent database tools & applications: hyperinformation access, data quality, visualization, automatic discovery,* New York, 1993, John Wiley & Sons.
20. Marcus A: Human communications issues in advanced UIs, *Communications of the Association of Computing Machinery* 36:101, 1993.
21. Huang HK, Taira RK: Infrastructure design of a picture archiving and communication system, *Am J Roentgenol* 158:743, 1992.
22. Best DE, and others: Review of the American College of Radiology–National Electrical Manufacturers Association standards activity, *Computer Methods Programs Biomed* 37:305, 1992.
23. ACR-NEMA: *Standards publication PS3.2: digital imaging and communications in medicine (DICOM),* Washington, DC, 1993, National Electric Manufacturers Association (NEMA).
24. Horii SC, Bidgood WD Jr: *DICOM: a standard for medical imaging (enabling technologies for high-bandwidth applications, Boston, MA, USA, 10–11 Sept. 1992),* 1993, Proceedings of the SPIE: The International Society for Optical Engineering.
25. Fisher HW: *Radiology departments: planning, operation, and management,* Ann Arbor, Mich, 1982, Edward Brothers.
26. Dwyer SJ III, Stewart BK, Spraggins TA: Modeling of analog film-file radiographic retrievals: a Markov chain, *Invest Radiol* 28:1144, 1993.
27. Moren B: RAID storage for imaging: what you need to consider, *Advanced Imaging* February: 14, 1993.
28. Chen PM, and others: RAID: high-performance, reliable secondary storage (redundant arrays of inexpensive disks), *Association of Computing Machinery Computing Surveys* 26:145, 1994.
29. Tighe LC: Digital archiving, *Medical Imaging* 9:52, 1994.
30. Frost MM, Honeyman JC, Staab E: Image archival technologies: PACS mini refresher course, *Radiographics* 12:330, 1992.
31. Giorgis TW, McDonough J: The technology behind 4-mm DAT drives, *Byte* 20:146, 1995.
32. Giorgis TW, McDonough J: DLT drives (digital linear tape), *Byte* 20:154, 1995.
33. Wah BW: File placement on distributed computer systems, *Computer* 17:23, 1984.
34. Sheng ORL, and others: *Design of knowledge-based image retrieval system: implications from radiologists' cognitive processes,* Newport Beach, Calif, 1992, Proceedings of the SPIE, Medical Imaging VI: PACS Design and Evaluation.
35. Piqueras J, and others: Worklists, preloading and archiving strategies: 3 years of clinical experience in the Barcelona PACS, *Medical Inf (Lond)* 19:123, 1994.
36. Gavish B, Sheng ORL: Dynamic file migration in distributed computer systems, *Communications of the Association of Computing Machinery* 33:177, 1990.
37. Buddhikot MM, Parulkar GM, Cox JR Jr: Design of a large scale multimedia storage server, *Computer Networks and ISDN Systems* 27:503, 1994.
38. Rosenfeld A, Kak AC: *Digital picture processing,* ed 2, vol 1, New York, 1982, Academic Press.
39. Sheinwald D: On the Ziv-Lempel proof and related topics, *Proceedings of the IEEE* 82:866, 1994.
40. Witten IH, Neal RM, Clearly JG: Arithmetic coding for data compression, *Communications of the Association of Computing Machinery* 30:520, 1987.
41. Wallace GK: The JPEG still picture compression standard (Joint Photographic Experts Group), *Communications of the Association of Computing Machinery* 34:30, 1991.
42. Pennebaker WB, Mitchell JL: *JPEG still image data compression standard,* New York, 1993, Van Nostrand Reinhold.
43. Le Gall D: MPEG: a video compression standard for multimedia applications, *Communications of the Association of Computing Machinery* 34:46, 1991.
44. Cooley JW, Lewis PAW, Welch PD: The fast fourier transforms algorithm: programming considerations in the calculation of sine, cosine and Laplace transforms, *Journal of Sound and Vibration* 12:315, 1970.
45. Ho BKT, and others: Design and implementation of a full-frame bit allocation image compression hardware module, *Radiology* 179:563, 1991.
46. Daubechies I: The wavelet transform, time-frequency localization and signal analysis, *IEEE Transactions on Information Theory* 36:961, 1990.
47. Antonini M, and others: Image coding using wavelet transform, *IEEE Transactions on Image Processing* 1:205, 1992.
48. Lucier BJ, and others: Wavelet compression and segmentation of digital mammograms, *J Digit Imaging* 7:27, 1994.
49. Chao W, and others: Implementation of system intelligence in a 3-tier telemedicine PACS hierarchical storage management system, *Proceedings of the SPIE* 2435:423, 1995.
50. Rector AL, and others: A framework for modeling the electronic medical record, *Methods Inf Med* 32:109, 1993.
51. Garfagni H, and others: MIMOSA: a functional model of the management of medical images, *Med Inf (Lond)* 19:95, 1994.
52. Chen PPS: The entity-relationship model: towards a unified view of data, *Association of Computing Machinery Transactions on Database Systems* 1:9, 1976.
53. Lindberg DAB, Humphreys BL, McCray AT: *The unified medical language system.* In van Bemmel JH, McCray AT, editors: *Yearbook of medical informatics,* Stuttgart, 1993, Schattauer.
54. US Department of Health and Human Services: *UMLS knowledge sources documentation (6th experimental edition),* 1995, National Institutes of Health, National Library of Medicine.
55. Gogolla M, Hohenstein U: Towards a semantic view of an extended entity-relationship model, *Association of Computing Machinery Transactions on Database Systems* 16:369, 1991.
56. Chu WW, Ieong IT, Taira RK: A semantic modeling approach for image retrieval by content, *VLDB Journal* 3:445, 1994.
57. Silberschatz A, Stonebraker M, Ullman J: Database systems: achievements and opportunities, *Communications of the Association of Computing Machinery* 34:110, 1991.
58. Fichman RG, Kemerer CF: Object-oriented and conventional analysis and design methodologies: comparison and critique, *IEEE Computer* October:22, 1992.
59. Kahn MG: Modeling time in medical decision-support programs, *Med Decis Making* 11:249, 1991.
60. Worboys MF: A unified model for spatial and temporal information, *Computer Journal* 37:26, 1994.
61. Gudivada VN, Raghavan VV: Design and evaluation of algorithms for image retrieval by spatial similarity, *Association of Computing Machinery Transactions on Information Systems* 13:115, 1995.
62. Chu WW, and others: *A temporal evolutionary object-oriented data model and its query language for medical image management,* San Mateo, Calif, 1992. Proceedings of the 18th International Conference on Very Large Database (VLDB) Conference.
63. Chu WW, and others: A unified timeline model and user interface for multimedia medical databases, *Comput Med Imaging Graph* 20, 1996.
64. Winsberg P: Legacy code: don't bag it, wrap it (application wrappers), *Datamation* 41:36, 1995.

65. Shahar Y, Musen MA: RESUME: a temporal-abstraction system for patient monitoring, *Comput Biomed Res* 26:255, 1993.
66. Hardman L, Bulterman DCA, van Rossum G: The Amsterdam hypermedia model: adding time and context to the Dexter model, *Communications of the Association of Computing Machinery* 37:50, 1994.
67. Dionisio JDN, Cardenas AF: Query M: a visual query language for multimedia. Timeline and simulation data, *Journal of Visual Languages and Computing* 7:377, 1996.
68. Sager N, Friedman C, Lyman MS: *Medical language processing: computer management of narrative data,* Reading, Mass, 1987, Addison-Wesley.
69. Haug PJ, Ranum DL, Frederick PR: Computerized extraction of coded findings from free-text radiologic reports, *Radiology* 174:543, 1990.
70. Do Amaral MB, Satomura Y: Structuring medical information into a language-independent database, *Med Inf (Lond)* 19:269, 1994.
71. Hripcsak G, and others: Unlocking clinical data from narrative reports: a study of natural language processing, *Ann Intern Med* 122:681, 1995.
72. Kofakis P, and others: Image archiving by content: an object-oriented approach, *Proceedings SPIE* 1234:275, 1990.
73. Tagare HD, and others: *A geometric indexing scheme for an image library.* In Lemke HU, and others, editors: *Proc CAR,* Berlin, 1991, Springer-Verlag.
74. Grosky WI: Image database management, *Advances in Computers* 35:237, 1992.
75. Chang SK, Hsu A: Image information systems: where do we go from here? *IEEE Transactions on Knowledge and Data Engineering* 4:431, 1992.
76. Orphanoudakis SC, Chronaki C, Kostomanolakis S: I2C: a system for the indexing, storage, and retrieval of medical images by content, *Med Inf (Lond)* 19:109, 1994.
77. Joseph T, Cardenas AF: PICQUERY: a high level query language for pictorial database management, *IEEE Transactions on Software Engineering* 14:630, 1988.
78. Gupta A, Weymouth T, Jain R: *Semantic queries with pictures: the VIMSYS model,* Barcelona, 1991, Proceedings 17th International Conference on Very Large Databases.
79. Weiland WJ, Shneiderman B: A graphical query interface based on aggregation/generalization hierarchies, *Information Systems* 18:215, 1993.
80. Chu WW, Cardenas AF, Taira RK: KMeD: a knowledge-based multimedia medical distributed database system, *Information Systems* 20:75, 1995.
81. Zloof MM: Query by example: a database language, *IBM Systems Journal* 16:324, 1977.
82. *Integration works user guide,* Los Angeles 1995, Data Integration Solutions Corporation.
83. Taira RK, and others: *CASE and object-oriented tools for rapid integration of HIS, RIS, and PACS,* 1994, Proceedings of the SPIE: Medical Imaging PACS: Design and Evaluation.
84. Shortliffe EH: *An integrated oncology workstation: final report,* Bethesda, Md, 1991, National Cancer Institute, NIH (in press).
85. Nygren E, Johnson M, Henriksson P: *Reading the medical record II: design of a human-computer interface for basic reading of computerized medical records, Comput Methods Programs Biomed* 39:1, 1992.
86. Kolari P, and others: CARTES: a prototype decision support system in oncology. Knowledge based systems in medicine: methods, applications and evaluation, *Proceeding of the Workshop 'System Engineering in Medicine* 148, 1991.
87. Enterline JP, and others: OCIS: 15 years' experience with patient-centered computing, *MD Comput* 11:83, 1994.
88. Dionisio JDN, and others: A multimedia database system for thermal ablation therapy of brain tumors, *J Digit Imaging* 10:21, 1997.

Part **III**

MR–GUIDED TREATMENT TECHNIQUES

Chapter 22

PRINCIPLES OF MR–GUIDED CRYOABLATION

John C. Gilbert, John Kurhanewicz

HISTORY OF CRYOSURGERY

Cryosurgery or cryosurgical ablation refers to therapeutic techniques in which tissues are destroyed *in situ* by freezing. Therapeutic use of low temperatures has been around for centuries. As early as 2500 BC, the Egyptians recommended cold compresses to treat compound skull fractures and infected wounds.[1,2] Hippocrates advocated the use of cold to control hemorrhage and reduce swelling.[3] Centuries later, William Harvey took Hippocrates' advice in treating his own gout with copious quantities of cold water.[4] Cold temperatures have also been used for anesthetics since an 11th century monk indicated their use for such purposes.[2,5] Refrigeration anesthesia was known to Italian physicians in the 16th and 17th centuries.[6] In the grisly world of early 19th century battlefield surgery, Napoleon's Surgeon General, Baron Dominique Jean Larrey, observed that amputations could be performed almost painlessly on soldiers who had laid in the snow for some time.[2,7,8]

Cryosurgery was first used as a therapeutic technique in 1845, when the English physician James Arnott[9,10] used local freezing to successfully treat melanoma by applying a solution of ice and brine at $-12°$ C. Arnott's success stimulated interest in low-temperature therapy, and by the 1930s, numerous successful applications had been reported in neurology and oncology. During the 1930s and 1940s, Temple Fay[11] treated more than 100 patients with advanced carcinomas, glioblastomas, or Hodgkin's disease using local or generalized freezing: 96% of patients received palliation, 8 patients with metastatic carcinoma survived longer than 5 years, and 1 patient survived more than 20 years after treatment. By the early 1950s, cryosurgery was being used as an adjunct to cardiac surgery[12,13] and was investigated[14] and applied clinically for treating patients with brain tumors.[15]

ADVANTAGES OF CRYOSURGERY

Several aspects of cryosurgery make it attractive as an interventional technique:

- Cryosurgery is an intrinsically focal therapy. Cryoprobes of various sizes are available ranging from small, thin probes approximately 3 mm in diameter to probes with diameters larger than 1 cm. There are many specialized probes designed for specific freezing applications. Using 3-mm liquid nitrogen- or compressed argon gas-cooled probes, a frozen region as large as 5 cm in diameter can be generated. Large and irregular freezing volumes can be achieved using multiple, independently controlled cryoprobes. For example, five or six 3-mm cryoprobes are frequently used for freezing the prostate. In the liver, cryosurgical ablation is frequently used to treat multiple metastatic sites in cases in which surgical resection would require removal of too much functioning organ.

- Larger tissue volumes can be treated cryosurgically than can be safely resected. Because the tissue is not removed, tumor margins that extend beyond an organ boundary can be treated effectively by freezing. For example, in metastatic prostate carcinoma in which the cancer has extended into the seminal vesicles, surgical resection is often contraindicated, whereas image-guided cryosurgical ablation can safely treat the entire volume of cancerous tissue.
- Cryosurgery is not dose limited. Unlike radiotherapy, cryosurgery has no dose limit because tissue outside the frozen region is not damaged. Therefore, cryosurgery can be performed multiple times if the disease recurs. For this reason, cryosurgery is often used as a salvage therapy when disease recurs after other techniques (e.g., radiation, resection) have failed.[16-20]
- Freezing produces sharp margins of destruction. The transition from completely necrotic to undamaged tissue occurs over a narrow range, usually less than 1 mm. The location of the necrotic boundary falls within the frozen region, where the thermal conditions are lethal to the tissue. Different tissues tend to exhibit different sensitivities to cold, so the location and width of the necrotic boundary depend somewhat on the tissue being frozen. The sharp margins of destruction allow damage to healthy tissue surrounding a solid tumor to be minimized. For instance, in the brain, which is very sensitive to freezing, the width of necrotic region can be as little as 30 cell diameters (approximately 200 μm), so brain tumors can be cryosurgically treated with good precision.
- Blood loss is minimal when treating tissues cryosurgically. Thin cryoprobes (approximately 3 mm) cause only a small amount of tissue damage along the wound tract. Because the tissue being frozen is not resected, large blood vessels remain intact. Although freezing damages the microvasculature, this internal hemorrhage tends to remain in the organ parenchyma. Some small amount of hemorrhage may occur from the puncture wound tract where the cryoprobe was inserted, but this bleeding can usually be controlled by applying pressure or inserting a hemostatic agent (e.g., an absorbable gelatin sponge) for highly vascularized tissues such as the liver. Puncture wound closure is generally accomplished with a single suture.
- Large vessels are not damaged by freezing. Large blood vessels are resistant to freezing and maintain their integrity after thawing. Gage and others[21,22] showed that large vessels are protected from freezing by their fibrous structure and by the warm blood flowing in them. The blood flow acts a heat sink to conduct the cold away from the vessel wall. As a result, nonresectable tumors abutting large blood vessels in the liver can be treated cryosurgically without damaging the vessels.[23-25]
- Peripheral nerves are resistant to freezing. Although freezing tends to damage axons because they are hydrophilic, the myelin sheaths are less easily damaged because they contain more lipid, which freezes at lower temperatures. If the myelin sheaths remain intact after cryosurgery, some axons can regenerate along this unobstructed path. Trumble and Whalen[26] showed that sciatic nerves recovered over 10 weeks after being frozen *in vivo*. Nerve regeneration may be helpful in preserving sexual function in patients who have undergone prostate cryosurgical ablation because the neurovascular bundle at the posterior of the prostate may recover. However, current data on this point are equivocal,[27-30] and more research is needed.

MECHANISMS OF DAMAGE

Tissue necrosis caused by freezing is a complex process involving the mechanisms of desiccation, crystallization, cell membrane rupture, intracellular denaturation of proteins, thermal shock, vascular stasis with intravascular thrombosis, and disturbances in enzyme metabolism. The mechanisms of tissue damage during freezing are similar in most tissues. During freezing, ice generally forms first within and propagates along the blood vessels, ducts, and intracellular spaces. For example, in the prostate or liver, these spaces would be the prostatic alveoli or bile ducts, respectively. The cells supercool and begin to freeze catastrophically only after the ice has surrounded them and the temperature is sufficiently low. Since ice cannot contain any solute, a hypertonic slush is pushed in front of the advancing freezing front. Thus, while the cells are cooling, they are subjected to a high extracellular concentration of solutes, which causes the cells to dehydrate to equilibrate the high osmotic potential between the frozen extracellular spaces and the unfrozen cells. This dehydration causes cellular damage because the cells become hypertonic. As a secondary effect, the blood vessels, ducts, alveoli, and other structures fill with fluid and expand before they also freeze. Because ice has a lower density than water, freezing results in greater expansion, causing physical damage to the vessels. Thus, tissue damage results from several factors, including the hypertonicity of the cells and the destruction of the microvasculature, ducts, and alveoli. Recrystallization during thawing (i.e., small ice crystals combining to make larger ones) may also be a significant mechanism of damage. Finally, ischemia, which occurs after thawing as a result of the damaged vasculature, is an additional mechanism of damage.

MODERN CRYOSURGERY

Modern cryosurgery began in the 1960s when Cooper and Lee[31] developed insulated cryoprobes for treating parkinsonism;

these cryoprobes used the recently developed vacuum technology and liquid nitrogen as a cryogen. Cooper placed cryoprobes stereotactically into the basal ganglia of patients through a burr hole in the skull; he monitored the freezing process indirectly by observing the patient's tremor at distant anatomical sites and stopped liquid nitrogen flow when the tremor reduced or disappeared. Although this technique did not become widely accepted, their development of cryosurgical devices and their work demonstrating the use of these devices for treating tumors stimulated much activity in cryosurgical treatment of cancerous tumors in various tissues, including the brain, liver, prostate, cervix, breast, skin, eye, and bone. Gage[32-34] provides an excellent review of the history and ongoing development of cryosurgy in the treatment of tissues.

MONITORING FREEZING

Thermocouples

A major concern from the inception of cryosurgical ablation as a therapeutic technique has been how to monitor the freezing process to ensure destruction of the target region while minimizing damage to the surrounding healthy tissues. Initial attempts to monitor freezing were limited to direct observation of the frozen region for surface freezing or to indirect assessment (e.g., Cooper's observation of a reduction of tremor in parkinsonism patients). Gonder, Soanes, and Schulman[35] monitored freezing of the prostate by palpating the prostate through the rectum during open perineal freezing of the gland. However, these techniques were not very accurate and were not sufficient for monitoring freezing of deep cutaneous lesions or sites within internal organs. The use of thermocouples, inserted into the tissue near the tumor margins, was one solution for monitoring freezing.[36] However, thermocouples can record only the temperature at specific points in the tissue, and monitoring of the entire freezing volume was inadequate using this technique.

Monitoring the temperature during cryosurgery is important because merely freezing the tissue to within a few degrees of 0° C is insufficient to cause necrosis. Temperatures of −20° C to −50° C for several minutes must be achieved for complete necrosis to occur. Thus, a certain amount of overfreezing is necessary to completely destroy the target volume. However, overfreezing can damage adjacent healthy tissue, which may cause adverse side effects. Because freezing occurs in three dimensions and can have irregular shapes, particularly when multiple cryoprobes are used, a more accurate technique for monitoring the frozen region was needed to improve accuracy.

Ultrasound monitoring

In the 1980s, technological improvements in ultrasound (US) imaging made small intraoperative US transducers available. This imaging technique could detect the location of the advancing freezing front when the transducer was placed on a nearby tissue surface.[37] This technique was first developed for freezing sites in the liver[38-41] and shortly thereafter was used for treating prostate cancer.[42-45] Current clinical techniques for treating liver and prostate cancer use intraoperative or transrectal US to monitor the freezing process.[44,46-50] The advantages of US for monitoring freezing are that it produces real-time images, it is easy to operate, US equipment is readily available, and equipment costs are relatively low. The disadvantages include its operation (the US transducer must be in complete contact with tissue near the cryoprobes) and its inability to image through bone or air so it cannot be used in all situations. In addition, the quality of the images obtained depends significantly on the operator of the equipment. Finally, only the edge of the freezing boundary nearest the transducer can be imaged; the rest of the frozen volume and any tissues behind it remain invisible in the acoustic shadow. For these limitations to be avoided, a monitoring technique that can image the entire frozen region in three dimensions is desirable for more accurate application of image-monitored cryosurgical ablation.

Magnetic resonance imaging monitoring

Interventional magnetic resonance imaging (MRI) can improve cryoablation procedures in several ways: first, MRI can image the entire frozen region and surrounding tissues during freezing. Because MRI uses the magnetic properties of hydrogen nuclei to create an image, the shadowing effects, which are a major limiting factor in US imaging, do not occur. Although in MR images, frozen tissue appears dark because its T2 is too short for there to be any detectable RF signal, the contrast between this dark image and the unfrozen tissue surrounding it makes the freezing boundary readily observable. Second, rapid high-resolution imaging sequences, such as fast spoiled gradient-recalled echo (FSPGR), can produce multiple slice images in seconds. Since the freezing interface moves through the tissue at velocities in the range of millimeters per minute, image updates of approximately 30 sec are adequate to monitor the freezing front in quasi–real-time. Finally, when multiple cryosurgical probes are used, freezing of the entire volume—including any potentially unfrozen islands of tissue that may be contained within the constellation of cryosurgical probes—can be observed using MRI. This ability may be advantageous when monitoring freezing around large blood vessels or around a warming catheter placed in the prostatic urethra to protect it during prostatic cryoablation.

Disadvantages of MRI guidance of cryosurgical ablation include the necessity to use MR-compatible instruments near the magnet bore and limited access to the patient in conventional high-resolution magnets. Therefore, MRI-guided cryosurgical ablation is best suited for interventional magnet systems with open access to the patient. However, at this writing, relatively few of these systems are available clinically. If asepsis is required during the procedure, interventional MR surgical suites may be required. Finally, although the cost of MR interventional cryoablation may be considerably less than that of surgical resection, it will most likely be more expensive compared with similar procedures using US guidance; the greater cost and accuracy of an MR interventional procedure should be considered when compared with the lower cost and accuracy of the US-guided procedure.

INTERVENTIONAL MAGNETIC RESONANCE–GUIDED CRYOSURGICAL ABLATION

Cryosurgical ablation using thin (approximately 3 mm in diameter) cryoprobes is a minimally invasive technique that is ideal in combination with MRI guidance for the focal treatment of cancerous tumors within the body. Although cryosurgery has flourished as a technique for treating tissues that are easily monitored visually (e.g., those on the skin and eye), its application to tissues within the body is limited by the ability to monitor the volume of frozen tissue, which is not observable to the naked eye. During cryosurgical ablation, or any tissue ablative technique, the goal is to treat just the target tissue and minimize damage to adjacent healthy tissue. Thus, monitoring the freezing process is essential.

Preliminary work

MRI monitoring of cryosurgical ablation is relatively new. This idea was first described by Isoda,[51,52] who monitored freezing in a gelatin phantom and in rat xenografts using MRI and computed tomography (CT). Isoda observed the disappearance of the frozen region in low–flip angle gradient echo images (100/18 msec, 60°) acquired every minute during freezing and thawing. He found that the frozen region was hypodense on enhanced CT images. In the rat xenografts, a higher intensity signal occurred immediately after thawing on spin-echo (1500/90 msec) and inversion recovery (IR) (1200/400 msec) images. Three years later, Matsumoto, Oshio, and Jolesz[53] used T1-weighted rapid acquisition with relaxation enhancement (RARE) (300/18 msec, 16 sec/image) sequences to depict the extent of thermal damage to rabbit liver from freezing- and laser-induced ablation techniques. They, too, reported a sudden signal intensity decrease in the frozen region caused by the disappearance of T2 in both *ex vivo* and *in vivo* rabbit liver. They quantified the change in T1 in the unfrozen tissue surrounding the frozen region and found a more-or-less linear signal intensity decrease of 0.7%/° C to 1.1%/° C over a temperature range of 10° C to 50° C. This decrease corresponded to an increase in T1 of 5 msec/° C (1% to 2%). In another set of experiments, they followed MRI-guided cryolesions in rabbit liver for up to 3 weeks after treatment to determine the physiologic sequelae after freezing. They found that the lesion size measured on MR images at the time of freezing was similar to the physical lesion size on postmortem evaluation, indicating that MR images obtained during freezing could adequately predict the area of final necrosis.[54]

Rubinsky, Gilbert, and others[45] showed the feasibility of MRI-guided cryosurgery in healthy rabbit brain and dog prostate in a preliminary study. In the rabbit brain, they used spin-echo sequences (400/33 msec) to monitor freezing as it progressed through the cingulate cortex and into the hippocampus. Freezing was accomplished using a Pyrex cryoprobe, which was placed on the surface of the cortex through a small (5-mm) burr hole in the skull. Four-slice spin-echo images were acquired every 2.5 min during freezing and thawing to track the progression of the freezing front. The animals were euthanized 4 h after the procedure. Histologic evaluation of the frozen lesion showed good correlation between the frozen and necrotic regions. The frozen region appeared to extend 1 to 2 mm beyond the necrotic region. The transition from necrotic to healthy tissue was very sharp and occurred over approximately 30 cell diameters (approximately 200 μm) in the pyramidal cell region of the brain.

In a more extensive study of MR-guided cryosurgery of the rabbit brain, Gilbert and others[55] showed the ability of MR to depict the extent of damage in brain after freezing by correlating findings from T2-weighted and Gd-DTPA enhanced T1-weighted spin-echo images with postmortem histologic slices. The results confirmed the 1- to 2-mm wide band of frozen but undamaged tissue at the periphery of the necrotic region. However, after thawing, T2-weighted spin-echo images (2000/100 msec) revealed a 2- to 3-mm wide band of higher signal intensity indicating the formation of edema around the cryolesion (Fig. 22-1). A similar enhancement was also seen in T1-weighted Gd-DTPA-enhanced spin-echo images (400/33 msec). These

A B C

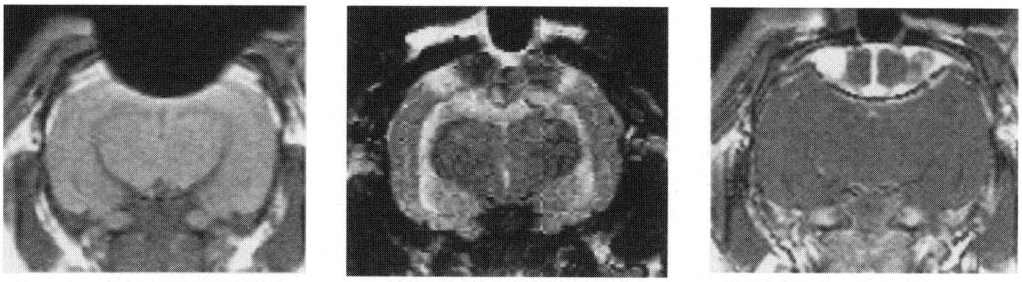

Fig. 22-1. Spin-echo (SE) images during and after cryosurgery of rabbit brain. **A,** T1-weighted SE (400/33 msec) at the end of freezing. **B,** T2-weighted SE (2000/100 msec) 13 min after the onset of thawing. **C,** T1-weighted SE (400/33 msec) 31 min after the onset of thawing and 9 min after injecting a single dose of Gd-DTPA to monitor blood-brain damage. An outline of the frozen region from panel **A** has been overlaid on panel **C.** At 31 min panel **C,** enhanced contrast was first seen at the margin of the cryolesion and in the cingulate gyrus. The central portion of the lesion was not as bright as the margin probably because Gd-DTPA could not reach the center of the lesion through the heavily damaged vasculature. The field of view was 3 × 3.5 cm.

results indicate the possibility of using imaging after cryotherapy to immediately assess cryosurgical damage.

Gilbert and others[56] also showed the accuracy with which MRI can monitor the progress of freezing in quasi–real-time. These experiments, carried out in healthy rabbit liver, showed the process of freezing as the freezing front moved outward through the liver parenchyma from the tip of a surface cryoprobe (Fig. 22-2, *A*). Each image (FSPGR, 13.68, 5 msec, 30°) represents an increment of 1 min. Figure 22-2, *B* shows the temperatures (in ° C) measured at the cryoprobe tip and on the opposite surface of the liver directly below the cryoprobe; the duty cycle (in %) of the cryovalve is also shown. Figure 22-2, *A* shows the time course of freezing as the size of the frozen region increased until the freezing front neared the posterior surface of the liver. Freezing was stopped just after the acquisition of image 6 before the entire thickness of liver was frozen. Fifteen minutes after thawing, the MR contrast in the frozen region appeared darker than in the surrounding, unfrozen liver. These researchers correlated the size of frozen region, determined from MR images at the end of freezing, with corresponding histologic slices and found that, although the freezing boundaries in the images and histologic slices corresponded, the boundary of necrosis was located 2 to 4 mm inside the freezing boundary. Freezing could be monitored with an accuracy of greater than 1 mm.

Also of interest in this study was that the freezing front continued to propagate 1 to 2 mm through the tissue after the liquid nitrogen flow was stopped, just after image 6 in Figure 22-2, *A* was acquired. This occurs because a finite amount of time (in this case almost 1 min) is needed for the temperature at the probe tip to climb to 0° C after liquid nitrogen flow ceases (see Fig. 22-2, *A*, *B*). During this time, the core of the frozen region was still considerably below 0° C and able to remove enough heat from the surrounding tissue for freezing to continue. Eventually, the freezing boundary stops and reverses direction as the tissue begins to thaw. The high-resolution images that MRI provides make it possible to monitor freezing because of this "thermal inertia." Although thermal inertia seldom accounts for residual frozen region growth of more than a few millimeters, it should be considered when performing cryosurgery. Second, liver *in situ* moves during respiration. In order to avoid image artifact caused by respiratory movement, the abdomen of the rabbit was opened and the liver immobilized on a plastic shelf. However, percutaneous interventional MRI-guided cryosurgical ablation of the liver would require motion artifact–reducing techniques.

Other contributions to the development of MRI-guided cryosurgical ablation have been made in the areas of (1) MRI-compatible devices, (2) thermal analyses of the freezing process[57-63] and techniques for estimating the temperature distribution in the frozen region,[57,64,65] (3) staging and identification of the spatial distribution of cancer using MR-based techniques,[66,67] (4) computer algorithms to help plan cryosurgical treatment,[68,69] and (5) automated control of the freezing process using MRI-guided feedback.[70,71]

Magnetic resonance–compatible devices

MR-compatible devices are required when working in or near the magnet bore. This requirement means that new devices for interventional MR techniques must be developed. One example of such a device is a combined cryoprobe and MR surface coil. Pease and others[72] developed a prototype device using acrylic and quartz that integrates a surface cryoprobe with a radiofrequency (RF) receiver coil for freezing deep lesions from the surface of tissue. This liquid nitrogen–cooled device was cylindrical, approximately 6 × 5 cm (diameter × height), and acrylic. A quartz window conducted the cold from the liquid nitrogen in the chamber to the tissue surface. A 6.2-cm diameter, single-turn RF surface coil made out of copper foil and tuned to the proton resonance frequency surrounded the device. The coil was used in transmit and receive modes. The device was tested in phantoms and on a rabbit thigh.[72] The advantage of integrating a surface coil with the freezing surface was that having the RF coil close to the cryoprobe surface meant that high-resolution images with high signal-to-noise ratios could be obtained. FSPGR images (30/4.3 msec) were acquired during freezing and thawing to monitor the freezing boundary as it progressed 6.2 mm into the underlying muscle. The spatial resolution of the images was 0.2 × 0.2 mm, with a 0.4-mm slice thickness. Although this device was a prototype, it shows the potential for new applications and hardware in MR-guided interventional cryosurgical ablation. MR-compatible freezing systems are being developed by some private companies.

Thermal analysis of the freezing process

Freezing of tissue can preserve and destroy tissue. This paradox is explained partially by understanding that at high subzero temperatures (near 0° C), the amount of destruction or preservation of cellular solutions depends greatly on the freezing rate and on the temperature to which the cells are frozen.[73-75] Considerable experimental work in cryobiology has shown that at high subzero temperatures, very slow (<10° C/min) and very fast (>80° C/min) rates of freezing cause the greatest destruction, whereas fewer cells are destroyed in-between.[73,74] Thus, the curve describing cellular destruction as a function of freezing rate looks "U shaped." The bottom of the "U" represents the freezing rate for least destruction (greatest preservation) of the cells. High and low freezing rates are best for destroying cells. Although during cryosurgical ablation of tissues a distribution of freezing rates occurs throughout the tissue, in practice the freezing rates usually encountered during clinical cryosurgical procedures tend to be very slow (approximately a few ° C/min).

Another principle helps mitigate the dependence of cellular destruction on freezing rate. As the temperature that tissues are exposed to decreases, so does the importance of the freezing rate on cellular destruction. Although this statement oversimplifies the situation, at low subzero temperatures (less than approximately −60° C), most organ tissues are destroyed regardless of the freezing rate. However, just inside the freezing boundary, which is just below 0° C, a portion of the tissue is only subjected to high subzero temperatures. As a consequence,

A

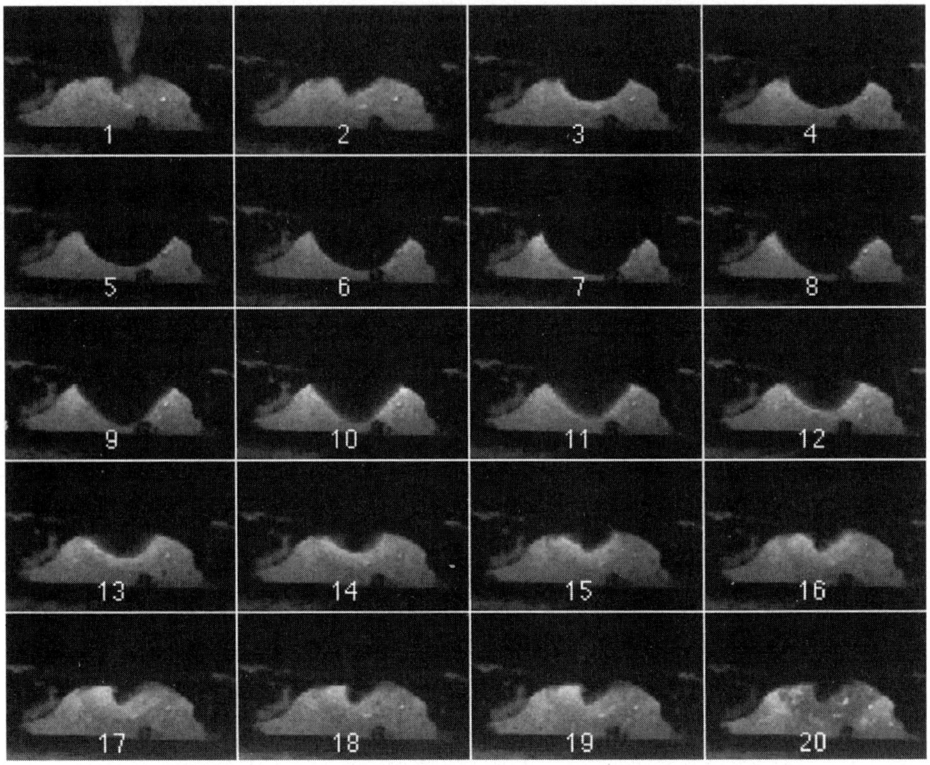

B

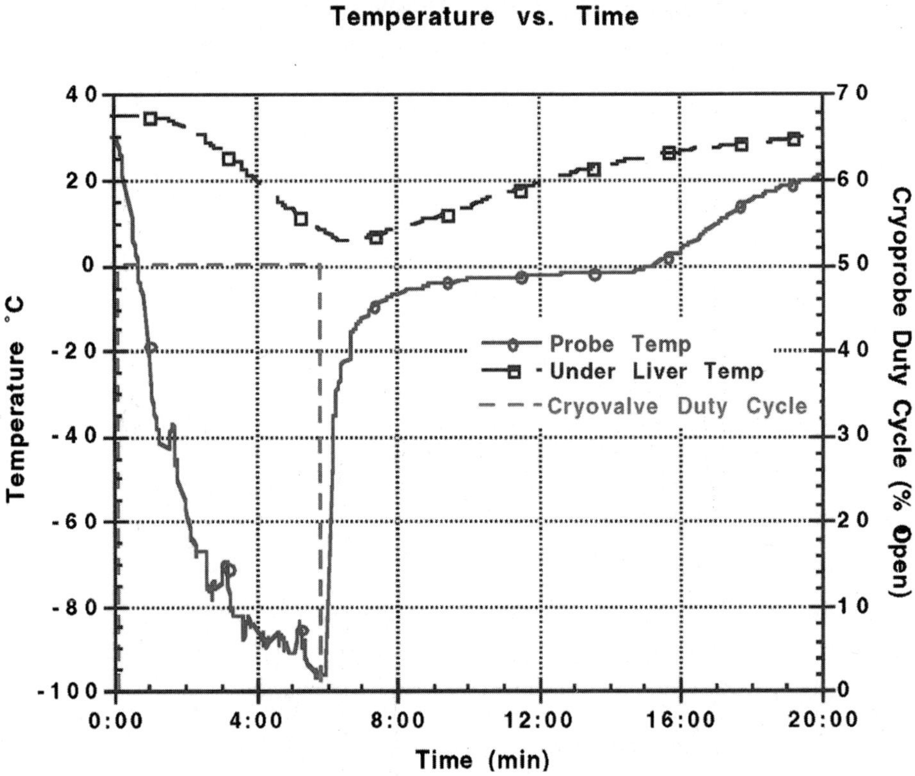

Fig. 22-2. A, Sequence of fast spoiled gradient-recalled echo images (13.68/5 msec, 30° flip angle, 5 slices, 4-mm slice thickness, 5-mm spacing; 256 × 192 matrix, 8-cm field of view acquired during freezing and thawing of rabbit liver. The time between images is 1 min. Liquid nitrogen flow was stopped just after image 6. The outline of the interior volume of the Pyrex cryoprobe is seen in image 1. Artifact from two thermocouples is present just below and to the left of the cryoprobe tip and to the right of center at the bottom surface of the liver. In image 20, acquired 15 min after thawing began, the change in tissue contrast represents the cryolesion, which was contained inside the maximum freezing boundary seen in image 7. **B,** Time course of the temperature during freezing and thawing of rabbit liver in **A.** Also shown is the duty cycle of the cryovalve (scale on the right-hand axis). (**A** From Gilbert JC, and others: *Mag Reson Imaging* 15:657, 1997.)

during cryosurgery, this region of tissue is usually not very damaged and may survive the freezing process. Thus, it is important to know how much tissue survives and where the necrotic boundary is relative to the freezing boundary.

The width of the frozen but undamaged region, which is just inside the freezing boundary, depends on several thermal factors (minimum temperature, exposure time, freezing rate) and on the type of tissue being frozen. For example, brain and liver tissue are more sensitive to cold than are muscle and prostate tissue, so the necrotic boundary is closer to the freezing boundary in brain and liver tissue than in muscle and prostate tissue. Local heating caused by blood flow and metabolism also affects the degree of necrosis. Since minimum temperature and exposure time are the two most controllable variables during a cryosurgical procedure, much of the cryosurgical literature has addressed the highest negative temperature necessary to cause complete necrosis;[36,62,64,76-84] temperatures from −15° C to −50° C have been cited as being lethal to tissue *in vivo.* The number of freeze/thaw cycles that the tissue experiences has also been shown to increase the amount of tissue destroyed in a frozen region.[85] Tissues *in situ* behave differently when frozen from tissues *in vitro* because of the presence of blood flow, metabolism, and surrounding tissues, therefore studies of freezing tissues *in vitro* may not be very useful in determining the precise conditions for complete tissue necrosis. Better data are required from tissues studied *in situ* to correlate the freezing and necrotic boundaries and the thermal conditions for necrosis. These studies would help determine the undamaged or partially damaged region just inside the freezing boundary.

Temperature determination in the frozen region

No current imaging technique (MRI, CT, US) can image inside frozen tissue. Since there is no measurable RF signal from the frozen region, MR-based temperature measurement techniques (e.g., diffusion, relaxation time, chemical shift) cannot be used for measuring the temperature in the frozen region during cryosurgery. To work around this problem, Hong, and others[57] developed a numerical technique to calculate the temperature in the frozen region rather than measure it directly or indirectly. This technique was based on the assumption that the frozen region is primarily ice and therefore has a uniform thermal conductivity. The calculated temperature could then be obtained from an analytic solution of the heat conduction equation (Laplace equation) in the frozen region

$$\nabla^2 T_f\,(x,y,z) = 0$$

where T_f is the temperature in the frozen region and x, y, and z are arbitrary coordinates in three dimensions. The boundary conditions required for solving the equation were (1) the temperature of the cryoprobe, which was measured with a thermocouple and (2) the thermal conditions at the boundary of the frozen region. If the boundary of the frozen region was adjacent to tissue, then it was assumed isothermal (constant temperature) and equal to 0° C by definition. If the boundary was adjacent to air, then it was assumed adiabatic (zero heat flux across the boundary). The geometry of the frozen region (including that of the freezing boundary) was obtained from spin-echo images (1135/28 msec) of the frozen region. Hong and others[57] validated their technique experimentally by comparing temperature measurements obtained from gelatin phantoms during MRI-guided freezing using a cryosurgical probe with their analytic results. The results of their analytic predictions were within a few percent of the measured temperatures.

Gilbert and others[56] extended the numerical technique of Hong and others[57] for calculating temperature in the frozen region to rabbit liver *in vivo.* They also correlated the locations of the freezing and necrotic boundaries. The necrotic boundary was determined from postmortem histologic slices corresponding with MR imaging planes. Equal temperature curves (isotherms) were overlaid on MR images of the frozen and necrotic regions to determine the range of thermal conditions under which the tissue was damaged (Fig. 22-3). The results of this correlation indicated that, on average, the margin of the cryolesion was located approximately 2 to 3 mm inside the boundary of the frozen region, which was equivalent to indicating that the necrotic boundary was located just inside the −5° C isotherm (Fig. 22-4). Knowing the location of the necrotic boundary can help guide the amount of overfreezing required during cryosurgical ablation. Although this work was conducted on rabbit liver, the technique is independent of tissue type and can be applied to any cryosurgically frozen tissue.

TREATMENT PLANNING

Magnetic resonance imaging/spectroscopic imaging staging and localization of prostate cancer for cryosurgical treatment planning

One advantage of MRI is that it provides excellent tissue contrast. Imaging studies performed before therapy can be used to develop a treatment plan for delivering a lethal amount of freezing to a desired target volume. Advance identification of the target volume will allow focal cryotherapy under MRI guidance to more accurately treat the cancer while minimizing damage to surrounding tissues. Kurhanewicz and others[66,67] developed a combined anatomic and metabolic MR imaging examination, which identifies the spatial distribution of cancer within the prostate and the extent of extracapsular disease (staging). Knowledge of the spread of cancer outside the prostate is critical for choosing an appropriate therapy (e.g., cryosurgery, brachytherapy, confomal radiation, resection, etc.). Currently, clinical staging is inaccurate, and understaging occurs in as many as 72% of patients thought to have localized disease by digital rectal examination[86] (Table 22-1). Staging of prostate cancer using transrectal ultrasound (TRUS), CT,[88,89] or whole-body MRI is unreliable.[87] However, the introduction of MR imaging using phased-array and endorectal coils has considerably improved the ability of MRI to be used for staging prostate cancer and thus represents an important advance in the management of prostate cancer.[90,91] The work by Schnall and others[90] and Kier, Wain, and Troiano[91] has demonstrated great potential for imaging

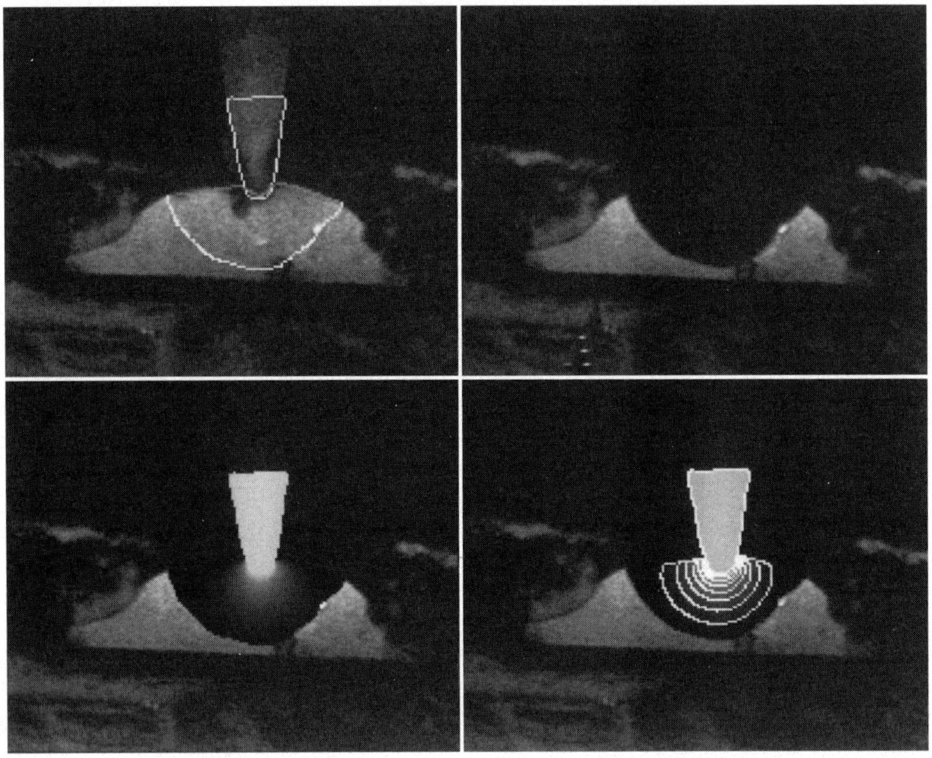

Fig. 22-3. Spoiled gradient-recalled echo images of a rabbit liver during a cryosurgical experiment. **A,** Before freezing with the thermal boundaries used for calculating the temperature distribution overlaid: adiabatic *(grey),* isothermal *(white)* (see text for a description of the calculation procedure). The cryoprobe can be seen because a few drops of water were poured into the glass cryoprobe before liquid nitrogen flow was started. **B,** Frozen region at the end of freezing. **C,** Composite image of the frozen region and the cryoprobe. The temperature as a function of position in the frozen region is shown in grey scale between the probe and freezing boundary (white, −97° C; black, −0.6° C). **D,** The same temperature distribution, except that isotherms in 10° C steps have been overlaid on the frozen region. (From Gilbert JC, and others: *Mag Reson Imag* 15:657, 1997.)

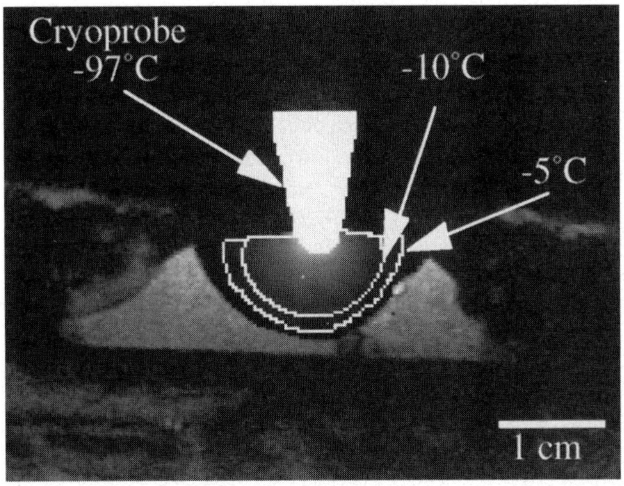

Fig. 22-4. Temperature distribution in the frozen region of rabbit liver from Figure 22-3 showing the −5° C and −10° C isotherms. The boundary of necrosis was sharp and located between these two isotherms. (From Gilbert JC, and others: *Mag Reson Imag* 15:657, 1997.)

Table 22-1. Staging accuracy for prostate cancer using current techniques

Technique	Overall accuracy (%)	ECE (%)	Reference
DRE	28		Zeitman and others[86]
TRUS	58	49 (25% SVI)	Rifkin[87]
CT	61–65		Hricak and others[88]; Platt, Bree, and Schwab[89]
MRI (whole-body)	69	22	Rifkin[87]
MRI (endorectal coil)	81	91	Hricak and others[92]
MRI/MRSI	91–95		Scheidler and others[67]

ECE—Extracapsular extension; DRE—digital rectal examination; TRUS—transrectal ultrasound; SVI—seminal vesicle invasion; CT—Computed tomography; MRI—magnetic resonance imaging; MRSI—magnetic resonance spectroscopic imaging.

using an endorectal and a phased-array coil, respectively, for improving the ability to stage local prostate cancer. More recently, detection of extracapsular extension and seminal vesicle invasion has markedly improved using fast spin-echo imaging with a pelvic phased-array and endorectal coil together.[92] Improved cancer staging is important for identifying patients who would benefit most from cryosurgery, e.g., patients with cancer in areas of the gland that are difficult to treat and patients with local spread of the disease beyond the prostatic capsule (local stage T3 disease).[19] However, planning focal cryosurgery requires accurate knowledge of the spatial extent of prostate cancer. MRI assessment of cancer within the gland is complicated by factors other than cancer that decrease signal intensity on T2-weighted imaging and indicate cancer (e.g., postbiopsy hemorrhage, chronic prostatitis, benign prostatic hyperplasia, intraglandular dysplasia, trauma, androgen deprivation therapy). These factors can limit definitive localization of prostate cancer by MRI alone and can, in some cases, lead to overestimation of tumor presence and extracapsular extension.[93-95]

Recent development of MR spectroscopic imaging[96] expands the diagnostic assessment of the prostate beyond the anatomic information provided by MRI alone.[66] MR spectroscopic imaging (MRSI) provides metabolic information throughout the prostate by detecting prostatic metabolites in the cytosol of prostatic cells. MRSI assesses normal glandular function by monitoring the concentration of the major prostatic secretory product citrate, which is normally high but decreases significantly in cancer, and phospholipid metabolism through the concentration of choline, which is normally low but increases if cancer is present. In a 3D ^{1}H MRSI study of 85 patients before undergoing radical prostatectomy, the feasibility of noninvasively assessing cancer extent was demonstrated based on metabolite levels at high spatial resolution (0.24 to 0.7 cc) in a clinically reasonable amount of time. The ratio of the peak areas of choline to citrate resonances in regions of cancer showed no overlap with normal peripheral zone values and only minimal overlap with benign prostatic hyperplasia (BPH) values.[66] However, since prostatic concentrations of choline and citrate are so low (millimolar concentration range) and because tissue water concentration, which for anatomic imaging is approximately 55 molar, there is an overall reduction in metabolite image resolution ($6.5 \times 6.5 \times 6.5$ mm, 0.24 cc voxels) compared with MRI. By combining the metabolic and anatomic data by overlaying the spectral data on the MR images, both the high sensitivity of MRI and the high specificity of MRSI can be used for identifying prostate cancer (Fig. 22-5).

In several recent studies, the addition of MRSI has significantly improved the localization of prostate cancer within the gland by excluding false-positive tumor sites identified on MR images. In a study of 62 patients, combined MRI/MRSI was performed before radical prostatectomy, and step-section histopathology of the gland was conducted afterward. In these patients, prostate cancer could be localized to a sextant of the prostate (i.e., left or right base, midgland, and apex).[67] The sensitivity and specificity of cancer localization could be adjusted to yield high values for both. If the evaluation of both MRI and MRSI indicated the presence of cancer, the specificity of cancer detection was as high as 91%. That is, if both MRI and MRSI findings are positive, cancer could be definitely diagnosed with a very high level of confidence. If the evaluation of either MRI or MRSI indicated the presence of cancer, the sensitivity of cancer detection was as high as 95%. Thus, if MRI or MRSI findings are positive for cancer, then there is a high level of confidence that all of the cancer present has been detected. This study indicates that the combined use of high-resolution anatomic and metabolic imaging allows sufficient noninvasive assessment of the spatial extent of prostate cancer for the planning of focal cryotherapy. Similar MRI/MRSI studies have been performed on other tissues, such as the liver[97] and brain,[98-101] and could potentially aid in cryosurgical planning in those tissues.

Computer algorithms for planning cryosurgical treatment

The ability to identify the spatial distribution of cancer in organ tissues raises the possibility of focal ablation using cryosurgery or other focal treatments. Once the target volume has been identified, the number of cryoprobes to be used must be selected and their arrangement determined. Keanini and Rubinsky[68] developed a computer program to minimize the amount of overfreezing by predicting the size of the frozen region given for an arrangement and size of multiple cryoprobes in a simulated prostate model.[68] The program inputs the probe diameters, the active freezing lengths, and the number of probes to be used and produces computer-generated maps estimating the amount of freezing, including isotherms, in a geometric model of the prostate. The results of such a simulation can be used to help suggest arrangements that maximize destruction in a particular area of the tissue. Arrangements of probes of different sizes and positions can also be simulated to determine the optimal conditions for focal destruction of tissue. This work, although preliminary, indicates the type of mathematical models of the freezing process that can assist in planning treatment. More sophisticated models that account for blood perfusion and metabolism could result in greater accuracy and clinical applicability in cryosurgical ablation of the prostate or other tissues.

Magnetic resonance imaging follow-up after cryosurgery

MRI can follow physiologic sequelae immediately after freezing. This ability can help estimate the volume of necrotic tissue during freezing and, thus, the effectiveness of the cryosurgery. In cryosurgical experiments conducted in canine prostates, the region of damage was visible in post-thawing images using both T2-weighted (5000/96 msec) fast spin-echo imaging sequences and Gd-DTPA contrast-enhanced T1-weighted (750/14 msec) FSPGR sequences. Damage was apparent in the images as a bright ring of high signal intensity surrounding the previously frozen region (Fig. 22-6). In the T2-weighted images, the enhanced signal indicated the presence

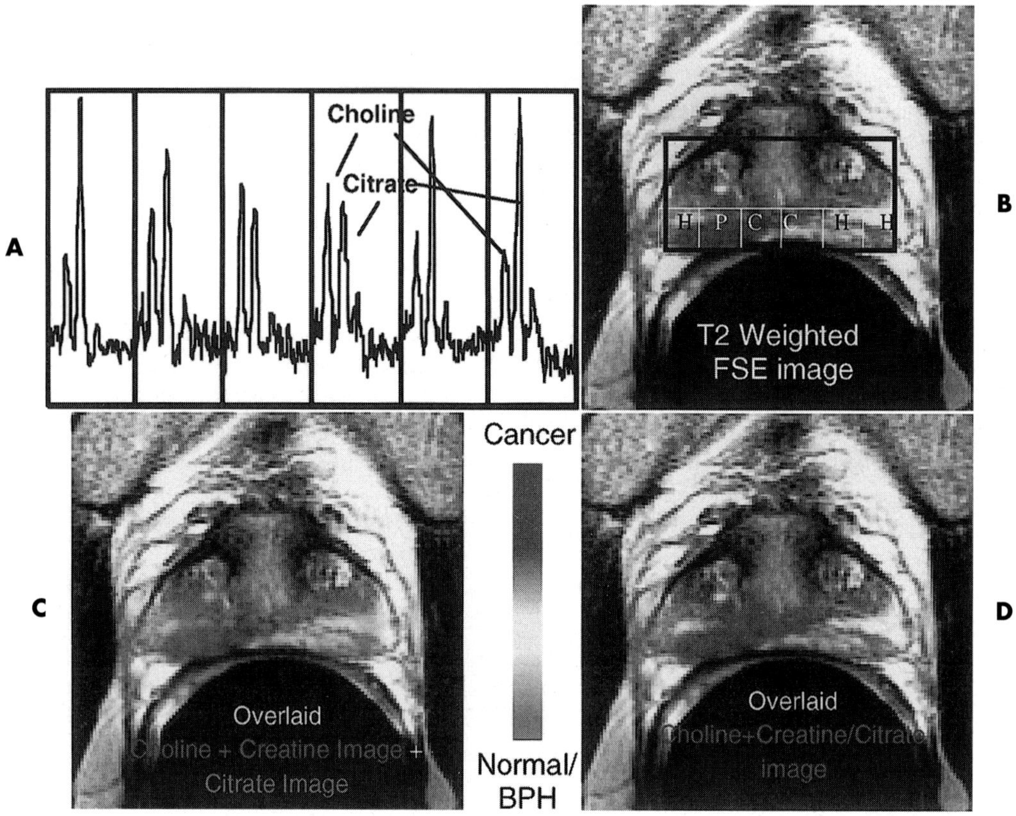

Fig. 22-5. Presentation of magnetic resonance spectroscopic imaging (MRSI) data. Metabolic information from MRSI sequence data can be presented as **A,** a single spectrum for each voxel of acquired data, **B,** a grid at the resolution of the metabolic data (0.24 cc voxels) overlying an anatomic image, or **C** and **D,** pseudocolored metabolic images (peak area maps) based on the relative concentrations of cellular metabolites. In **B,** each voxel is labeled based on the metabolic data: *C*—probable cancer (choline + creatine/citrate ratio > 3 std dev of normal values); *P*—possible cancer (either a choline + creatine/citrate ratio > 2 std dev of normal values, or a two-fold citrate reduction relative to normal); *H*—healthy. In **C,** the peak area images for citrate and choline + creatine are overlaid on the T2-weighted anatomic images. In **D** the choline + creatine/citrate ratio image is thresholded. See Color Plate 13.

of edema just inside the freezing boundary (Fig. 22-6, *D*). In the contrast-enhanced T1-weighted images, a bright ring also formed at the location of the freezing boundary 10 to 15 min after administering a single dose of Gd-DTPA (0.1 mmol/kg). In this case, the signal enhancement was caused by pooling of the contrast medium at the periphery of the necrotic region. The center of the region showed less signal enhancement. This appearance can be explained as follows. In healthy prostatic tissue, the entire gland enhances only slightly in the presence of Gd-DTPA because the contrast medium remains in the bloodstream in low concentration. However, the Gd-DTPA leaks out of the damaged blood vessels and pools in the damaged region, causing marked MR signal enhancement (Fig. 22-6, *F*). Since freezing tends to damage the vasculature completely in the center of the lesion but less at the necrotic boundary, less enhancement is likely to be observed in the center because the Gd-DTPA has to diffuse into the center of the lesion, which is a slow process. At the boundary, the Gd-DTPA only has to leak out of the damaged vasculature, which occurs rapidly. The amount of signal enhancement next to the cryoprobe in Figure 22-6, *F* may have been caused by leakage along the cryoprobe from where it pierced the boundary of the cryolesion. Thus, increased signal intensity near the freezing boundary indicates the location of the freezing-damaged vasculature. The relationship between the location of the damaged vasculature and the necrotic boundary remains to be documented.

Magnetic resonance imaging/spectroscopic imaging follow-up after cryosurgery

Combined high-resolution MRI/MRSI will probably have its greatest impact in the assessment of recurrent prostate cancer after failed cryosurgery and in the selection and planning of additional therapy. Even when the goal of cryosurgery is total ablation of the entire prostate, as is currently the case using TRUS-guided cryosurgery, this goal is not achieved in many patients, who often have a detectable prostate-specific antigen (PSA) level months after treatment. Although a detectable PSA level after cryosurgery indicates residual prostate tissue, it is not specific for

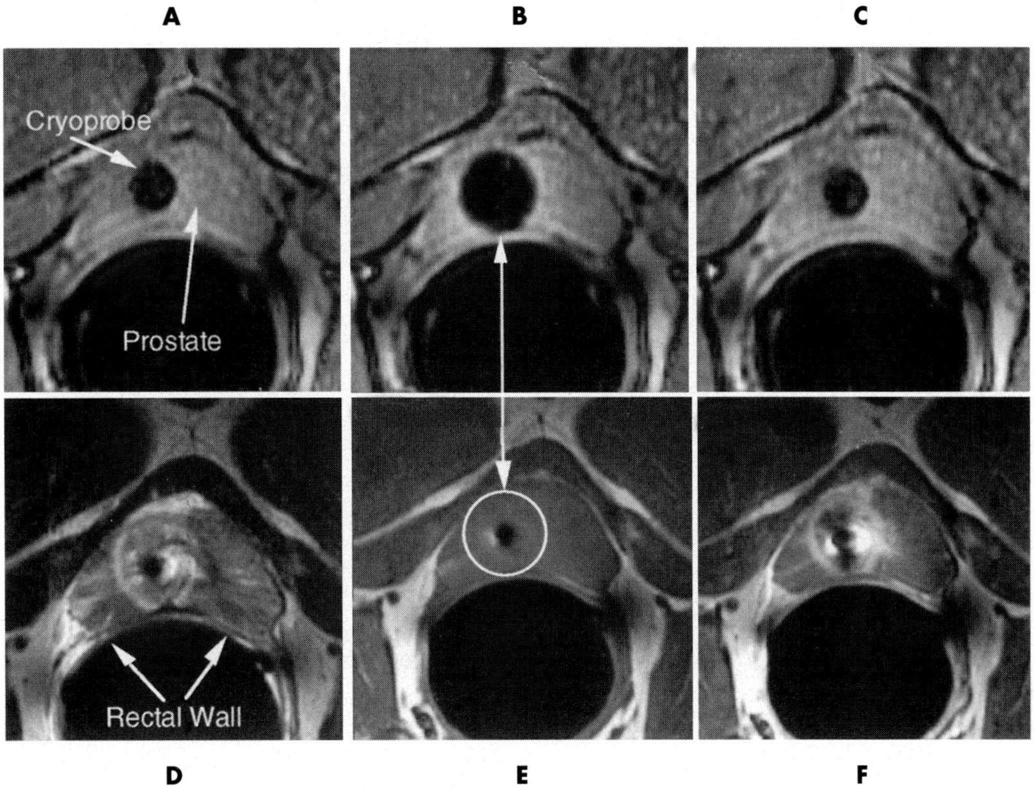

Fig. 22-6. Axial section of a dog prostate before, during, and after freezing. The cryoprobe is seen as the *dark circle* just off center. Monitoring of freezing using fast spoiled gradient recalled echo images (9.1/4.2 msec; 6sec/slice acquisition time) before freezing: **A,** before freezing, **B,** at the end of freezing, and **C,** just after thawing. **D,** After thawing, T2-weighted (5000/96 msec), **D,** and **E,** T1-weighted (750/14 msec) spin-echo images show evidence of damage, though the contrast in **E** was poor. **D** shows edema at the boundary of the cryolesion. 15 to 20 min after injecting Gd-DTPA, signal enhancement is seen at the boundary of the cryolesion in **F** indicating vascular damage. The boundaries of edema seen in **D** and **E,** and Gd-DTPA enhancement seen in **F** were contained within the outline of the frozen region.

cancer. When the goal is to ablate only a portion of the prostate, the use of PSA is even more problematic. However, PSA velocity (the rate of PSA change over time) after cryosurgery may still be useful in assessing cancer progression, but not all PSA elevations imply that current disease is still present.[19,46,102]

Destruction of the prostatic architecture by the freezing process makes detection of residual cancer by TRUS or MRI extremely difficult. Residual prostate cancer after unsuccessful cryosurgery may be missed or understaged because TRUS used for biopsy guidance cannot discriminate between viable tumor, inflammation, and necrosis.[103] Additionally, high-resolution MRI alone is of little use in assessing the presence and extent of residual cancer after the effects of freezing the gland.[94] The positive (44%) and negative (57%) predictive values for detecting cancer after cryosurgery were significantly lower than pretreatment values of 86% and 92%, respectively.[94]

In a study of 25 prostate cancer patients before and 6 months after cryosurgery, MRSI was able to discriminate regions of residual tumor from both BPH and necrosis in patients after unsuccessful cryosurgery.[104] The ratio of choline plus creatine to citrate in regions of histologically confirmed BPH (0.61 ± 0.21, 52 voxels) and cancer (2.4 ± 1.0, 65 voxels) after cryosurgery was not significantly different from that before therapy, but the ratio was significantly different from that of necrosis and each other. Images of the ratio of choline plus creatine to citrate (appropriately thresholded and overlaid in color on T2-weighted images) yielded an estimate of the spatial extent of prostate cancer and BPH after cryosurgery (Fig. 22-7). These studies suggest that combined MRI/MRSI can provide a noninvasive assessment of the presence and location of residual cancer after unsuccessful cryosurgery and can identify successful cryosurgery in patients who had an elevated PSA level caused by benign or normal tissue.[103,104] This unique information helps guide biopsies and plan additional therapy.

Automated magnetic resonance image–guided control of freezing

An interesting aspect of interventional MRI and focal cryosurgical ablation is the possibility of performing computer-automated MR image-guided control of freezing. Pease and others[7] developed software and hardware that demonstrated the possibility of freezing with an automated control system that used MR image guidance in a feedback loop to control the freezing front trajectory. They tested the system in gelatin

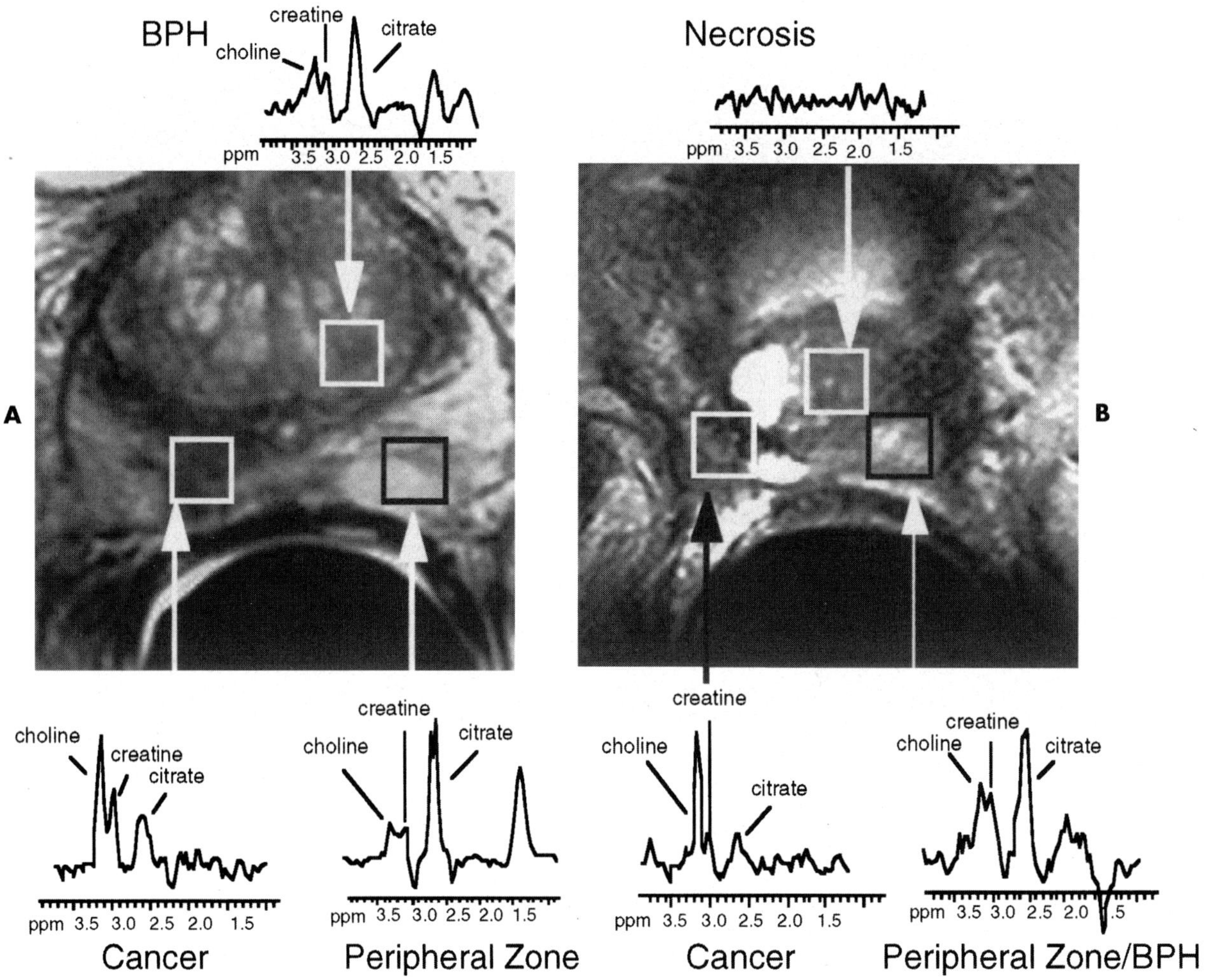

Fig. 22-7. Axial T2-weighted prostate images from a patient with prostate cancer **A,** before cryosurgery and **B,** 6 months after cryosurgery. Selected voxels from a three-dimensional magnetic resonance spectroscopic imaging data set indicate that after cryosurgery, residual cancer can be discriminated from other viable tissues (healthy tissue and benign prostatic hyperplasia) and from necrotic tissue that has not been sloughed off by the immune system.

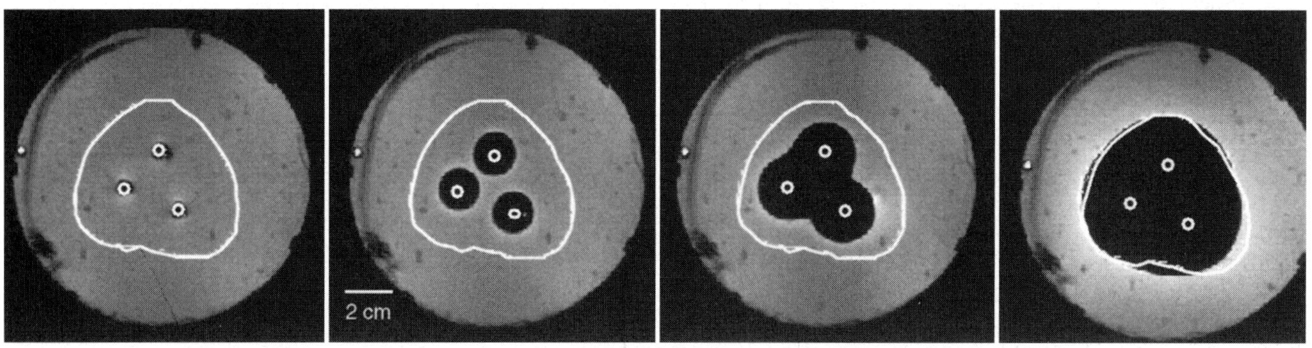

Fig. 22-8. Spoiled gradient-recalled echo (14/5 msec) images of a gelatin phantom frozen using three cryosurgical probes under automated magnetic resonance image (MRI) feedback control. **A,** The target region was drawn on **A,** (white—region of interest) before freezing. A computer-optimization procedure was used to set the initial freezing parameters. During freezing, MR images of the freezing boundary acquired every 30 sec were processed in real-time to determine the location of the boundary relative to the target. Freezing lasted approximately 7 min.

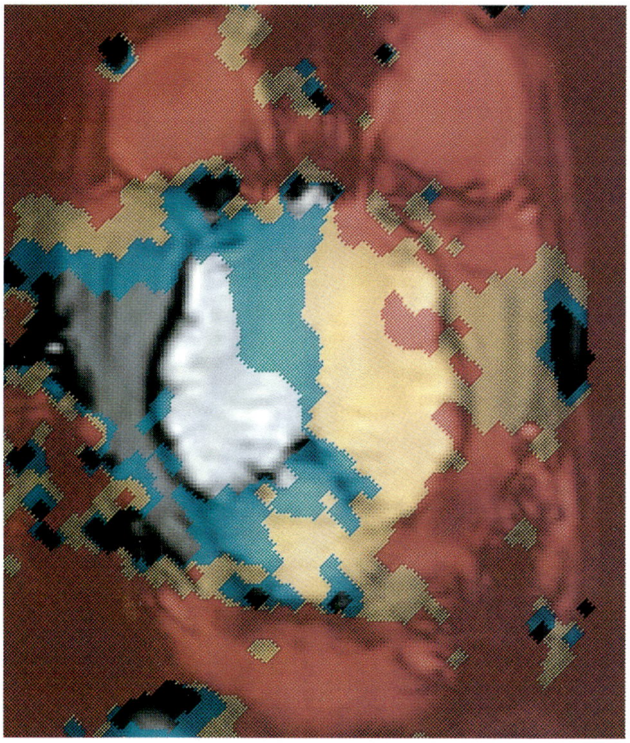

Color Plate 1: An example of magnetic resonance (MR) thermometry during brain hypothermia in a cat. The scan plane is approximately axial and the orbits are visible toward the top of the image. Blood entering the cat's right carotid artery has been chilled and is preferentially cooling this hemisphere. Translucent color overlays are applied to the image to depict local temperature. In this example *red tinted* tissue is warmer than 36° C, *yellow tinted* tissue is between 33° C and 36° C, and *blue tinted* tissue is between 30° C and 33° C. Temperatures less than 30° C have no color overlay, revealing the underlying grey-scale MR image. (See also Fig. 5-3.)

A

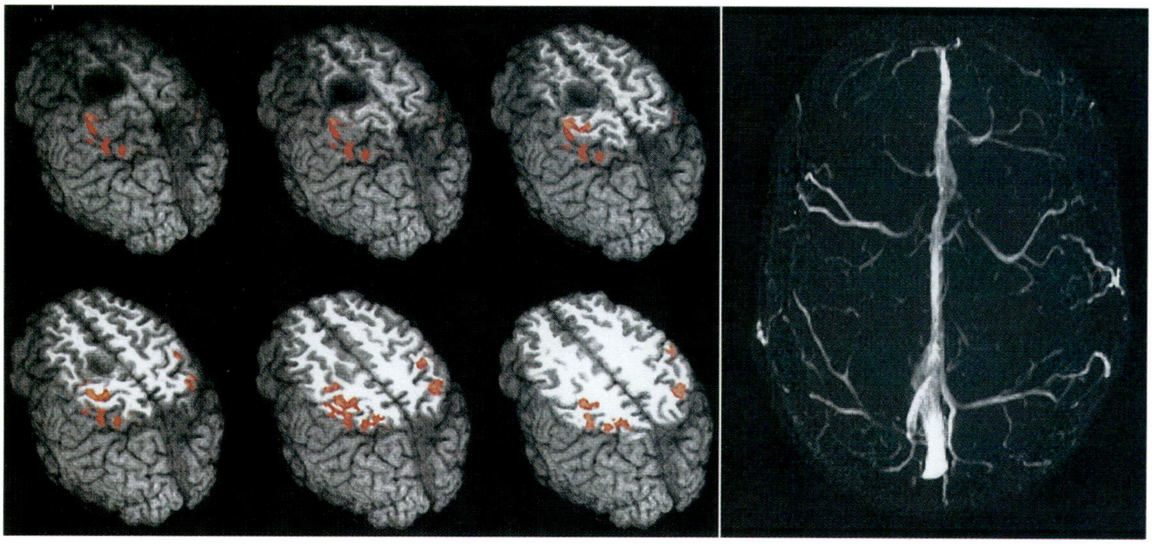

B

Color Plate 2: A brain activation map **A,** during a finger tapping exercise and **B,** a venogram obtained before tumor resection. Similar brain activation maps were acquired for tongue and toe motion. These studies revealed a vein overlying the lesion and the close proximity of the motor strip to the lesion. However, overlap of the motor cortex with the lesion was not apparent, and thus full resection was possible. (See also Fig. 5-11.) (Courtesy of C.L. Truwit, University of Minnesota.)

A 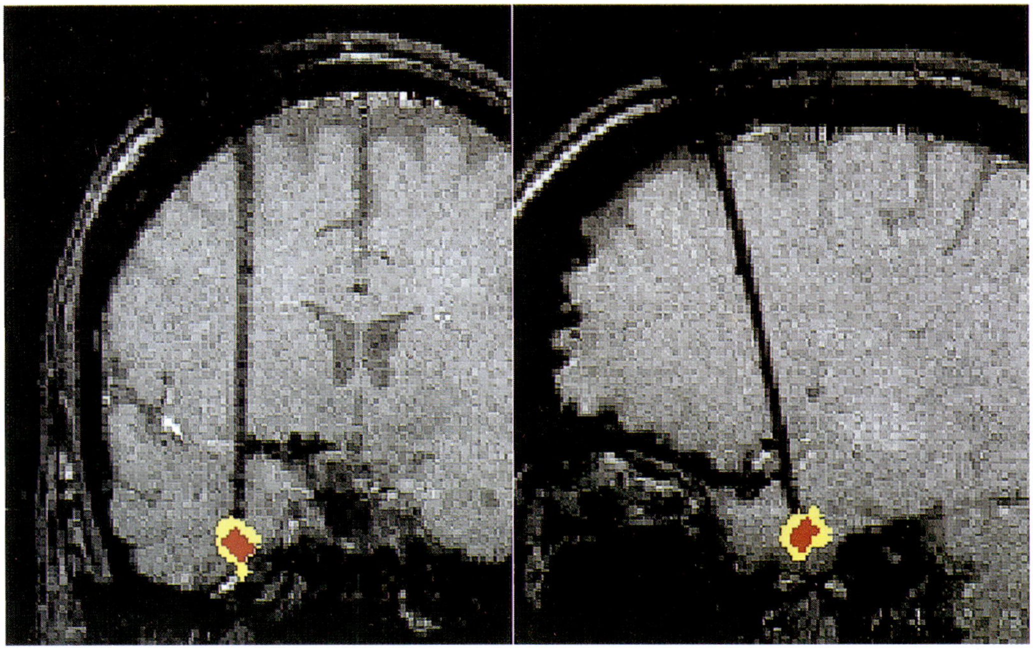 B

Color Plate 3: Laser ablation of a deep brain astrocytoma was monitored with magnetic resonance thermometry. Scan planes approximating **A,** coronal and **B,** sagittal views show the laser track, and the color overlay indicates the region experiencing temperature rise. (See also Fig. 5-12.) (From Stollberger R, and others: Temperature monitoring of interstitial thermal tissue coagulation using MR phase images, *J Magn Reson Imaging* 8:188, 1998.)

A 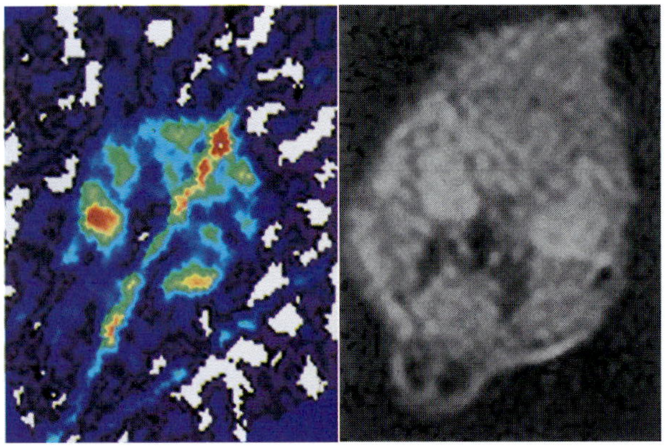 B

Color Plate 4: Contemporaneous **A,** Positron emission tomography scan and **B,** magnetic resonance image acquired from a rat's brain *in vivo.* (See also Fig. 18-3.)

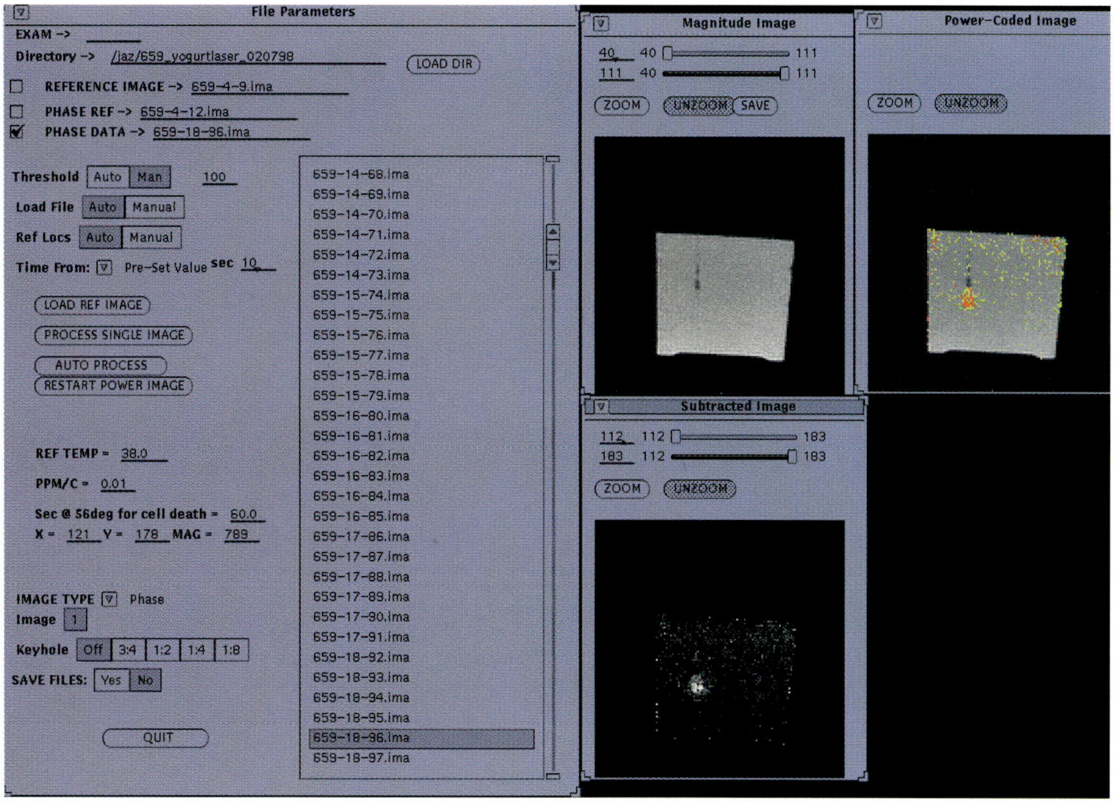

Color Plate 5: This computer display package allows real-time visualization of heat lesions. Temperature maps are generated from phase images and displayed in color for ease of visualization. User interaction is minimal and involves only identification of the reference image before the dynamic ablation procedure. In addition to the temperature maps, the integral under the temperature-time curve is also displayed because this parameter is an indicator of cell death. The map of this integral is also displayed in color superimposed on the original images. (See also Fig. 19-2.)

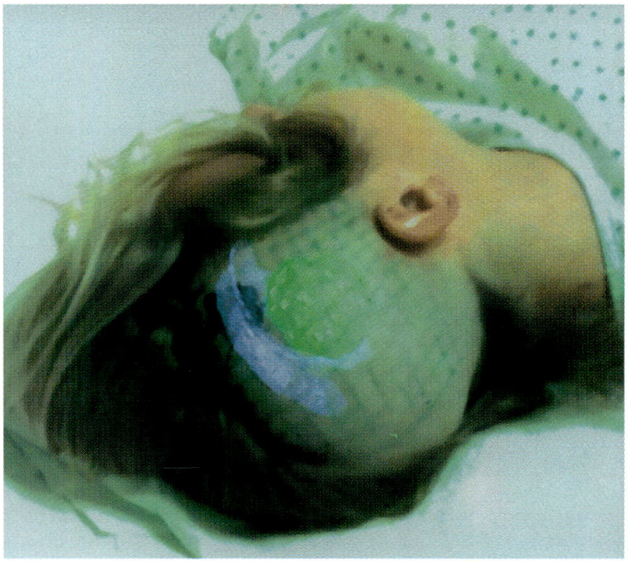

Color Plate 6: Magnetic resonance image reconstruction with the patient on the operating table shows a brain tumor and the ventricles overlaid onto a live video of the patient. (See also Fig. 20-1.) (From Grimson, and others: An automated registration method for frameless stereotaxy, *Image Guided Surgery and Enhanced Reality Visualization,* April, 1996.)

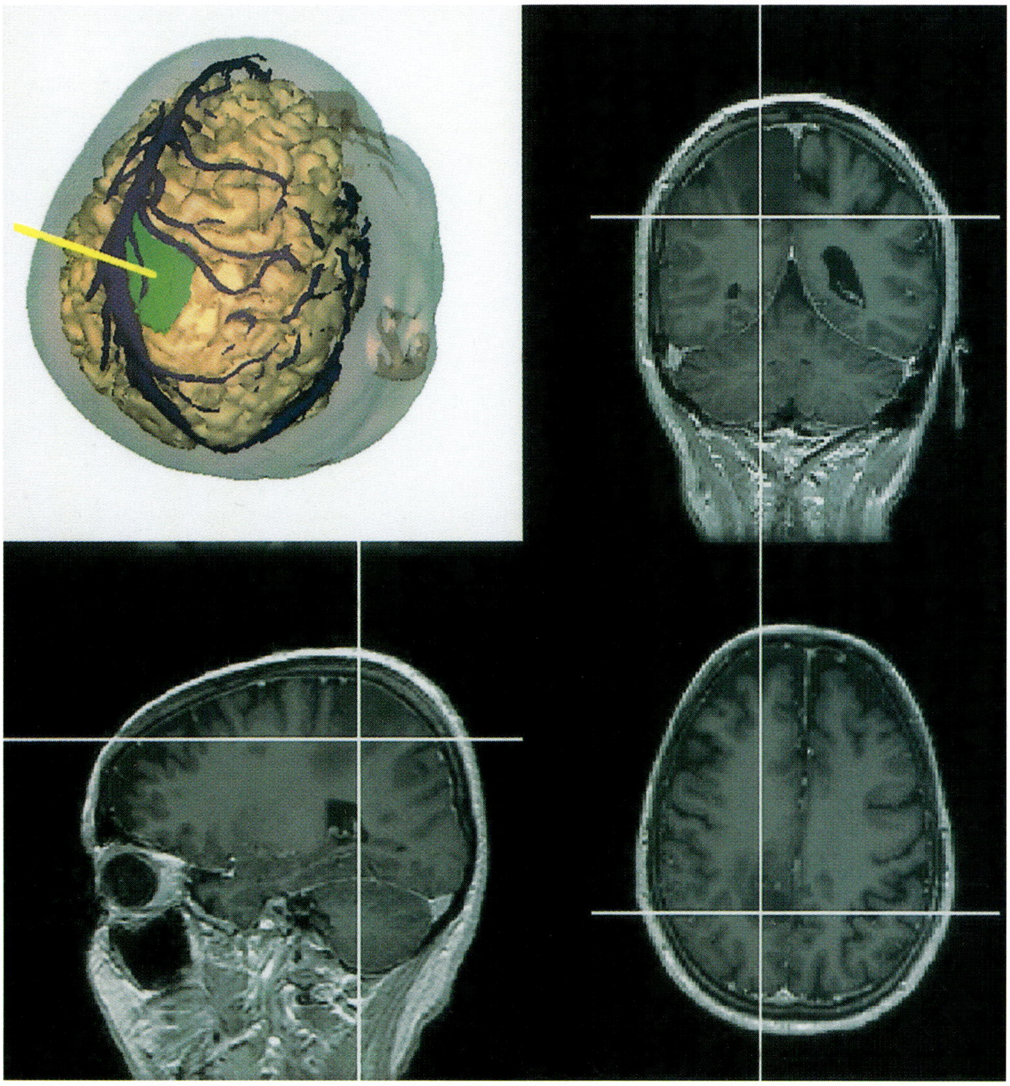

Color Plate 7: Tracking of a surgical probe. A three-dimensional graphic reconstruction of the patient's head displays the position of the probe and three cross-sectional slices of the patient's magnetic resonance data. *Crosshairs* denote the probe's tip. (See also Fig. 20-2.)

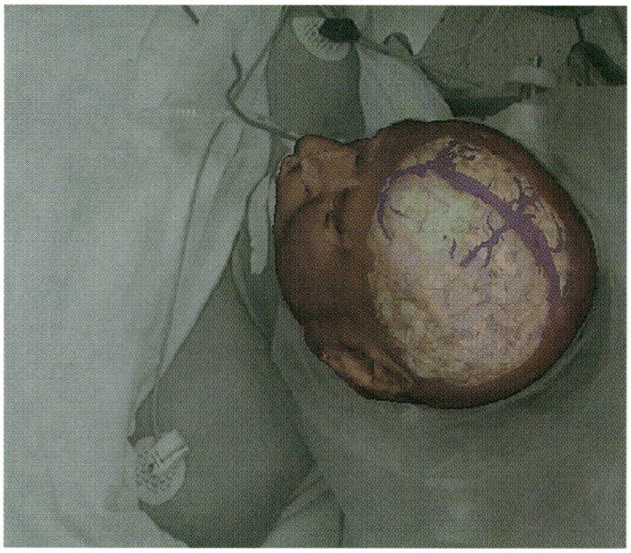

Color Plate 8: Magnetic resonance image reconstruction with the patient on the operating table shows an overlay of the skin, skull, and internal structures onto a live view of the patient. (See also Fig. 20-3.)

A

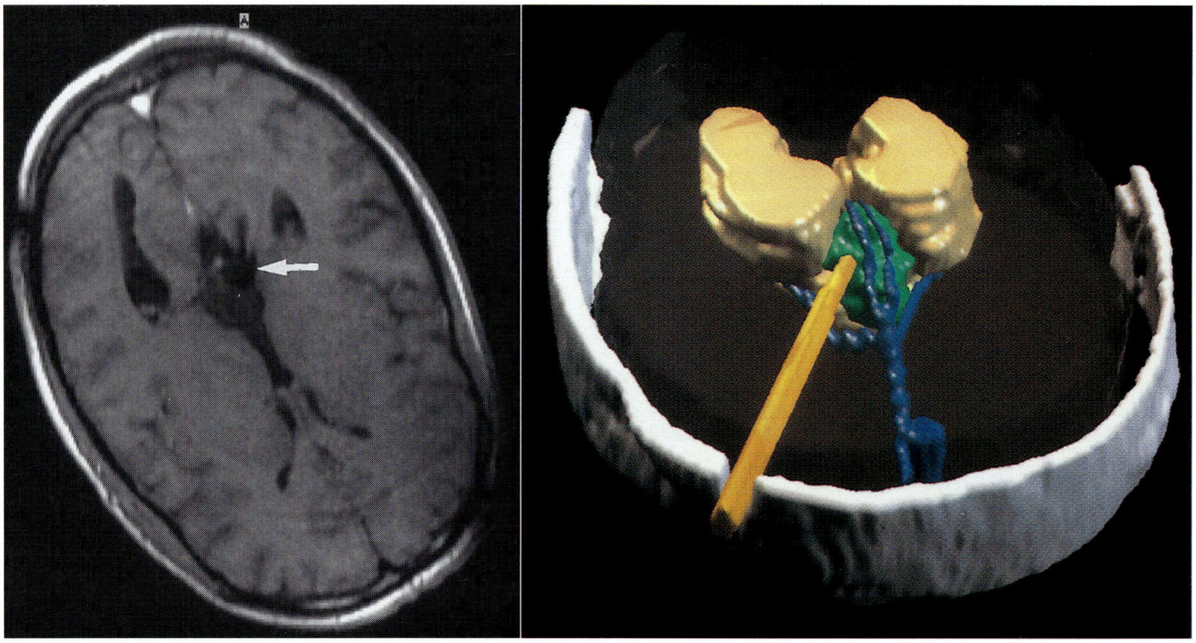

B

Color Plate 9: Image-guided drainage of a pineal cyst using magnetic resonance image guidance. **A,** The tip of the biopsy needle is guided into the pineal cyst (*arrow* shows the needle artifact). **B,** For better visualization, three-dimensional rendering from the volumetric dataset shows the cyst, thalami, and surrounding veins For hemorrhage to be avoided, the needle was introduced between the internal cerebral vein and the vein of Rosenthal. (See also Fig. 20-6.) (From Jolesz FA, and others: Image-guided procedures and the operating room of the future, *Radiology* 204:601, 1997.)

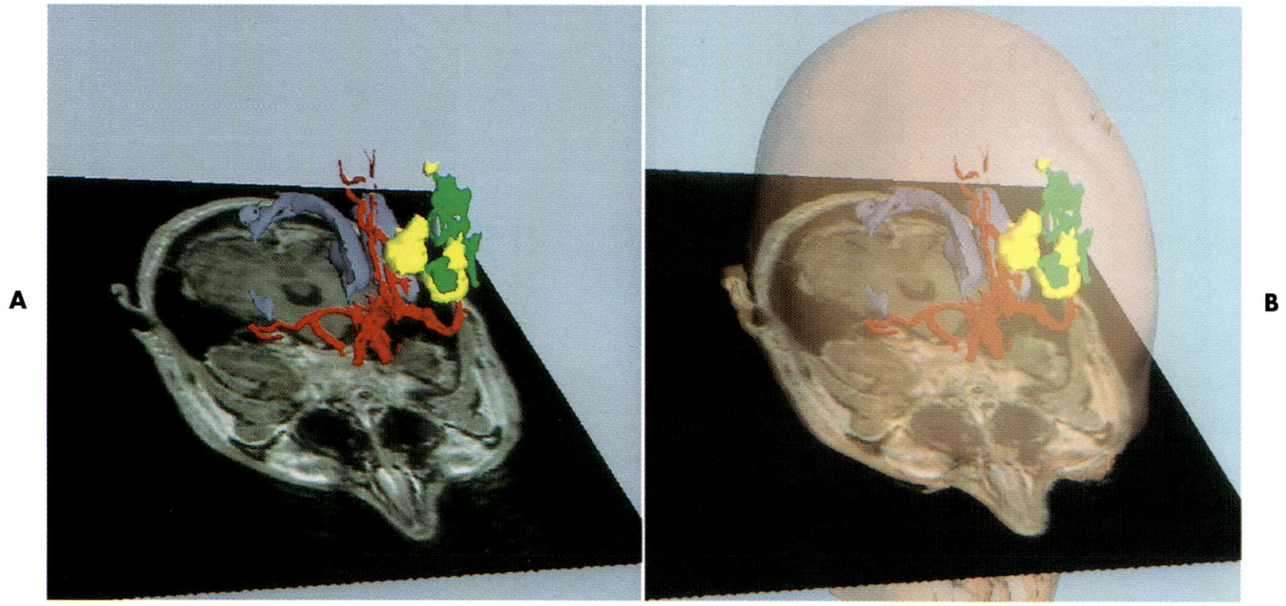

Color Plate 10: Multimodality image in three-dimensional graphics display. **A,** An axial magnetic resonance image (MRI) spoiled gradient-recalled (SPGR) echo sequence with a vessel model extracted from MR angiography and a tumor modeled from gadolinium-enhanced SPGR. **B,** The same axial MRI (SPGR) and a skin model extracted from MRI (SPGR). (See also Fig. 20-9.)

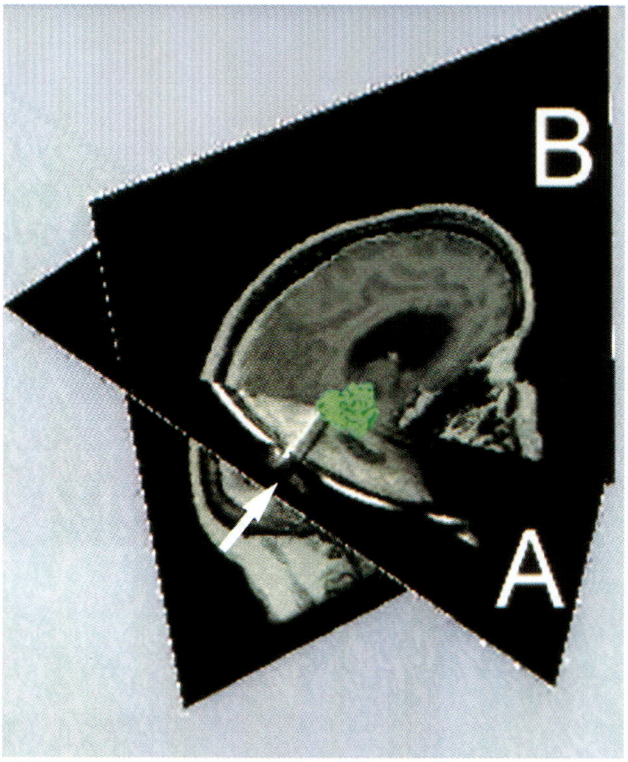

Color Plate 11: Three-dimensional graphics interface for better spatial recognition and access to registered preoperative magnetic resonance image (MRI). **A,** Intraoperative MRI with biopsy needle *(arrow)* and **B,** preoperative MRI are fused and displayed together. (See also Fig. 20-10.) (From Hata N, and others: Registration of pre-operative and intra-operative images for MR-guided therapy, *SPIE* [in press].)

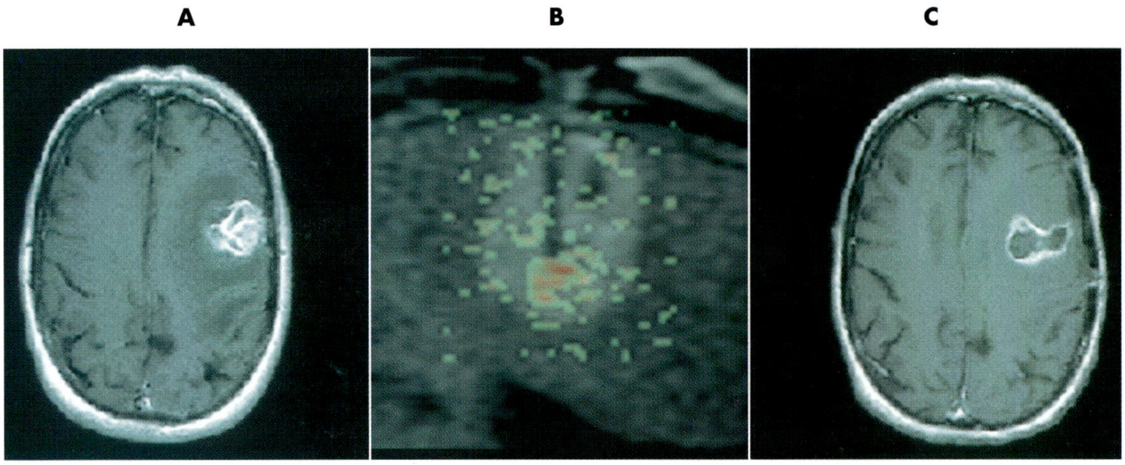

Color Plate 12: Interstitial laser therapy for brain tumors. **A,** T1-weighted (repetition time [TR], 500 msec; echo time [TE], 20 msec) contrast-enhanced image acquired with a 1.5-T scanner before the procedure showed the enhanced brain tumor. **B,** Thermal monitoring of interstitial neodymium-yttrium-garnet laser therapy with pixel subtraction of T1-weighted fast spin echo images (TR, 400 msec; TE 17 msec) acquired within the open magnet during a 4-W power deposition. Changes in signal intensity around the laser fiber were color-encoded in red. **C,** T1-weighted (TR, 500 msec; TE, 20 msec) contrast-enhanced image at 1.5-T 24 hours after laser management. Note the lack of enhancement within the tumor. The ring enhancement around the coagulated tumor is consistent within the breakdown of the blood-brain barrier. (See also Fig. 20-12.) (**A, C,** From Kettenbach J, and others: MRI paper #976243, monitoring and visualization techniques for MR-guided laser ablation in open MR-system.)

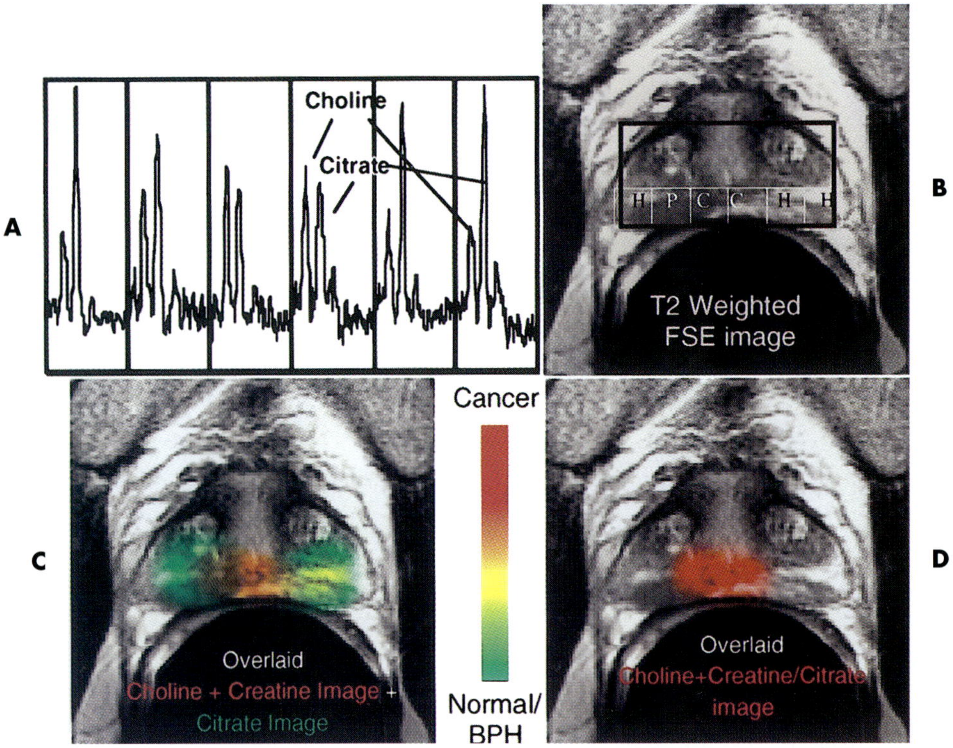

Color Plate 13: Presentation of magnetic resonance spectroscopic imaging (MRSI) data. Metabolic information form the MRSI sequence data can be presented as **A,** a single spectrum for each voxel of acquired data. **B,** a grid at the resolution of the metabolic data (0.24 cc voxels) overlying an anatomic image, or **C** and **D,** pseudocolored metabolic images (peak area maps) based on the relative concentration of cellular metabolites. In **B,** each voxel is labeled based on the metabolic data. C—probable cancer (choline + creatine/citrate ratio >3 std dev of normal values); P—possible cancer (either a choline + creatine/citrate ratio >2 std dev of normal values, or a two-fold citrate reduction relative to normal); H—healthy. In **C,** the peak area images for citrate and choline + creatine are overlaid on the T2-weighted anatomic images. In **D** the choline + creatine/citrate ratio image is thresholded. (See also Fig. 22-5.)

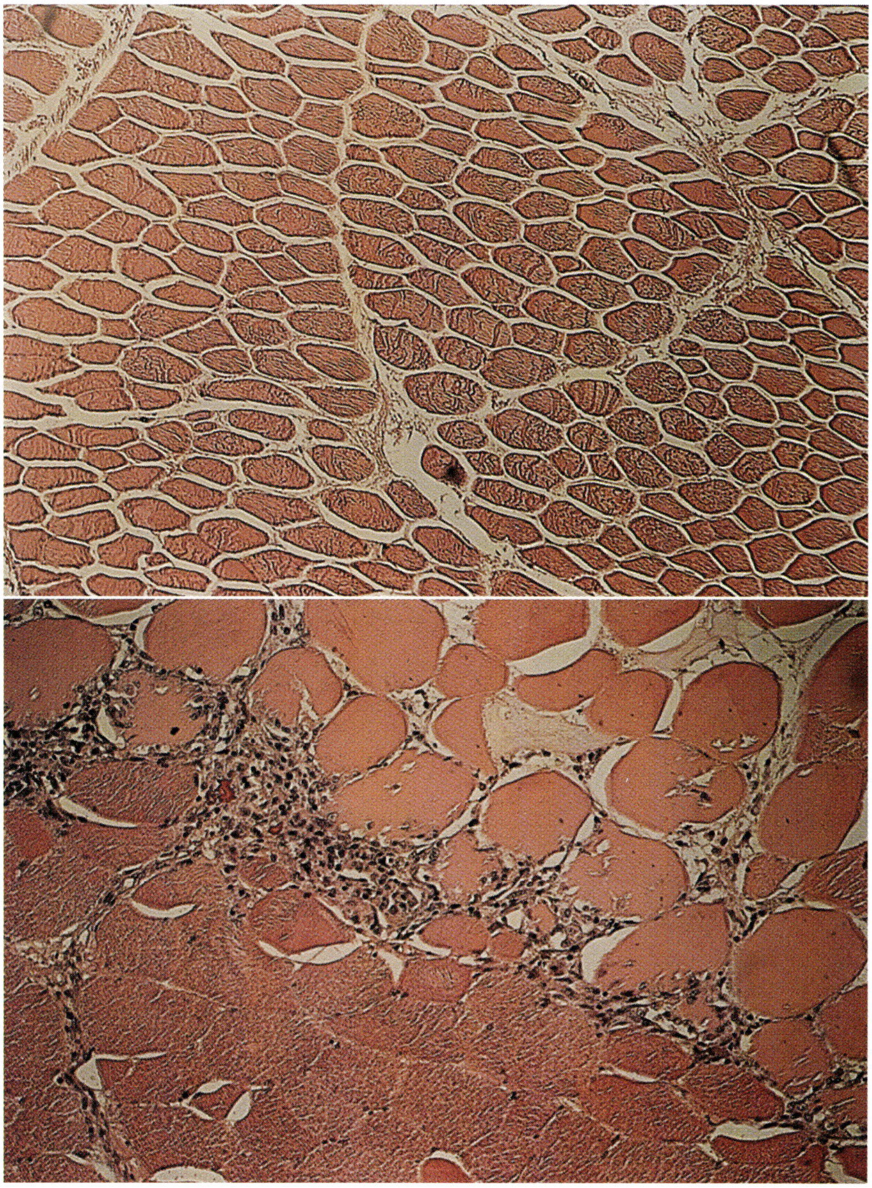

A

B

Color Plate 14: A, Pathologic specimen of the paraspinal muscle of a New Zealand rabbit obtained after completion of the ethanol injection and magnetic resonance scan and stained with hematoxylin-eosin. This image shows healthy-appearing muscle with no definite histologic abnormalities. **B,** Pathologic specimen of the paraspinal muscle of a New Zealand rabbit obtained 5 days after ethanol injection shows the typical findings seen in coagulative necrosis and a peripheral inflammatory fibrovascular response. (See also Fig. 26-2.)

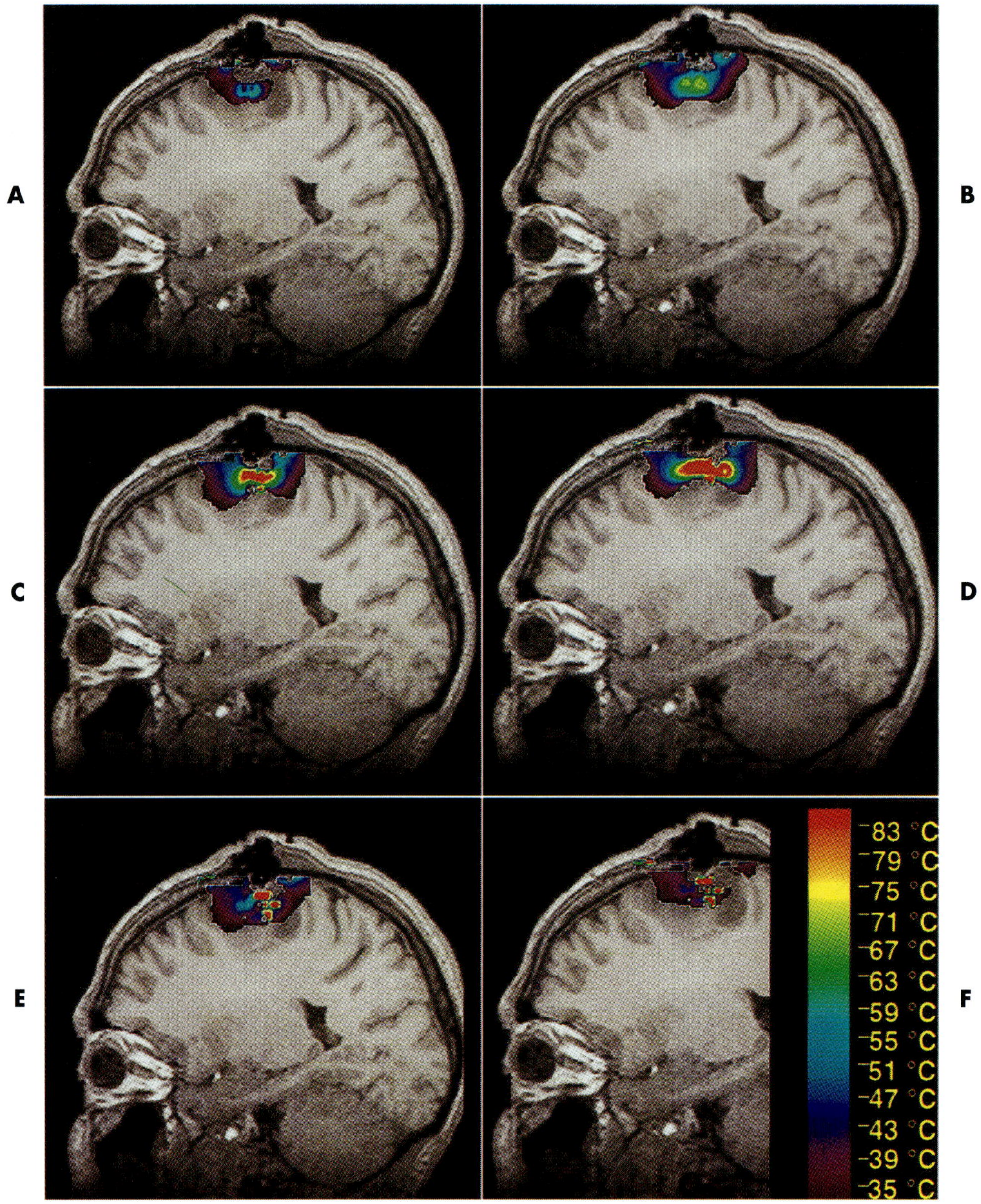

Color Plate 15: Postprocessed phase-sensitive two-dimensional fast low-angel shot images acquired and displayed during and after laser-induced thermometry (LITT). The calculated temperatures are color-coded (bottom right), gradually increasing the heat-affected zone with increasing maximum temperatures. **A** to **D,** Images acquires during LITT 1, 4, 8, and 10 minutes after starting the laser therapy. **E** and **F,** Temperature distribution 2 and 4 minutes after switching off the laser. The temperature returned to baseline values. However, some scattered pixels remain unchanged during cooling. (See also Fig. 29-2.)

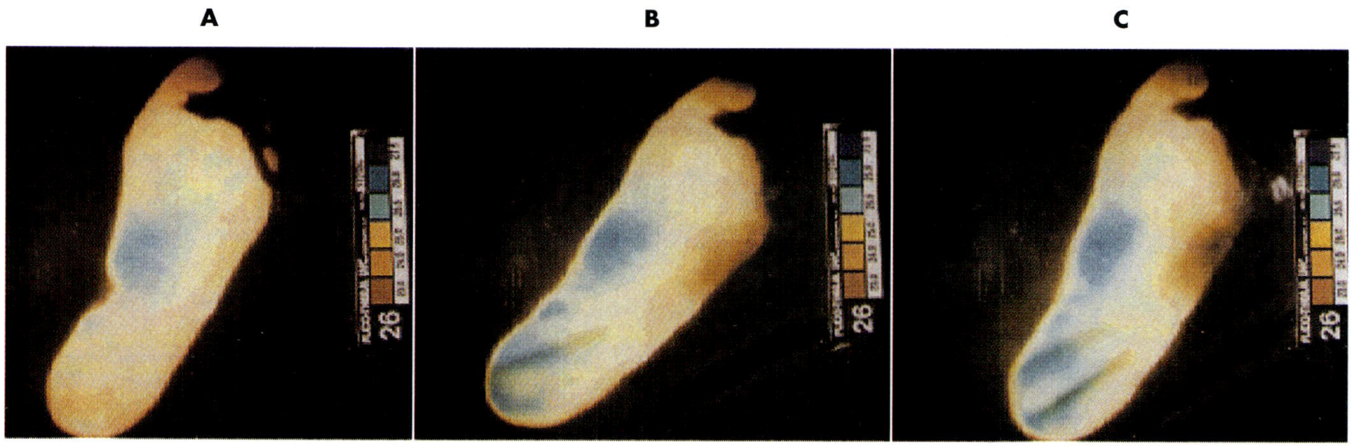

Color Plate 16: Thermosensitive liquid crystal film allows display of temperature changes of the foot. **A,** before; **B,** 2 minutes after; and **C,** 5 minutes after sympathectomy. (See also Fig. 32-2.)

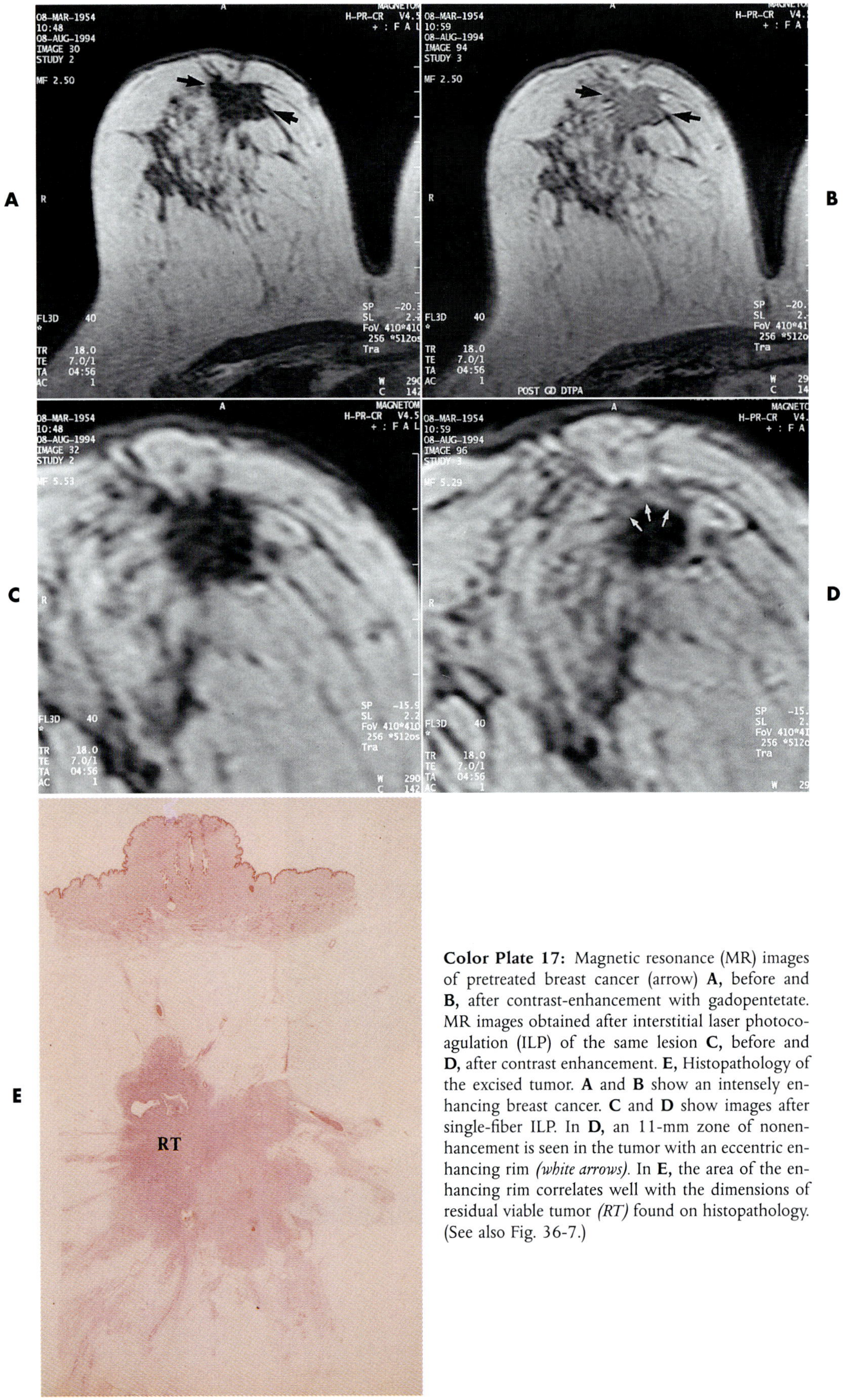

Color Plate 17: Magnetic resonance (MR) images of pretreated breast cancer (arrow) **A,** before and **B,** after contrast-enhancement with gadopentetate. MR images obtained after interstitial laser photocoagulation (ILP) of the same lesion **C,** before and **D,** after contrast enhancement. **E,** Histopathology of the excised tumor. **A** and **B** show an intensely enhancing breast cancer. **C** and **D** show images after single-fiber ILP. In **D,** an 11-mm zone of nonenhancement is seen in the tumor with an eccentric enhancing rim *(white arrows).* In **E,** the area of the enhancing rim correlates well with the dimensions of residual viable tumor *(RT)* found on histopathology. (See also Fig. 36-7.)

A

B

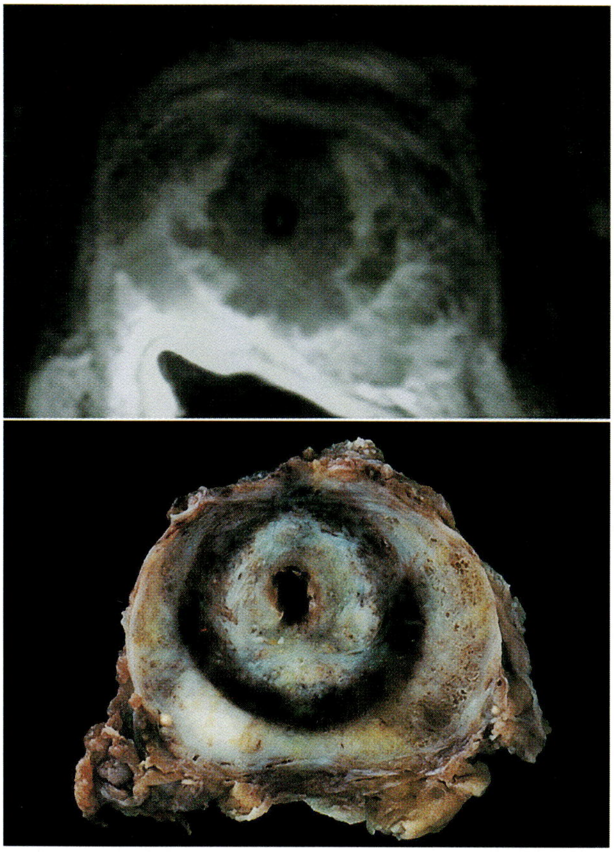

Color Plate 18: Magnetic resonance imaging findings in a patient with prostate cancer after sidefire laser ablation. **A,** Endorectal axial, T1-weighted, gadolinium-enhanced spin-echo image was obtained 3 days after ablation. The central necrotic periurethral zone is hypointense, whereas the marginal zone shows inhomogeneous contrast enhancement. **B,** Resected prostate 4 days after laser ablation. Macroscopic specimen confirms periurethral necrosis with a hemorrhagic marginal zone. (See also Fig. 42-5.) (From Huch Böni, and others: Laser ablation-induced changes in the prostate: findings at endorectal MR imaging with histologic correlation, *Radiology* 202:232, 1997. Used with permission.)

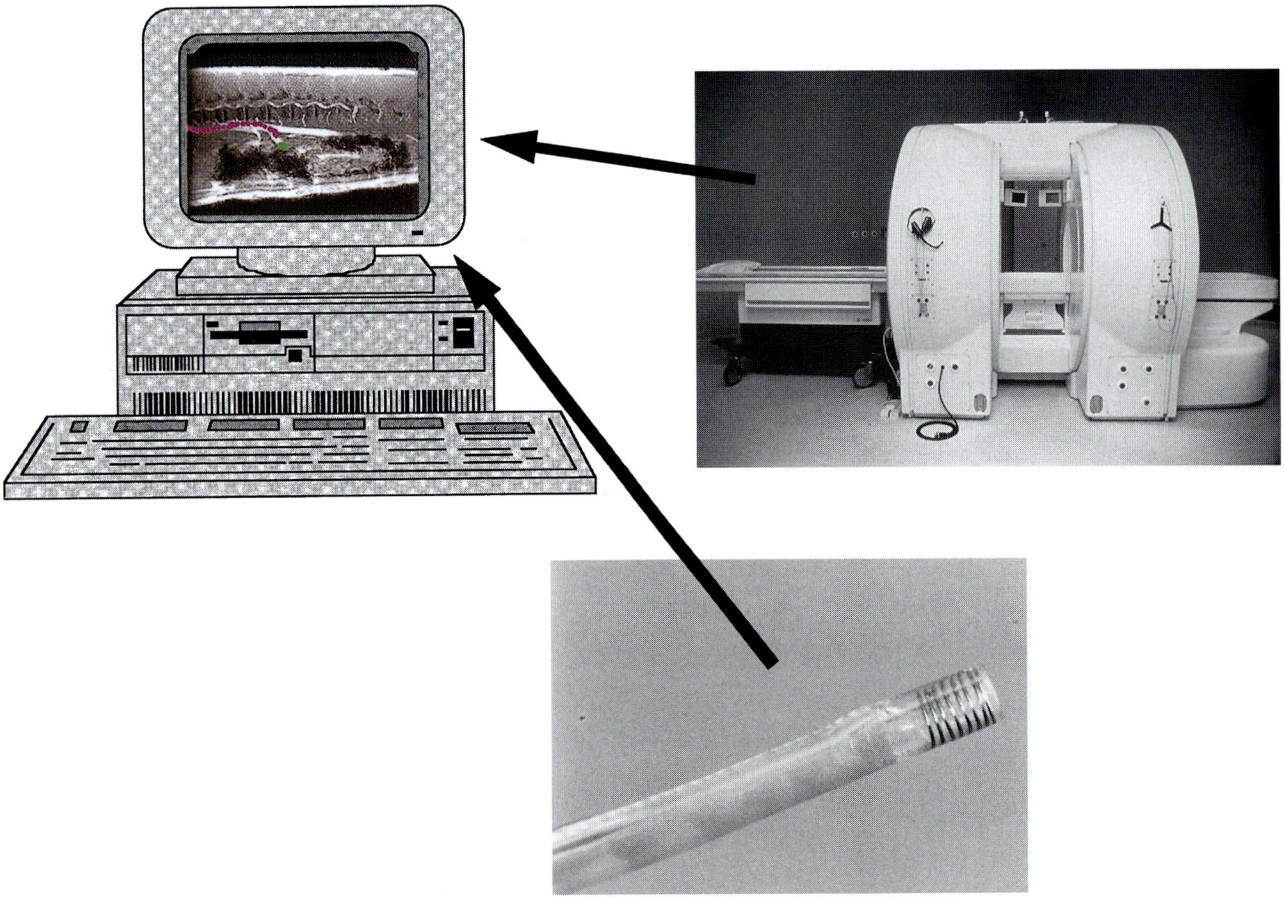

Color Plate 19: Set-up used for instrument tracking combining a magnetic resonance road map with a tip localization point whose position can be updated in real-time. The tip of the catheter has been placed in the superior mesentric artery. (See also Fig. 44-2.) (From Debatin JF, Adam G, editors: *Interventional magnetic resonance imaging,* Heidelberg, 1998, Springer-Verlag.)

A

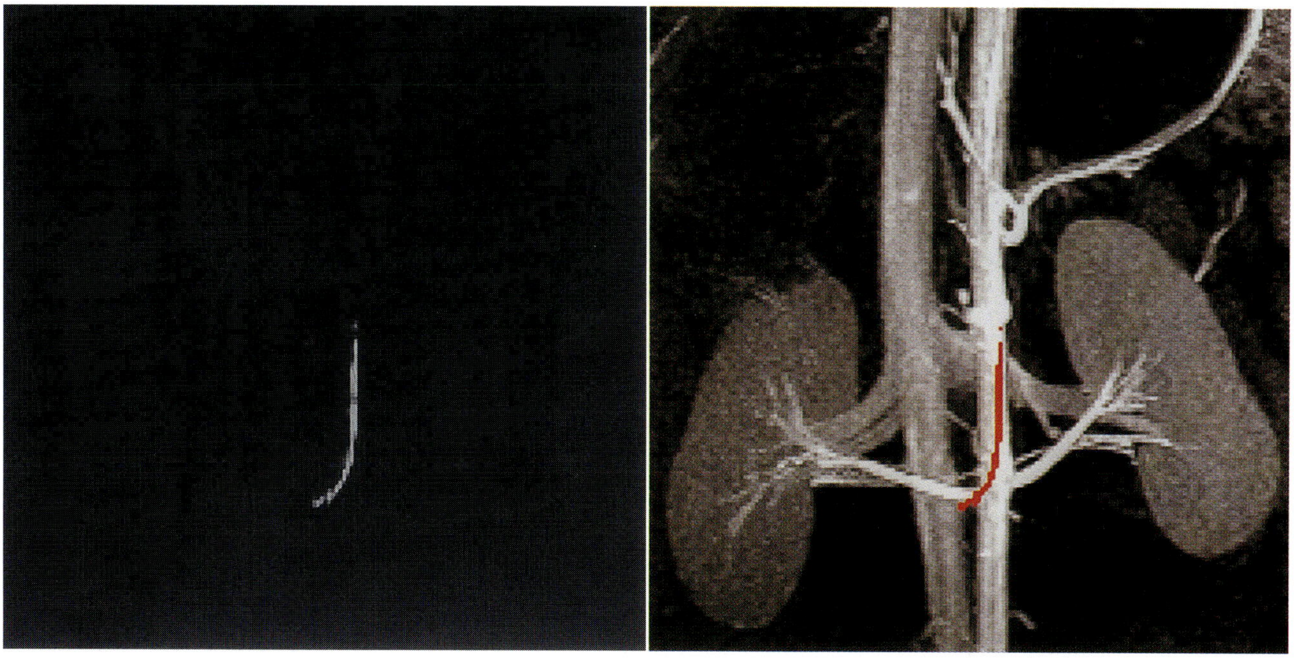

B

Color Plate 20: Image from a profiling coil shows the distal end of a prototype guidewire **A,** without being superposed on a road map and **B,** after being superposed on a road map, where the track of the instrument is color coded. (See also Fig. 44-5.)

A

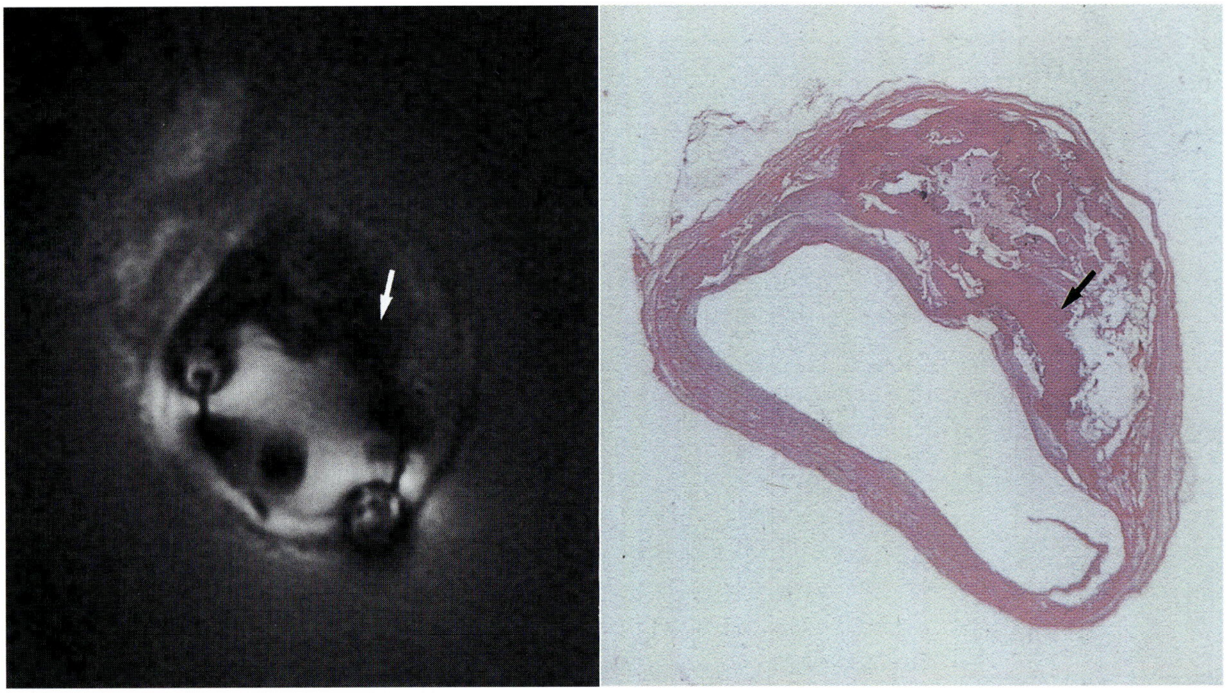

B

Color Plate 21: Ex vivo plaque shows calcification *(arrow)* on **A,** a T2-weighted image correlating to calcification in the **B,** histologic sections. (See also Fig. 44-6.) (From Zimmerman GG, and others: Intravascular MR imaging of the atherosclerotic plaque: ex vivo analysis of human femoral arteries with histologic correlation, *Radiology* 204: 771, 1997.)

phantoms.[71] An edge detection routine was used to locate the freezing front during freezing in real-time from FSPGR images (14/5 msec) acquired at 15-sec intervals. The location of the freezing front was then fed back to the control system, which adjusted the flow of liquid nitrogen to the cryoprobe. The automated control system was based on the theoretical control principle of a self-tuning regulator. In this system, the cost factor (error function) was defined as the difference between the location of the target and the actual freezing boundaries. The control system attempted to minimize this cost factor to achieve an optimal target freezing zone. In numerical simulations using a single cryosurgical probe, Pease and others showed that an ice front with a cylindrical symmetry can be accurately controlled using this MR image-guided feedback scheme.

Pease and others also extended this work to three independently controlled cryosurgical probes arrayed in several configurations and provided a complete description of the control system and its mathematical foundation.[70] The same principle of a self-tuning regulator that they used for a single probe was used for three probes. For the single probe case, freezing was radially symmetric so the problem could be reduced to one dimension. For the three-probe case, the problem to be solved was one in two dimensions. The system was tested in gelatin phantoms to demonstrate feasibility (Fig. 22-8). In the implementation of this system, a target region was drawn on an MR image of the gelatin phantom acquired before freezing (Fig. 22-8, *A*). The system was then turned on, and liquid nitrogen began flowing to the probes. Single-slice FSPGR images (14/5 msec) were acquired every 30 sec, and the mathematical calculations (edge detection and optimization routines) were conducted in real-time. Temperatures measured at each of the cryoprobes were used to calculate the appropriate amount of liquid nitrogen flow to the cryoprobes. When the control system determined that the frozen and target boundaries were as close as possible, the control system maintained that freezing volume for 10 min to demonstrate the ability of the control system to freeze and maintain a defined volume. This groundbreaking work demonstrates that MR image-guided freezing is possible. For such an automated control system to be implemented in a clinical setting more research is required such as extending freezing in two dimensions to freezing in three dimensions.

CONCLUSIONS

The advantages of interventional MRI-guided cryosurgical ablation of tumors have been discussed. The factors that make focal cryosurgical ablation particularly well suited to interventional MR guidance include (1) the ability of MRI to image the entire volume of tissue during freezing with high accuracy and in real-time, (2) the easy detection of the freezing boundary under MRI, (3) the sharp, definable margins of necrosis that cryosurgical freezing produces, (4) the ability to detect and stage cancers using combined MRI and MRSI and use this information for planning focal treatment and follow-up, (5) the ability of MRI to assess the effectiveness of treatment immediately after thawing, and (6) the possibility of controlling the freezing process automatically.

The combination of these factors with the emerging ability to determine the location and distribution of cancer tumors using MR spectroscopic imaging makes it possible to treat cancerous tumors focally. MRI-guided focal cryoablation is likely to take its place with other emerging interventional focal therapies as these technologies develop and more interventional magnets become available. Although this technique is still at the research stage, only a few technical details remain to be solved for this technique to be applied in a clinical setting. Most of these details involve developing MR-compatible devices (e.g., cryoprobes, freezing devices, patient positioning equipment, accessory hardware). The development of an MR-compatible cryosurgical system is currently underway. Imaging sequences must also be optimized for lower field interventional magnet systems, but MRI-guided cryosurgical ablation has great potential to improve patient care as this minimally invasive therapy evolves.

REFERENCES

1. Brested JH: *The Edwin Smith surgical papyrus.* In *The University of Chicago Oriental Institute Publications Vol III,* vol. 2, plate IV, Chicago, 1930, University of Chicago Press.
2. Rand RW, Rinfret AP, von Leden H: *Cryosurgery,* Springfield, Ill, 1968, CC Thomas.
3. Brock A: *Airs, waters and places.* In *Greek medicine: being extracts illustrative of medical writers from Hippocrates to Galen,* London, 1929, EP Dutton & Co (Translated by AJ Brock).
4. Aubrey J: *Brief lives: William Harvey,* London, 1949, Secker and Warburg.
5. Grattan JHG: *Anglo-Saxon magic and medicine,* London, 1952, Oxford University Press.
6. Davidson M: The evolution of anesthesia, *Br J Anaesth* 31:134, 1959.
7. Ablin RJ: *Handbook of cryosurgery,* New York, 1980, Marcel Dekker.
8. Larrey DJ, Mercer: *Surgical memoirs of campaigns of Russia, Germany and France,* Philadelphia, 1832, Carrey and Lea.
9. Arnott J: *On the treatment of cancer by the regulated application of an anesthetic temperature,* London, 1851, J Churchill.
10. Arnott J: *On the present state of therapeutic inquiry,* London, 1845, J Churchill.
11. Fay T: Experiences with refrigeration of the human brain, *J Neurosurg* 16:239, 1959.
12. Bailey CP, and others: Cardiac surgery under hypothermia, *J Thorac Cardiovasc Surg* 27:73, 1954.
13. Lewis FJ, Tanfic M: Closure of atrial septal defects with the aid of hypothermia: experimental accomplishments and the report of one successful case, *Surgery* 33:52, 1953.
14. Rosomoff HL, Holaday DA: Cerebral blood flow and cerebral oxygen consumption during hypothermia, *Am J Physiol* 179:85, 1954.
15. Botterell EH, and others: Hypothermia and interruption of carotid, or carotid and cerebral circulation, in the surgical management of intracranial aneurysms, *J Neurosurg* 13:1, 1956.
16. Cespedes RD, and others: Long-term followup of incontinence and obstruction after salvage cryosurgical ablation of the prostate: results in 143 patients, *J Urol* 157:237, 1997.
17. Corral DA, Pisters LL, von Eschenbach AC: Treatment options for localized recurrence of prostate cancer following radiation therapy, *Urol Clin North Am* 23:677, 1996.
18. Lee F, and others: Cryosurgery of prostate cancer: use of adjuvant hormonal therapy and temperature monitoring. A one year follow-up, *Anticancer Res* 17:1511, 1997.

19. Miller R Jr, and others: Percutaneous, transperineal cryosurgery of the prostate as salvage therapy for post radiation recurrence of adenocarcinoma, *Cancer* 77:1510, 1996.
20. Pisters LL, and others: The efficacy and complications of salvage cryotherapy of the prostate, *J Urol* 157:921, 1997.
21. Gage AA, Fazekas G, Riley EJ: Freezing injury to large blood vessels in dogs: with comments on the effect of experimental freezing of bile ducts, *Surgery* 61:748, 1967.
22. Riley EE, Fazekas G, Gage AA: Freezing of blood vessels and bile ducts without excision, *Surg Forum* 16:141, 1965.
23. Onik G, and others: Ultrasound-guided hepatic cryosurgery in the treatment of metastatic colon carcinoma: preliminary results, *Cancer* 67:901, 1991.
24. Onik GM, and others: Cryosurgery of liver cancer, *Semin Surg Oncol* 9:309, 1993.
25. Ravikumar TS: The role of cryotherapy in the management of patients with liver tumors, *Adv Surg* 30:281, 1996.
26. Trumble TE, Whalen JT: The effects of cryosurgery and cryoprotectants on peripheral nerve function, *J Reconstr Microsurg* 8:53, 1992.
27. Garnick MB, Fair WR: Prostate cancer: emerging concepts. Part II, *Ann Intern Med* 125:205, 1996.
28. Chaikin DC, and others: Erectile dysfunction following minimally invasive treatments for prostate cancer, *Urology* 48:100, 1996.
29. Stamey TA, and others: Morphometric and clinical studies on 68 consecutive radical prostatectomies, *J Urol* 139:1235, 1988.
30. Robinson JW, Dufour MS, Fung TS: Erectile functioning of men treated for prostate carcinoma, *Cancer* 79:538, 1997.
31. Cooper I, Lee A: Cryothalamectomy: hypothermic congelation: A technical advance in basal ganglia surgery, *J Am Geriatr Soc* 9:714, 1961.
32. Gage A: Current progress in cryosurgery, *Cryobiology* 25:483, 1988.
33. Gage A: Cryosurgery in the treatment of cancer, *Surg Gynecol Obstet* 174:73, 1992.
34. Gage AA: Progress in cryosurgery, *Cryobiology* 29:300, 1992.
35. Gonder M, Soanes W, Schulman S: Cryosurgical treatment of the prostate, *Invest Urol* 3:372, 1966.
36. Zacarian SA: How accurate is temperature monitoring in cryosurgery and is there an alternative? *J Dermatol Surg Oncol* 6:627, 1980.
37. Onik G, and others: Ultrasonic characteristics of frozen liver, *Cryobiology* 21:321, 1984.
38. Gilbert J, and others: Ultrasonic characterization of a cryosurgical process in gelatin, *Cryobiology* 21:715, 1984 (abstract).
39. Gilbert JC, and others: Real time ultrasonic monitoring of hepatic cryosurgery, *Cryobiology* 22:319, 1985.
40. Onik GM, and others: Ultrasonic monitoring of hepatic cryosurgery: preliminary report on an animal model, *Cryobiology* 21:715, 1984 (abstract).
41. Onik G, and others: Sonographic monitoring of hepatic cryosurgery in an experimental animal model, *Am J Roentgenol* 144:1043, 1985.
42. Onik G, and others: US characteristics of frozen prostate, *Radiology* 168:629, 1988.
43. Onik G, and others: Percutaneous transperineal prostate cryosurgery using transrectal ultrasound guidance: animal model, *Urology* 37:277, 1991.
44. Onik GM, and others: Transrectal ultrasound-guided percutaneous radical cryosurgical ablation of the prostate, *Cancer* 72:1291, 1993.
45. Rubinsky B, and others: Monitoring cryosurgery in the brain and prostate with proton NMR, *Cryobiology* 30:191, 1993.
46. Bahn DK, and others: Prostate cancer: US-guided percutaneous cryoablation. Work in progress, *Radiology* 194:551, 1995.
47. Lee F, and others: US-guided percutaneous cryoablation of prostate cancer, *Radiology* 192:769, 1994.
48. Onik G, and others: *Percutaneous Prostate cryoablation,* St Louis, 1994, Quality Medical Publishing.
49. Zippe CD: Cryosurgical ablation for prostate cancer: a current review, *Semin Urol* 13:148, 1995.
50. Zippe CD: Cryosurgery of the prostate: techniques and pitfalls, *Urol Clin North Am* 23:147, 1996.
51. Isoda H: Sequential MRI and CT monitoring in cryosurgery: an experimental study in polyvinyl alcohol gel phantom, *Nippon Igaku Hoshasen Gakkai Zasshi* 49:1096, 1989.
52. Isoda H: Sequential MRI and CT monitoring in cryosurgery: an experimental study in rats, *Nippon Igaku Hoshasen Gakkai Zasshi* 49:1499, 1989.
53. Matsumoto R, Oshio K, Jolesz FA: Monitoring of laser and freezing-induced ablation in the liver with T1-weighted MR imaging, *J Magn Reson Imaging* 2:555, 1992.
54. Matsumoto R, and others: MR monitoring during cryotherapy in the liver: predictability of histologic outcome, *J Magn Reson Imaging* 3:770, 1993.
55. Gilbert JC, and others: *NMR monitored cryosurgery in the rabbit brain,* Berlin, 1992, Proceedings of The Society for Magnetic Resonance in Medicine.
56. Gilbert JC, and others: Temperature determination in the frozen region during cryosurgery of rabbit liver using magnetic resonance image analysis, *Magn Reson Imaging* 15:657, 1997.
57. Hong J, and others: MR imaging assisted temperature calculations during cryosurgery, *Magn Reson Imaging* 12:1021, 1994.
58. Rubinsky B, Pegg DE: A mathematical model for the freezing process in biological tissue, *Proc R Soc Lond [Biol]* 234:343, 1988.
59. Rubinsky B, Eto TK: Heat transfer with phase transition in biological materials, *Cryo-Letters* 10:153, 1989.
60. Rubinsky B: The energy equation for freezing of biological tissue, *ASME Trans J of Heat Trans* 111:988, 1989.
61. Rubinsky B, Eto TK: *Heat transfer during freezing of biological materials.* In *Annual review of heat transfer,* vol 3, New York, 1990, Hemisphere Publishing.
62. Rubinsky B, Onik G: Cryosurgery: advances in the application of low temperatures to medicine, *Int J Refr* 14:1, 1991.
63. Rubinsky B: *Thermodynamics and heat transfer in cryosurgery.* In *Percutaneous prostate cryoablation,* St Louis, 1994, Quality Medical Publishing.
64. Gilbert JC, and others: *MR image analysis for assessing the temperature distribution in a cryosurgical frozen region,* New York, 1996, Proceedings of the 4th Scientific Meeting of the International Society for Magnetic Resonance in Medicine (abstract).
65. Gilbert JC, and others: MRI-monitored cryosurgery in the rabbit brain, *Magn Reson Imaging* 11:1155, 1993.
66. Kurhanewicz J, and others: Three-dimensional H-1 MR spectroscopic imaging of the in situ human prostate with high (0.24-0.1-cm (3)) spatial resolution, *Radiology* 198:795, 1996.
67. Scheidler J, and others: *Combined MR imaging and H1 spectroscopic imaging in prostate cancer localization: correlation with step section pathology,* Chicago, 1997, Proceedings of the RSNA.
68. Keanini RG, Rubinsky B: Optimization of multiprobe cryosurgery, *J Heat Tran - ASME Trans* 114:796, 1992.
69. Reference deleted in pages.
70. Pease G: *Magnetic resonance image-guided control of cryoablation,* Berkeley, Calif, 1995, University of California Berkeley (PhD dissertation).
71. Pease GR, and others: MR image-guided control of cryosurgery, *J Magn Reson Imaging* 5:753, 1995.
72. Pease GR, and others: An integrated probe for magnetic resonance imaging monitored skin cryosurgery, *J Biomech Eng* 117:59, 1995.
73. Mazur P, and others: *Interaction of cooling rate, warming rate and protective additives on the survival of frozen mammalian cells.* In *The Frozen Cell,* London, 1970, J Churchill.
74. McGrath JJ, Cravalho EG, Huggins CE: An experimental comparison of intracellular ice formation and freeze thaw survival of HeLa S-3 cells, *Cryobiology* 12:540, 1975.
75. Merryman MT: *Cryobiology,* London, 1966, Academic Press.
76. Cozzi PJ, and others: Critical temperature for in vivo cryoablation of human prostate cancer in a xenograft model, *Br J Urol* 77:89, 1996.
77. Dow JA: Effects of surgical capsular temperature on cryosurgery of the prostate, *J Urol* 100:66, 1968.
78. Dow JA, Coughlin JD, Waterhouse K: Lethal freezing temperatures of the surgical capsule and cryosurgery of the prostate, *J Urol* 104:459, 1970.

79. Dow JA, Waterhouse K: An experimental study in lethal freezing temperatures of the prostate gland, *J Urol* 103:454, 1970.
80. Gage AA, Caruana J Jr, Montes M: Critical temperature for skin necrosis in experimental cryosurgery, *Cryobiology* 19:273, 1982.
81. Gage AA, and others: Tissue impedance and temperature measurements in relation to necrosis in experimental cryosurgery, *Cryobiology* 22:282, 1985.
82. Rivoire ML, and others: Hepatic cryosurgery precision: evaluation of ultrasonography, thermometry, and impedancemetry in a pig model, *J Surg Oncol* 61:242, 1996.
83. Steed J, and others: Correlation between thermosensor temperature and transrectal ultrasonography during prostate cryoablation, *Can Assoc Radiol J* 48:186, 1997.
84. Tatsutani K, and others: Effect of thermal variables on frozen human primary prostatic adenocarcinoma cells, *Urology* 48:441, 1996.
85. Wong WS, and others: Cryosurgery as a treatment for prostate carcinoma: results and complications, *Cancer* 79:963, 1997.
86. Zietman AL, and others: Adjuvant irradiation after radical prostatectomy for adenocarcinoma of prostate: analysis of freedom from PSA failure, *Urology* 42:292, 1993.
87. Rifkin M: Comparison of magnetic resonance imaging and ultrasonography in staging early prostate cancer: results of a multi-institutional cooperative trial, *Invest Radiol* 26:1024, 1991.
88. Hricak H, and others: Prostatic carcinoma: staging by clinical assessment, CT, and MR imaging, *Radiology* 162:331, 1987.
89. Platt JF, Bree RL, Schwab RE: The accuracy of CT in the staging of carcinoma of the prostate, *Am J Roentgenol* 149:315, 1987.
90. Schnall MD, and others: Prostate cancer: local staging with endorectal surface coil MR imaging, *Radiology* 178:797, 1991.
91. Kier R, Wain S, Troiano R: Fast spin-echo MR images of the pelvis obtained with a phased-array coil: value in localizing and staging prostatic carcinoma, *Am J Roentgenol* 161:601, 1993.
92. Hricak H, and others: Carcinoma of the prostate gland: MR imaging with pelvic phased-array coils versus integrated endorectal—pelvic phased-array coils, *Radiology* 193:703, 1994.
93. White S, and others: Prostate cancer: effect of postbiopsy hemorrhage on interpretation of MR images, *Radiology* 195:385, 1995.
94. Kalbhen CL, and others: Prostate carcinoma: MR imaging findings after cryosurgery, *Radiology* 198:807, 1996.
95. Chen M, and others: Hormonal ablation of prostatic cancer: effects on prostate morphology, tumor detection, and staging by endorectal coil MR imaging, *Am J Roentgenol* 166:1157, 1996.
96. Brown TR, Kincaid BM, Ugurbil K: NMR chemical shift imaging in three dimensions, *Proc Natl Acad Sci U S A* 79:3523, 1982.
97. Thomsen C: Quantitative magnetic resonance methods for in vivo investigation of the human liver and spleen: technical aspects and preliminary clinical results, *Acta Radiol Suppl* 401:1, 1996.
98. Barker PB, Lee RR, McArthur JC: AIDS dementia complex: evaluation with proton MR spectroscopic imaging, *Radiology* 195:58, 1995.
99. Graham GD, and others: Early temporal variation of cerebral metabolites after human stroke: a proton magnetic resonance spectroscopy study, *Stroke* 24:1891, 1993.
100. Hetherington H, and others: Proton nuclear magnetic resonance spectroscopic imaging of human temporal lobe epilepsy at 4.1 T, *Ann Neurol* 38:396, 1995.
101. Wald LL, and others: Proton spectroscopic imaging of the human brain using phased array detectors, *Magn Reson Med* 34:440, 1995.
102. Connolly JA, and others: Prostate-specific antigen after cryosurgical ablation of the prostate: defining the appropriate response, *Urol Clin North Am* 24:415, 1997.
103. Parivar F, and others: Detection of locally recurrent prostate cancer after cryosurgery: evaluation by transrectal ultrasound, magnetic resonance imaging, and three-dimensional proton magnetic resonance spectroscopy, *Urology* 48:594, 1996.
104. Kurhanewicz J, and others: Prostate cancer: metabolic response to cryosurgery as detected with 3D H-1 MR spectroscopic imaging, *Radiology* 200:489, 1996.

Chapter 23

PRINCIPLES OF MR–GUIDED LASER THERAPY

Martyn Paley, Margaret A. Hall-Craggs, Stephen G. Bown

Newly developed technology to precisely locate laser applicators and monitor their thermal effects under noninvasive magnetic resonance (MR) guidance may revolutionize minimally invasive therapy of breast, liver, and prostate tumors and many other regions of the body.[1–38]

Precise visual definition of target lesions with high spatial and contrast resolution; the ability to accurately visualize and guide the approach of applicators to the target under MR fluoroscopy in three dimensions; and implementation of rapid MRI sequences, which are sensitive to increasing temperature when combined with newly developed open MR systems, provide a near-optimal solution for this new approach to surgical intervention.[39–51]

Advances in image–guided biopsy techniques may confirm pathology and allow subsequent interventional procedures to be performed while the patient remains in the image–guided operating suite, thus reducing delays in treatment.

Processing algorithms, which can interpret changes in images during treatment, will become increasingly important, providing feedback to the therapeutic system to control the amount and distribution of energy to accurately and completely destroy lesions. This capability will be possible only after rigorous correlation between changes observed on MRI and corresponding histopathology is validated in many clinical cases.

This chapter reviews the current status of therapeutic laser tools and MR guidance systems and provides a few possible directions for future development.

DIODE LASER SYSTEMS FOR INTERVENTIONAL MAGNETIC RESONANCE IMAGING

Since lasers were introduced in 1963 for eye surgery, clinical applications for lasers range from cosmetic surgery and precise bloodless cutting for routine surgery to interstitial therapy of tumors *in situ.* Introduction of compact diode-based lasers (Fig. 23-1) weighing only 30 kg has changed the practical and economical basis for lasers in medicine, resulting in a much wider diffusion of the technology. Previously, medical lasers were expensive devices weighing more than 150 kg that were usually restricted to a single location and required water cooling.[52–63]

Single-diode or two-dimensional (2D)-diode laser arrays are available with reliable power output up to 60 W for clinical use. Wavelength coverage is from 650 to 2000 nm. Shorter wavelength diode devices are not readily available, although prototype devices operating at 630 nm have been constructed. The wavelength of operation depends on the exact chemical and physical composition of the semiconductor. Aluminum-gallium-arsenide (Al-Ga-As) diode lasers produce wavelengths of 760 to 900 nm depending on the relative amounts of Al and Ga in the active layer of the diode. At a wavelength of 900 to 1100 nm, indium-gallium-arsenide (In-Ga-As) lasers are used. Below a wavelength of 760 nm, aluminum-gallium-indium-phosphide (Al-Ga-In-P) lasers emit 600 to 690 nm. Diode lasers can also

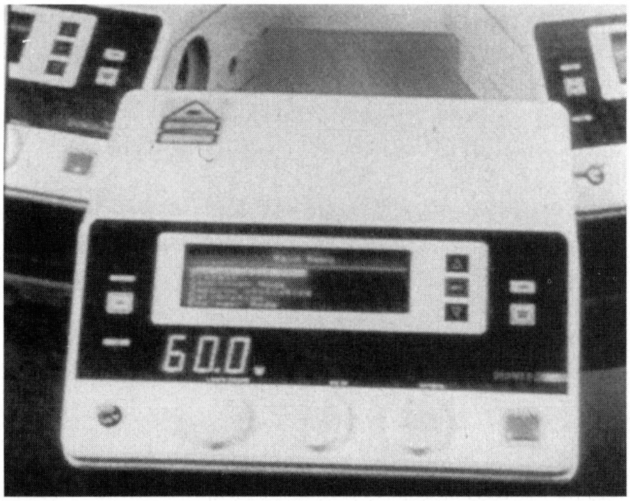

Fig. 23-1. Diomed diode laser (Diomed, Cambridge, United Kingdom).

be used to optically pump conventional lasers, such as neodymium:yttrium-aluminum-garnet (Nd:YAG) lasers, operating at 1064 nm rather than at the wavelength of traditional arc lamps, resulting in increased efficiency, wavelength, and power conversion. Nonlinear optical systems may be used to quarter or halve the wavelength of operation, resulting in an Nd:YAG laser that can provide light at 266 or 532 nm.

Diode lasers are manufactured from epitaxial-layer semiconductor wafers designed to have very highly defined spectral, spatial, and temporal characteristics. Coupling the light from the laser diodes into a fiberoptic delivery system requires very precise optical engineering. Most commercial lasers have built-in power meters, which can assess output. However, to ensure safe operation, an external calibration system (e.g., a spectroradiometer) should be used. An integrating sphere traceable to national standards to ensure light delivered at the end of the fiberoptic system has the desired spectral radiance.

Establishing the optimal operating wavelength and power versus time characteristic (which leads to absorbed energy dose) for various laser treatments has a priority in research. The temperature that the tissue reaches depends on a balance of the input power multiplied by the optical to thermal transfer efficiency minus the heat extracted through thermal diffusion in the tissue and conductive cooling by the blood system. Thermal conductivity depends on the precise physical structure of the tissue being treated and differs between healthy and cancerous tissue.[58] The heat transfer process in tissue can be mathematically modeled[11] to produce a treatment plan, but the situation *in vivo* is complicated and real-time changes in thermally sensitive images can better guide the treatment process in practice.

Typical treatment of a large liver metastasis requires 10 to 20,000 J of energy at 805 nm delivered into the lesion over 500 sec. Shorter duration, high-power treatments have been tried but result in vaporization of tissue and intense charring in the local vicinity of the probe tip, which reduces the overall lesion size produced. Not all light energy is converted into heat because some energy is lost in reflection up the fibers and through inelastic light scattering. Vaporization of tissue by high-power deposition can also cause small explosions, which can be very dangerous.

If the laser applicator is located near a major blood vessel, then the vessel may be occluded, resulting in a marked change in heating characteristics. Before occlusion, blood vessels can carry heat far from the treatment site, resulting in thermal effects along the course of the blood vessels. In the liver, heat seems to diffuse rapidly through fatty tissue. Microbubbles of steam caused by local tissue boiling have been produced in some experiments.[17] Local charring of tissue may also occur at the fiber tip, and the residual gases produced may exit up the fibers and into the operating room. This possibility suggests that good air extraction should always be used in MR–guided laser therapy suites.

In some experiments using MR guidance, a diode laser (Diomed, Cambridge, UK) capable of producing 25 W at 805 nm has been used. This output is usually split into four or eight plastic optical fibers of 0.4 mm in diameter using one or more prismatic optical coupling devices. These devices should be well aligned, clean, and dust-free to avoid power loss. Fibers should be carefully cleaved to interface with the beam splitters and provide high optical efficiency. Each fiber continuously delivers 3 to 4 W of power and is individually calibrated for power output before use. A low-power red light output mode allows the surgeon to visualize the precise position of the output beam for locating the fibers.

Several safety precautions should be implemented when using lasers in a clinical setting. The laser features a foot switch, which requires continuous operator pressure, and an audible alarm to ensure that personnel are aware that the laser is activated. A timer on the laser output ensures that exposures are not excessive. A special laser-controlled area with warning signs and physical barriers is required to prevent unauthorized personnel from entering the suite. All staff in the controlled area and the patient should be provided with glasses of high optical density, which effectively filter the wavelength in use.

LASER APPLICATORS AND GUIDANCE SYSTEMS FOR LASER THERAPY

Interstitial laser photocoagulation is an invasive technique that requires puncturing the organ (usually under local anesthetic) and locating the laser applicator in the target lesion. Typically, a laser applicator will consist of an MR-compatible biopsy needle (e.g., 18 gauge, Cook, Bjeverskov, Denmark) with a polytef oversheath (e.g., Secalon-T, Viggo-Spectromed, Swindon, UK) and a fine fiberoptic passed through the needle. A micropore adhesive tape tag is used to anchor the fiber to the needle and sheath to prevent slippage of the fiber with patient motion. This tag also allows measurement of distance when performing pullbacks (see below). Tape secures the bundle of fiberoptics to the patient bed to prevent tangling when the patient is moved in and out of the magnet.

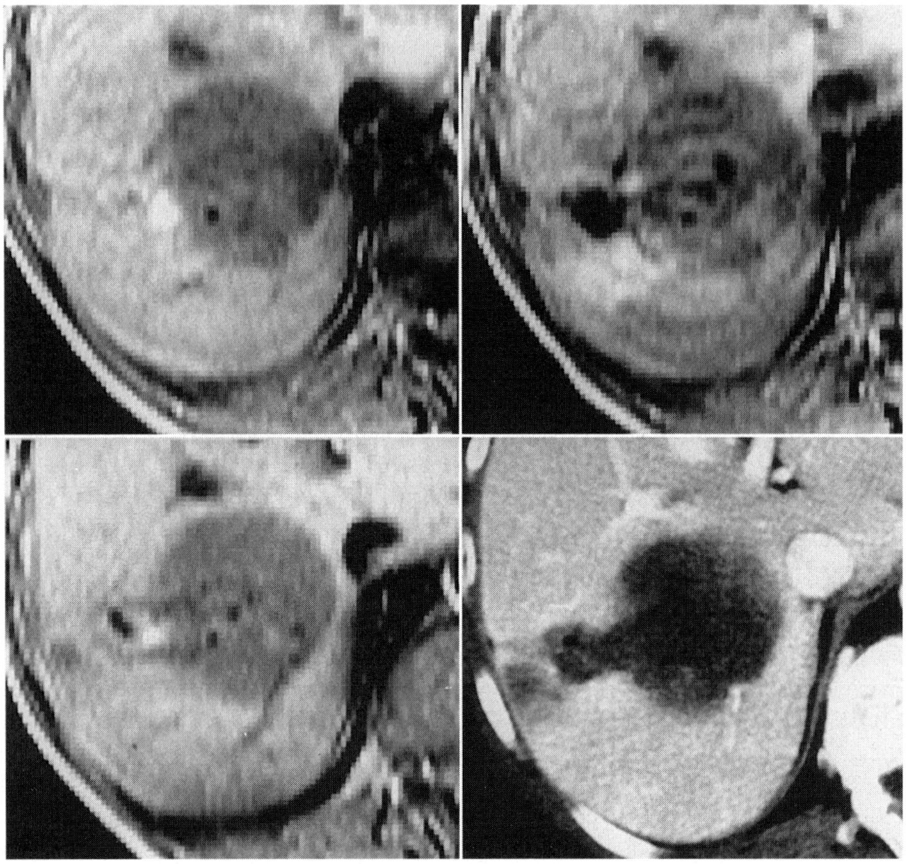

Fig. 23-2. Magnetic resonance images acquired at peak burn for treatment of a patient with liver metastasis with three pullbacks and 24-hrs after procedural computed tomography. (From Roberts HRS, and others: Magnetic resonance imaging control of laser destruction of hepatic metastases: correlation with post-operative dynamic helical CT, *J Min Invas Ther and All Tech,* 6: 53, 1997.)

Several approaches on how to couple light into the tissue exist. Some researchers use a focusing lens (typically 1 to 2 mm in diameter) at the tip of the fiberoptical system, which delivers the energy into a well-defined conical region.[20] Diffuser-tip fibers have also been used. However, laser energy deposition appears to be primarily a thermal process. A precharred bare fiber can provide equal thermal results at considerably lower cost and with a smaller fiber diameter (0.4 mm), allowing use of a finer needle gauge with considerably less discomfort for the patient. Each fiber produces a region of thermal damage, which approximates to a 3D Gaussian distribution and typically extends 10 to 15 mm about the tip.

Larger volume lesions can be treated using the pullback technique, in which the fibers are inserted to the distal side of the tumor and the first treatment initiated. After completion of the energy deposition (typically over 500 sec or longer), each fiber is pulled out by 1 cm and the treatment repeated. This procedure is then iterated until the entire lesion and safety margin have received thermal energy (Fig. 23-2). Occasionally, this approach requires repositioning of the fibers; however, the procedure often can be completed with one set of needle insertions.

The applicators are usually introduced into the patient under ultrasound (US) guidance. Some investigators perform the entire procedure using MR guidance. The sheath, needle, and fiber are inserted until the sheath reaches the margin of the tumor. The sheath has two purposes: to protect healthy tissue from being seeded with cancerous cells on retraction of the needle and fiber and to provide mechanical support and anchorage for the fiber once the MR-compatible needle has been withdrawn. MR-compatible needles produce a considerable artifact near the tip, making precise visualization of signal changes caused by thermal effects very difficult to observe; thus, the needles are usually withdrawn. New materials for manufacturing MR-compatible needles (e.g., carbon fiber tubes) may solve this problem. The fibers can also be coated with magnetite markers or small superferromagnetic particles to allow direct visualization of the fiber without the presence of a needle.[64]

US systems can be used near the MR system if a long cable is used. US images can be acquired[65] in the MRI field with no degradation of image quality. This ability allows the high temporal resolution and ease of spatial location of US for applicator positioning to be advantageously combined with the high contrast and spatial resolution of MRI for thermal monitoring.

MR-compatible optical guidance systems are an alternative approach to localizing the laser applicator. These systems use a pair of infrared light-emitting diodes (LEDs) attached to a probe, which the physician holds and to which the applicator device may be attached. The light from the LEDs is picked up by spatially sensitive photodetectors, which can calculate the exact 3D location of the probe with respect to a fixed coordinate system (often based at the center of the magnet). From these data, the MR system can be set to acquire oblique images perpendicular and parallel to the plane of the probe, allowing the clinician to readily locate the probe. The positional information may also be used to reformat previously acquired high-resolution 3D images to present a high-resolution 2D image of the required plane in the case of stationary organs.

MR-compatible stereotactic localization frames, which control needle angulation and trajectory, may be used to assist in placing applicators. They require MR reference markers, which are visible in all image planes. They are more useful in relatively static organs (e.g., brain, prostate), in which previously acquired high-resolution images may help guidance.

INTERVENTIONAL MAGNETIC RESONANCE SYSTEMS

Interventional MRI–guided laser therapy can be performed on a conventional tunnel MRI unit.[66] In practice, however, adequate assessment of the patient during the procedure may be difficult. Additional pain control and anesthesia during the procedure often result in considerable delays because of the need to re-establish the image plane after repositioning the patient.

New open-aperture magnets specifically designed for interventional use have largely solved these problems. Most of these systems currently operate at 0.5 T or below and feature less than state-of-the-art imaging performance using gradient systems of 15 mT/m or less. Newer interventional MRI systems with various field strengths, magnet geometries, and lower costs are under investigation and should be available soon.[39–42]

Interventional MRI systems typically feature in-room monitors, which allow the physician to control the scanner and view the acquired images in almost real-time while seated next to the patient. Special lighting systems provide good visibility of the patient, and MR-compatible monitoring and anesthesia equipment allow good patient care during the procedure.

Diode laser systems produce radiofrequency (RF) interference during operation (even in standby mode) and cannot be used in the suite during imaging. Typically, the laser is situated outside the MR room, and long fibers (10 to 15 m) are fed through a wave guide into the MR suite. Good communication between the laser operator and the interventional MR physician is required unless the laser can be activated remotely (which has obvious safety implications).

Acoustic noise from the MR system becomes important when physicians and technologists are working continually within the imaging environment; care should be taken to ensure that safe working limits are not exceeded. The staff will receive some exposure to RF energy, especially on systems that use a whole-body transmitting coil, although this exposure is usually less than the recommended SAR limits. It may be precautionary to devise some form of integrating RF exposure badge, similar to x-ray badges, for staff exposed daily on a long-term basis. Long-term exposure to fringe static and oscillating magnetic fields is unlikely to give rise to health hazards, but this situation is new and should be carefully monitored.

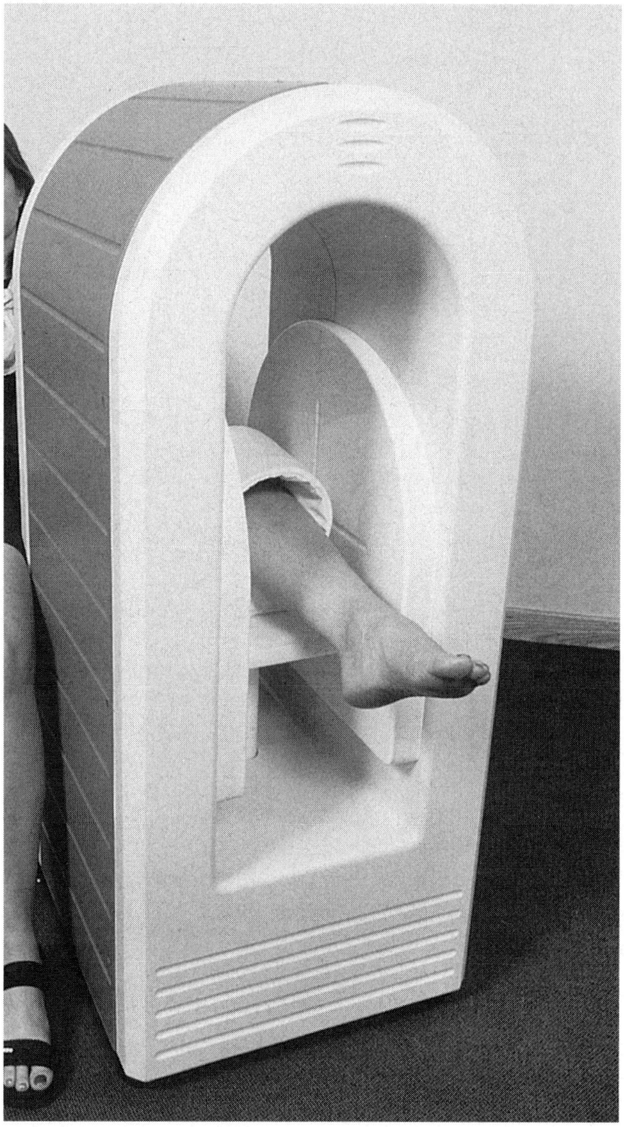

Fig. 23-3. This specialized interventional magnetic resonance imaging system is limited to extremity body parts.

Use of dedicated MR systems for specific parts of the body can help reduce many potential long-term exposure hazards associated with interventional MRI and can provide better access to the patient with reduced operating costs (Fig. 23-3).

MAGNETIC RESONANCE IMAGING SEQUENCES FOR LASER THERAPY MONITORING

An advantage of MRI is high sensitivity to many physical parameters; the many imaging sequences available allow contrast to be optimized for a particular situation. Imaging sequences for interventional laser monitoring should meet the following requirements:

A 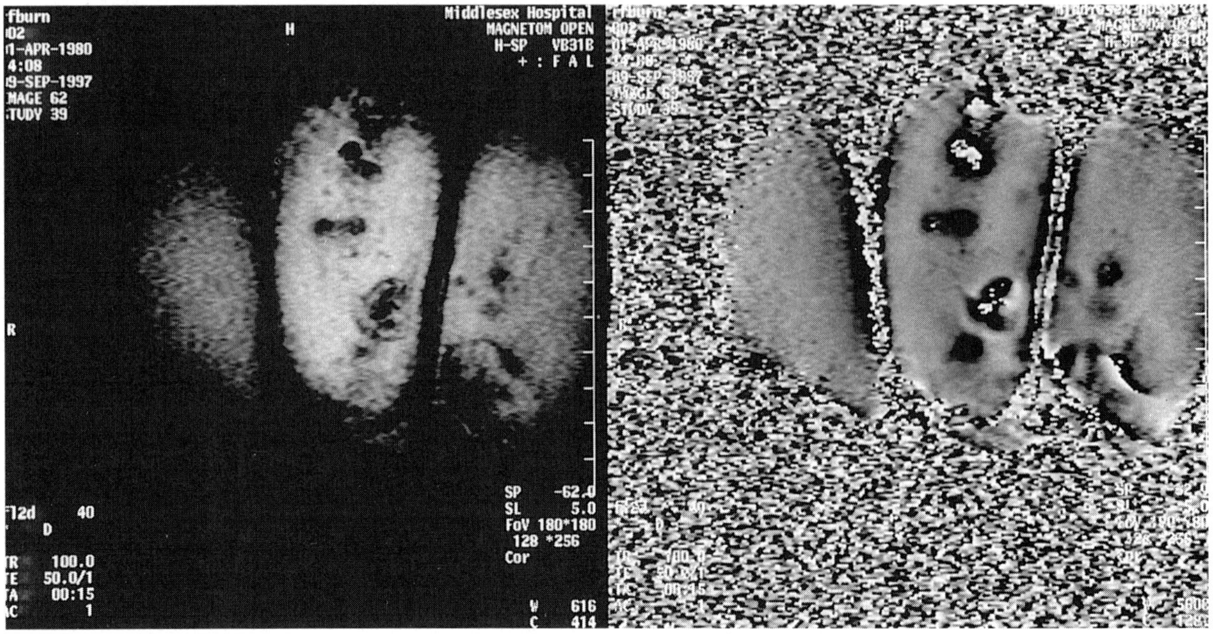 B

Fig. 23-4. A, Gradient echo with heavy T2*-weighting (repetition time, 100 msec; echo time, 50 msec) acquired from a thermal injury (laser) in chicken muscle at 0.2 T. **B,** The corresponding phase map.

1. High temporal resolution of 30 sec per sequence allows 20 to 30 images to be acquired during a thermal procedure, which is usually adequate. For needle localization, time resolution (including image reconstruction and display) of less than 0.5 sec is required.
2. Moderate spatial resolution typically involves 1- to 2-mm in-plane resolution and 3- to 7-mm slice resolution for interventions in the body. Fibers tend to move in and out of plane because of respiration, so acquisition of three to four adjacent planes is usually required for each image.
3. High contrast resolution differentiates the lesion from healthy tissue for needle localization, unless the needles were positioned under US or computed tomography guidance.
4. High thermal sensitivity involves an increasing T1 relaxation time as the lesion evolves, resulting in a loss of signal on a T1-weighted sequence. This process is somewhat complicated because at higher temperatures (approximately 60° C) the tissue starts to coagulate as proteins denature, and there are subsequent changes in proton density and nonlinear changes in T1.
5. Low sensitivity to susceptibility effects for needle location requires that the needle artifact depend on the needle susceptibility, magnetic field strength, the needle angle with respect to the main field direction, the direction of frequency encoding, and the imaging sequence frequency bandwidth.
6. High sensitivity to susceptibility and relaxation effects for monitoring intraprocedural changes in the blood is required. As blood is heated, the state of iron atoms in hemoglobin may change, altering relaxivity. Intracellular deoxyhemoglobin reduces signal on T1-weighted images, whereas intra- and extracellular methemoglobin increases signal. These contrast mechanisms compete with the thermal change in T1 to modify image contrast, and they may give unpredictable results depending on the details of the imaging sequence.
7. Low sensitivity to bulk patient motion requires breathhold imaging sequences for procedural monitoring, as long as the patient remains conscious and alert enough to comply.

The imaging sequences that best suit most of these requirements are rapid fast low-angle shot (FLASH) and fast imaging with steady-state precision (FISP), which produce T1 and T2* contrast with low motion artifact and allow three to four planes to be acquired within the breathhold time window of 15 to 30 sec with relatively high spatial and contrast resolution. In turbo format, these sequences are also useful for needle guidance to the target, with scan times of less than 1 sec. Figure 23-4 illustrates a thermal burn monitored by a heavily T2*-weighted sequence acquired on an open MR system at 0.2 T. T1-weighting provides a much weaker effect at this field strength.

Echoplanar imaging, although faster in principle, has several drawbacks for interventional use. It is oversensitive to susceptibility and current-generation MR-compatible needles produce excessive artifact. It also has poor signal-to-noise ratio, especially at low field strength, and is unavailable on some first-generation interventional MRI systems.[67]

Spin-echo imaging, especially in turbo mode, is less sensitive to susceptibility artifacts while retaining T1 thermal sensitivity; it is also useful for needle artifact reduction. Use of high-

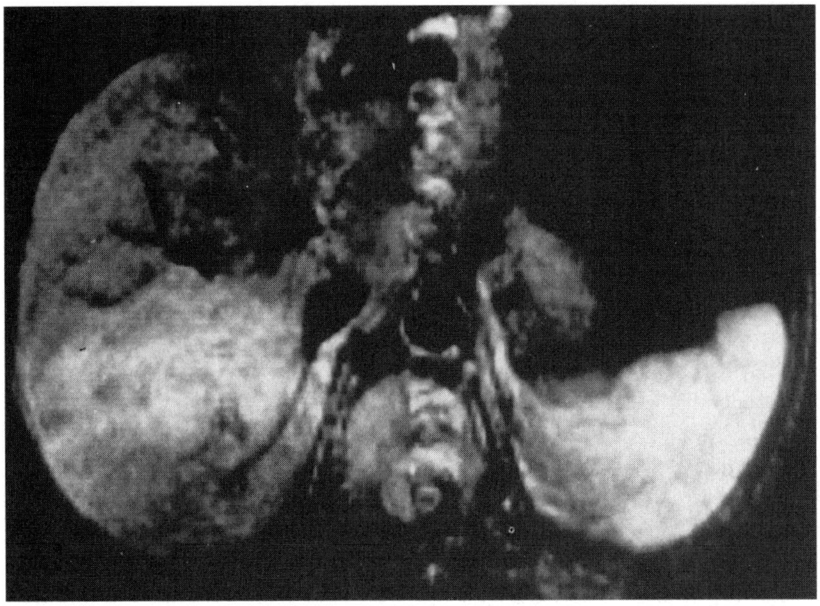

Fig. 23-5. A 24-hr postprocedure short TI inversion recovery image of a patient with laser-treated liver metastasis.

resolution spin-echo images is common after completion of needle localization to confirm the tip positioning. Spin-echo imaging appears to be less useful for thermal monitoring in human liver because of competing contrast from thermal and blood-related mechanisms, which appear to cancel out signal changes. Good results have been shown in rodent models with a high-intensity signal rim developing after the laser is switched off, which marks the region of necrosis.[66,68] This difference between the signal changes on spin-echo in rodents and humans may reveal more detailed physical and biochemical mechanisms involved in thermal changes.

In general, inversion recovery sequences take too long for procedural monitoring (except for some exotic turbo forms) but can be extremely useful for postprocedural monitoring. Short TI inversion recovery (STIR) images are particularly useful for highlighting edematous versus thermal changes after therapy (Fig. 23-5).

Gadopentetate (Gd-DTPA) T1 contrast agent is sometimes used during the thermal procedure. Gd-DTPA is extremely useful for postprocedural monitoring, and the results correlate well with other imaging techniques (e.g., computed tomography) to delineate the region of thermal necrosis.

TEMPERATURE MEASUREMENT AND ERRORS

The aim of interstitial laser therapy is to raise the temperature of the lesion to greater than 60° C while producing minimal effects within healthy tissue. The use of changes in MRI to produce spatially localized temperature maps around the fiber tips would be very useful. MR signal changes are nonlinear over the required temperature range because of several factors, including thermal tissue denaturation. Reversible quasilinear effects may occur over a temperature range of approximately 20° C greater than body temperature; however, above this range, nonlinear behavior introduces measurement errors.[69]

The most direct method to measure temperature is to insert fine thermocouples with fiberoptics to measure the temperature,[15] although such a system should be made MR compatible if procedural imaging is required. Also, the coverage and exact location of the thermocouples are difficult to ascertain.

An approximately linear change in tissue T1-relaxation time with temperature[70] provides the basis for the MRI signal reduction on heating. A linear change in T1 implies an exponential change of T1-weighted signal with temperature, but over the limited temperature range this change approximates to a linear change in signal with temperature. Other methods investigated in this temperature range are diffusion-based sequences;[71] proton chemical shift–based sequences, which use the small change in proton chemical shift with temperature;[72] and the related phase mapping technique. MR thermometry is covered in detail in Chapter 13.

Because true temperature calibration cannot easily be achieved, it is essential to correlate thermal changes on the images with histopathologic results so a marker of adequate management may be obtained.[68]

IMAGE PROCESSING METHODS FOR MONITORING LASER THERAPY

Advances in processing algorithms and computing horsepower have led to an explosion in applications for image processing and display in image–guided therapy. Perhaps the most simple application is the use of pre-acquired high-resolution 3D datasets with multiplanar reformatting software to provide quasi–real-time updates of patient anatomy based on a localization device, which provides spatial position information. This technology is available and works relatively well in fairly static organs, such as the brain.[73,74] However, where considerable motion occurs in the body because of the respiratory cycle and where changes in tissue morphology and structure arise because of the effects of the thermal laser procedure (swelling, displacement, denaturing), the pre-acquired images are soon out of date.

In an attempt to overcome these problems, image registration schemes to align image sets acquired at different times are being investigated. Simple approaches treat tissue as a rigid body and apply simple rotation and translation operators to minimize the least squares difference between the two datasets in 3D. Sophisticated interpolation schemes, such as 'sinc' interpolation, reduce quantification of the data.[75] These algorithms have been improved and can be completed in almost real-time on very high-power workstations. However, the situation is more complicated as tissue warps and changes elastically and nonelastically. Which elements of treated tissue correspond with the original untreated tissue are difficult to determine.

Registration and subtraction of pre- and postcontrast injection images is particularly useful in breast imaging, in which small amounts of patient movement can produce dramatic changes in subtraction quality. This drawback is especially important when small malignant lesions near fatty tissue are missed if accurate registration is not performed.[76] Changes with laser management lead to additional problems, which can sometimes be avoided with image registration.

Colored overlays of calculated data spatially registered onto the original high-resolution images are being used increasingly. For example, the temperature phase mapping method produces temperature distribution overlays.[20] This technique is easy to implement in software and can provide precise information to help the interventional physician to decide when to terminate treatment.

A major goal of image processing is to be able to automatically classify different types of tissue. Several schemes have been proposed based on edge detectors, pattern recognition algorithms, and scatter plot analysis. Scatter plot analysis is particularly useful for MRI data because MRI can acquire images with independent contrast behavior from the same plane. This approach allows a multidimensional histogram analysis of pixel values to be calculated, which provides a better separation of tissue clusters.[77,78]

An example of an automated classification is the computer laser assisted surgical system (CLASS) methodology, which has been validated in phantoms and in an extensive study of atrophy in patients with human immunodeficiency virus and acquired immunodeficiency syndrome and in control patients.[79] This methodology is particularly useful for monitoring longitudinal changes after therapy and can provide accurate volumetric changes in lesions. For monitoring laser therapy, the MR acquisition sequence should be adapted to use pairs of rapidly acquired 2D images from the same slice with different contrast behavior. For example, pairs of FLASH and FISP images can provide well-separated tissue clusters for the CLASS image processing algorithm to estimate thermal changes automatically. In principle, these data can be combined with previously analyzed spatial information on the target lesion to provide feedback to control management delivery. For a full discussion of all image processing strategies related to interventional MR, please see Chapter 20.

IN VIVO STUDIES OF MAGNETIC RESONANCE–GUIDED LASER THERAPY

Establishing the correct power and time characteristics for delivering laser energy to achieve complete tumor necrosis is important for creating adequate treatment plans for laser therapy of lesions *in vivo.* To establish whether necrosis has occurred, histopathology should be performed on resected samples of tissue that had received laser treatment. A sensitive way to make this determination is through use of nicotinamide adenine dinucleotide phosphate–diaphorase staining of resected sections.[18,68]

FLASH images of a resected rat liver are shown in Figure 23-6, *A,* and the corresponding diaphorase-stained section is shown in Figure 23-6, *B.* Figure 23-7 shows the correlation of the diameter of the region of signal reduction on T1-weighted spin-echo and gradient echo with the diaphorase-negative region from lesions created in 17 resected healthy rat livers after treatment with 1 W of laser power at 805 nm for 510 sec delivered through one fiber. The correlation coefficient was $r^2 = 0.95$ ($P < 0.001$); the gradient echo technique showed excellent agreement between the edge of the lesion at the end of MRI (defined as signal reduction greater than 5% from the mean before start of treatment) and the region of tissue necrosis.[68] Similar results for spin-echo images had a correlation coefficient of $r^2 = 0.88$ ($P < 0.001$).

A 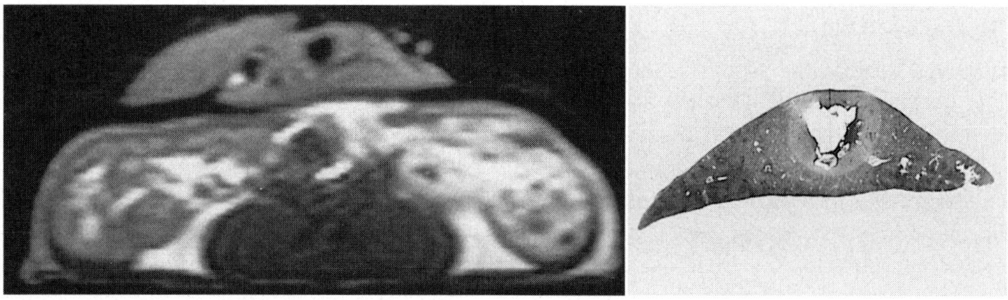 B

Fig. 23-6. A, A fast low-angle shot image and **B,** a diaphorase-stained section of laser-treated normal rat liver.

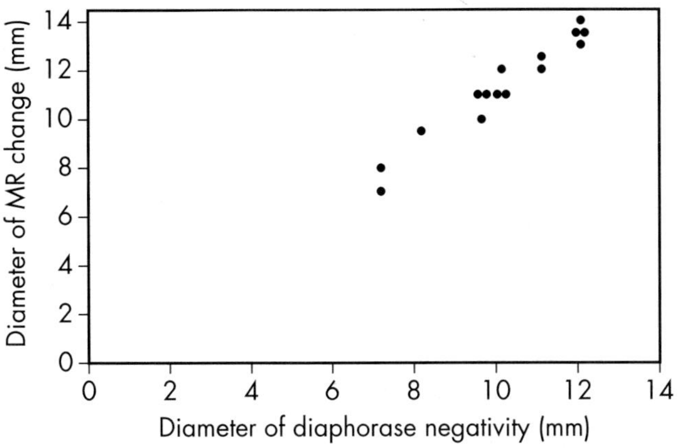

Fig. 23-7. The diameter of the lesion on T1-weighted fast low-angle shot images correlates with the diameter of the diaphorase-negative region for laser-treated normal rat liver.

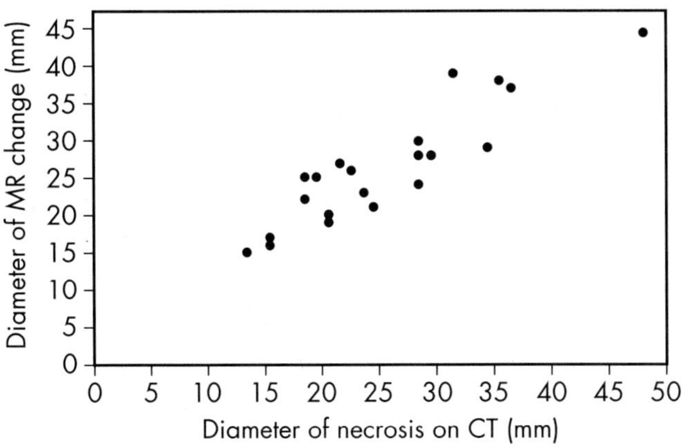

Fig. 23-8. The diameter of a signal change region on fast low-angle shot images correlates with that on a 24-hr delayed computed tomography scan of a patient with liver metastases.

Figure 23-8 shows correlation of the diameter of signal change caused by laser therapy on FLASH images of metastases from colorectal primaries in human liver with the extent of tumor necrosis assessed by the gold standard dynamic computed tomography at 24 hr. Each treatment used 1.5 W of power at 805 nm for 500 sec. The correlation coefficient was $r^2 = 0.83$ ($P < 0.001$) for 22 applications in seven patients. Good agreement was seen between the two methods for measuring thermal damage to metastatic lesions[66] and good validation was provided for the use of FLASH MRI to monitor laser therapy in liver metastases.

REFERENCES

1. Mumtaz H, and others: Laser therapy for breast cancer: MR imaging and histopathologic correlation, *Radiology* 200:651, 1996.
2. Harries SA, and others: Interstitial laser photocoagulation as a treatment for breast cancer, *Br J Surg* 81:1617, 1994.
3. Muller-Lisse GU, and others: MRI monitoring before, during and after interstitial laser-induced hyperthermia of benign prostatic hyperplasia: initial clinical experiences, *Radiologe* 36:722, 1996.
4. Flynn RJ, and others: Endoscopic laser ablation of the prostate (ELAP): changes in magnetic resonance imaging and clinical outcome at 1 year, *Br J Urol* 78:747, 1996.
5. Mueller-Lisse UG, and others: Postoperative MRI in patients undergoing interstitial laser coagulation thermotherapy of benign prostatic hyperplasia, *Comput Assist Tomogr* 20:273, 1996.
6. Tazaki H, Nakashima J, Nakagawa K: MRI evaluation of cavitation induced by laser prostatectomy, *J Endourol* 9:171, 1995.
7. Tazaki H, and others: Magnetic resonance imaging following microwave thermotherapy, laser ablation and transurethral resection in patients with BPH, *J Urol (Paris)* 34:105, 1995.
8. McNicholas TA, Steger AC, Bown SG: Interstitial laser coagulation of the prostate: an experimental study, *Br J Urol* 71:439, 1993.
9. Amin Z, Lees WR, Bown SG: Technical note: interstitial laser photocoagulation for the treatment of prostatic cancer, *Br J Radiol* 66:1044, 1993.
10. Fried MP, and others: Dynamic T1-weighted magnetic resonance imaging of interstitial laser photocoagulation in the liver: observations on in vivo temperature sensitivity, *Lasers Surg Med* 18:410, 1996.
11. Vogl TJ, and others: Laser-induced thermotherapy of liver metastases with MRI control: prospective results of an optimized therapy procedure, *Radiologe* 35:188, 1995.
12. Roberts HR, and others: Dynamic magnetic resonance control of interstitial laser photocoagulation therapy of colorectal hepatic metastases, *Lancet* 343:1221, 1994.
13. Amin Z, Bown SG, Lees WR: Local treatment of colorectal liver metastases: a comparison of interstitial laser photocoagulation (ILP) and percutaneous alcohol injection (PAI), *Clin Radiol* 48:166, 1993.
14. Masters A, and others: Interstitial laser hyperthermia: a new approach for treating liver metastases, *Br J Cancer* 66:518, 1992.
15. Steger AC, and others: Multiple-fibre low-power interstitial laser hyperthermia: studies in the normal liver, *Br J Surg* 79:139, 1992.
16. Masters A, Steger AC, Bown SG: Role of interstitial therapy in the treatment of liver cancer, *Br J Surg* 78:518, 1991.
17. Amin Z, and others: Hepatic metastases: interstitial laser photocoagulation with real-time US monitoring and dynamic CT evaluation of treatment, *Radiology* 187:339, 1993.
18. Amin Z, and others: Computed tomography-pathologic assessment of laser-induced necrosis in rat liver, *Invest Radiol* 28:1148, 1993.
19. Menovsky T, and others: Interstitial laser thermotherapy: developments in the treatment of small deep-seated brain tumors, *Surg Neurol* 46:568, 1996.
20. Kahn T, and others: Laser-induced interstitial induced hyperthermia of cerebral tumors with nuclear magnetic resonance tomography control, *Radiologe* 36:713, 1996.
21. Scholz M, and others: MRI–guided endoscopy in the brain: a feasibility study, *Minim Invasive Neurosurg* 39:33, 1996.
22. Kahn T, and others: MRI–guided laser-induced interstitial thermotherapy of cerebral neoplasms, *J Comput Assist Tomogr* 18:519, 1994.
23. Roux FX, and others: Stereotaxic laser interstitial thermotherapy: a new alternative in the therapeutic management of some brain tumors, *Neurochirurgie* 38:238, 1992.
24. Kelly PJ, Regli L, al Rodhan NR: Carbon dioxide laser and stereotaxic craniotomy, *Neurochirurgie* 38:208, 1992.
25. Sargeant IR, and others: Radiotherapy enhances laser palliation of malignant dysphagia: a randomised study, *Gut* 40:362, 1997.
26. Jager L, and others: Initial results with MRI-controlled laser-induced interstitial thermotherapy of head and neck tumors, *Radiologe* 36:236, 1996.
27. Vogl TJ, and others: MR–guided laser-induced thermotherapy in tumors of the head and neck region: initial clinical results, *Rofo Fortschr Geb Rontgenstr Neuen Bildgeb Verfahr* 163:505, 1995.
28. Sculpher MJ, and others: A cost analysis of Nd:YAG laser ablation versus endoscopic intubation for the palliation of malignant dysphagia, *Eur J Cancer* 31A:1640, 1995.
29. Castro DJ, and others: Metastatic head and neck malignancy treated using MRI guided interstitial laser phototherapy: an initial case report, *Laryngoscope* 102:26, 1992.

30. Loizou LA, and others: A prospective comparison of laser therapy and intubation in endoscopic palliation for malignant dysphagia, *Gastroenterology* 100:1303, 1991.
31. Lufkin RR, and others: Interventional magnetic resonance imaging in the head and neck, *Top Magn Reson Imaging* 2:76, 1990.
32. Ahmad A, Roberts C, Herderick EE: High resolution MR imaging and localization of laser-induced thermal injury in the vascular wall, *J Magn Reson Imaging* 6:868, 1996.
33. Sargeant IR, and others: Laser ablation of upper gastrointestinal vascular ectasias: long term results, *Gut* 34:470, 1993.
34. Brookes JA, Lees WR, Bown SG: Interstitial laser photocoagulation for the treatment of lung cancer. *Am J Roentgenol* 168:357, 1997.
35. Sargeant IR, and others: Radiation enhancement of laser palliation for advanced rectal and rectosigmoid cancer: a pilot study, *Gut* 34:958, 1993.
36. Loizou LA, Grigg D, Boulos PB, Bown SG: Endoscopic Nd:YAG laser treatment of rectosigmoid cancer, *Gut* 31:812, 1990.
37. Hendrich C, and others: Magnetic resonance imaging and temperature measurement in cartilage following laser therapy, *Orthopade* 25:17, 1996.
38. Castro WH, and others: Changes in the lumbar intervertebral disk following use of the Holmium-Yag laser: a biomechanical study, *Z Orthop Ihre Grenzgeb* 131:610, 1993.
39. Schoenenberger AW, and others: Puncture with an open-sided, interventional MRI system: illustration with a case report, *Radiologe* 36:705, 1996.
40. Silverman SG, and others: Design and implementation of an interventional MR imaging suite, *Am J Roentgenol* 168:1465, 1997.
41. Frahm C, Kloess W, Gehi HB, Weiss HD: A new laser puncture guidance device for CT- and MRT- guided punctures of the trunk, *Rofo Fortschr Geb Rontgenstr Neuen Bildgeb Verfahr* 163:73, 1995.
42. Silverman SG, and others: Interactive MR–guided biopsy in an open-configuration MR imaging system, *Radiology* 197:175, 1995.
43. Anzai Y, and others: Nd:YAG interstitial laser phototherapy guided by magnetic resonance imaging in an ex vivo model: dosimetry of laser-MR-tissue interaction, *Laryngoscope* 101:755, 1991.
44. Pushek T, and others: Dynamic MRI–guided interstitial laser therapy: a new technique for minimally invasive surgery, *Laryngoscope* 105:1245, 1995.
45. Schwarzmaier HJ, Kahn T: Magnetic resonance imaging of microwave induced tissue heating, *Magn Reson Med* 33:729, 1995.
46. Jolesz FA, Blumenfeld SM: Interventional use of magnetic resonance imaging, *Magn Reson Q* 10:85, 1994.
47. Demongeot J: Computer-assisted surgery: assessment and perspectives, *Chirurgie* 120:19, 1994.
48. Gewiese B, and others: Magnetic resonance imaging-controlled laser-induced interstitial thermotherapy, *Invest Radiol* 29:345, 1994.
49. Cline HE, and others: Magnetic resonance–guided thermal surgery, *Magn Reson Med* 30:98, 1993.
50. Castro DJ, Saxton RE, Lufkin RB: Interstitial photoablative laser therapy guided by magnetic resonance imaging for the treatment of deep tumors, *Semin Surg Oncol* 8:233, 1992.
51. Masters A, Bown SG: Interstitial laser hyperthermia in tumour therapy, *Ann Chir Gynaecol* 79:244, 1990.
52. Carbatzas C, and others: Nd:YAG laser treatment for bleeding from radiation proctitis, *Endoscopy* 28:497, 1996.
53. Menovsky T, and others: Interstitial laser thermotherapy in neurosurgery: a review, *Acta Neurochir (Wien)* 138:1019, 1996.
54. Fried MP, Jolesz FA, Morrison PR: Image guidance with laser applications, *Otolaryngol Clin North Am* 29:1063, 1996.
55. Black PM, Guttmann C, Jolesz F: Present and future applications of lasers in neurosurgery, *Keio J Med* 42:169, 1993.
56. Higuchi N, and others: Magnetic resonance imaging of the acute effects of interstitial neodymium:YAG laser irradiation on tissues, *Invest Radiol* 27:814, 1992.
57. Masters A, Bown SG: Interstitial laser hyperthermia, *Semin Surg Oncol* 8:242, 1992.
58. Steger AC, and others: Ultrasound features of low power interstitial laser hyperthermia, *Clin Radiol* 46:88, 1992.
59. McKenzie AL: Physics of thermal processes in laser-tissue interaction, *Phys Med Biol* 35:1175, 1990.
60. Hillenkamp F: Laser radiation tissue interaction, *Health Phys* 56:613, 1989.
61. Colles MJ: Medical lasers, *J Biomed Eng* 10:569, 1988.
62. Pearce JA: Laser applications in clinical medicine, *Med Instrum* 21:209, 1987.
63. Stein BS: Laser physics and tissue interaction, *Urol Clin North Am* 13:365, 1986.
64. Paley M, and others: High magnetic susceptibility coatings for visualisation of optical fibres used in MR guided laser therapy on a specialized interventional MRI system, *Eur Radiol* 1997 (in press).
65. Paley M, and others: *Combined MR imaging and ultrasound for interventional procedure monitoring,* Vancouver, 1997, ISMRM, Proceedings of the 5th Scientific Meeting.
66. Roberts HRS, and others: Magnetic resonance imaging control of laser destruction of hepatic metastases: correlation with post-operative dynamic helical CT, *J Min Invas Ther and All Tech* 6:53, 1997.
67. Cohen MS, Weisskoff RM: Ultra-fast imaging, *Magn Reson Imaging* 9:1, 1991.
68. Roberts HRS, and others: Magnetic resonance imaging of interstitial laser photocoagulation of normal rat liver: imaging-histopathological correlation, *J Min Invas Ther and All Tech* 6:41, 1997.
69. Young IR, and others: Further observations on the measurement of tissue T1 to monitor temperature in vivo by MRI, *Magn Reson Med* 31:342, 1994.
70. Dickinson RJ, and others: Measurement of changes in tissue temperature using MR imaging, *J Comput Assist Tomogr* 10:468, 1986.
71. Le Bihan D: Diffusion, perfusion and functional magnetic resonance imaging, *J Mal Vasc* 20:203, 1995.
72. Young IR, and others: An evaluation of the effects of susceptibility changes on the water chemical shift method of temperature measurement in human peripheral muscle, *Magn Reson Med* 36:366, 1996.
73. Cline HE, and others: Three-dimensional segmentation of MR images of the head using probability and connectivity, *J Comput Assist Tomogr* 14:1037, 1990.
74. Cline HE, and others: 3D surface rendered MR images of the brain and its vasculature, *J Comput Assist Tomogr* 15:344, 1991.
75. Kassam A, Wood ML: Fourier registration of three-dimensional brain MR images: exploiting the axis of rotation, *J Magn Reson Imaging* 6:894, 1996.
76. Davey M, and others: *Detecting breast cancer: registration of pre- and post contrast 3D data sets,* Vancouver, 1997, Proc ISMRM, 5th Scientific Meeting.
77. Kikinis R, and others: Computer-assisted interactive three-dimensional planning for neurosurgical procedures, *Neurosurgery* 38:640, 1996.
78. Vaidyanathan M, and others: Comparison of supervised MRI segmentation methods for tumor volume determination during therapy, *Magn Reson Imaging* 13:719, 1995.
79. Paley MN, and others: Cerebrospinal fluid-intracranial volume ratio measurements in patients with HIV infection: CLASS image analysis technique, *Radiology* 190:879, 1994.

Chapter 24

PRINCIPLES OF MR–GUIDED RADIOFREQUENCY ABLATION

Jeffrey L. Duerk, Jonathan S. Lewin, Yiu Cho Chung

Advances in imaging and interventional technology have profoundly impacted patient diagnosis and management over the past decade. For cancer diagnosis, interventional imaging–based diagnostic procedures, including percutaneous and stereotactic biopsy, have decreased the need for surgery and reduced patient morbidity, mortality, and expense. For management of cardiac arrhythmias, destruction of anomalous conduction pathways via catheter-based procedures has reduced patient morbidity. For patients with uncontrollable tremor, minimally invasive destruction of foci in the brain has improved patients' daily functioning.[1–3] Similar approaches have been used successfully for patients with intractable pain.[4,5]

Over the past several years, new methods for minimally invasive procedures using radiofrequency (RF) energy under magnetic resonance imaging (MRI) guidance to destroy localized regions of the body have been developed to manage cancer, alleviate pain, reduce tremor, and eliminate cardiac conduction abnormalities. This new interventional minimally invasive treatment technology may prolong life while reducing the morbidity and cost associated with local therapy, thus significantly altering medical care in many patients.

This chapter provides an overview of hyperthermia via RF thermal ablation and recent exciting innovations through the use of MR-guided observation and monitoring of localized tissue destruction. An example in a cancer patient defines some key clinical issues. Basic principles of cell death by temperature and hyperthermia physics are described. An overview of RF ablation systems is provided in the context of RF thermal modeling and treatment planning. Unique challenges of RF ablation in the MRI environment are also discussed.

CLINICAL EXAMPLE: REGIONAL METASTATIC CANCER

Local control of regional metastatic cancer is a significant and important component of cancer therapy for many tumors. In many patients, regional metastasis may be the only life-threatening component of their disease. For example, of the

160,000 Americans newly diagnosed with colorectal carcinoma each year, approximately 24,000 have metastases at the time of diagnosis, approximately 40,000 subsequently develop metastases, and approximately 80,000 die of metastatic disease.[6,7] In 20% to 30% of these patients, metastasis is initially confined to the liver,[6,7] and for many, progressive involvement is the sole determinant of survival.[6,8–11]

Patients with metastatic disease may have three forms of local cancer control: surgical resection, intra-arterial chemotherapy, and radiotherapy. Each form has cumulative side effects. For patients who are surgical candidates, resection of liver metastases significantly increases survival. However, the repeated trauma and morbidity may reach a point where further resection becomes a risk greater than the immediate threat of disease. The radiation and chemotherapy dose to other organs is cumulative, limiting safe treatment. However, many patients are not candidates for surgical resection, radiation, or chemotherapy and thus have no treatment options. An effective alternative to surgery, radiotherapy, and chemotherapy must be developed to control regional cancer. This chapter reviews a new method of MRI-guided RF ablation of tissue for treatment of cancer as well as tremor and pain.

Over the past decade, other minimally invasive methods for local cancer therapy without imaging guidance have been advocated, including cryotherapy, alcohol injection, and laser heating. These ablative techniques are problematic in immediately visualizing the effects of treatment.

More recently, these limitations are being overcome by combining the advantages of a minimally invasive method of tissue destruction with the ability to interactively observe and direct the procedure under MRI guidance to ensure complete destruction of the specified tissue. The major difference between MR-guided ablation and these non–image-guided techniques is that a lower-morbidity alternative to surgery that increases survival, particularly in certain types of cancer with regional patterns of spread, may be possible. Thus, development of this technique has great potential to alter the natural history of metastatic (and perhaps multifocal primary) disease and significantly improve the poor prognosis for these patients. Extension to other treatments, beyond cancer, is expected.

BASIC PRINCIPLES OF CELL DEATH BY TEMPERATURE

This chapter considers two forms of hyperthermia: chronic or long-duration low-temperature elevation–based methods for killing cells (i.e., classic hyperthermia) and acute or short-duration high-temperature methods (hereafter, cell ablation). The difference generally lies in the invasiveness of the procedure: to obtain high temperature changes localized to small regions in the body, acute methods often rely on minimally invasive methods for introduction of the energy delivery source.

Cells die when exposed to high thermal dose. At a fixed temperature, the fraction of surviving cells decreases as time increases. At a fixed time, the fraction of surviving cells decreases as the temperature increases. For example, at 42.5° C, virtually all cells survive for 10 min, whereas 0.1% of mammalian cells in culture (Chinese hamster CHO line) survive a 300-min exposure; this 0.1% survival is also obtained after approximately 10 min at 46.5° C. Although the cell survival curves for ionizing radiation and heat exposure have similar shape, the energy involved in cell inactivation is 1000 times greater for thermal mechanism than for x-rays. This finding suggests separate mechanisms for cell killing.

The actual neoplastic cell response to thermal challenge in hyperthermia should be considered. First, unlike healthy tissue, the vast yet less organized and less efficient capillary network in many tumors is usually fully dilated. As such, the tumor has limited ability to change its blood flow to respond to hyperthermia. Even at baseline, tumor heat dissipation by blood flow is less than and slower than that of healthy tissue, which often leads to increased tumor temperatures. Furthermore, tumor vasculature is more sensitive to damage at increased temperature than are healthy cells. Thus, as injury occurs, the inefficient vasculature network becomes even less efficient, dissipates less heat, and allows temperatures to increase further with additional injury ensuing. Thus, tumor blood flow may decrease during temperature elevation, whereas flow in healthy tissue increases.[12]

However, at increased temperature in thermal ablation, other processes may be involved in cell death. The activation energy of the chemical process responsible for cell death varies dramatically near 42° C, indicating different mechanisms above or below this temperature or development of thermotolerance over the extended hyperthermia durations required. Similarity between activation energy for protein denaturation and activation energy for heat cytotoxicity (from Arrhenius equation) led to the hypothesis that the target for heat cell killing may be a protein (e.g., structural, chromosomal, nuclear, repair enzymes, membrane).[12] The overall response is modulated by other factors, such as pH, hypoxia, and availability of nutrients. For cells undergoing hyperthermia, a thermotolerance may develop but is unlikely to occur for cells undergoing acute temperature (>20° C) changes as occur in most RF (or other) thermal therapies used in interventional MRI.

Classic hyperthermia (e.g., temperature change of 5° C to 10° C over 1 to 2 hr) exploits the different temperature sensitivity between healthy and malignant cells. This extended temperature elevation makes whole-body hyperthermia possible. However, ablation (temperature change of 20° C or more over seconds to 30 min) kills healthy and malignant cells identically. As such, localization is required. For both methods, the temperature rise not the heat deposition ultimately kills the cells.

RADIOFREQUENCY ABLATION SYSTEMS AND THEIR APPLICATION

This chapter discusses only RF ablation systems that rely on electromagnetic through-space propagation (propagating electric field) or on interstitial electrode placement (near electric field).

Through-space transmission systems

Microwave and high-frequency (approximately 27 MHz to 2.5 GHz) ablation systems, which generate high-frequency current oscillations in the tissue by through-space propagation into the conductive medium of the body, have been developed. Radiating systems include coaxial TEM systems; rectangular waveguide systems, in which the patient lies across two apertures in the walls of a rectangular waveguide; and annular arrays of RF applicators arranged around the body.[13] In phased-array systems, focusing is obtained (in principle) by altering the magnitude and phase of the RF current to each array element, thus achieving constructive interference of the electromagnetic fields at the site of the tumor. General difficulties in the use of broadcast versions of microwave hyperthermia include limited and nonuniform spatial power dissipation caused by skin depth effects and additional dielectric induced spatial nonuniformities and hot spots.

Interstitial electrode hyperthermia systems

Direct interstitial methods permit use of lower-frequency electromagnetic fields to reduce the extent of nonuniform heating problems. Frequencies from 0.5 to 27 MHz have been applied in direct interstitial thermal RF ablation of tissues. In these methods, electrodes are put in direct contact with the tumor to be ablated, most commonly via minimally invasive percutaneous electrode insertion.

RF thermal ablation systems typically use an RF power source ranging from 50 to 100 W of deliverable power and an instrumented electrode (e.g., a probe), which looks similar to a biopsy needle with wires attached. Closer inspection reveals no central cannula, a sealed tip, and insulation along much of the shaft. A few millimeters to a few centimeters of the electrode remain uninsulated, allowing RF current to flow into the surrounding tissue. A dispersive ground pad is placed on the patient, remote to the lesion site. Heat is then generated by ohmic or resistive heating from ionic movement and measured by thermal sensors in the probes.

At the wavelengths involved (frequency < 30 MHz), the body can typically be considered an infinite conductive medium; the current density is highest at the electrode and decreases further from the probe. The probe tip temperature increases from heat that flows back onto its surface; ohmic heating of the probe does not occur because the probe's resistance is much less than that of the tissue. Because current is delivered directly to the tissue, the total delivered power to the tissue (tumor and surrounding) is known. Energy delivery is controlled by the variable output current level, I, the tissue's resistance, R, (power $= I^2R$), and the duration of ablation.

Microwave RF ablation systems with direct capacitive coupling to the patient (i.e., the patient is part of the circuit and current path between adjacent electrodes) and interstitial microwave systems, which do not require a ground pad, are also available.

Theory

Why does a small change in current have a potentially significant change in lesion size during RF ablation? Why are tissue perfusion, thermal conductivity, and electrical conductivity of tissue important in thermal ablation? Understanding of virtually all electromagnetic phenomena, including RF thermal ablation in tissues, begins with Maxwell's equations. For the absorbed power in tissue to be determined, the electric potential field should be established by considering the current source (e.g., probes) in the tissue. Inclusion of the current source in the standard form of the H and E field relationship gives rise to:

(1)

$$\nabla \times H = (\sigma + j\omega\epsilon)E + J_{probe}$$
$$\nabla \times E = -j\omega\mu H$$

where E is the vector electric field (the interaction field around charged particles), H is the magnetic field vector (the interaction field around moving charged particles), σ is the tissue conductivity, ϵ is the tissue permitivity, μ is the tissue magnetic permeability, j is $\sqrt{-1}$, ω is the frequency of the RF oscillation, and J is the current density from the probe.[14]

At the RF frequencies used for interstitial hyperthermia (e.g., approximately 500 KHz), the wavelength is sufficiently long (>6 m) so the magnetic field in the second equation can be neglected.[15] Similarly, the ratio of $\omega\epsilon/\sigma$ is sufficiently small that a quasistatic approximation can be assumed.[16] That is, wavelength effects can be ignored, and the temporal response can be assumed to be in constant phase with respect to the applied current. Many accepted limitations of high frequency and microwave methods for hyperthermia (e.g., poor penetration, hot spots at fat-water boundaries) can be traced to the short wavelength and high frequencies used (> 400 MHz to 2.5 GHz). Thus, nonquasistatic solutions to Maxwell's equations and the dielectric properties of tissues should be considered.[17]

The quasistatic approximation allows

(2)

$$E = -\nabla V$$

where V is the electric potential. Furthermore, if J, the current density, is expressed as a general complex quantity ($J = \kappa E$; k = complex admittance), then

(3)

$$\nabla \cdot J + \nabla \cdot J_{probe} = 0$$
$$-\nabla \cdot \kappa \nabla V + \nabla \cdot J_{probe} = 0$$

If V is known, the volume power density in the tissue can be calculated from

(4)

$$\dot{\omega} = \frac{1}{2}\sigma|\mathrm{E}|^2 = \frac{1}{2}\frac{\sigma}{|\kappa|^2}|J|^2 \text{ (watt/m}^3\text{)}$$

where the specific absorption rate (SAR, in W/kg) is then calculated from $\dot{\omega}/\rho$ and ρ is the tissue mass density.[14,18] SAR, well known to mid- and high-field MRI users, provides a measure of the RF energy deposition per kilogram of tissue.

These equations indicate that the power delivered to each gram of tissue is proportional to the tissue conductivity and the square of the current density in that tissue. Current leaves the probe (electrode) and disperses throughout the tissue. As such, the concentration of current (i.e., current density) is highest near the electrode and decreases further from it. If the total current (and, hence, current density) is doubled, the local SAR will quadruple.

Power delivery to the tissue does not directly indicate how the local temperature will vary spatially around the probe. For local temperature increases in tissue to be determined, the bioheat equation should be solved. The principle of conservation of energy applied to any location within tissue is:[19,20]

$$\rho c \frac{dT(\vec{r})}{dt} = (\dot{Q}_P + \dot{Q}_m) + (\dot{Q}_{c\,in} - \dot{Q}_{c\,out}) + (\dot{Q}_{b\,in} + \dot{Q}_{b\,out}) \quad (5)$$

Here, $\dot{Q}_P$ is the conversion of electromagnetic energy into thermal energy (i.e., $\rho \times$ SAR), $\dot{Q}_m$ is the rate of development of thermal energy (typically insignificant), $\dot{Q}_c$ is the conduction of thermal energy into and out of the tissue at location (r), and $\dot{Q}_b$ is the thermal energy delivered and removed by the blood.

If the tissue is assumed to have constant thermal conductivity, k,[20] it can be shown that

$$\rho c \frac{dT(\vec{r})}{dt} = (\dot{Q}_P + \dot{Q}_m) + k\nabla^2 T + (\dot{Q}_{b\,in} + \dot{Q}_{b\,out}) \quad (6)$$

Normally, the flowing blood is assumed to arrive at arterial temperature (Ta) at a perfusion rate given by $\dot{w}$ and leaves at the local temperature T. As such

$$\rho c \frac{dT(\vec{r})}{dt} = (\dot{Q}_P + \dot{Q}_m) + k\nabla^2 T + \dot{w} c_b (Ta - T) \quad (7)$$

where c_b is the blood's specific heat. During ablation, T is greater than Ta. Substituting the RF application into the equation and allowing the metabolic production of heat to be negligible in comparison, the ablation energy deposition yields

$$\rho c \frac{dT(\vec{r})}{dt} = \frac{1}{2}\sigma |E|^2 + k\nabla^2 T + \dot{w} c_b (Ta - T) = \frac{1}{2}\frac{\sigma}{|k|^2}|J|^2 + k\nabla^2 T + \dot{w} c_b (Ta - T) \quad (8)$$

This equation can be interpreted as the time rate of change of temperature at location r is proportional to the square of the current density (RF energy deposition) plus the heat removal caused by perfusion from blood flow plus the diffusion of heat out of the location. This relationship allows appreciation of the experimentally observed difficulty of increasing the temperature and ablating tissues having higher blood flow, lower density, lower specific heat and/or lower conductivity when compared with average tissue. The importance of the local current density is restricted to power delivery to the first few millimeters adjacent to the electrode; beyond that, other mechanisms such as heat conduction become important.[21]

Local E fields are insufficient for determining the local temperature rise. Rather, properties such as thermal conductivity, blood flow, and temperature at the boundary of the nearby tissue will also affect local alteration of temperature. Clearly, the spatial heating pattern will depend on the current density (J), which in turn is dependent on the size and shape of the probe. Although the rate of blood perfusion to tissues varies widely across different organs, it is relatively constant in a given organ type (approximately constant locally) over small temperature changes but can vary significantly in tumors. The low variation in perfusion in healthy tissue provides initial motivation for developing thermal treatment planning systems; spatial variation at higher temperatures in healthy tissue and heterogeneity in tumors will complicate this task.

PARAMETERS AFFECTING LESION SHAPE

One difficulty in the development of RF thermal therapy treatment planning is the many tissue parameters that need to be known to accurately determine the time course of the developing spatial temperature profile. These parameters include tissue conductivity, tissue density, perfusion, specific heat, and location and blood flow in large vessels. Furthermore, these parameters should be known initially and as a function of time and temperature.

Nonetheless, much experimental literature guides understanding of the impact of nontissue parameters that influence the lesion's size and shape. Under various controlled conditions, it has been shown that:[22,23]

- Tissue charring from excessive local temperature increases, and formation of gas caused by temperatures greater than that of vaporization of water should be avoided for patient safety (e.g., hematoma, embolism).
- Lesion shapes are similar to oblate spheroids.
- The aspect ratio of the lesions (length to width) gradually decreases throughout the ablation, indicating that the lesions become progressively more spheroidal over the ablation duration.
- The length of the lesion is approximately twice the length of the exposed portion of a straight cylindrical electrode with sharp tip.[23,24]
- Lesion diameter increases with decreased probe gauge (approximately 1 cm for a 20-gauge needle during 6-min 80° C ablation in *ex vivo* calf liver).
- For constant-tip temperature during ablation, lesion volume increases with ablation time up to a plateau near 13 min (70° C to 90° C). The plateau is reached when an energy balance is obtained throughout the volume in which current flows. Clinically, total ablation times in the liver may exceed 30 min at 50 W.
- For fixed ablation time, lesion size increases with tip temperature; lesion size increases with the size of the equilibrium or basal temperature. That is, the higher the basal temperature (i.e., the temperature of the body as a heat sink), the larger the lesion. This aspect is easy to understand in terms of the energy balance (Equation 8) de-

scribed earlier. The temperature gradient to the boundary conditions is reduced at higher basal temperature; as such, the region falling within the temperature required for cell death and necrosis is greater.

- Variable lesion shapes (e.g., cones, dumbbells) can be created by using multiple electrode arrays or by varying the position of the probe and its withdraw velocity throughout the ablation time.[23]
- The lesion volume increases with use of multiple source arrays provided that the spacing is less than approximately 1.5 cm,[26] whereas the shape of a lesion depends on the spatial arrangement (e.g., spheres, cubes).
- The lesion volume can be increased through the use of a chilled saline perfused electrode, which allows greater power deposition before tissue charring.[27]

These results are likely to be useful guidelines for an *in vivo* ablation paradigm provided that the temperature rise at the probe tip is well controlled and does not lead to charring or vaporization. *In vivo* lesions are likely smaller than *ex vivo* lesions because perfusion effects are absent in *ex vivo* samples.[23] Similar results to those reported in the liver have been obtained in the myocardium, albeit with smaller electrodes, lower power settings, and shorter ablation times as required to ablate only localized conduction pathways.[28] More detailed descriptions of clinical MRI-guided RF thermal ablation can be found in Chapters 29 and 39.

Although the source electrode (i.e., probe) is critical in successful RF thermal ablation, the ground (or dispersive) electrode also affects the formed lesion, albeit indirectly if located remotely. The location of the dispersive electrode has no significant effect on the impedance, voltage, current delivery, and tip temperature during ablation. However, doubling its size may reduce the impedance and yield higher current density and increased tip temperatures, particularly if the initial probe-ground impedance is greater than 100Ω.[29]

In summary, a lesion's size depends on current density, tissue density, conductivity, and thermal conductivity. Lesion size is also influenced by duration of RF exposure (until thermal equilibrium is obtained), tip temperature, and probe size.[30] Size of the ground pad can also have an effect, albeit typically to a lesser extent than other parameters.

APPLICATIONS OF RADIOFREQUENCY ABLATION

The goal of any method for high temperature thermal therapy is to create localized temperature increases in the tumor to greater than 57° C to 60° C while simultaneously restricting the temperature in healthy tissues to normal ranges. Various applications for RF tissue ablation have been developed.

Brain and neurologic lesion generation

Initial methods for developing electric current–based lesions in neurologic tissues used DC currents.[31]However, inconsistent lesion size, dependence on electrolysis and subsequent gas formation, dependence on anatomic tissue planes, and vascular interruptions made the method impractical. Development of RF methods that relied on ohmic heating from ionic motion of electrolytes began overcoming this limitation.

RF thermal lesions have been generated in various brain and neurologic applications.[32] RF ablation techniques have been used to eliminate trigeminal neuralgia, in the ventrolateral thalmus to abolish tremor, in the cingulum to alleviate pain,[33] in thalomotomy,[31,34] in cervical cordotomy,[35,36] in pallidotomy,[37] in the treatment of advanced Parkinson's disease, and in the treatment of intractable seizures.[38]

Myocardial ablation

RF thermal ablation has been used most extensively in the treatment of various cardiac conditions. Cardiac arrythmias from multiple abnormal conduction pathways have also been treated successfully with RF ablation, typically under fluoroscopic guidance. Several recent examples exist.[39–46]

Tumor ablation

Recent reports show various applications in which RF energy deposition, via direct interstitial electrode placement, has been used successfully in curative and palliative treatment of cancer patients. The feasibility of the use of MR-guided RF ablation for treatment of brain lesions was shown in 1995.[30]

Abdominal tumors have also been treated with RF thermal therapy. These efforts have primarily been directed toward the treatment of liver metastases.[47–50] More recently, this treatment method was extended to use in MRI for localization and treatment monitoring.[51]

Modeling and treatment planning

With such well-described physical and physiologic phenomena in place and such wide-ranging clinical applications, various hyperthermia modeling programs have evolved. The most notable are those at Duke University, Stanford University,[53] Dartmouth College,[54] University of Wisconsin,[55] and University Hospitals Utrecht, The Netherlands.[56,57] All rely on formulation of energy deposition via Maxwell's equations and use of some form of the bioheat equation.

Methods of finite element analysis and treatment planning or modeling include use of uniform grids of points and the dielectric properties of the tissues,[57] use of surface patches to generate the finite element array from computed tomography data with extensive emphasis on result visualization,[54] and use of a frequency-dependent finite difference time domain method using a series of modeled phased-array antennas.[53] Tissue injury and modeling have also been developed to predict transient response of the temperature field in RF thermal ablation[58] and incorporate the influence of blood flow in large vessels.[59] Specific constraints imposed in myocardial ablation caused by the presence of significant blood flow, the torso, and myocardial tissue have also been formulated.[60] More recently, analytic solutions and experimental expectations have been compared with actual RF thermal lesions and used in patient trials.[16]

Full realistic and reliable methods for thermal treatment planning analogous to radiation treatment planning, which includes "a realistic 3D model of a patient including all the important inhomogeneities"[61] have to be achieved. Graphical user interfaces, models of multiple sources (196 temperature probes), and three-dimensional temperature mapping via thermocouple arrays represent a close approximation to the current state-of-the-art[62] in hyperthermia modeling, although accuracy remains to be verified.

INTERVENTIONAL MAGNETIC RESONANCE IMAGING RADIOFREQUENCY ABLATION CONSIDERATIONS

The success of RF ablation depends on ensuring that the RF probe is inserted in the lesion and not in tissue that is to be spared. Recently, interventional MRI use of RF ablation has predominantly used two approaches to localize the probe: stereotactic frames and frameless image-guided localization.

Stereotactic systems

Stereotactic frames are restricted to use in brain lesions. Use of stereotactic frames requires an initial set of images to be obtained before probe localization. This image set is acquired with an MR-compatible ring attached to the patient's head. The image data set is analyzed to determine the coordinates of fiducial locations on the frame and coordinates of the tumor. From these data, the coordinates of the lesions and the desired probe insertion angles[30] are determined, the patient is sedated, and a burr hole for biopsy and RF electrode insertion is made in the skull. The probe is then inserted as prescribed.

Frameless guidance

Stereotactic frames are not feasible in soft tissues (often no rigid structure for attachment) or in organs that undergo significant motion throughout insertion. In frameless stereotaxy, the actual coordinates of the lesion are irrelevant. Instead, near real-time images are acquired, which show the probe tip and tumor simultaneously through use of MRI's multiple-angle oblique imaging capabilities. Location of the insertion site and insertion trajectory can be determined by the interventionalist before the procedure via MR-compatible markers (in simplest form, fluid-filled syringes) or via localization systems that convert, for example, optical information on the location and orientation of an instrumented wand directly to the MRI system to adjust upcoming scan planes to follow the probe.[51] Recent advent of patient-accessible MRI systems has greatly facilitated the use of frameless stereotactic methods in interventional MRI.

Electrode and system issues

Noise

One challenge for the use of RF electromagnetic energy for thermal ablation of tumors is minimization of its interaction with the MR imager. After all, the MR imager is designed to detect extremely small time-varying magnetic fields and, as such, may detect any spurious fields generated in the frequency range of the imager, reducing image quality. For example, a 500-KHz RF generator has its 17th harmonics at 8.5 MHz (approximately 0.2 T), the 42nd harmonic at approximately 21 MHz (approximately 0.5 T), the 85th harmonic at 42.5 MHz (1.0 T), and the 128th harmonic at 64 MHz (1.5 T). Distortions to the waveform resulting from imperfections in generating a pure sine wave may broaden the spectrum around these harmonics and lead to spurious interference on imagers operating near these frequencies. RF ablation systems that operate at other frequencies will likely have similar problems, particularly because higher power levels (approximately 100 W) are being used.

Recently, researchers have successfully modified 500-KHz ablation units for use at 0.2 T. The Case Western Reserve University group used a switching circuit to open the thermocouple, RF electrode, and ground connections to the patient immediately before data sampling and restored them on completion of sampling. Duty cycles (ratio of ablating time to total time) of 60% to 90% or more have been obtained.[63]

Susceptibility

Basis of susceptibility effects

A second system factor that affects MR-guided RF thermal ablation image quality is the magnetic susceptibility[64] and potentially conductivity of the probe. Magnetic susceptibility (X) is used to relate the amount of magnetization caused by the magnetic induction field ($M = XH$: $X = \mu_r - 1$ where μ_r is the material magnetic permeability). Differences in X (ΔX) lead to spatial distortions of the applied magnetic field, which increase signal loss in image acquisitions via decrease in T2, or lead to image distortions. The amount of image distortion in the read or slice select direction is dependent on the difference in X, the magnetic field, and the read or slice gradient strength.[65]

The distortion, Δy, is dependent on the susceptibility difference, ΔX, the static magnetic field, B_o and the read gradient strength G, by:

$$\Delta y \propto \frac{\Delta X B_0}{G}$$

Thus, the same value of ΔX will produce different effects at different magnetic fields. The distortion will be inversely proportional to the pixel bandwidth in the read or slice-select direction. The distortion and added induced field inhomogeneity in Hertz will be less at lower fields.

Probe materials

Materials used to construct the RF probe for interventional MRI should be biocompatible and have minimal effect on image quality (distortions, local signal loss). The MR-guided biopsy literature provides guidance.[66,67] Commonly, RF ablation probes are made of metals (e.g., titanium, titanium alloys, alloys with high nickel content), which are biocompatible and have low magnetic susceptibility compared with conventional stainless steel.

Implications for needle insertion trajectory

The susceptibility artifact of an RF probe, with vastly different magnetic susceptibility from tissue, is dependent on the orientation of the probe to the magnetic field. In comparison with the distortions resulting from biopsy needles in MRI, the effect is minimum when the probe is parallel to the field and maximum when perpendicular.[67,68] The effect is greatest in gradient echo acquisitions, moderate in spin-echo acquisitions, and least in turbo spin-echo acquisitions.

The susceptibility artifact of increased local field inhomogeneity resulting from RF probes is neither good nor bad. During frameless stereotaxy, the interventionalist relies on the signal void to exaggerate the size of the device and provide a margin of safety for guidance near critical structures. Without the susceptibility artifact, probe visualization would depend solely on displacement of protons from the voxel (i.e., probe, not water in voxel). With many probes having a diameter smaller than 1 mm and voxel sizes greater than this amount, relying strictly on proton displacement from voxels will be insufficient. In image guidance, presence of susceptibility artifact is important.

Effect on temperature monitoring sequences

Guidance is only one aspect of interventional MRI RF thermal therapy. Effort is underway to develop temperature-sensitive pulse sequences that rely on proton chemical shift variation with temperature (approximately 0.01 ppm/°C). [69] In these gradient echo pulse sequences, variation in the local magnetic field inhomogeneity from the RF probe can cause signal loss in the tissue immediately adjacent to the probe and can thereby prevent observation of the tissue undergoing the greatest temperature change. Phase difference methods cannot be used to overcome this limitation; with no signal to measure, no phase can be determined.[70] In areas beyond the signal loss, the field inhomogeneity from the probe is constant between acquisitions and does not typically impact on phase difference methods for temperature estimation.

CONCLUSIONS

RF thermal ablation in interventional MRI uses induced electric fields from interstitial electrodes to create ohmic heating in tissue. The power deposition is proportional to the square of the local E field (or current density), whereas the actual temperature change is a function of tissue parameters, including thermal conductivity, electrical conductivity, perfusion, and local heat sinks, such as large vessels. Effective use of RF thermal ablation in interventional MRI relies on meeting the challenges of monitoring probe placement, progression of thermal lesion development, and accurately mapping or predicting local temperature changes. Understanding the manifestation of susceptibility artifacts in interventional MRI through studies of MRI-compatible biopsy needles has proven useful.

Unlike earlier antenna-based methods of RF (and microwave heating), direct interstitial methods at low frequencies (<1 MHz) avoid limitations of differential effects across changing dielectric properties in tissues (e.g., hot spots). The ability to vary the output power, monitor tip temperature, and detect tissue impedance suggestive of effective ablation make RF thermal ablation a useful technique to include in the armamentarium for local control of cancer.

REFERENCES

1. Sweet WH, Mark VH, Hamlin H: Radiofrequency lesions in the central nervous system of man and cat: including case reports of eight bulbar pain-tract interruptions, *J Neurosurg* 17:213, 1960.
2. Tew JM, Kller JT: *The treatment of trigeminal neuralgia by percutaneous radiofrequency technique.* In Keener EB, editor: *Clinical neurosurgery,* Baltimore, 1977, Williams & Wilkins.
3. Laitinen LV, Bergenheim AT, Hariz MI: Leksell's posteroventral pallidotomy in the treatment of Parkinson's disease, *J Neurosurg* 76:53, 1992.
4. Siegfried J: 500 percutaneous thermocoagulation of Gasserian ganglion for trigeminal pain, *Surg Neurol* 126, 1977.
5. Hitchcock ER, Teixeira MJ: A comparison of results from center-median and basal thalamotomies for pain, *Surg Neurol* 15:341, 1981.
6. Niederhuber JE, Ensminger WD: *Treatment of metastatic cancer to the liver.* In De Vita VT Jr. Hellman S, Rosenberg SA, editors: *Cancer: principles and practice of oncology,* ed 4, 1993.
7. Alexander HR, and others: Regional treatment strategies for unresectable primary or metastatic cancer confined to the liver, *Principles and Practice of Oncology Update* 10:1, 1996.
8. NIH Consensus Conference: Adjuvant therapy for patients with colon and rectal cancer, *JAMA* 264:1444, 1990.
9. Wood CB, Gillis CR, Blumgart LH: A retrospective study of patients with liver metastases from colorectal cancer, *Clin Oncol* 2:285, 1976.
10. Lise M, and others: Colorectal metastases to the liver: present status of management, *Dis Colon Rectum* 35:688, 1990.
11. August DA, Sugarbaker PH, Ottow RT: Hepatic resection of colorectal metastases, *Ann Surg* 201:210, 1985.
12. Hall EJ: *Hyperthermia in radiobiology for the radiologist,* ed 4, Philadelphia, 1994, JB Lippincott.
13. Bardati F, and others: SAR optimization in a phased array radiofrequency hyperthermia system, *IEEE Trans Biomed Eng* 42:1201, 1995.
14. De Bree J, Van der Koikk JF, Lagendijk JJW: A 3D SAR model for current source interstitial hyperthermia, *IEEE Trans Biomed Eng* 43:1038, 1996.
15. Plonsey RB: *Bioelectric phenomenon,* New York, 1969 McGraw Hill.
16. Strohbenm JD, Lynch DF, Paulsen KD: *Hyperthermic oncology.* In Susahara T, Saito M, editors: *Special plenary lectures: plenary lectures and symposium and workshop summaries,* vol 2, New York, 1989 Taylor and Francis.
17. Paglione RW: *Power deposition with microwaves.* In Nussbaum SH, editor: *Physical aspects of hyperthermia,* New York, 1982. The American Institute of Physics.
18. Iskander MF: *Physical aspects and methods of hyperthermia production by RF currents and microwaves.* In Nussbaum SH, editor: *Physical aspects of hyperthermia,* New York, 1988, American Institute of Physics.
19. Roemer RB: *Heat transfer in hyperthermia treatments: basic principles and applications in biological, physical and clinical aspects of hyperthermia,* New York, 1988, American Institute of Physics.
20. Nussbaum GH: *Conceptual outline of hyperthermia physics,* New York, 1982, The American Institute of Physics.
21. Wittkampf FHM: Temperature response in radiofrequency catheter ablation, *Circulation* 86:1648, 1992.
22. Goldberg SN, and others: Tissue ablation with radiofrequency: effect of probe size, gauge, duration and temperature, *Acad Radiol* 3:212, 1996.
23. Chung YC, Duerk JL, Lewin JS: Generation and observation of radio frequency thermal lesion ablation for interventional MRI, *Invest Radiol* 32:466, 1997.
24. Goldberg SN, and others: Tissue ablation with radiofrequency: effect of probe size, gauge, duration and temperature on lesion volume, *Acad Radiol* 2:399, 1995.
25. Goldberg SN, and others: Tissue ablation with radiofrequency using multiprobe arrays, *Acad Radiol* 2:670, 1995.
26. Reference deleted in pages.
27. Goldberg NH, and others: Radiofrequency tissue ablation: increased lesion diameter with a perfusion electrode, *Acad Radiol* 3:636, 1996.
28. Wittkampf FHM, Hauer RNW, Robles de Medina EO: Control of radiofrequency lesion size by power regulation, *Circulation* 80:962, 1989.

29. Nath S, and others: Effects of dispersive electrode position and surface area on electrical parameters and temperature during radiofrequency ablation, *Am J Cardiol* 77:765, 1996.
30. Anzai Y, and others: Preliminary experience with MR guided thermal ablation of brain tumors, *Am J Neuroradiol* 16:39, 1995.
31. Cosman ER, Cosman BJ: *Methods of making nervous system lesions.* In Williams RH, Rengachary SS, editors: *Neurosurgery,* New York, 1984, McGraw Hill.
32. Aranow S: The use of radiofrequency power in making lesions in the brain, *J Neurosurg* 17:431, 1960.
33. Hassenbusch SJ, Pillary PK, Barnett GH: Radiofrequency cingulotom for intractable cancer pain using stereotactic guided by magnetic resonance imaging, *Neurosurgery* 27:220, 1990.
34. Cosman ER, Nashold BS, Ovelman-Levitt J: Theoretical aspects of radiofrequency lesions in the dorsal root entry zone, *Neurosurgery* 15:945, 1984.
35. Rosomoff HL, Brown CJ, Sheptak P: Percutaneous radiofrequency cervical cordotomy: technique, *J Neurosurg* 23:414, 1965.
36. Lin PM, Gildenberg PL, Polakoff PP: Anterior approach to percutaneous lower cervical cordotomy, *J Neurosurg* 25:55, 1966.
37. Baron MS and others: Treatment of advanced Parkinson's disease by posterior GPI pallidotomy: 1 year results of a pilot study, *Ann Neurol* 40:355, 1996.
38. Patil AA, Andrews R, Torkelson R: Stereotactic volumetric radiofrequency lesioning of intracranial structures for control of intractable seizures, *Stereotact Funct Neurosurg* 64:122, 1995.
39. Prystowsky EN: Atrioventricular node reentry: physiology and radiofrequency ablation, *PACE Pacing Clin Electrophysiol* 20:552, 1997.
40. Simons GR, Klein GJ, Natale A: Ventricular tachycardia: pathophysiology and radiofrequency catheter ablation, *PACE Pacing Clin Electrophysiol* 20:534, 1997.
41. Vijgen J, and others: Tachycardia-induced cardiomyopathy secondary to right ventricular outflow tract ventricular tachycardia: improvement of left ventricular systolic function after radiofrequency catheter ablation of the arrhythmia, *J Cardiovasc Electrophysiol* 8:445, 1997.
42. Mangru NN, Young ML, Wolff GS: Radiofrequency catheter ablation of a verapamil-sensitive ventricular tachycardia, *Pediatr Cardiol* 18:235, 1997.
43. Kottkamp H, and others: Radiofrequency catheter ablation of the anterosuperior and posteroinferior atrial approaches to the AV node for treatment of AV nodal reentrant tachycardia: techniques for selective ablation of "fast" and "slow" AV node pathways, *J Cardiovasc Electrophysiol* 8:451, 1997.
44. Menz V, and others: Right ventricular radiofrequency ablation of ventricular tachycardia after myocardial infarction, *PACE Pacing Clin Electrophysiol* 20:1727, 1997.
45. Singh B, and others: Radiofrequency catheter ablation of accessory pathways in with congenital heart disease, *Indian Heart J* 49:198, 1997.
46. Van Hare GF: Indications for radiofrequency ablation in the pediatric population, *J Cardiovasc Electrophysiol* 8:952, 1997.
47. McGahan JP, and others: Treatment of liver tumors by percutaneous radiofrequency electrocautery, *Semin Interven Radiol* 10:143, 1993.
48. McGahan JP, and others: Hepatic ablation using radiofrequency electrocautery, *Invest Radiol* 25:267, 1990.
49. Rossi S and others: Percutaneous RF interstitial thermal ablation in the treatment of liver cancer, *Am J Roentgenol* 167:759, 1996.
50. Solbiati L, and others: Percutaneous US-guided radio-frequency tissue ablation of liver metastases: treatment and follow-up in 16 patients, *Radiology* 202:195, 1997.
51. Lewin JS, and others: Interactive MR-guided radiofrequency interstitial thermal ablation of abdominal tumors: clinical trial for evaluation for safety and feasibility, *J Magn Reson Imaging* 1998 (in press).
52. Reference deleted in pages.
53. Sullivan DM, Ben-Yosel R, Kapp DS: Stanford 3D hyperthermia treatment planning system: technical review and clinical summary, *Int J Hyperthermia* 9:627, 1993.
54. Paulsen KD: *Finite element modeling of hyperthermia delivery: the Dartmouth experience in hyperthermic oncology 1992*, vol 2, in Gerner EW, Cetas TC, editors: Arizona Board of Regents, Library of Congress No. 1021–9625, pp. 267–269, 1993.
55. Robbins HI: *Whole body hyperthermia: the University of Wisconsin Clinical Cancer Center experience*, New York, 1982, The American Institute of Physics.
56. Crezee J, Lagendijk JJW: Experimental verification of bioheat transfer theories: measurement of temperature profiles around large artificial vessels in perfused tissues, *Phys Med Biol* 6:843, 1991.
57. De Bree J, Van der Koijk JF, Lagendijk, JJW: A 3-D model for current source interstitial hyperthermia, *IEEE Trans Biomed Eng* 43:1038, 1996.
58. Hayes LJ, and others: Prediction of transient temperature fields and cumulative tissue destruction for radiofrequency heating of a tumor, *Med Phys* 12:684, 1985.
59. Lagendisk JJW: The influence of blood flow in large vessels on the temperature distribution in hyperthermia. 17–23.
60. Shahidi AV, Savard P: A finite element model for RF ablation of the myocardium, *IEEE Trans Biomed Eng* 41:963, 1994.
61. Cheng YC, and others: Calculated RF electric field and temperature distributions in RF thermal ablation: comparison with gel experiments and liver imaging, *J Magn Reson Imaging* 1998 (in press).
62. Lagendijk JJW, and others: Interstitial hyperthermia and treatment planning: the 27 MHz multi-electrode current source method, *Nucletron-Oldelft Activity Report* 6:83, 1995.
63. Zhang Q, and others: A method for simultaneous RF ablation and magnetic resonance imaging, *J Magn Reson Imaging* 1998 (in press).
64. Shenk JF: The role of magnetic susceptibility in magnetic resonance imaging: MRI magnetic compatibility of the first and second kind, *Med Phys* 23:815, 1996.
65. Ludeke KM, Roschmann R, Tischler R: Susceptibility artifacts in NMR imaging, *Magn Reson Imaging* 3:329, 1985.
66. Ladd ME, and others: Biopsy needle susceptibility artifacts, *Magn Reson Med* 36:646, 1996.
67. Lewin JS, and others: Needle localization in MR-guided biopsy and aspiration: effects of field strength, sequence design and magnetic field orientation, *Am J Roentgenol* 166:1337, 1996.
68. Moscatel MA, Shellock FG, Morisoli SM: Biopsy needles and devices: assessment of ferromagnetism and artifact during exposure to a 1.5T MR system, *J Magn Reson Imaging* 5:369, 1995.
69. Harth T, and others: Determination of laser-induced temperature distributions using echo shifted TurboFlash, *Magn Reson Med* 38:238, 1997.
70. Conturo TE, Smith GD: Signal to noise in phase angle reconstruction: dynamic range extension using phase reference offsets, *Magn Reson Med* 15:420, 1990.

Chapter 25

PRINCIPLES OF MR–GUIDED FOCUSED ULTRASOUND

Kullervo Hynynen, Ferenc A. Jolesz

The only noninvasive method to allow highly localized tissue destruction deep in the body is ultrasound (US) or shockwaves, its extreme form. Use of US in focal tissue coagulation was shown in the 1940s and was followed by extensive research that led to clinical tests of focused US surgery in brain disorders.[1,2] These early experiments did not, however, lead to the use of US in routine practice because of the lack of image guidance and the complexity of the procedure. Recent success with minimally invasive surgeries has led to renewed interest in focused US surgery in combination with online image guidance and monitoring. The first commercial clinical devices used diagnostic US to aim the therapeutic beam to the target volume. These devices have been tested in treatment of the eye,[3] prostate,[4] and bladder and kidney[5] with encouraging results. The clinical results have also shown variability between patients, indicating the need for online monitoring of the US exposures. Currently, only magnetic resonance imaging (MRI) provides potential exposure quantification. This chapter discusses the basic principles of focused US and the use of MRI to guide energy delivery. A more detailed description of the history of focused US surgery with references for studies not covered in this chapter may be found in several review articles.[6–10]

PROPAGATION THROUGH TISSUE

US is a form of vibrational energy (at a frequency greater than 20,000 Hz) that is propagated as a mechanical wave by the motion of molecules within the medium. For therapeutic purposes, the US frequency is typically 0.5 to 10 MHz. A continuous US wave propagating in a tissue causes the tissue molecules to form compressions and refractions such that the molecules oscillate around their rest position. This oscillation results in a pressure wave that propagates with the particle disturbance. The speed of the propagating wave (v) is independent of the frequency and is approximately 1500 m/sec in soft tissues and water. The distance between the molecules in the same phase of motion (e.g., the distance between two compressions) is the wavelength. The wavelength (λ) can be calculated from the speed of sound and from the frequency (f):

$$\lambda = v/f$$

For example, the wavelength in soft tissues at 1 MHz is about 1.5 mm and at 2 MHz is about 0.75 mm.

US can be generated by piezoelectric transducers, which are driven by a radiofrequency (RF) voltage at the frequency of the desired sound wave. The thickness of the piezoelectric element changes proportionally to the amplitude of the applied voltage. The electrical signal is thus converted to mechanical motion of the same frequency. The piezoelectric element is most often made of ceramic polycrystal that can be manufactured in a desired shape, such as a plate to generate planar waves or a spherically curved bowl to generate focused fields. The resonant

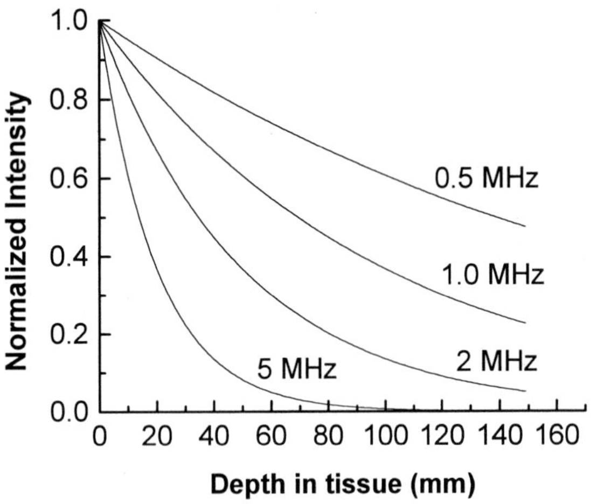

Fig. 25-1. Theoretical ultrasound intensity versus depth in tissue at different frequencies. The beam is assumed to be a collimated plane wave, and the tissue attenuation is assumed to be 5 Np/m/MHz.

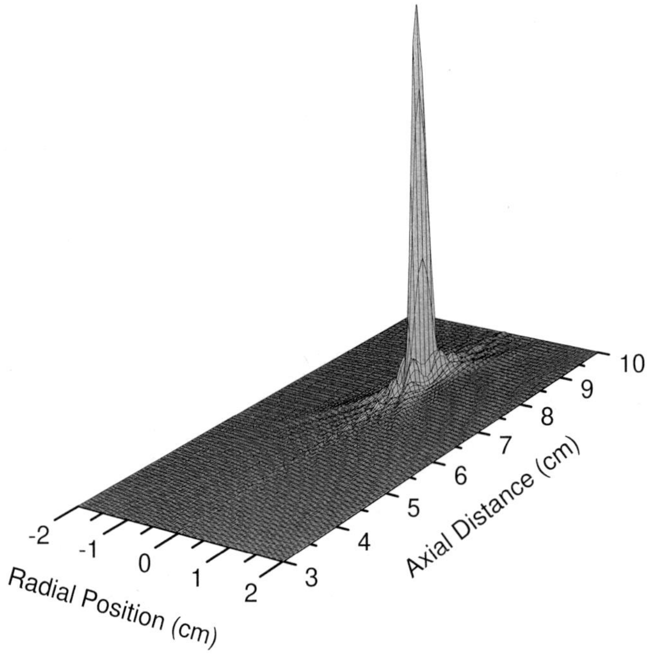

Fig. 25-2. A surface plot shows the ultrasound intensity distribution from a spherically curved focused transducer (diameter, 10 cm; radius of curvature, 8 cm; frequency, 1.5 MHz) calculated in tissue.

frequency of the transducer is determined by its thickness. For therapy purposes, the transducer is driven at the frequency that maximizes power output. The generated acoustic power is directly proportional to the driving RF power. Thus, the transducer can be calibrated and the desired acoustic output can be generated by controlling the RF signal. A typical therapy transducer converts 50% to 90% of the RF power to acoustic power.

As the US energy passes through tissue, it is attenuated according to an exponential law. The rate of energy flow through a unit area normal to the direction of wave propagation is called the *acoustic intensity.* At 1 MHz, the US wave is attenuated approximately 50% while it propagates through 7 cm of tissue. At 2 MHz, the wave is reduced to approximately 25% of its initial value by the same tissue. The attenuated energy is translated to temperature elevation in the tissue (Fig. 25-1).[11]

US is effectively transmitted from one soft-tissue layer to another with a small (few percent) amount of wave reflected back. At soft-tissue–bone interfaces, approximately one third of the incident energy is reflected back at normal incidence. In addition, the amplitude attenuation coefficient of US is approximately 10 to 20 times higher in bone than in soft tissues. This difference causes the transmitted beam to be absorbed rapidly, resulting in a hot spot at the bone surface.[12,13] At soft-tissue–gas interfaces, all of the energy is reflected back.

FOCUSED BEAMS

Similar to optics, the US beams can be focused by using focused radiators, lenses, or reflectors. The wavelength limits the size of the focal region, and the sharpness of the focus can be described by the half-intensity beam width ($d_{1/2}$) estimated by:

$$d_{1/2} = 1.41\lambda\ (R/2a)$$

where R is the radius of curvature and 2a is the diameter of the transducer.[14] A focal diameter of 1 mm can be achieved in practice at 1.5 MHz with a sharply focused transducer. The focus is typically 5 to 20 times longer than the diameter. The axial length of the focus ($d_{1/2ax}$) can be approximated by:

$$d_{1/2ax} = 7.1\lambda\ (R/2a)^2$$

Because the US beam is transmitted from an applicator that is several centimeters in diameter, the US intensity at the millimeter size focal spot can be several hundred times higher than in the overlying tissues. Similarly, the US exposure drops off rapidly across the focus, thus limiting the high US exposure to the focus (Fig. 25-2).

Similar focusing can be achieved by using transducer arrays that are driven with signals having the proper phase difference to obtain a common focal point (electrical focusing).[15] Large arrays allow multiple focal points to be induced simultaneously.[16,17] Large tissue volumes can thus be exposed with optimized energy-deposition patterns.[18,19]

TISSUE EFFECTS

The US beam can interact with tissue by elevating the temperature caused by energy absorption from the wave. The temperature elevation during short (a few seconds) sonications closely follows the US field distribution. At longer exposures, the thermal conduction and perfusion smooth the temperature distribution, resulting in less sharp gradients and more variable temperature elevation. The variability in the temperature elevation is induced by the increased influence of blood flow and perfusion on the heat transfer. Because blood flow varies according to location and tissue, the temperature distribution becomes unpredictable. In addition, tissue close to large blood vessels will be cooled by the flow if the energy delivery is slow. Short exposures can coagulate tissues next to the large blood vessels, as has been shown by theoretical models and *in vivo* animal experiments.[20–22] Therefore, exposures of 10 sec or less should be used to reduce the variability caused by blood flow and perfusion.

Different degrees of thermal damage to the tissue depend on the temperature reached and the duration of the exposure. The effect of elevated temperature on cells and tissues is a nonlinear function of time and temperature.[23–26] For exposures of a few seconds, temperatures greater than approximately 60° C are needed to cause irreversible tissue damage.[27] The elevated temperature can block microvasculature and stop blood perfusion in the coagulated tissue volume. Occlusion of surgically exposed veins by thermal effects of US has been shown.[28] The temperature elevation may also be useful in localizing gene therapy.[29] When the temperatures reach 100° C, the tissue water boils, resulting in gas formation. The gas blocks the propagation of the US beam and significantly modifies the energy deposition pattern.

Although US surgery has mainly exploited thermal effects so far, it can also induce mechanical tissue destruction if high-pressure amplitudes that induce gas bubbles are used.[30–32] The high-pressure wave causes these bubbles to expand and collapse. The collapse of the bubbles causes shock waves with high pressures and shear forces that can cause direct mechanical damage to the tissue. This phenomenon is called *transient or inertial cavitation.* The US exposures that induce cavitation often also induce tissue temperature elevation; thus, the thermal and mechanical effects are difficult to separate. Use of short bursts of high-pressure amplitudes allows the thermal effects to be minimized or eliminated; various mechanical effects have been observed. Histologic studies have shown that cavitation can break the blood-brain barrier, cause selective vascular damage, and generate tissue necrosis[33] and noninvasive occlusion of deep arteries.[34] In addition, animal tumor studies have shown that focused US-induced cavitation can activate certain chemicals.[35] The disruption of arteriosclerotic plaques and the formation of thrombi are also cavitation-mediated events.[36,37] High-amplitude focused US beams can also be distorted to shock waves at the focus;[38] thus, they may potentially influence cell membrane permeability[39] in a manner similar to shock waves generated by pulsed laser exposures.[40] An increase in blood vessel permeability has been shown in muscle tissue *in vivo.*[41] The use of mechanical effects may offer new therapeutic options.

ADVANTAGES AND DISADVANTAGES OF FOCUSED ULTRASOUND

The main advantages of using focused US are that it is noninvasive and can be focused. These advantages allow deep targets to be precisely destroyed without damaging overlying or surrounding tissues. These characteristics also make it possible to deliver the energy fast, thus minimizing the effects of perfusion and thermal conduction and resulting in sharp temperature gradients and accurate tissue coagulation. The fast energy delivery also allows use of MRI temperature-sensitive sequences without motion artifacts or signal changes induced by edema or perfusion changes that could reduce the accuracy of the temperature estimates.

The main disadvantages of focused US are its need for an acoustic window and its small focal size. The strong attenuation in bones and reflection from gas interfaces limit the use of US to sites that offer a soft-tissue window for the beam propagation. US propagation through overlying tissues limits the amount of energy transfer to deep tissues and allows only target volumes up to 3 to 4 cm to be coagulated in a 1- or 2-hr treatment session.[42] This size is larger if the target volume is more superficial. Larger tumors can be treated in multiple settings or by extending the treatment time.

THE ROLE OF MAGNETIC RESONANCE GUIDANCE

Recently, several groups[43–52] have tested the use of MRI to guide and monitor the focused US exposures. These studies have shown that temperature-sensitive MRI sequences can detect the temperature elevations at levels that do not induce histologic or physiologic tissue damage.[53] Thus, the location of the focus can be detected at low powers to verify that the targeting is accurate. Temperature-sensitive sequences allow the achieved focal temperature and the thermal exposure to be estimated. This feature can be useful in ensuring that the target volume is adequately covered. The tissue changes induced by the sonications can be detected using MRI. T1- and T2-weighted images can have signal intensity changes caused by tissue damage. Similarly, the tissue volume with coagulated capillaries can be detected by using contrast agent uptake.[45]

Good temperature resolution has been obtained using the proton resonance frequency. Changes in the proton resonance frequency linearly relate to temperature and can be mapped by using changes in phase images.[54–56] The disadvantage of the frequency shift technique is its insensitivity to temperature changes in fat. Based on *in vitro* studies of different soft tissues by Kuroda and others,[57] the maximum variations in the temperature dependency of the proton frequency in tissues are small enough to ensure that temperatures between 60° C and 100° C are reached during the 10-sec therapy exposures. The temperature history can be used to calculate the biologic effect or thermal dose induced by US exposure (Fig. 25-3).[58] In addition, the imaging can be used to monitor normal tissue temperatures for safety.

Some uncertainty still exists in the temperature coefficient of the proton resonant frequency shift, and more experiments in different tissues, especially tumors, are required. In addition, the coefficient may be dependent on the shape of the heating field.[59] In these calibration experiments, an invasive probe should be inserted in the tissue. Care should be used in selecting the probes because US-induced artifacts are present in the temperature readings. Some probes (e.g., many fiberoptic probes) are encased in plastic sleeving that absorbs US more than the surrounding tissue, causing artificially high temperatures. This artifact can be several degrees.[60] Generation of shear waves at the probe tissue interface causes a temperature artifact

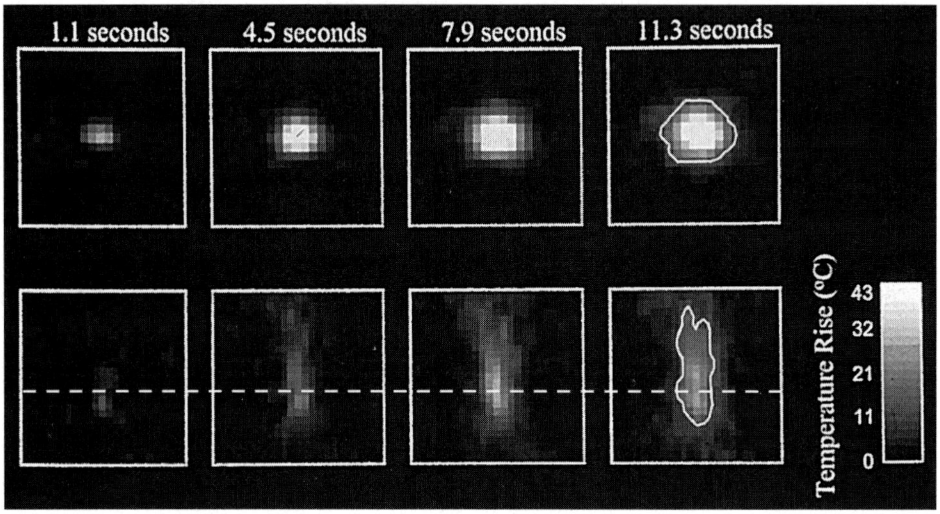

Fig. 25-3. The temperature distribution derived from the phase difference maps in a tumor of the thigh in a rabbit during and after a 10-sec sonication *in vivo.* The *top row* shows the maps across the focus, and the *bottom row,* along the axis of the beam. The *contour line* in the last image shows the boundary of the tissue coagulation estimated from the temperature maps. The *dotted line* on the images in the bottom row shows the focal depth of the transducer. The phase images were obtained using a fast spoiled gradient-recalled echo sequence, (repetition time, 26.6 msec; echo time, 12.8 msec; flip angle, 30°; matrix size, 256 × 128; field of view, 16 cm; slice thickness, 3 mm). (From McDannold N, and others: MRI evaluation of thermal ablation of tumors with focused ultrasound, *J Mag Res Imag,* 1998 (in press).)

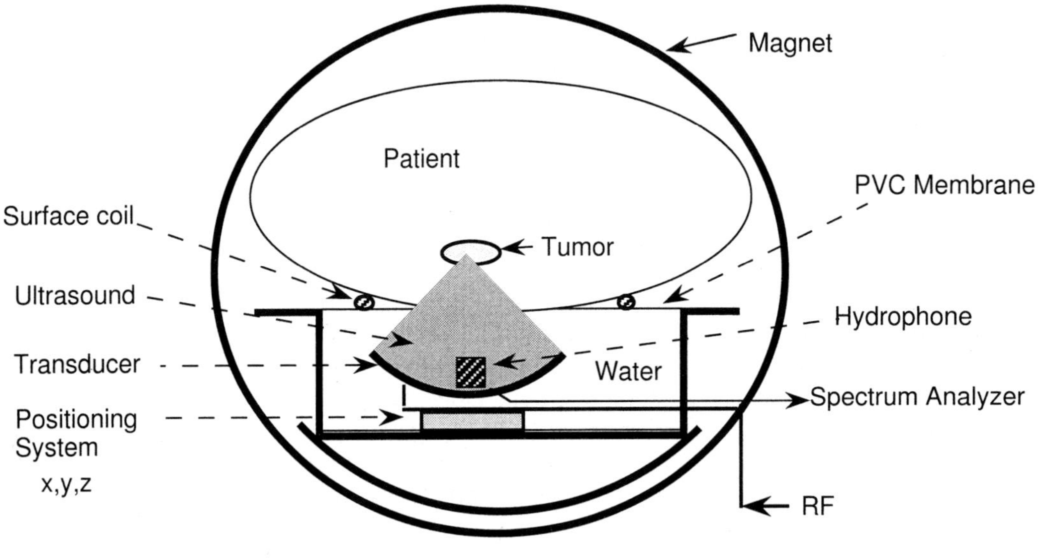

Fig. 25-4. The clinical prototype magnetic resonance image–guided focused ultrasound system manufactured by General Electric Medical Systems.

(viscous heating).[61] The probe size is typically similar to the wavelength and can thus distort the energy deposition pattern.[60] Generally, the artifacts can be minimized by using uninsulated small-diameter probes oriented parallel with the beam. In addition, the power should be briefly switched off before temperature measurement to allow the viscous heating artifact to decay. Therefore, caution is warranted when invasive temperature measurements are performed in US field.

A CLINICAL MAGNETIC RESONANCE–GUIDED ULTRASOUND SYSTEM

The prototype MR–guided US device was manufactured for surgery of breast tumors by General Electric Medical Systems and CRD (Milwaukee, Wis) in collaboration with Brigham & Women's Hospital (Fig. 25-4). The US fields were generated by one focused, air-backed transducer that was mounted in a standard MRI table. The transducer could be moved by a computer-

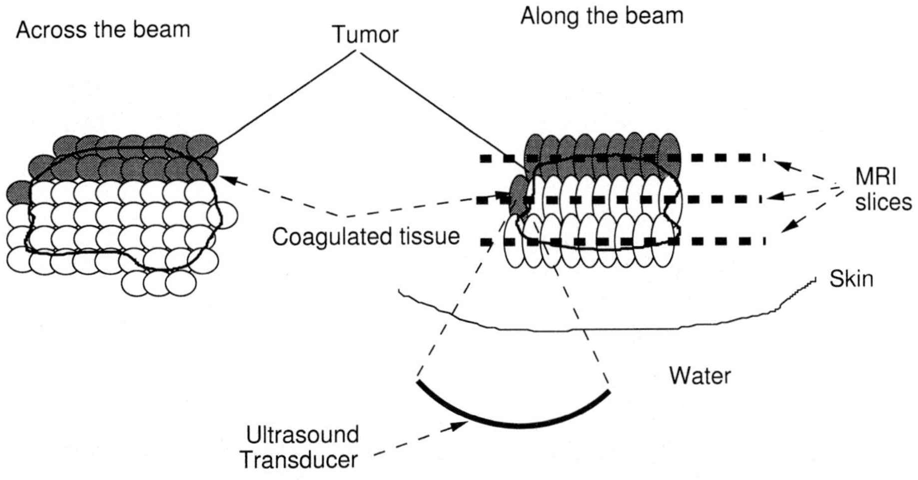

Fig. 25-5. The use of multiple sonications to coagulate a tumor.

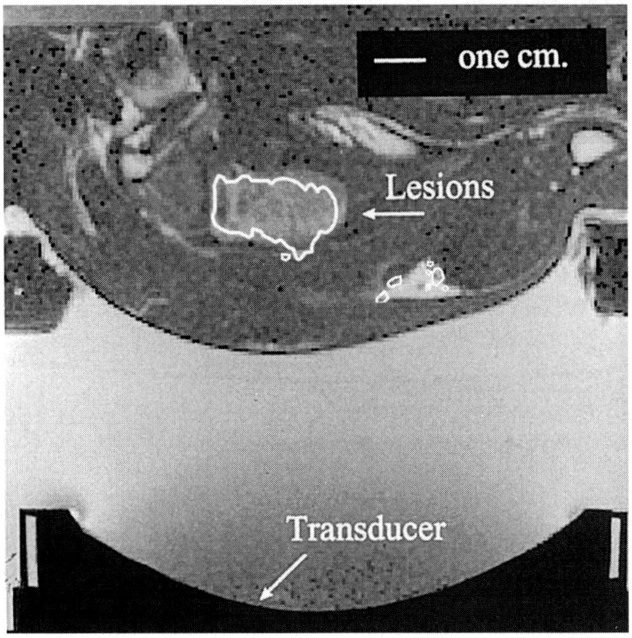

Fig. 25-6. A T2-weighted image along the beam axis shows the focused transducer and a rabbit thigh muscle that was sonicated *in vivo* using seven sonications placed next to each other (center to center spacing, 3 mm). The time delay between the sonications was 50 sec.

controlled positioning device in the *x*, *y*, and *z* directions in the waterbath, which acts as a coupling medium. In this prototype, the positioning was done by a hydraulic system. The latest version uses piezoelectric servo motors mounted at the end of the scanner table. A workstation that controls the transducer motion is programmed to aim the US beam at a location defined on an MRI scan.[47,49] A hydrophone next to the therapy transducer or in the middle of it detected cavitation. The collapse of gas bubbles is associated with wide-band noise emission that can be detected when the hydrophone signal is analyzed by a spectrum analyzer.[62]

During typical treatment, the target volume is outlined on a series of MRI scans. The workstation registers the target, aims the focus to that location, sonicates a low-power test pulse, and transfers the temperature-sensitive image obtained during the sonication. If the location of the temperature elevation is not overlapping with the target volume, a correction can be made and the test pulse resonicated to verify the alignment accuracy. After the test pulses, the complete target volume is sonicated using multiple high-power pulses placed so that the coagulated volumes overlap. Figures 25-5 and 25-6 illustrate this principle. The ability of this method to treat tumors has been tested by treating healthy tissues[46,47] and implanted tumors in rabbits.[63] The clinical testing of this system in the treatment of the fibroadenoma of breast is in progress. It is too early to make any conclusions on the clinical efficacy or toxicity of treatment (Fig. 25-7).

CLINICAL POTENTIAL

The proposed US surgery could replace some present tumor surgeries. Potential sites should have a soft-tissue window, which allows passage of the US beam without passing through gas or bone. In addition to the breast, some liver tumors could

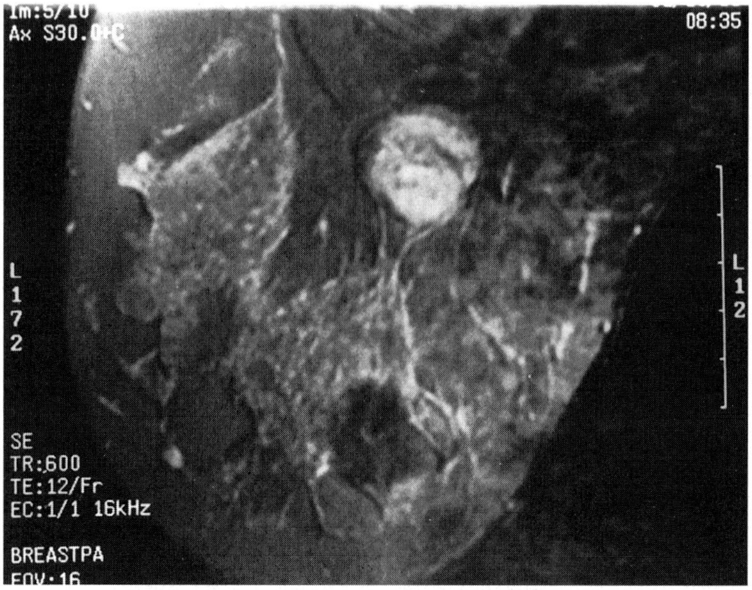

Fig. 25-7. An axial T1-weighted fast spin-echo image (repetition time, 600 msec; echo time, 12 msec; echo train length, 4; one data acquisition; field of view, 16 cm; slice thickness, 5 mm) with contrast of the sonicated breast 7 days after treatment, (sonicated tumor (*lower*) and untreated tumor (*top*)). (From Hynynen K, and others: A clinical noninvasive MRI monitored ultrasound surgery method, *Radiographics* 16:185, 1996.)

be treated with MR–guided focused US. Secondary liver cancer is a common problem with a poor prognosis. However, treatment of liver tumors is complicated by ribs and abdominal gas, which limit the available US window. In addition, the movement of the liver with breathing should be compensated. Prostate cancer, benign prostatic hyperplasia, and bladder and kidney tumors could be technically easier targets for MR–guided US. Many prostate tumors could be reached through the US window created by a full bladder or specially developed rectal applicators.[64] Bladder and kidney tumors could be reached using external US applicators. As in early clinical trials, deep target volumes in the brain can also be reached by US if a piece of skull is removed. The development of large phased-arrays may allow correction of the US beam distortion caused by skull bone[65–67] and adequate focus of the energy for trans skull-brain therapy.[67] This possibility would allow some brain tumors and functional disorders that can be visualized by MRI to be treated using focused US.

Blood vessel occlusion is useful for treating arteriovenous malformations in different parts of the body and for treatment of some tumors with an identifiable blood supply. It may also be useful for controlling abdominal, peritoneal, and pelvic hemorrhage and in the treatment of some trauma victims. Similarly, the experimental evidence that MR–guided and monitored focused US can modify the permeability of blood vessels and cell membranes may make it a key tool in targeted drug delivery and gene therapy.

CONCLUSIONS

Focused high-power US beams are well-suited for noninvasive local concentration of thermal or mechanical energy. The feasibility of guiding and monitoring the thermal energy deposition using MR has been shown in animals and in clinical settings, and this technique shows promise for tumor coagulation. However, more clinical testing and device development are needed before routine clinical use of this technique.

REFERENCES

1. Fry WJ, and others: Ultrasonic lesions in the mammalian central nervous system, *Science* 122:517, 1955.
2. Fry WJ, Fry FJ: Fundamental neurological research and human neurosurgery using intense ultrasound, *IRE Trans Med Electron* 7:166, 1960.
3. Coleman DJ, and others: Therapeutic ultrasound in the treatment of glaucoma, *Ophthalmology* 92:339, 1985.
4. Sanghvi NT, and others: Noninvasive surgery of prostate tissue by high-intensity focused ultrasound, *IEEE Trans Ultrason Ferroelectr Freq Contr* 43:1099, 1996.
5. Vallancien G, and others: Focused extracorporeal pyrotherapy: feasibility study in man, *J Endourology* 6:173, 1992.
6. Sanghvi NT, Hawes RH: High-intensity focused ultrasound, *Experim Investig Endoscopy* 4:383, 1994.
7. Sanghvi NT, Hynynen K, Lizzi FL: New developments in therapeutic ultrasound, *IEEE Trans Biomed Eng* 15:83, 1996.
8. Hill CR, ter Haar GR: Review article: high intensity focused ultrasound. Potential for cancer treatment, *Br J Radiol* 68:1296, 1996.
9. ter Haar GR: Ultrasound focal beam surgery, *Ultrasound Med Biol* 21:1089, 1995.
10. Crum LA, Hynynen K: Sound therapy, *Physics World* 9:28, 1996.
11. Wells PNT: *Biomedical ultrasound,* Boston, 1977, Academic Press.
12. Lehmann JF, and others: Heating produced by ultrasound in bone and soft tissue, *Arch Phys Med Rehabil* 48:397, 1967.
13. Hynynen K, DeYoung D: Temperature elevation at muscle-bone interface during scanned, focussed ultrasound hyperthermia, *Int J Hyperthermia* 4:267, 1988.
14. Hunt JW: *Principles of ultrasound used for generating localized hyperthermia.* In Field SB, Franconi C, editors: *Physics and technology of hyperthermia,* Boston, 1987, Martinus Nijhoff.
15. Ebbini ES, Cain CA: Multiple-focus ultrasound phased-array pattern synthesis: optimal driving-signal distributions for hyperthermia, *IEEE Trans Ultrason Ferroelectr Freq Contr* 36:540, 1989.
16. Fan X, Hynynen K: A study of various parameters of spherically curved phased arrays for noninvasive ultrasound surgery, *Phys Med Biol* 41:591, 1996.

17. Wan H, and others: Ultrasound surgery: comparison of strategies using phased array systems, *IEEE Trans Ultrason Ferroelectr Freq Contr* 43:1085, 1996.
18. Fjield T, Hynynen K: The combined concentric-ring and sector-vortex phased array for MRI guided ultrasound surgery, *IEEE Trans Ultrason Ferroelectr Freq Contr* 44:1157, 1997.
19. Hutchinson EB, Hynynen K: Intracavitary phased arrays for non-invasive prostate surgery, *IEEE Trans Ultrason Ferroelectr Freq Contr* 43:1032, 1996.
20. Dorr LN, Hynynen K: The effect of tissue heterogeneities and large blood vessels on the thermal exposure induced by short high power ultrasound pulses, *Int J Hyperthermia* 8:45, 1992.
21. Yang R, and others: Liver cancer ablation with extracorporeal high-intensity focused ultrasound, *Eur Urol* 23(suppl 1):15, 1993.
22. Kolios MC, Sherar MD, Hunt JW: Blood flow cooling and ultrasonic lesion formation, *Med Phys* 23:1287, 1996.
23. Moritz AR, Henriques FCJ: Studies of thermal injury: II. The relative importance of time and surface temperature in the causation of cutaneous burns, *Am J Pathol* 23:695, 1947.
24. Crile G: The effect of heat and radiation on cancers implanted on the feet of mice, *Cancer Res* 23:372, 1963.
25. Sapareto SA, Dewey WC: Thermal dose determination in cancer therapy, *Int J Radiat Oncol Biol Phys* 10:787, 1984.
26. Landry J, Marceau N: Rate-Limiting events in hyperthermic cell killing, *Radiat Res* 75:573, 1978.
27. Lele PP: *Threshold and mechanisms of ultrasonic damage to organized animal tissues,* Rockville, Md, 1977 Proceedings of a Symposium on Biological Effects and Characterization of Ultrasound Sources.
28. Delon-Martin C, and others: Venous thrombosis generation by means of high-intensity focused ultrasound, *Ultrasound Med Biol* 21:113, 1995.
29. Moonen C, and others: MRI–guided focused ultrasound as a potential tool for control of gene therapy, *Eur Radiol* 7:1165, 1997.
30. Coakley A: Acoustical detection of single cavitation events in a focused field in water at 1 MHz, *J Acoust Soc Am* 49:792, 1971.
31. Frizzell LA, and others: Involvement of ultrasonically induced cavitation in the production of hind limb paralysis of the mouse neonate, *J Acoust Soc Am* 74:1062, 1983.
32. ter Haar GR, and others: Ultrasonically induced cavitation in vivo, *Br J Cancer* 45:151, 1982.
33. Vykhodtseva NI, Hynynen K, Damianou C: Histologic effects of high intensity pulsed ultrasound exposure with subharmonic emission in rabbit brain in vivo, *Ultrasound Med Biol* 21:969, 1995.
34. Hynynen K, and others: Noninvasive artery occlusion using MRI guided focused ultrasound, *Ultrasound Med Biol* 22:1071, 1996.
35. Umemura S, and others: Sonochemical activation of hematoporphyrin: a potential modality for cancer treatment, *Proc IEEE Ultrasonics Symp* 955, 1989.
36. Siegel RJ, and others: Percutaneous ultrasonic angioplasty: initial clinical experience, *Lancet* 772, 1989.
37. Rosenschein U, and others: Experimental ultrasonic angioplasty: disruption of atherosclerotic plaques and thrombi in vitro and arterial recanalization in vivo, *IEEE Trans Ultrason Ferroelectr Freq Contr* 43:1043, 1990.
38. Carstensen EL, and others: Finite amplitude effects on thresholds for lesion production in tissues by unfocused ultrasound, *J Acoust Soc Am* 70:302, 1981.
39. Kim HJ, and others: Ultrasound-mediated transfection of mammalian cells, *Hum Gene Ther* 7:1339, 1996.
40. Doukas AG, Flotte TJ: Physical characteristics and biological effects of laser-induced stress waves, *Ultrasound Med Biol* 22:151, 1996.
41. Bednarski MD, and others: In vivo target-specific delivery of macromolecular agents with MR–guided focused ultrasound, *Radiology* 204:263, 1997.
42. Fan X, Hynynen K: Ultrasound surgery using multiple sonications: treatment time considerations, *Ultrasound Med Biol* 22:471, 1996.
43. Hynynen K, and others: MRI–guided noninvasive ultrasound surgery, *Med Phys* 20:107, 1993.
44. Darkazanli A, and others: On-line monitoring of ultrasound surgery with MRI, *J Magn Reson Imaging* 3:509, 1993.
45. Hynynen K, and others: The usefulness of contrast agent and GRASS imaging sequence for MRI guided noninvasive ultrasound surgery, *Invest Radiol* 29:897, 1994.
46. Hynynen K, and others: MR monitoring of focused ultrasonic surgery of renal cortex: experimental and simulation studies, *J Magn Reson Imaging* 5:259, 1995.
47. Hynynen K, and others: A clinical noninvasive MRI monitored ultrasound surgery method, *Radiographics* 16:185, 1996.
48. Cline HE, and others: Magnetic resonance guided thermal surgery, *Magn Reson Med* 31:628, 1993.
49. Cline HE, and others: A focused ultrasound system for MRI guided ablation, *Radiology* 194:731, 1995.
50. Suzuki T, and others: MRI monitoring during high-intensity focused ultrasound treatment, *Proc SMR 3rd Meeting* 10652:1177, 1995.
51. Stepanow B, and others: Fast MRI temperature monitoring: application in focused ultrasound therapy of malignant tissue in vivo, *Proc SMR 3rd Meeting* 1065:1172, 1995.
52. Smith NB, and others: Experimental verification of theoretical in vivo ultrasound heating using cobalt detected magnetic resonance, *IEEE Trans Ultrason Ferroelectr Freq Contr* 42:489, 1995.
53. Hynynen K, and others: Thermal effects of focused ultrasound on the brain: determination with MR imaging, *Radiology* 204:247, 1997.
54. Cline HE, and others: Simultaneous magnetic resonance phase and magnitude temperature maps in muscle, *Magn Reson Med* 35:309, 1996.
55. Chung A, and others: Optimization of spoiled gradient-echo phase imaging for in vivo localization of focused ultrasound beam, *Magn Reson Med* 36:745, 1996.
56. Cline HE, and others: Simultaneous magnetic resonance phase and magnitude temperature maps in muscle, *Proc SMR 3rd Meeting* 1065:1174, 1995.
57. Kuroda K, and others: Water proton magnetic resonance spectroscopic imaging, *Biomedical Thermology* 13:43, 1995.
58. Chung A, and others: Quantification of thermal exposure using proton resonance frequency shift, *Proc SMR 4th Meeting* 3:1751, 1996 (abstract).
59. Stollberger R, and others: Influence of the temperature dependent susceptibility on monitoring of interstitial tissue coagulation using the proton resonance frequency method, *Proc SMR 4th Meeting* 1963, 1997 (abstract).
60. Hynynen K, Edwards DK: Temperature measurements during ultrasound hyperthermia, *Med Phys* 16:618, 1989.
61. Fry WJ, Fry RB: Determination of absolute sound levels and acoustic absorption coefficients by thermocouple probes-experiment, *J Acoust Soc Am* 26:311, 1954.
62. Hynynen K: The threshold for thermally significant cavitation in dog's thigh muscle in vivo, *Ultrasound Med Biol* 17:157, 1991.
63. McDannold N, and others: MRI evaluation of thermal ablation of tumors with focused ultrasound, *J Magn Reson Imaging* 8:91, 1998.
64. Hutchinson EB, Dahleh M, Hynynen K: MRI feedback control for phased array prostate hyperthermia, *IEEE Ultrasonics Symp* 2:1285, 1996.
65. Smith SW, and others: *Some advances in acoustic imaging through skull.* In Hazzard DG, Litz ML, editors: *Symposium on biological effects and characterizations of ultrasound sources,* Rockville, Md, 1977, U.S. Department of Health, Education, and Welfare, Food and Drug Administration.
66. Thomas J-L, Fink MA: Ultrasonic beam focusing through tissue inhomogeneities with a time reversal mirror: application to transskull therapy, *IEEE Trans Ultrason Ferroelectr Freq Contr* 43:1122, 1996.
67. Hynynen K, Jolesz FA: Demonstration of potential noninvasive ultrasound brain therapy through intact skull, *Ultrasound Med Biol* 34:275, 1998.

Chapter 26

PRINCIPLES OF MR–GUIDED ETHANOL ABLATION

Alexandra R. Borges, David S. K. Lu

Ethyl alcohol (ethanol) has been used extensively in a clinical setting as a sclerosing and embolic agent. Selective injections into the arterial or venous system have found wide application in vascular therapy for sclerosis of esophageal varices and embolization of bronchial, hepatic, and renal arteries.[1] More recently, ethanol was found to be an effective agent for tumor ablation when injected percutaneously into neoplastic tissues. The most thorough investigation and application has been in the ablation of hepatic tumors, although other neoplasms, including thyroid, parathyroid, renal, and suprarenal tumors, are also amenable to this type of therapy.[2–5]

Ethanol ablation is easily performed, inexpensive, safe, and valuable in patients who are not surgical candidates. In the liver it has been used with varying success rates in the management of hepatocellular carcinoma (HCC), adenomatous hyperplasia, and metastases.[6–8]

Imaging is crucial for the performance and posttherapy evaluation of this form of management. The goals of imaging include identification of the lesion or lesions to be managed, delivery of the therapeutic agent without damage to adjacent structures, and detection of residual or recurrent tumor. Although magnetic resonance imaging (MRI) has been used primarily in postablation evaluation of lesions, the advent of interventional MRI guidance has revealed potential use for guiding needle placement and for monitoring the diffusion of ethanol and subsequent histopathologic effects of the ablative procedure.

MOLECULAR BASIS OF ETHANOL CYTOTOXICITY

Ethanol enters cells by diffusion, producing cell dehydration and protein denaturation, which lead to coagulation necrosis, similar to that seen in other types of chemical injury.[7] In this type of necrosis, nucleolysis occurs with preservation of the cellular membranes, which permits recognition of the cellular outlines and tissue architecture.[9] The mechanism of protein denaturation is not fully understood. Dehydration leads to decreased solubility, delaying the proteolysis by lysosomal enzymes and preserving an eosinophilic coagulate for several days. Ultimately, the coagulated cells undergo liquefaction and are removed by fragmentation and phagocytosis. Fibrotic changes ensue, with replacement of the necrotic tissue. In addition, alcohol produces ischemic changes via damage to the endothelial lining of vessels, with subsequent thrombosis and vascular occlusion.[7]

CLINICAL APPLICATION

The broadest application of percutaneous ethanol ablation (PEA) has been for management of liver tumors. The choice of management depends on several factors, including the severity of underlying liver disease and the number, size, and location of the lesions.[6,7,10–13] Many patients are not surgical candidates because of poor liver function reserve related to cirrhosis or because of the presence of multiple lesions involving both hepatic lobes. Ethanol ablation is associated with minimal morbidity and does not damage healthy liver parenchyma.[6,7,10–14] HCC is a soft tumor typically surrounded by hard cirrhotic parenchyma, which allows for selective diffusion of ethanol into the neoplastic tissue. Once recurrence occurs, this technique can be used repeatedly without increased risk.[6,7]

Many authors now consider PEA the management of choice for adenomatous hyperplasia and solitary HCC less than 3 cm in cirrhotic livers. In these cases, PEA has proven as safe if not safer than surgery with the same survival rates.[6,7,10–14] Surgery, however, remains the management of choice in noncirrhotic patients. For HCC greater than 3 cm or for multiple lesions, a combination of transarterial chemoembolization and PEA may be considered. The efficacy of ethanol ablation in liver metastases is much lower than that in primary tumors. This difference appears to be caused by the irregularity of ethanol diffusion in metastatic lesions, which have a more heterogeneous architecture and firmer consistency.[6,7] Other interventional therapies, (e.g., radiofrequency ablation, interstitial laser photocoagulation) show better results in the management of metastasis.[15,16]

TECHNIQUE

PEA is a safe and easy technique that can be performed on an outpatient basis under local anesthesia. Sedatives and analgesics can be given before therapy as needed.[6,7,10–14] Usually, more than one session is performed to complete the management. The amount of ethanol injected depends on the number and size of the lesions (approximately 2 to 12 ml of 95% ethanol).

In the first session, the needle is inserted into the center of the lesion, and the ethanol is injected until a homogeneous distribution of the ethanol throughout the lesion is noted. This approach may require several passes at slightly different sites.

Recent studies have proven the efficacy of ethanol at lower concentrations and lower volumes with a reduced rate of complications and adverse effects.[14,17,18] These adverse effects are usually mild and include pain and moderate fever. The effect on liver function is minimal (e.g., elevation of serum transaminases) or absent. More serious complications are rare and include hepatic infarct, portal vein thrombosis, bile duct damage, peritoneal bleeding, pleural effusion, and pneumothorax.*

IMAGING GUIDANCE

Ablation of tumors by percutaneous ethanol injection requires adequate imaging guidance and monitoring to ensure delivery of an adequate amount of ethanol into the target lesion without damaging the surrounding tissues. For this purpose, imaging guidance should allow identification of the lesions and the injected ethanol and should differentiate necrotic tissue, residual tumor, and surrounding viable tissue. Several imaging techniques have been used, including conventional and Doppler ultrasound (US), enhanced computed tomography (CT), CT arterioportogram, CT after iodized oil injection, angiography, and more recently, MRI.[8,19,20–23]

US has been the most commonly used imaging modality because of its availability, low cost, and real-time capability. However, US suffers limitations in guidance and in evaluation of therapy. US has a low sensitivity for the detection of small HCC in cirrhotic livers, is suboptimal in monitoring alcohol diffusion in the lesion, and may unreliably differentiate necrotic tumor from viable tumor (both hypoechoic). The only reliable indicator of effective management is reduced tumor size.

Color Doppler has proven valuable in the assessment of hypervascular lesions, particularly in detecting residual or recurrent tumor and in decreasing the false-negative rate of US. Any Doppler signals recognized in the lesion should be considered viable tumor and necessitate further management. However, the absence of vascularity on Doppler US does not guarantee the absence of viable tumor, and further investigation with enhanced CT or dynamic MRI is necessary. Using sonographic monitoring at the beginning of therapy can identify the ethanol as hyperechoic material flowing from the needle tip, which is distinct from hypoechoic tumoral tissue. Soon after the injection, however, the margins of this hyperechoic zone become indistinct, and the bright hyperechogenicity begins to obscure the lesion and the needle tip position.[7,8,24] CT is superior to US in determining the exact extent of ethanol diffusion as the alcohol appears markedly hypodense and distinct from the unmanaged tissue. Dynamic-enhanced CT is very useful in evaluating the therapeutic effect of PEA. It depicts lesions managed by ethanol ablation as hypodense nonenhancing areas, whereas residual tumor appears as a hypervascular enhancing region. Drawbacks to CT guidance, including the use of ionizing radiation, limitation to one imaging plane, and the lack of real-time capabilities, make this technique time consuming and cumbersome as a guiding method.[7,19]

TECHNIQUE AND ADVANTAGES OF MAGNETIC RESONANCE IMAGING GUIDANCE

MRI guidance can overcome most limitations of other imaging modalities. The development of open scanners, rapid sequences permitting almost real-time imaging (MRI fluoroscopy), and high contrast resolution make MRI a very appealing technique for guidance of several interventional procedures.[23,25–27] In the field of ethanol ablation, MRI has been used primarily in the follow-up of patients with liver tumors managed by PEA. However, recent investigations have also shown its potential for guiding and monitoring this type of therapy. This task requires MRI-compatible needles and an in-room MR-compatible liquid crystal display monitor, which allows the radiologist to visualize the needle without leaving the room, thereby permitting fine adjustments in needle position.[28–30]

Few investigations have studied the dynamic tissue signal changes that occur over time after ethanol injection.[20,31] In one study in which ethanol was injected into the paraspinal muscle of the New Zealand white rabbit, fast spin-echo T2-weighted images showed initial hyperintensity at the site of the injection that progressively enlarged but was followed in minutes by a zone of hypointensity, which enlarged over the subsequent hours,

*Refs. 6, 7, 10–14, 17, 18.

surrounded by a hyperintense rim. The authors theorized that the initial hyperintensity represented the ethanol (fluid), whereas the subsequent hypointensity represented the ensuing dehydration and eventual coagulative necrosis (Figs. 26-1, 26-2).[20]

In another study, ethanol was injected in a tissue phantom (*ex vivo* sheep liver) (Fig. 26-3) and into *in vivo* porcine liver. Serial fast spin-echo T2-weighted images showed an enlarging hypointense lesion that corresponded to a discolored and indurated lesion on gross pathology and showed marked architectural distortion on histology (Fig. 26-4).[31]

In both studies, the T1-weighted sequences (T1 spin-echo and T1 gradient-recalled echo; the latter has better temporal resolution in the range of seconds) showed enlarging hypointensities at the injection site. Whether different tissue undergoes different T2 signal changes or different rates of signal changes after ethanol injection is unclear (Fig. 26-5). Because the temporal resolution of clinically useful T2-weighted sequences is in the range of minutes, the initial transient T2 hyperintensity may not be as clinically relevant, whereas T2 hypointensity may be an ideal marker for the zone of ethanol effect because it would contrast well against the T2 hyperintensity of most tumors. For the same reason, the T1 hypointensity of ethanol is not as clinically useful because most tumors are hypointense on T1-weighted images. However, as faster scanners and pulse sequences become capable of monitoring T2 signal changes with temporal resolution in the range of seconds, very early signal abnormalities may become more important.

In the MR follow-up of ethanol-managed HCC, use of gadolinium for separating managed tumor from residual unmanaged tumor is under debate.[32–35] Not all authors agree that residual T2 hyperintensity is a reliable sign of residual or recurrent tumor. Some believe that areas of coagulative necrosis may manifest as hyperintensity on T2-weighted images, rendering them indistinguishable from viable tumor. In this instance, dynamic contrast-enhanced MRI may help differentiate necrosis from viable tumor. Contrast enhancement is used by

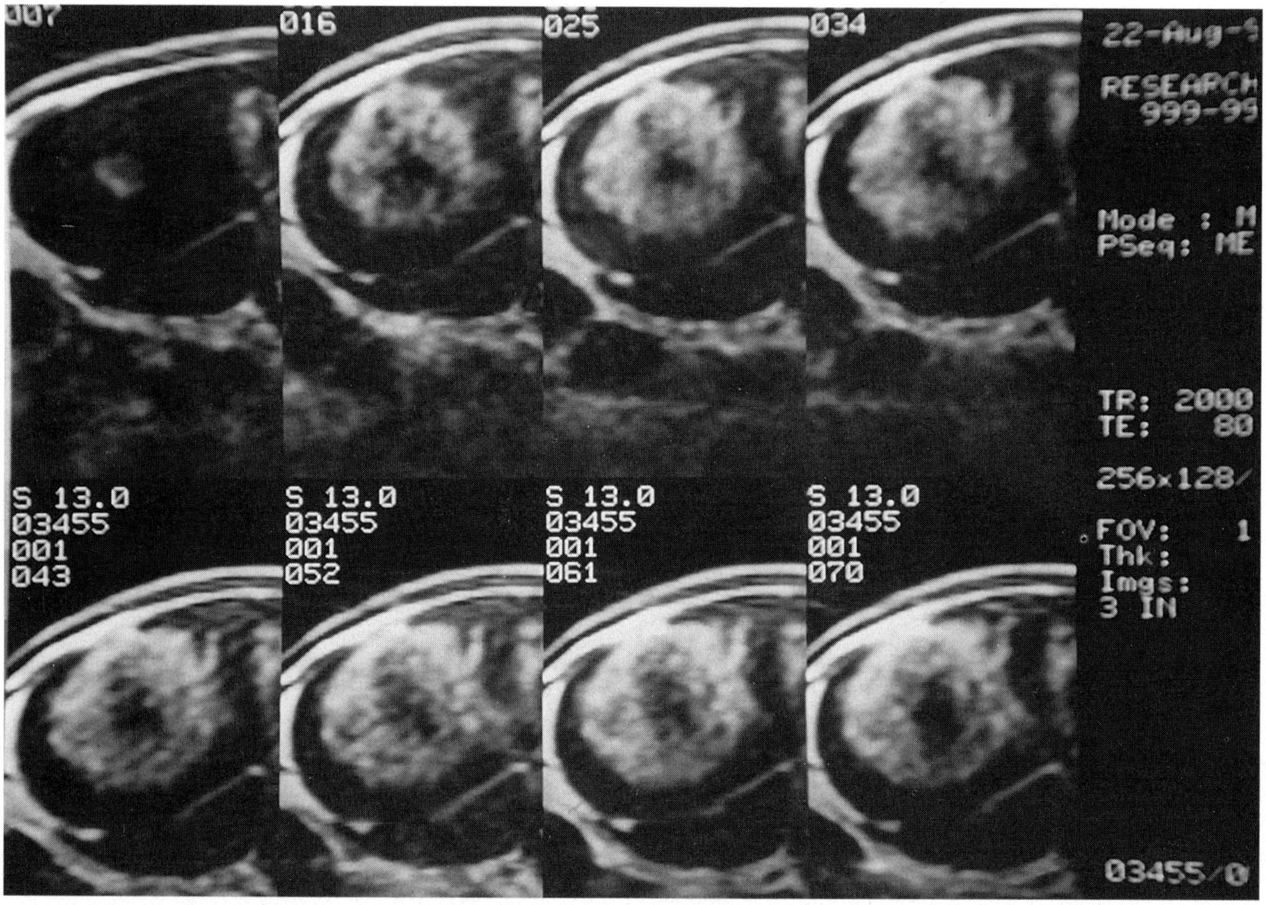

Fig. 26-1. Sequential spin-echo T2-weighted images of the paraspinal muscles in a New Zealand rabbit *in vivo* (from left to right and top to bottom the images were obtained at 2-min intervals during and after ethanol injection). The initial region of hyperintensity corresponds to the presence of the injected fluid, and the subsequent growing area of hypointensity corresponds to cellular dehydration in the early stages and to coagulative necrosis in the latter stages.

most authors in post management follow-up.[33–35] Residual tumor and inflammatory tissue may present as areas of enhancement; the former is seen early as a crescentic or globular area of enhancement, whereas the latter shows delayed rim enhancement. The necrotic tissue appears as a nonenhancing area replacing the primary site of tumor.

For the purpose of intraprocedural monitoring of PEA ablation, gadolinium injection is not an option because its effect is too transient and it cannot be administered repeatedly. Therefore, during ablation, T2 hyperintensity is a useful guide in defining the extent of the tumor; ideally, all hyperintense areas should be rendered hypointense by the ethanol to complete the ablation. In the few patients with dysplastic nodules or fat containing HCC that shows hyperintensity on T1-weighted images, the T1 prolongation effect of ethanol may help separate managed and unmanaged tumors.

Text continued on p. 251

A

B

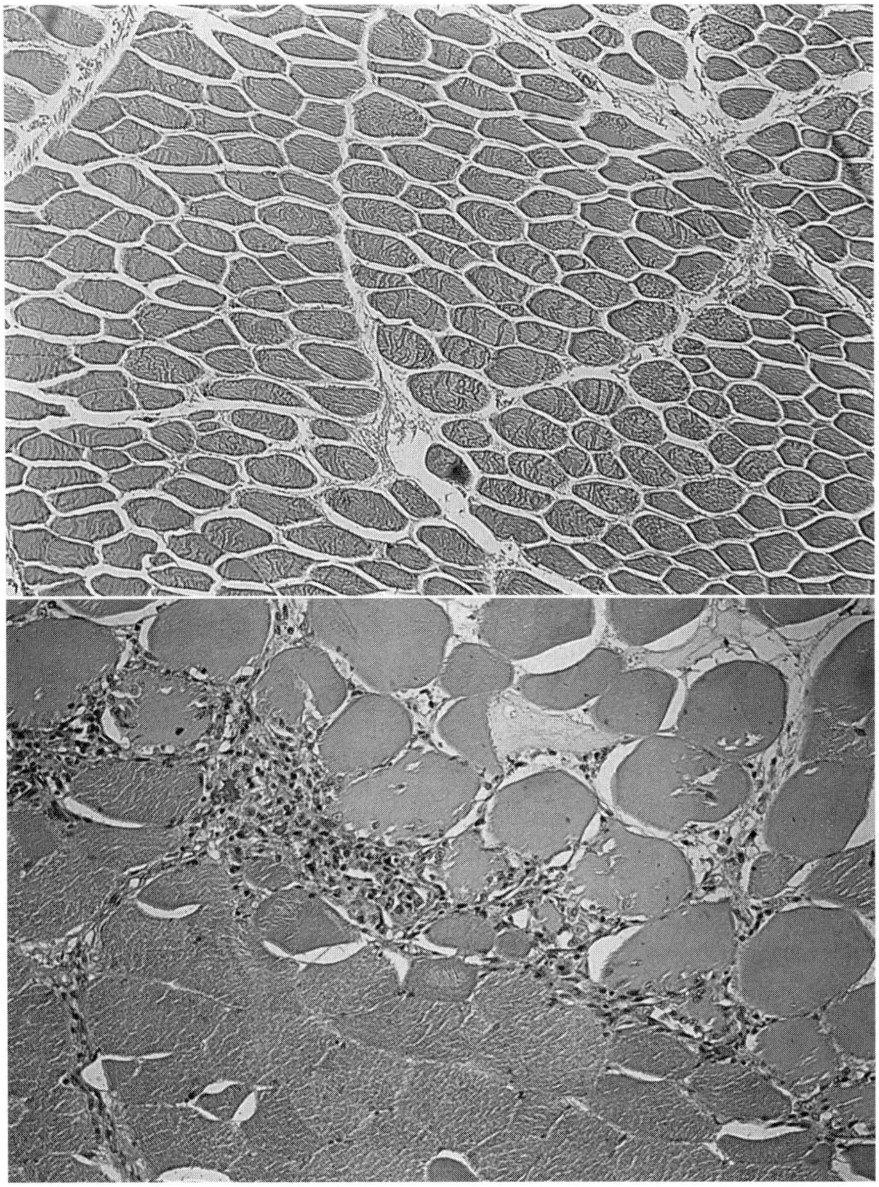

Fig. 26-2. A, Pathologic specimen of the paraspinal muscle of a New Zealand rabbit obtained immediately after completion of the ethanol injection and magnetic resonance scan (Fig. 26-1) and stained with hematoxylin-eosin. This image shows healthy-appearing muscle with no definite histologic abnormalities. **B,** Pathologic specimen of the paraspinal muscle of a New Zealand rabbit obtained 5 days after ethanol injection shows the typical findings seen in coagulative necrosis and a peripheral inflammatory fibrovascular response. See Color Plate 14.

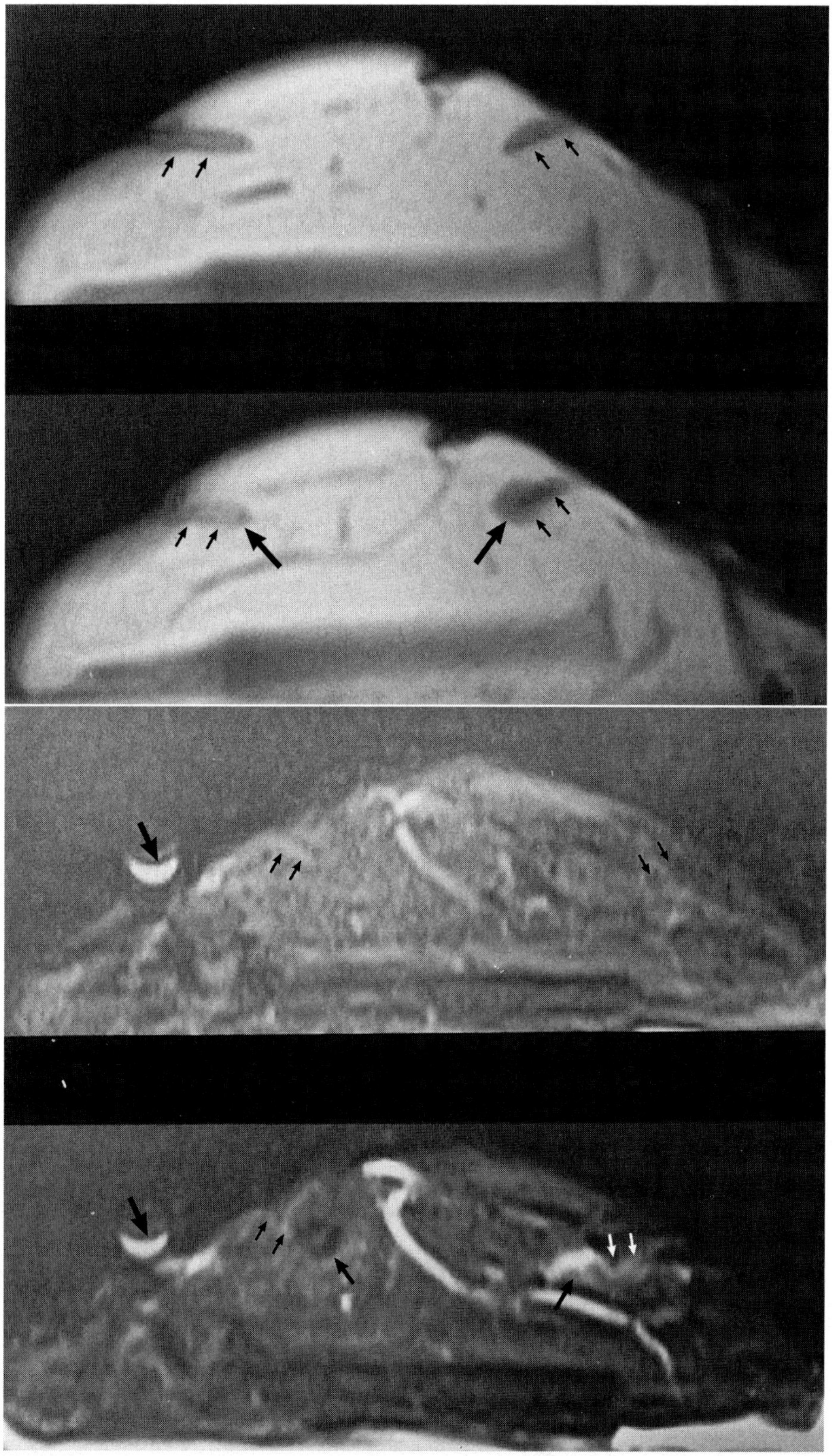
A
B

Fig. 26-3. Tissue phantom study. Two 22-gauge magnetic resonance–compatible needles *(small arrows)* were placed into *ex vivo* sheep liver. **A,** T1-weighted fast low-angle shot and **B,** T2-weighted fast spin-echo images showing preinjection *(top)* and postinjection *(bottom)* appearance of 10 ml of ethanol (left needle) and normal saline (right needle). Note the hypointense effect of ethanol *(midsized black arrow)* on the liver tissue on both sequences. Saline injection produced no T1 signal change and mild irregular T2 hyperintensity at the tip of the needle, with probable diffusion into an adjacent vessel *(small arrows)*. The signal of free-standing 96% ethanol *(large arrow)* in the vial is hypointense on T1- and hyperintense on T2-weighted images when compared with the liver phantom.

A

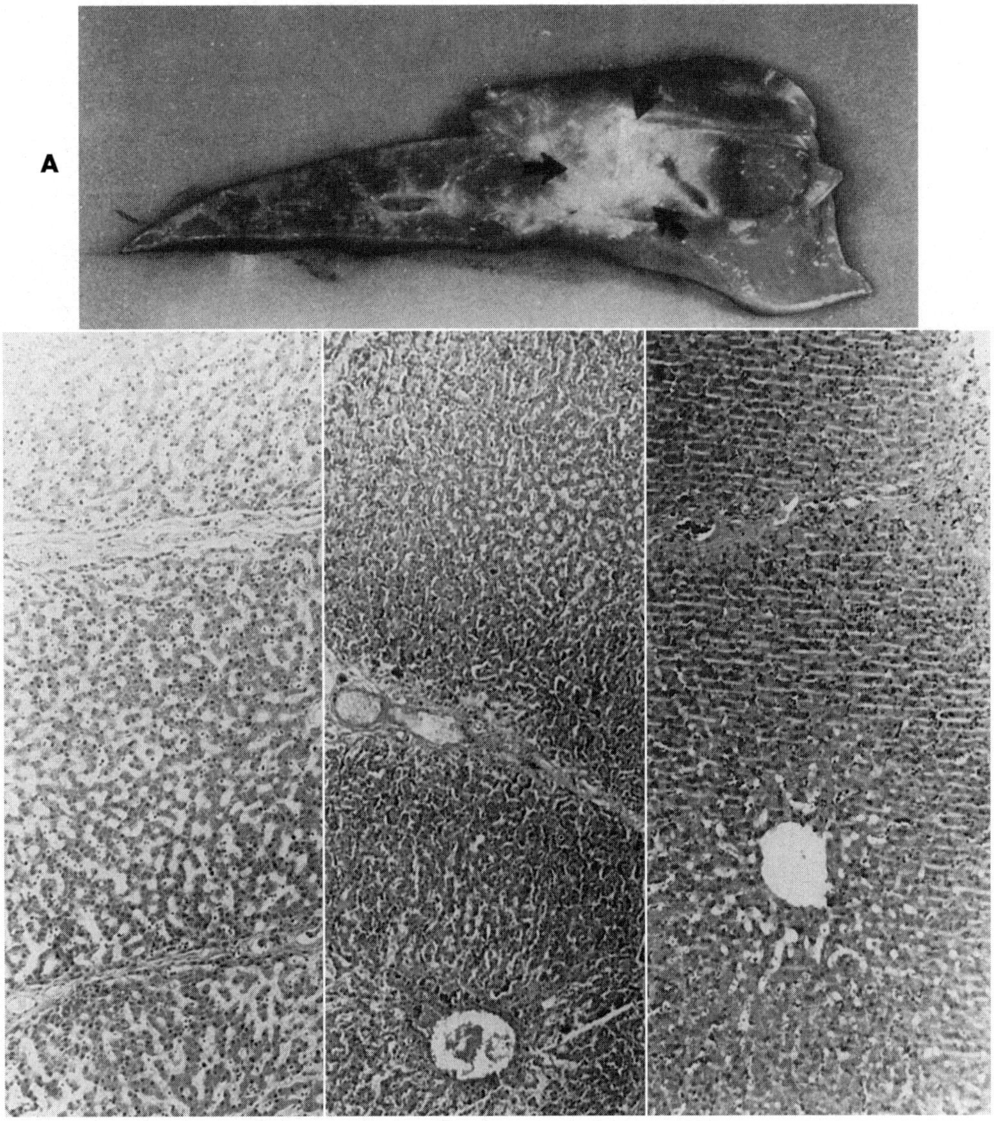

B C D

Fig. 26-4. **A,** Gross pathologic specimen of the right lobe of the pig liver shows a grey area corresponding to the ethanol-infiltrated area *(arrows)*. This area corresponds to the lesion seen on magnetic resonance imaging. Histologic appearance (low-power magnification) of **B,** ethanol-infiltrated liver; **C,** saline-infiltrated liver; and **D,** healthy liver. Note the diffuse-marked sinusoidal dilation in the ethanol-infiltrated liver and the minimal sinusoidal dilation in the saline-infiltrated liver as compared with the healthy liver.

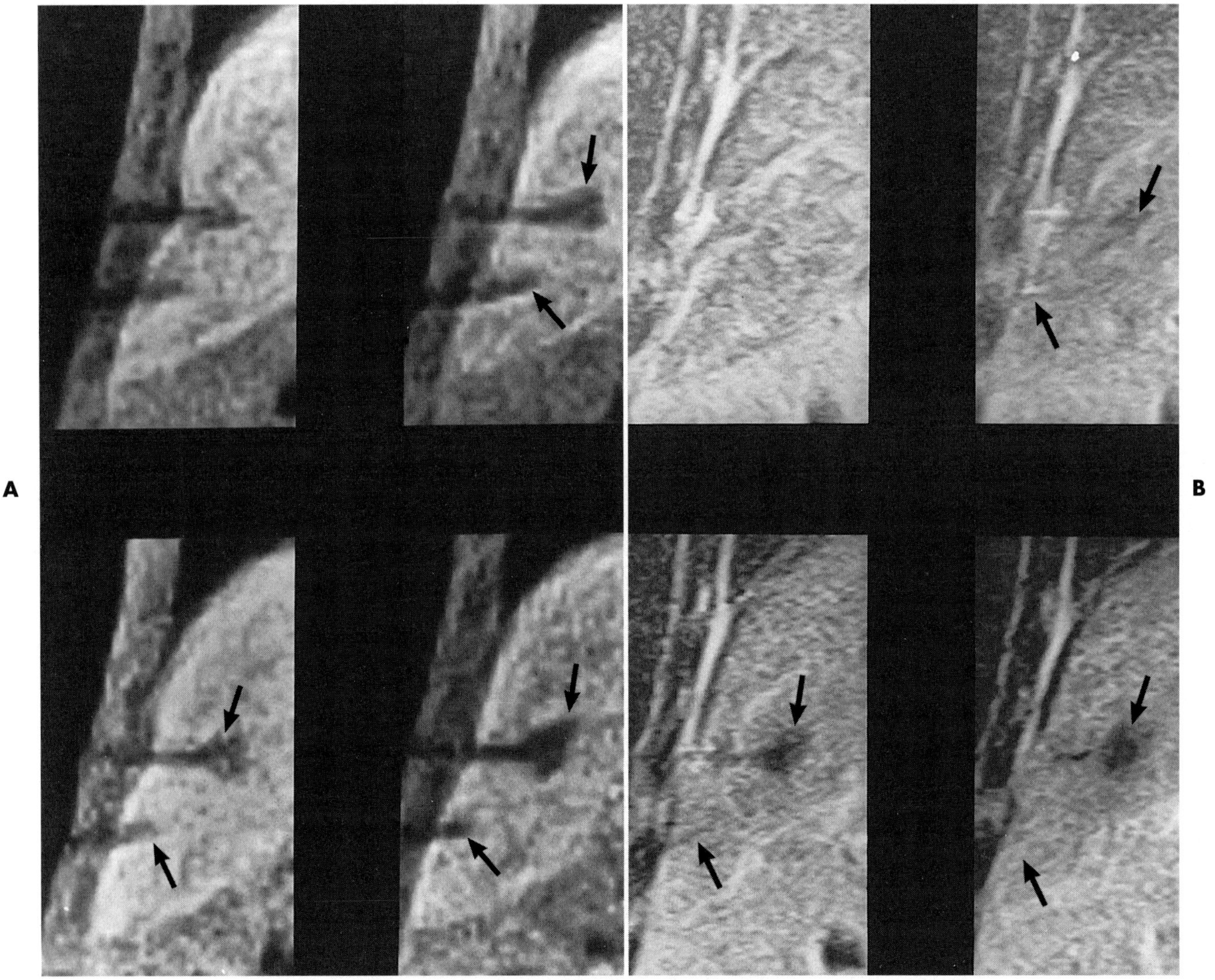

Fig. 26-5. *In vivo* pig study. Two 22-gauge magnetic resonance–compatible needles have been placed by magnetic resonance guidance into the right lobe of the liver and imaged in the coronal plane. **A,** T1-weighted fast low-angle shot and **B,** T2-weighted fast spin-echo images show the preinjection appearance *(top left)* and appearance after 1-ml *(top right),* 5-ml *(bottom left),* and 10-ml *(bottom right)* injections of 96% ethanol (top needle) and saline (bottom needle). Note the growing hypointensity at the ethanol-infused site (*upper arrow*) and the lack of any signal change at the saline-infused site *(lower arrow)* on all sequences. Note also the excellent needle visualization by the T1-weighted fast low-angle shot compared with the T2-weighted fast spin-echo sequence.

CONCLUSIONS

MRI shows promise as a sensitive and accurate technique for intra- and postprocedural monitoring of PEA. Although continued investigations are needed, preliminary data show MR's capability to depict tissue changes that occur with ethanol injection. One challenge is the development of faster pulse sequences for true real-time intraprocedural monitoring. In combination with the open access to the patient afforded by open-configuration scanners, clinical MR-guided ethanol ablation of tumors may become an established therapeutic technique.

REFERENCES

1. Miyazono N, and others: Transcatheter arterial renal and adrenal embolization with iohexol-ethanol solutions: animal experimental study and clinical application, *Invest Radiol* 31:755, 1996.
2. Regge D, and others: Interventional radiology of the adrenal glands, *Minerva Endocrinol* 20:15, 1995.
3. Park JH, and others: Transcatheter arterial embolization of unresectable renal cell carcinoma with a mixture of ethanol and iodized oil, *Cardiovasc Intervent Radiol* 17:323, 1994.
4. Livraghi T, and others: Percutaneous ethanol injections in the treatment of autonomous thyroid nodules: 4 years' experience, *Minerva Endocrinol* 18:187, 1993.
5. Inoue H, and others: Transcatheter arterial ablation of aldosteronomas with high-concentration ethanol: preliminary and long-term results, *Am J Roentgenol* 168:1241, 1997.
6. Liu CL, Fan ST: Nonresectional therapies for hepatocellular carcinoma, *Am J Surg* 173:358, 1997.
7. Bartolozzi C, Lencioni R: Ethanol injection for the treatment of hepatic tumours, *European Radiology* 6:682, 1996.
8. Lencioni R, and others: Management of adenomatous hyperplastic nodules in the cirrhotic liver: US follow-up or percutaneous alcohol ablation? *Abdom Imaging* 18:50, 1993.
9. Robbins SL: *Pathologic basis of disease,* ed 5, Philadelphia, 1994, WB Saunders.
10. Livraghi T, and others: Percutaneous ethanol injection in the treatment of hepatocellular carcinoma in cirrhosis: a study on 207 patients, *Cancer* 69:925, 1992.
11. Shiina S, and others: Percutaneous ethanol injection therapy of hepatocellular carcinoma: analysis of 77 patients, *Am J Roentgenol* 155:1221, 1990.
12. Shiina S, and others: Percutaneous ethanol injection therapy for hepatocellular carcinoma: results on 146 patients, *Am J Roentgenol* 160:1023, 1993.
13. Livraghi T, and others: Percutaneous ethanol injection of hepatic tumors: single session therapy with general anesthesia, *Am J Roentgenol* 161:1065, 1993.
14. Redvanly RD, and others: Malignant hepatic tumors: safety of high-dose percutaneous ethanol ablation therapy, *Radiology* 188:283, 1993.
15. Anzai Y, and others: MR imaging-guided interstitial Nd:YAG laser phototherapy: dosimetry study of acute tissue damage in an in vivo model, *J Magn Reson Imaging* 1:553, 1991.
16. Matsumoto R, Oshio K, Jolesz FA: Monitoring of laser and freezing induced ablation in the liver with T1W MR imaging, *J Magn Reson Imaging* 2:555, 1992.
17. Tapani E, and others: Toxicity of ethanol in low concentrations: experimental evaluation in cell culture, *Acta Radiol* 37:923, 1996.
18. Giorgio A, and others: One-shot percutaneous ethanol injection of liver tumors under general anesthesia: preliminary data on efficacy and complications, *Cardiovasc Intervent Radiol* 19:27, 1996.
19. Amin Z, Lees WR, Bown SG: Hepatocellular carcinoma: CT appearance after percutaneous ethanol ablation therapy, *Radiology* 188:882, 1993.
20. Anzai Y, and others: Dynamic MRI monitoring of percutaneous ethanol injection: preliminary study in the experimental in-vivo model (unpublished data).
21. Sironi S, and others: Small hepatocellular carcinoma: MR follow-up of treatment with percutaneous ethanol injection, *Radiology* 187:119, 1993.
22. Lencioni R, Caramella D, Bartolozzi C: Response of hepatocellular carcinoma to percutaneous ethanol injection: CT and MR evaluation, *J Comput Assist Tomogr* 17:723, 1993.
23. Dumoulin CL, Souza SP, Darrow RD: Real time position monitoring of invasive devices using magnetic resonance, *Magn Reson Med* 29:411, 1993.
24. Livraghi T, and others: US guided percutaneous ethanol injection of small hepatic and abdominal tumors, *Radiology* 161:309, 1986.
25. Lufkin R, and others: MR body atereotaxis: an aid for MR-guided biopsies, *J Comput Assist Tomogr* 12:1088, 1988.
26. Sinha S, Sinha U, Lufkin R, Hanafee W: Pulse sequence optimization for use with a biopsy needle in MRI, *Magn Reson Imaging* 7:575, 1989.
27. Silverman SG, and others: Interactive MR-guided biopsy in an open-configuration MR imaging system, *Radiology* 197:175, 1995.
28. Lufkin R, Layfield L: Coaxial needle system of MR and CT-guided aspiration cytology, *J Comput Assist Tomogr* 13:1105, 1989.
29. Lufkin RB, and others: A technique for MR-guided needle placement, *Am J Roentgenol* 151:193, 1988.
30. Adam G, and others: Interventional magnetic resonance: initial clinical experience with a 1.5-tesla magnetic resonance system combined with c-arm fluoroscopy, *Invest Radiol* 32:191, 1997.
31. Lu DS, and others: MR-guided percutaneous ethanol ablation of liver tissue in a 2-T open MR system: preliminary study in porcine model, *J Magn Reson Imaging* 7:303, 1997.
32. Nagel HS, Bernardino ME: Contrast-enhanced MR imaging of hepatic lesions treated with percutaneous ethanol ablation therapy, *Radiology* 189:265, 1993.
33. Kubata Y, and others: Validity of MR imaging for monitoring effects of percutaneous ethanol injection for HCC, *Hepatogastroenterology* 36:262, 1989.
34. Sironi S, and others: Small hepatocellular carcinoma treated with percutaneous ethanol injection: unenhanced and gadolinium enhanced MR imaging follow-up, *Radiology* 192:407, 1994.
35. Bartolozzi C, and others: Treatment of hepatocellular carcinoma with percutaneous ethanol injection: evaluation of contrast enhanced MR imaging, *Am J Roentgenol* 162:827, 1994.

Part IV

CLINICAL APPLICATIONS

Chapter 27

INTRAOPERATIVE MRI FOR NEUROSURGERY

Thomas M. Moriarty, Ferenc A. Jolesz, Eben Alexander, III, Philip E. Stieg, Eric J. Woodard, Richard Schwartz, Peter M. Black

Intraoperative magnetic resonance imaging (MRI) may be most significant in the field of neurosurgery. One 0.5-T system for intraoperative MRI (Signa SP, General Electric, Milwaukee, Wis), designed in collaboration with the Brigham & Women's Hospital (Boston, Mass), is being applied in image-guided neurosurgery. This chapter summarizes the role of intraoperative MRI in image-guided neurosurgery, current applications of intraoperative MRI for various neurosurgical diseases, and the potential role of intraoperative MRI for minimally invasive image-guided neurosurgery.

IMAGE-GUIDED NEUROSURGERY

Over the past decade, a distinct field of neurosurgery, image-guided neurosurgery, has evolved through advances in neuroimaging, computer science, and stereotactic neurosurgery. Conceptually, the goal of image-guided neurosurgery brings the "vision" of powerful neuroimaging technologies into the operating room by taking advantage of principles of computer science and engineering. Through the use of various computer-enhanced intraoperative displays and surgical interfaces, image-guidance technologies are being used for neurosurgical navigation through intracranial (and spinal) space, for refined localization of neural structures, and for enhanced differentiation of normal and diseased tissues. The goals of image-guided technology are to make neurosurgery safer and more precise, as well as to broaden the scope of surgically treatable pathology.

The field of image-guided neurosurgery has been driven forward by technologic developments. From the first use of a stereotactic atlas and the stereotactic frame[1] through the development of frame-based stereotactic surgery,[2–7] computer-assisted neurosurgery,[8–12] and stereotactic radiosurgery,[13–15] the foundation for interactive image-guided neurosurgery[16] and frameless stereotaxy[17–21] was laid. These advances have attempted to bring the anatomic and pathologic detail of preoperatively acquired neuroimages into the operating room to guide surgery. These systems have been applied to relatively simple neurosurgical procedures (e.g., brain biopsies, placement of catheters and probes) and have been proven to aid in more complex three-dimensional (3D) procedures (e.g., tumor resection, epilepsy surgery, stereotactic radiosurgery).

A significant limiting factor in all conventional image-guided neurosurgery is that images are not updated intraoperatively without moving the patient to an imaging device. In open surgery, the brain and pathology of interest can shift substantially as the operation proceeds,[22–24] thereby negating the value of the enhanced information in the images guiding the surgery. Painstaking efforts can be made to prevent such shifts, or intraoperative recalibrations can be performed. However, image-guided technologies should provide seamless, reliable information to help the surgeon perform better. If the surgeon must rely on skill and experience to overcome the possible deficiencies of the neuronavigational aid, the need for the technology is hard to defend.

Intraoperative MRI permits image-guided surgery in an environment in which high-resolution neuroimaging is available throughout the entire operation.[25–27] Interventional MR in the operating suite offers three unique advantages: (1) continuous access to high-resolution multi planar MRI, (2) an integrated neuronavigational aid, and (3) a virtual 3D digital operative environment.

MAGNETIC RESONANCE IMAGING

MRI offers several advantages for imaging the central nervous system and for image-guided therapy.[28–36] MRI provides excellent tissue contrast to define normal structures and to identify pathology. The ability to acquire multiplanar and 3D volume images allows for an immediate appreciation of 3D anatomic relationships. The spatial resolution of MR is at least at the millimetric range using conventional coils, which is within the rigorous demands for application accuracy in stereotactic neurosurgery.[6,22] The temporal resolution of MR continues to increase with fast and ultrafast imaging sequences, permitting near real-time tracking of physiologic motion, movement of instruments, and changes induced by therapy.[37–45] In addition to structural imaging, MR can also monitor several functional characteristics of tissues. At this time, MR monitoring of temperature and thermal therapy is well understood and practiced.[30,31,46–48] MR monitoring of tissue perfusion, vascular flow, and physiologic activation (functional MR) is possible, and its routine implementation is likely in the near future.[49,50]

Other imaging modalities for intraoperative monitoring and image-guided surgery have been used but are somewhat limited in practice.[18,51] Fluoroscopy gives excellent real-time imaging but lacks 3D detail and subjects operative personnel and the patient to ionizing radiation. Intraoperative computed tomography (CT) gives 3D information but also generates ionizing radiation; also, the patient should be moved in and out of the imaging bore. Ultrasound provides excellent real-time imaging of soft-tissue pathology; however its spatial resolution and tissue discrimination are less than ideal. It is also a very operator-dependent imaging modality.

This information led to the concept of MRI devices engineered so that a surgeon or interventional radiologist could have access to the patient while performing continuous high-resolution MRI. In a collaborative project between General Electric Medical Systems and the Brigham & Women's Hospital, a prototype interventional open MRI was developed and installed in the Brigham & Women's Hospital. The intraoperative MR suite (also referred to as *open-configuration MR, magnetic resonance image therapy [MRT], or Signa SP),* is based on a cryogenless, 0.5-T open-configuration superconducting magnet (NbSn, General Electric Medical Systems, Milwaukee, Wis) (see Chapter 3). The unit is integrated into a fully equipped operating room, which conforms to Massachusetts' regulatory standards for operating rooms. The imager is a fully functional, 0.5-T, multiplanar, high-resolution, whole-body imaging system. A linear imaging volume 30 cm in diameter at the center of the imager's axis is used. The coil housings are separated by 56 cm, allowing two surgeons free access to a patient positioned at the center of the field of view. Patient positioning is flexible. All conventional approaches to intracranial and intraspinal pathology can be accomplished in the scanner.

Imaging is driven by one of two processes: Signa or interactive, real-time imaging. Through the standard Signa console, electronics, and software, the system can acquire all conventional multiplanar MRI scans, including T1, T2, proton, 3D volume, and MR angiography or venography, with equivalent resolution and acquisition times to those of General Electric 0.5-T diagnostic scanners. Interactive imaging allows the surgeon to prescribe single-slice images in any specified orientation while performing surgery in the scanner. This imaging mode uses an optical digitizer 3D tracking system (Flashpoint, Integrated Technologies, Boulder, Colo), which is integrated into the scanner. Specialized image guidance software, implemented on a SUN 4/670 workstation (Sun Microsystems, Mountain View, Calif), allows the surgeon to use this system in a manner analogous to an ultrasound probe to obtain single MR images. This system can also be used to plan the direction and movement of instruments through image space and physical space, effectively acting as a frameless stereotactic device.

The optical tracking system is based on three high-resolution, linear charge coupled device video cameras rigidly fixed to the bore of the magnet over the imaging region. These cameras track the movement of small light-emitting diodes (LEDs) mounted on instruments in the imaging space. Various software choices allow the surgeon to define points in physical space and image space relative to the LED-mounted instrument.

Conventional head coils and spine coils, which would impede surgical access to the patient, have been replaced by new flexible surface coils, which function both as transmit and receive coils. These pliable devices, which can be wrapped in a sterile fashion, are applied to the body surface and secured circumferentially with Velcro straps. Various sizes and shapes of these coils have been designed to accommodate different surgical approaches. Most intracranial pathology can be addressed using one medium-sized flexible coil.

Because the center of the intraoperative MR suite is a fully functional MR imaging device, all conventional MR imaging sequences can be used. Currently, fast spin-echo (FSE) sequences provide adequate temporal resolution for frameless stereotactic applications. Gradient echo sequences can also be used but with less image clarity.[25,52–57] 3D spoiled gradient refocused (SPGR) volumes are used for open craniotomy and lesion resections. Furthermore, as novel surgical and interventional applications are explored, MR pulse sequences can be developed to exploit the sensitivity, including such techniques as dynamic imaging,[39,41,45,43] MR fluoroscopy,[37,40,44] keyhole imaging,[38] and adaptive imaging.[58–63]

Instrumentation for the intraoperative MR suite was initially a problem in the application of intraoperative MRI for neurosurgery. Because the MRI system generates a substantial static magnet field, all instruments to be used in the room could not be ferromagnetic. Also, any instrument to be placed within the imaging volume would have to be composed of relatively inert materials that would not yield significant image artifacts.

Currently, two classes of instruments are recognized: field compatible or image compatible. Field-compatible tools will not move in the magnetic field. Image-compatible tools, if positioned within the imaging volume, do not induce any distortion in the image. Thus, tools such as the high speed drill (modified Midas Rex, Ft. Worth, Tex) and surgical hand tools (e.g., curettes, Penfields, needle holders), which will never be used during imaging, can be made of stronger materials, such as low-grade stainless steel.

For image-compatible tools, the degree of image distortion created by any instrument is a function of its magnetic susceptibility, size, shape, and orientation in the magnetic field. Thus, tools intentionally left in the imaging volume, such as a brain retractor blade or brain biopsy needles, are composed of materials specific to the intended purpose. The retractor blade need not be seen in the image, so materials with very low magnetic susceptibility (e.g., plastic, graphite) should be used. The biopsy needle should be very strong and rigid and should be seen clearly without significantly altering the image. Current biopsy needles are composed of titanium alloys (Elekta Instruments, Atlanta, Ga). Intraoperative MRI-compatible instruments for most conventional neurosurgical procedures are now commercially available.

CURRENT NEUROSURGICAL APPLICATIONS

Intraoperative MRI has been integrated into the management of neurosurgical disease at the Brigham & Women's Hospital in the following areas to date: (1) stereotactic brain biopsy and stereotactic placement of catheters, (2) image-guided craniotomy for tumor resection, (3) image-guided laser ablation of brain tumors, (4) transsphenoidal resection of pituitary lesions, and (5) image-guided spine surgery.

The brain biopsy is an essential component of management of intracranial mass lesions. Conceptually, brain tissue should be sampled through the least destructive and safest means possible, ideally permitting the patient to return home as quickly as possible. Toward these ends, the standard of care for intracranial biopsy has become frame-based stereotaxy. The most common systems used are the Cosman-Roberts-Wells Radionics (Burlington, Mass) and the Leksell system (Electra AB, Sweden),[5,6] in which a preoperative enhanced cranial CT (or MRI) is obtained with a rigid frame and fiducial cage affixed to the patient's head. A simple computer program calculates the relative location of the lesion to the relative position of the bars of the fiducial cage and then translates these data into a coordinate scheme to place a biopsy needle through a small burr hole into the lesion and to obtain a sample. Patients generally remain in the hospital for 24 hr of observation or undergo postoperative neuroimaging to confirm the location of the biopsy and assess for intracranial bleeding. Stereotactic brain biopsy, as performed using intraoperative MRI, is advantageous in that preoperative imaging, the surgical procedure, and postoperative imaging are performed at the same sitting (Fig. 27-1). At the Brigham & Women's Hospital, more than 70 brain biopsies have been performed using intraoperative MRI.

The accuracy and predictability of various frame-based stereotactic devices have been assessed; however, even in the best circumstances, errors up to 1.7 cm have been reported.[6,22–24] Therefore, successful biopsy of small targets, targets adjacent to critical structures, or targets in cerebrospinal fluid spaces can be difficult. Success is confirmed by clear pathological diagnosis or postoperative neuroimaging. In an open-configuration MR, intraoperative MR images annotated to mark the entry site and pathway of the biopsy needle to the target are used. Serial images are acquired as the needle is passed to the target. Any aberration from the intended pathway is clearly seen by divergence of the needle artifact and annotation. The needle can be removed, reoriented, and easily passed to the target.

In addition, all brain biopsies performed under conventional circumstances are confirmed to be lesional tissue by intraoperative consultation with the neuropathologist. Because such a preliminary diagnosis by frozen section may be difficult and time consuming, the surgeon is often requested to perform multiple biopsies to obtain adequate tissue for confirmation. Each request for tissue lengthens the procedure and adds a sense of doubt about the accuracy of the biopsy. Repeated biopsies of lesions in or adjacent to critical brain structures may not be advisable or even possible. In an open-configuration MR, intraoperative images will provide unambiguous confirmation that the biopsy needle is located in the lesion. Therefore, the cost and time of an intraoperative frozen section are avoided.

The reported rate of intracranial hemorrhage with stereotactic brain biopsy ranges from 0% to 11.5%.[64–68] Usually, major hemorrhages are diagnosed by emergency postoperative CT, and, if necessary, the patient should be transported back to the operating room. This procedure requires time, which is valuable in the setting of an expanding hematoma. In an open-configuration MR, biopsy-related hemorrhage will be immediately apparent and can be quickly addressed. Extending an incision and turning a craniotomy to evacuate a clot can be simply performed in the scanner.

Stereotactic placement of catheters and probes can also be accomplished in an intraoperative MRI with preoperative imaging, intraoperative confirmation of placement, and postoperative evaluation of the procedure. At the Brigham & Women's Hospital, intraoperative MRI has been used to place catheters and drain several tumor cysts and arachnoid cysts.

The real strengths and potential of the intraoperative MR are found in volumetric applications of the system. At the Brigham & Women's Hospital, intraoperative MRI has been used in more than 140 craniotomies for tumor and vascular lesions. Intraoperative imaging is used to localize the lesion, plan the craniotomy, and navigate toward the lesion. This technique results in a less-invasive approach to intracranial lesions than is afforded by conventional stereotaxy (Fig. 27-2). Using various image acquisitions, usually T2-weighted and gadolinium-enhanced T1-weighted images, the borders of a lesion can be

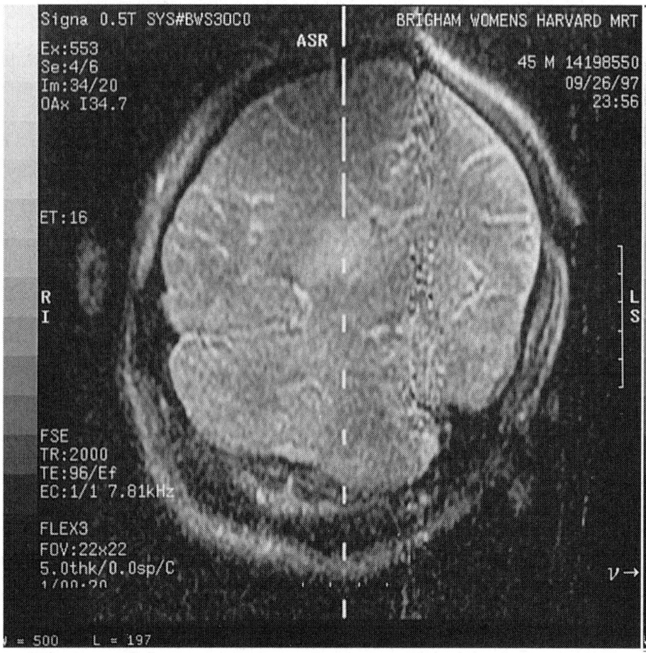

A

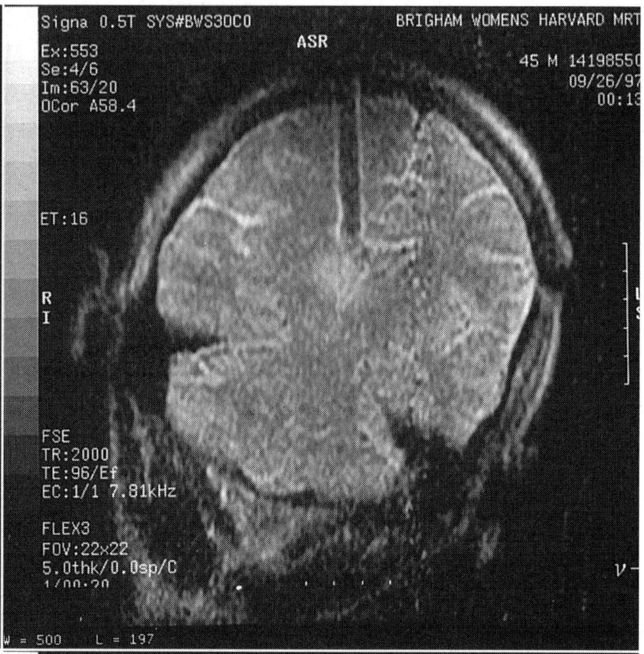

B

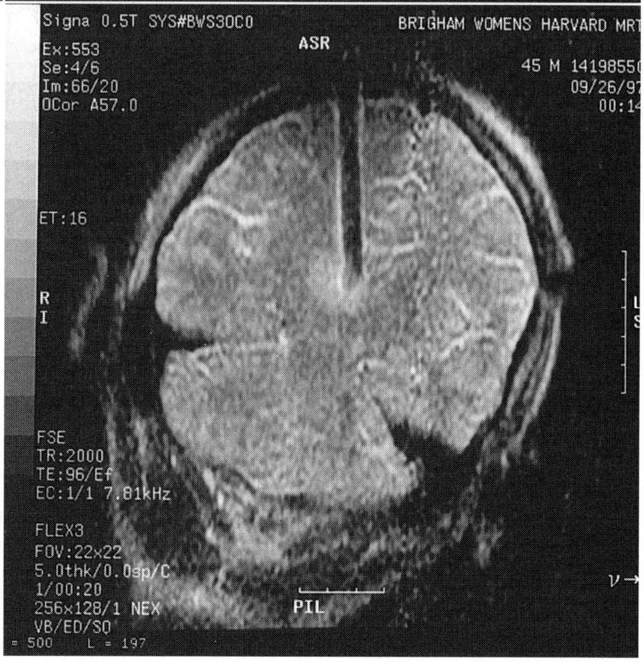

C

Fig. 27-1. An interactive T2-weighted image during stereotactic brain biopsy of a small deep lesion. **A,** The *dotted line* shows the proposed trajectory for the biopsy needle. **B,** The needle is passed to the lesion. **C,** The needle is seen in the lesion.

radiographically defined. Serial imaging can then be used to monitor the progress of lesion resection. Intraoperative MRI has been helpful in the resection of low-grade glial lesions, which may be difficult to differentiate from healthy brain tissue by visual or tactile cues. It is also extremely helpful for large lesions, in which the debulking process may lead to a significant shift of intracranial contents, so that the preoperative anatomy defined by conventional image-guided technologies may no longer be accurate (Fig. 27-3).

A number of image-guided spine procedures have been performed to date at the Brigham & Women's Hospital in the intraoperative MRI. These have included lumbar and cervical laminectomies for decompression, microdiscectomy, anterior cervical discectomy with interbody fusion—with and without anterior plate fixation—and cervical syringostomy. Imaging has been most useful for assessing the extent and adequacy of neural element decompression, localization, and trajectory planning for spinal instrumentation. As with cranial surgery,

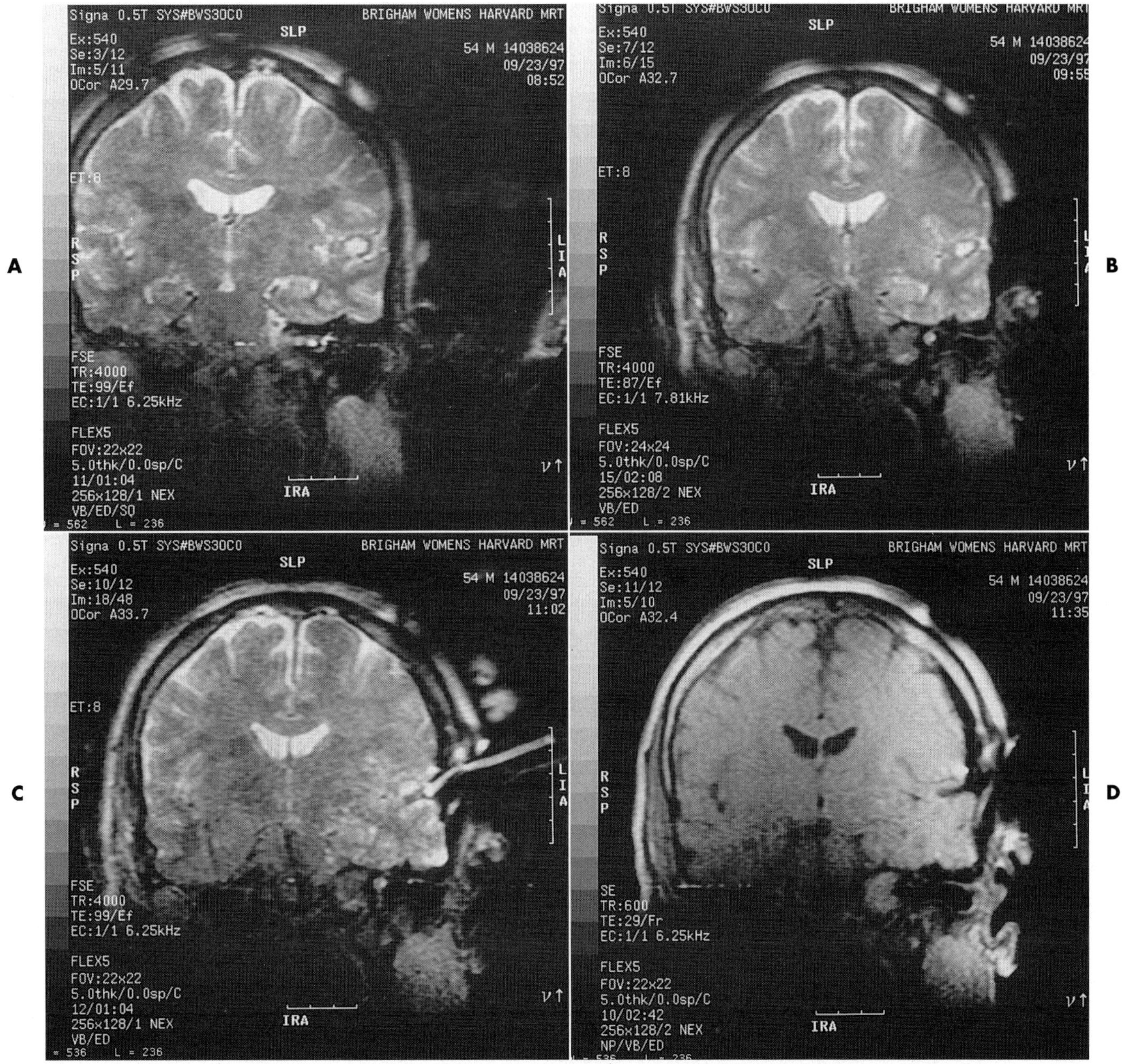

Fig. 27-2. Image-guided resection of a small brain lesion. A 54-year-old man with new-onset seizures is found on diagnostic magnetic resonance imaging to have a small arteriovenous malformation in the left temporal lobe. This diagnosis was confirmed by angiography. **A,** Representative T2-weighted coronal image was used for planning the craniotomy. **B,** A T2-weighted coronal image was acquired after the craniotomy began. **C,** An intraoperative image was acquired during resection of the lesion. **D,** A T1-weighted image was acquired after complete removal of the lesion.

however, the lack of adequate operating instrumentation currently remains a primary limitation in the extent and scope of applying this technology to spinal procedures.

FUTURE OF INTRAOPERATIVE MAGNETIC RESONANCE IMAGING IN NEUROSURGERY

Intraoperative MRI is a remarkable tool for image-guided conventional neurosurgery.[27] However, it also has great potential for novel minimally invasive therapy for complex neurosurgical disease. The major future directions for intraoperative MRI in neurosurgery are interstitial thermal therapies, endoscopy, and MR physics.

Intraoperative MRI should have a major effect on the development of thermal therapies for brain and spine lesions. Another ideal volumetric application of intraoperative MRI is interstitial thermal therapy. Interstitial laser treatment of brain

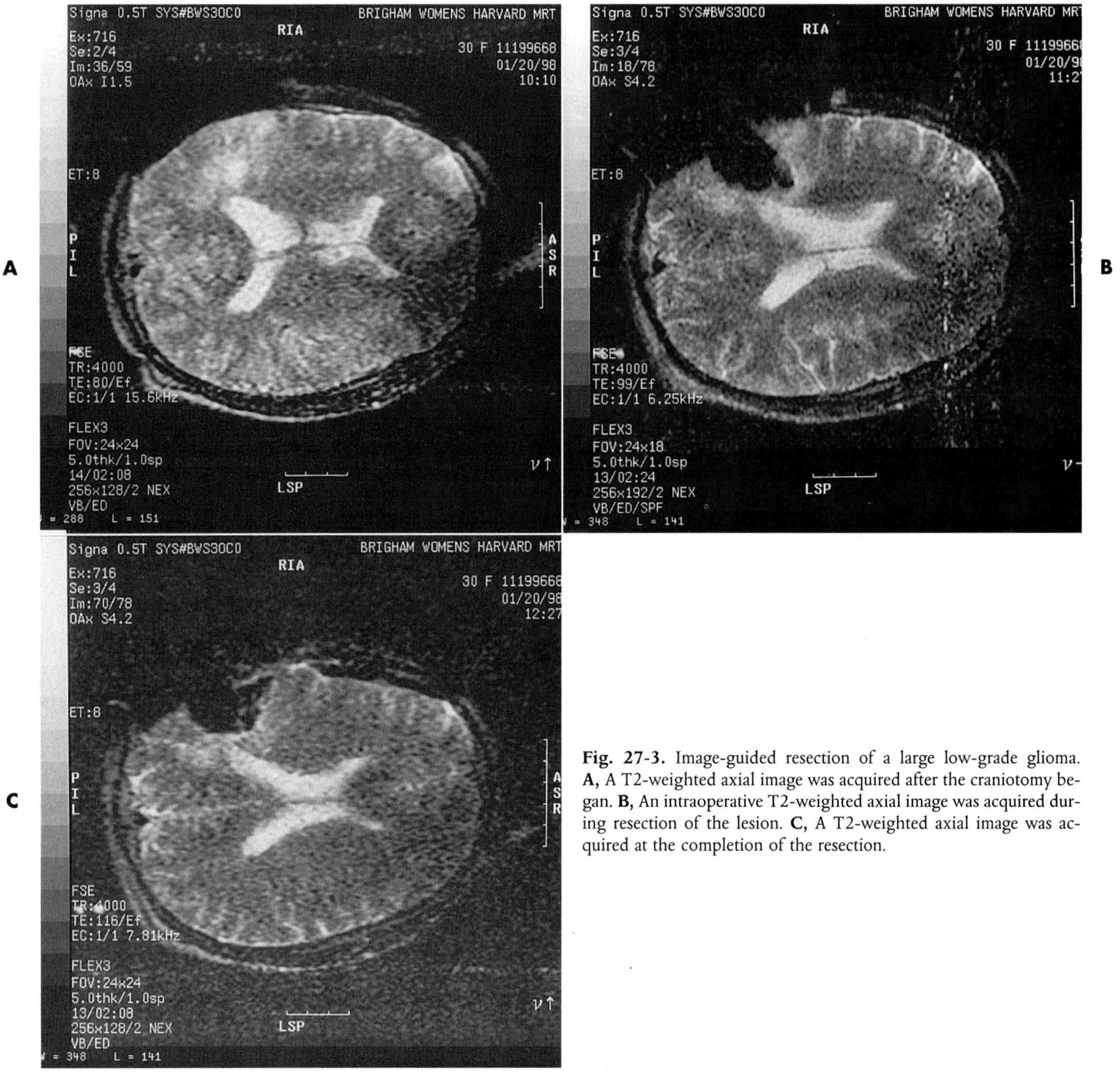

Fig. 27-3. Image-guided resection of a large low-grade glioma. **A,** A T2-weighted axial image was acquired after the craniotomy began. **B,** An intraoperative T2-weighted axial image was acquired during resection of the lesion. **C,** A T2-weighted axial image was acquired at the completion of the resection.

tumors has had varied success over the years. The most significant shortcoming of this technique has been the inability to monitor the extent of therapy in any way other than an empirical way. MRI offers the ability to quantitatively monitor small changes in temperature. Thus, interstitial laser therapy for focal lesions can be accomplished with exacting precision. Because MR can monitor small changes in tissue temperatures and can clearly differentiate heated tissue from ablated tissue, MR can be used to differentiate transient changes from permanent changes in treated tissues. Thus, use of lasers, radiofrequency, cryoprobes, and focused ultrasound in neurosurgery should be re-explored. For example, intraoperative MRI could be used to localize a target for thermal ablation, accurately guide the thermal probe to the location, and monitor the deposition of heat or cold in brain tissue over the course of the treatment. Conceptually, this approach should work well for true anatomical localization for functional neurosurgery (e.g., pallidotomy, thalamotomy). Alternatively, intraoperative MRI could be used to monitor the progression of a surface laser in 3D during microsurgical resection of a craniocervical junction tumor, thus adding one more "sense" to the surgeon's toolkit.

The integration of endoscopy with intraoperative MRI could have a dramatic effect on minimally invasive neurosurgery. Currently, endoscopy provides magnification and illumination over a very small region. Its greatest limitations are that it should be used in open spaces (e.g, ventricles, subarachnoid cisterns) and requires significant hands-on training, particularly in cases of distorted anatomy. Neuroendoscopy would be greatly enhanced by intraoperative MRI. With an MR-compatible endoscope, the surgeon's view would be illuminated and magnified, and cross-sectional MR images of the brain would be referenced to the tip of the endoscope during surgery. The MR image would be a clear roadmap for navigating with the endoscope, thus simplifying the orientational complexities of neuroendoscopy. MR would also allow the surgeon to approach intraparenchymal lesions with an endoscope by allowing visualization beyond the view of the scope.

As clinical applications of intraoperative MRI increase, understanding and exploitation of MR physics will continue to improve, thereby enabling further applications of intraoperative MRI. Over the next few years, developments will make functional MRI, real-time MR angiography, and MR fluoroscopy available for image-guided neurosurgery.

REFERENCES

1. Horsley V, Clark R: The structure and functions of the cerebellum examined by a new method, *Brain* 31:45, 1908.
2. Brown R: A stereotactic head frame for use with CT body scanners, *Invest Radiol* 14:300, 1979.
3. Olivier A, Peters T, Bertrand G: Stereotactic system and apparatus for use with magnetic resonance imaging, computerized tomography and digital subtraction imaging, *Appl Neurophysiol* 48:94, 1985.
4. Lunsford L, Martinez A, Latchaw R: Stereotaxic surgery with a magnetic resonance- and computerized tomography-compatible system, *J Neurosurgery* 64:872, 1986.
5. Lunsford L: *Modern stereotactic neurosurgery,* Boston, 1988, Martinus Nijhoff.
6. Galloway R, Maciunas R: Stereotactic neurosurgery, *Crit Rev Biomed Eng* 18:181, 1990.
7. Alexander E III, and others: Magnetic resonance image-directed stereotactic neurosurgery: use of image fusion with computerized tomography to enhance spatial accuracy, *J Neurosurg* 83:271, 1995.
8. Maroon J, and others: Intracranial biopsy assisted by computerized tomography, *J Neurosurg* 46:572, 1977.
9. Shelden C, and others: Development of a computerized microstereotaxic method for localization and removal of minute CHS lesions under direct 3-D vision: technical report, *J Neurosurg* 52:21, 1980.
10. Kelly P, and others: Computer assisted stereotaxic laser resection of intra-axial brain neoplasms, *J Neurosurg* 64:427, 1986.
11. Kelly PJ, and others: Imaging-based stereotaxic serial biopsies in untreated intracranial glial neoplasms, *J Neurosurg* 66:865, 1987.
12. Kelly PJ: Volumetric stereotactic resection of intra-axial brain mass lesions, *Mayo Clin Proc* 63:1186, 1988.
13. Leksell L: The stereotaxic method and radiosurgery of the brain, *Acta Chir Scand* 102:316, 1951.
14. Winston KR, Lutz W: Linear accelerator as a neurosurgical tool for stereotactic radiosurgery, *Neurosurgery* 22:454, 1988.
15. Alexander E III, Loeffler JS, Lunsford LD: *Stereotactic radiosurgery,* New York, 1993, McGraw-Hill.
16. Maciunas RJ, and others: A technique for interactive image-guided neurosurgical intervention in primary brain tumors, *Neurosurg Clin N Am* 7:245, 1996.
17. Roberts D, and others: A frameless stereotaxic integration of computerized tomographic imaging and the operating microscope, *J Neurosurg* 65:545, 1986.
18. Berger M: Ultrasound-guided stereotaxic biopsy using a new apparatus, *J Neurosurg* 50:550, 1986.
19. Barnett G, and others: Intraoperative localization using an armless, frameless stereotactic wand, *J Neurosurg* 78:510, 1993.
20. Olivier A, and others: Frameless stereotaxy for surgery of the epilepsies: preliminary experience, *J Neurosurg* 81:629, 1994.
21. Gleason P, and others: Video registration virtual reality for frameless stereotacic surgery, *Stereotact Funct Neurosurg* 62, 1995.
22. Nuata HJW: Error assessment during "image guided" and "imaging interactive" stereotactic surgery, *Comput Med Imaging Graph* 18:279, 1993.
23. Walton L, and others: A phantom study to assess the accuracy of stereotactic localization, using T1-weighted magnetic resonance imaging with the Leksell stereotactic system, *Neurosurgery* 38:170, 1996.
24. Bucholz R, and others: Estimation of inaccuracy caused by tissue shift using an optically tracked intraoperative ultrasound device, *Computer Aided Surgery* 1998 (in press) (abstract).
25. Schenck J, and others: Superconducting open-configuration MR imaging system for image-guided therapy, *Radiology* 195:805, 1995.
26. Moriarty TM, and others: Magnetic resonance-imaging therapy (MRT): intraoperative MRI, *Neurosurg Clin N Am* 7:323, 1996.
27. Black P, and others: The development and implementation of intraoperative MRI and its neurosurgical applications, *Neurosurgery* 41:831, 1997.
28. Lufkin R, and others: A technique for MR-guide needle placement *Am J Radiol* 151:193, 1988.
29. Mountz JM, and others: Thallium-201 tumor/cardiac ratio estimation of residual astrocytoma, *J Neurosurg* 68:706, 1988.
30. LeBihan D, Delannoy J, Levin RL: Effects related to temperature changes during MR imaging, *J Magn Reson Imaging* 171:853, 1989.
31. Bleier A, and others: Real-time magnetic imaging of laser heat deposition in tissue, *Magn Reson Med* 21:132, 1991.
32. Cline HE, and others: MR-guided focused ultrasound surgery, *J Comput Assist Tomogr* 16:956, 1992.
33. Crim JR, and others: Diagnosis of soft tissue masses with MR imaging: can benign masses be differentiated from malignant ones? *Radiology* 195:581, 1992.
34. Cline HE, and others: Magnetic resonance thermal guided surgery, *Magn Reson Med* 30:98, 1993.
35. Schwartz MS, and others: *Reoperation following radiosurgery of glioblastoma: impact on survival and neurologic status.* In Alexander E III, and others editors: *Radiosurgery,* Basel, 1995, Karger.
36. Kikinis R, and others: Computer assisted interactive three-dimensional planning for neurosurgical procedures, *Neurosurgery* 38:640, 1996.
37. Riederer SJ, and others: MR fluoroscopy: technical feasibility, *Magn Reson Med* 8:1, 1988.
38. Wright RC, and others: Realtime MR fluoroscopic data acquisition and image reconstruction, *Magn Reson Med* 12:407, 1989.
39. Haacke EM, Liang Z-P, Izen SH: Constrained reconstruction: a superresolution, optimal signal-to-noise alternative to the Fourier transform in magnetic resonance imaging, *Med Phys* 16:388, 1989.
40. Holsinger AE, and others: Realtime interactive magnetic resonance imaging, *Magn Reson Med* 14:547, 1990.
41. Cohen MS, Weisskoff RM: Ultra-fast imaging, *Magn Reson Imaging* 9:1, 1991.
42. Brummer ME, and others: *Composite k-space windows (keyhole techniques) to improve temporal resolution in a dynamic series of images following contrast administration.* In *SMRM conference abstracts,* 1992.
43. van Vaals JJ, Tuithof HH, Dixon WT: *Increased time resolution in dynamic imaging.* In *10th SMRI conference abstracts,* 1992.
44. Xiang QS, Henkelman RM: Dynamic image reconstruction: MR movies from ghosts, *J Magn Reson Imaging* 2:679, 1992.
45. Chenevert TL, Pipe JG: *Dynamic 3D imaging at high temporal resolution via reduced k-space sampling.* In *SMRM conference abstracts,* 1993.
46. Jolesz FA, and others: MR imaging of laser tissue interactions, *Radiology* 168:249, 1988.
47. Jolesz FA, and others: Response to and control of destructive energy by magnetic resonance, *Invest Radiol* 24:1024, 1989.
48. Higuchi N, and others: MRI of the acute effects of interstitial neodymium: YAG laser on tissues, *Invest Radiol* 27:814, 1992.

49. Moonen CT, and others: Functional magnetic resonance imaging in medicine and physiology, *Science* 250:53, 1990.
50. Bullock PR, and others: Dynamic imaging of contrast enhancement in brain tumors, *Magn Reson Med* 19:293, 1991.
51. Lunsford LD, Albright L: Intraoperative imaging with a therapeutic computed tomographic scanner, *Neurosurgery* 15:559, 1984.
52. Frahm J, Haase A, Matthaei D: Rapid NMR imaging of dynamic processes using the FLASH technique, *Magn Reson Med* 3:321, 1986.
53. Haase A: Snapshot flash MRI: application to T1, T2, and chemical shift imaging, *Magn Reson Med* 13:77, 1990.
54. Mulkern RV, and others: Phase encode order and its effect on contrast and artifact in single shot RARE sequences, *Med Phys* 18:1032, 1991.
55. Oshio K, Feinberg DA: GRASE imaging: a novel fast MRI technique, *Magn Reson Med* 20:344, 1991.
56. Chien D, Edelman RR: Ultrafast imaging using gradient echoes, *Magn Reson Q* 7:31, 1991.
57. Jolesz FA, Jones KM: *Fast spin-echo imaging of the brain.* In Yuh WTC, editor: *Topics in magnetic resonance imaging: magnetic resonance techniques in brain neoplasms and pediatrics,* 1993.
58. Ehman RL, Felmlee JP: Adaptive technique for high-definition MR imaging of moving structures, *Radiology* 173:255, 1989.
59. Healy DM, Weaver JB: Two applications of wavelet transform in magnetic resonance imaging, *IEEE Trans Inform Theory* 38:840, 1992.
60. Cao Y, Levin DN: MR imaging with spatially variable resolution, *J Magn Reson Imaging* 2:701, 1992.
61. Weaver JB, and others: Wavelet-encoded MR imaging, *Magn Reson Med* 24:275, 1992.
62. Cao Y, Levin DN: Feature-recognizing MRI, *Magn Reson Med* 30:305, 1993.
63. Panych LP, Jakab PD, Jolesz FA: An implementation of wavelet encoded MRI, *J Magn Reson Imaging* 3:649, 1993.
64. Heilbrun MP, Roberts TS, Apuzzo MLJ: Preliminary experience with Brown-Roberts-Wells (BRW) computerized tomography stereotaxic guidance system, *Neurosurgery* 59:217, 1983.
65. Luzzati R, and others: Stereotactic brain biopsy in human immunodeficiency virus-infected patients, *Arch Intern Med* 156:565, 1996.
66. Chimowitz MI, Barnett GH, Palmer J: Treatment of intractable arterial hemorrhage during stereotactic brain biopsy with thrombin: report of three patients, *J Neurosurg* 74:301, 1991.
67. Levy RM, and others: The efficacy of image-guided stereotactic brain biopsy in neurologically symptomatic acquired immunodeficiency syndrome patients, *Neurosurgery* 30:186, 1992.
68. Bernstein M, and others: *Complications and failures of stereotactic biopsy of brain lesions,* CNS 1994 Annual Meeting, 1994.

Chapter 28

MRI-GUIDED BRAIN BIOPSY AND STEREOTACTIC PROCEDURES

Volker M. Tronnier, Andreas Staubert, Michael Knauth

Initiated by Clarke and Horsley[1] in 1906, stereotactic methodology has been used by neurosurgeons to map image space onto physical space. Although earlier attempts were made to operate following brain maps,[2,3] Clarke and Horsley used a cartesian coordinate system for the first time. The first operation in humans was performed more than 40 years later in 1947 by Spiegel and others.[4] Construction of stereotactic systems has followed the same principle, with a reference system fixed to the patient's body serving as a mechanical platform for an aiming device that guides surgical tools to an intended target. This target is calculated in relation to external or internal landmarks visible on the different imaging modalities as ventriculography, computed tomography (CT), or magnetic resonance imaging (MRI). Two-dimensional (2D) projectional ventriculography is replaced in most centers by computerized 3D reconstructions of slices from the CT or directly nonreformatted 3D images from MRI. One major advantage of the modern imaging techniques is the use of the same cartesian coordinates as in stereotaxy. New imaging modalities and computer techniques led to a resurgence of stereotaxy in the 1980s and 1990s.

Despite these modern imaging and computer techniques, frame-based stereotaxy as the gold standard for target accuracy is still a point-based, single-trajectory technique, making new calculations necessary if other entry points, target points, or trajectories are chosen. Sharp fixation of a frame to the skull is uncomfortable for the patient, and any dislocation of the frame disrupts the relationship of the reference system to the chosen target. Another disadvantage of frame-based stereotaxy, especially in open neurosurgical procedures, is the bulky frame, often limiting the surgeon's access to the operative field. Therefore, frameless procedures were developed with surface markers or a surface-matching algorithm, allowing determination of the head orientation and location of an extra- or intracranial target. Different neuronavigational systems, based on passive robotic pointers, rely on angle detectors in articulated arms,[5–11] which are mechanically linked to the digitizing system and nonlinked systems, and on detection of optical,[12] sonic,[13–15] or magnetic[16] signals generated by special emitters. These different systems are used to guide special probes, common surgical instruments, endoscopes, or even the operating microscope in the surgical field. Based on the advances in computer technology, these navigational systems are compatible with the different imaging modalities. In addition to CT and MRI, angiography, magnetoencephalography, and positron emission tomography data can be integrated with the

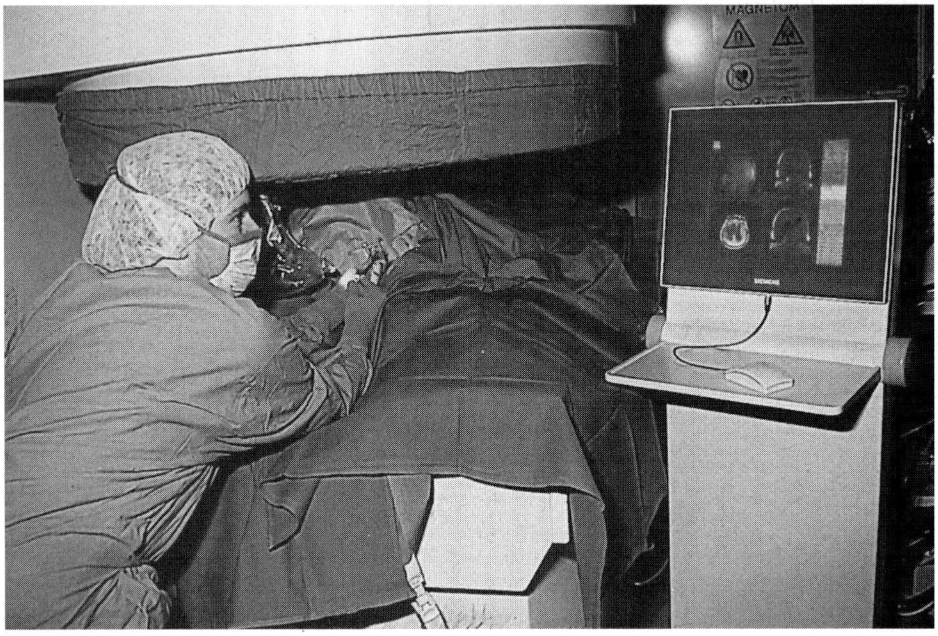

Fig. 28-1. Interventional procedures can be monitored with a magnetic resonance–compatible in-room liquid crystal display monitor.

surgical planning to provide intraoperative guidance. The surgeon obtains a view of the real-time position of the instrument in relation to the target region. However, these neurosurgical navigational systems have major drawbacks. Arm-based systems are bulky and often limited in the range of the operational field. Optical systems with light-emitting diodes need a camera array and an unobstructed path for detecting the infrared light. Sonic digitizers determine the position by measuring the time of flight of sound to an array of microphones; unobstructed or undisturbed connections are absolutely necessary. Magnetic digitizers superimpose a magnetic field on the surgical field. Position can be determined by a probe that measures the gradients in the magnetic field. However, the homogenicity of the magnetic field is often disturbed by ferromagnetic instruments and electromagnetic radiation, limiting the accuracy of such systems.

Also, this kind of computer-assisted surgery or interactive image-guided surgery is based on preoperative data sets. Any anatomic distortion created by the surgery (e.g., by loss of cerebrospinal fluid or insertion of brain spatulas) is not taken into account. Description of these approaches as "real-time image-guided surgery" is therefore incorrect, and many neurosurgical groups are looking for a solution. Intraoperative CT as a possible solution to overcome these disadvantages was developed by Lunsford, Parrish, and Albright[17,18] and Okudera, Takemae and Kobayashi.[19] Several groups have tried to integrate intraoperative ultrasound for image correction[14] and most recently introduced intraoperative MRI.[20–22] This chapter focuses on the latter technique and describes the different approaches of intraoperative MRI in image-guided surgery with special respect to biopsy and stereotactic procedures.

MAGNETIC RESONANCE SCANNERS

Percutaneous biopsies in different body regions guided by MRI using conventional MR systems have been reported.[23–28] Also, reports on therapeutic interventional procedures, especially laser ablation, have recently been published.[29–32] The advantages of MRI compared with ultrasound and CT are obvious. In addition to multiplanar capabilities, high spatial resolution, and excellent soft-tissue contrast, the absence of ionizing radiation makes MR guidance for brain biopsies and interventions an attractive alternative. The possibility to monitor therapy by near real-time MRI and temperature-sensitive MR sequences is very appealing.[33–35]

The problem of limited patient access with conventional MR scanners has been solved by the introduction of dedicated open MR systems based on different concepts and principles for use in neurosurgical cases (see Chapters 1 through 5). These open scanners allow wide patient access to monitor anesthesia and to perform neurosurgical interventions and even open neurosurgical procedures. In addition to dedicated MR scanners, developed with additional accessories to perform open neurosurgical resection of brain tumors and other lesions, many general purpose open MR scanners can be used for brain biopsies and other interventional procedures. For biopsies and other stereotactic procedures to be performed, special requirements (e.g., an in-room monitor [Fig. 28-1], fast MR sequences to monitor an instrument advancing through the brain to a desired target) are needed.

INSTRUMENTATION

MR-compatible instruments are required to perform any procedure in a magnetic field. Moving or torquing of the instrument, which may harm the patient, should be ruled out, and distortions of the magnetic field should be avoided to minimize imaging artifacts by the different tools.

The first MR-compatible needles for biopsies were designed a decade ago.[23,25] Today, ceramic, carbon fiber, plastic, and titanium needles are available.[36] Unlike body regions where freehand biopsies are performed under imaging control, the skull

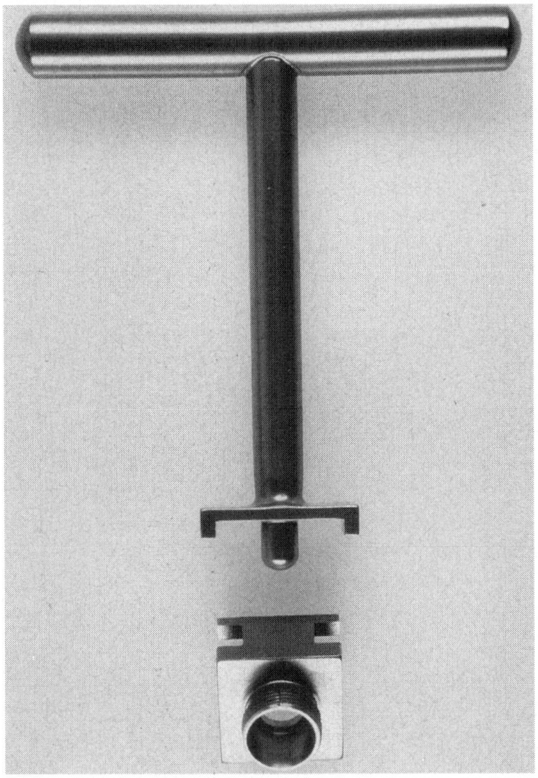

Fig. 28-2. The Heidelberg Intervention Trajector (Pilling-Weck GmbH, Karlstein, Germany) has a handle and fixation plate with a thread for a 14-mm drill.

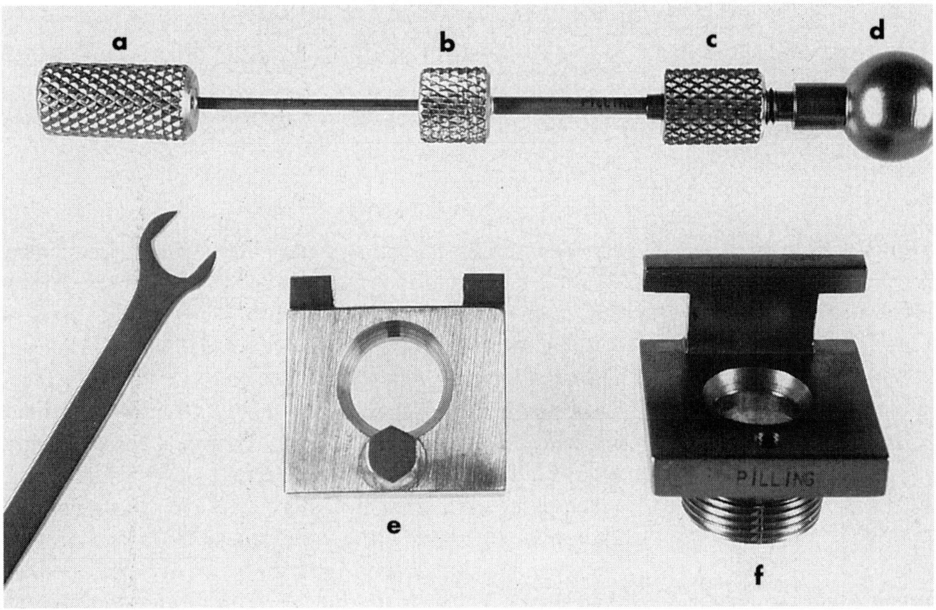

Fig. 28-3. Different parts of the Heidelberg Intervention Trajector (Pilling-Weck GmbH, Karlstein, Germany): stylet *(a),* guiding cannula *(b),* fixation screw *(c)* for guiding cannula (depth fixation), sphere *(d)* for angulation with central bore, fixation plate *(e)* for sphere (angulation fixation), and fixation plate with burrhole thread *(f).*

offers the possibility to mount a positioning device for safe introduction and advancement of the instrument to the desired target. In common stereotaxy, this positioning was provided by the head frame, fixed sharply to the skull, and an aiming bow. However, the goals of interventional MRI are to be as least invasive as possible and to perform the procedure in a frameless manner using local anesthesia.

Different burrhole–mounted devices have been constructed (Heidelberg Intervention Trajector, Pilling Weck GmbH, Karlstein, Germany; Snapper Stereoguide, Magnetic Vision GmbH, Rüti, Switzerland), which allow the secure fixation of a biopsy needle or aspiration catheter with an angulation in a certain range. Although the Magnetic Vision system is guided by a navigation system using light-emitting diodes, which allow the surgeon to plan the exact localization of the burr hole according to the chosen trajectory and straight insertion of the needle, the Heidelberg Intervention Trajector uses an integrated gadolinium-filled wand and a bored sphere that allows angulation from $-20°$ to $20°$ in each direction (Figs. 28-2 and 28-3). The Heidelberg Intervention Trajector integrates a 1-mm biopsy cup

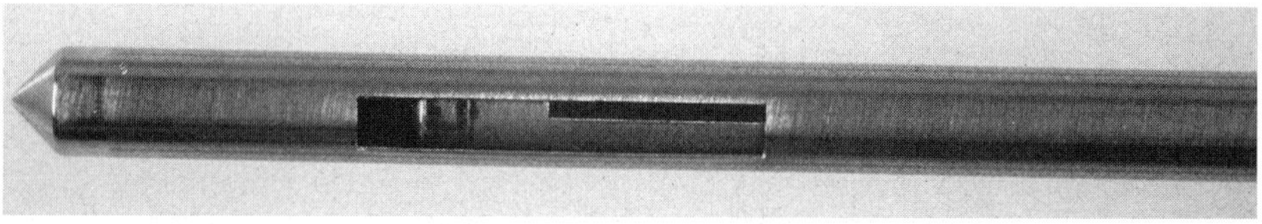

Fig. 28-4. The Heidelberg Brain Biopsy cannula (Somatex, Medizintechnische Instrumente GmbH, Berlin, Germany), based on the side-cutting and aspiration principle has a side cutting window (titanium).

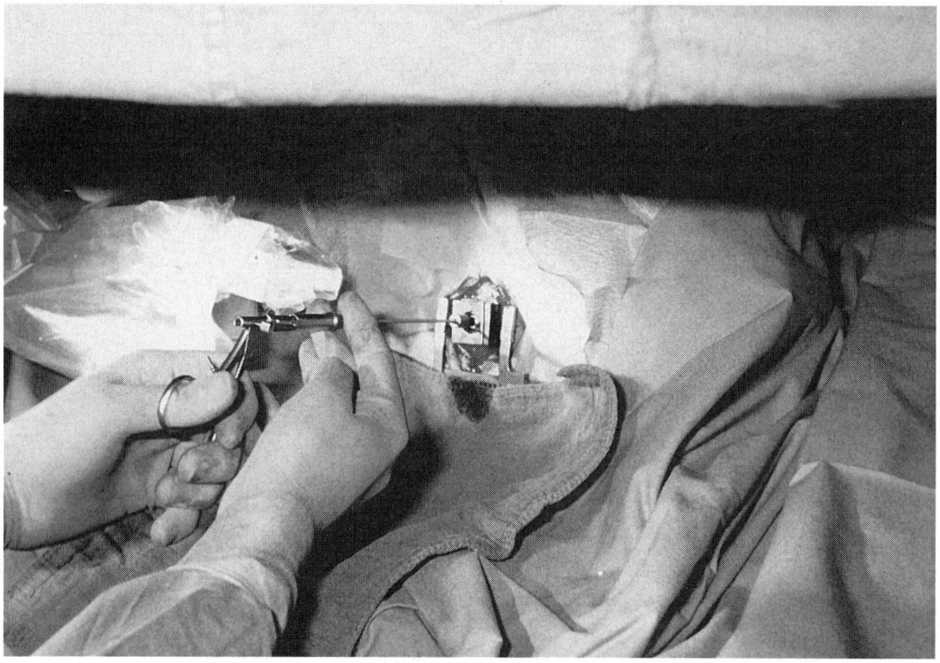

Fig. 28-5. The Heidelberg Intervention Trajector (Pilling-Weck GmbH, Karlstein, Germany) is screwed into the skull.

forceps, allowing the operator to take biopsies from small lesions in delicate areas. The Magnetic Vision System and the Heidelberg Brain Biopsy Cannula (Somatex, Medizintechnische Instrumente GmbH, Berlin, Germany) are based on the side-cutting and aspiration principle (Fig. 28-4) and have coaxial plastic or titanium cannulas with a side window for taking small cores of tissue by aspiration and cutting of the specimen.

TECHNIQUE FOR ON-LINE MAGNETIC RESONANCE–GUIDED INTERVENTIONS IN THE MAGNETOM OPEN

For the technique for on-line MR–guided interventions in the Magnetom Open (Siemens AG, Erlangen, Germany), the patient is positioned on the MR table in a supine position. The head is situated in the commercially available headcoil, which allows access to standard stereotactic approaches (precoronal, parietal, and temporal). For other lesions (e.g., infratentorial), a multipurpose ring-shaped coil is used. The lesion is first shown with a gadolinium-enhanced T1-weighted image (spin-echo; repetition time, 570 msec; echo time, 15 msec; two acquisitions; 19 slices; 5-mm slice thickness; acquisition time, 3:15 sec; 256 × 256 matrix) or a T2 proton density image (spin-echo; repetition time, 4000 msec; echo time, 26 msec; two acquisitions; acquisition time, 5:13 sec; 256 × 256 matrix). The entry point and the trajectory are planned with two orthogonal laser beams or a gadolinium-filled wand and a fast imaging with steady-state precession (FISP)-2D sequence (gradient echo; repetition time, 17.8 msec; echo time, 8.1 msec; one acquisition; 256 × 256 matrix; 2.5 msec/image). After the slice position and orientation are determined, the patient is moved outside the 20-m T line, and a burrhole craniotomy is performed using conventional drills and electrocautery. A titanium wound retractor is inserted, and the burrhole mounted cannula holder (Heidelberg Intervention Trajector, Pilling-Weck GmbH, Karlstein, Germany) (Fig. 28-5) is screwed into the skull. The patient is brought back into the scanner in the same position, and the procedure (e.g., biopsy, catheter placement) is continued under almost real-time conditions (one image every 2 sec) using a FISP 2D sequence. Biopsies can be taken from different tumor areas, and cysts or absesses can be emptied under real-time conditions (Figs. 28-6 and 28-7). At the end of the procedure, another T1-weighted image is performed. Major intraoperative complications such as hemorrhages may be detected immediately.

A

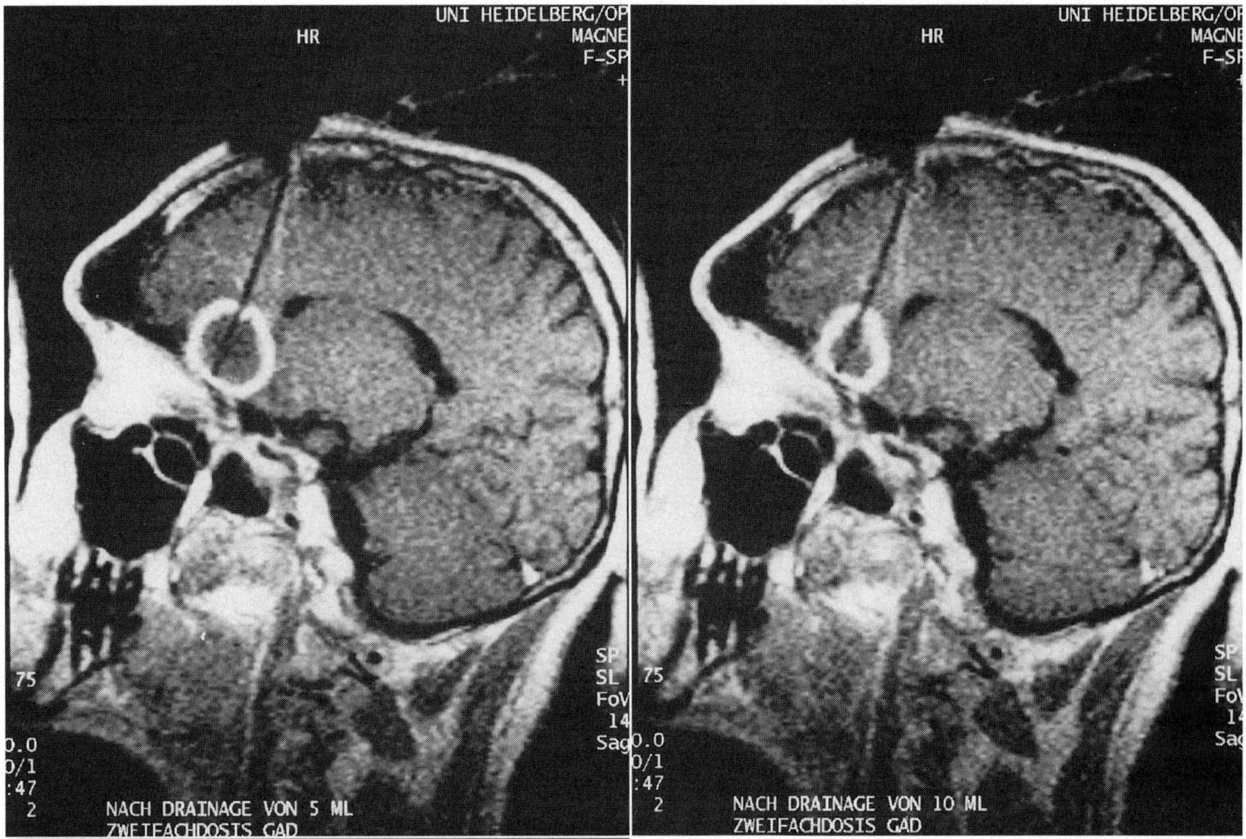

B

C

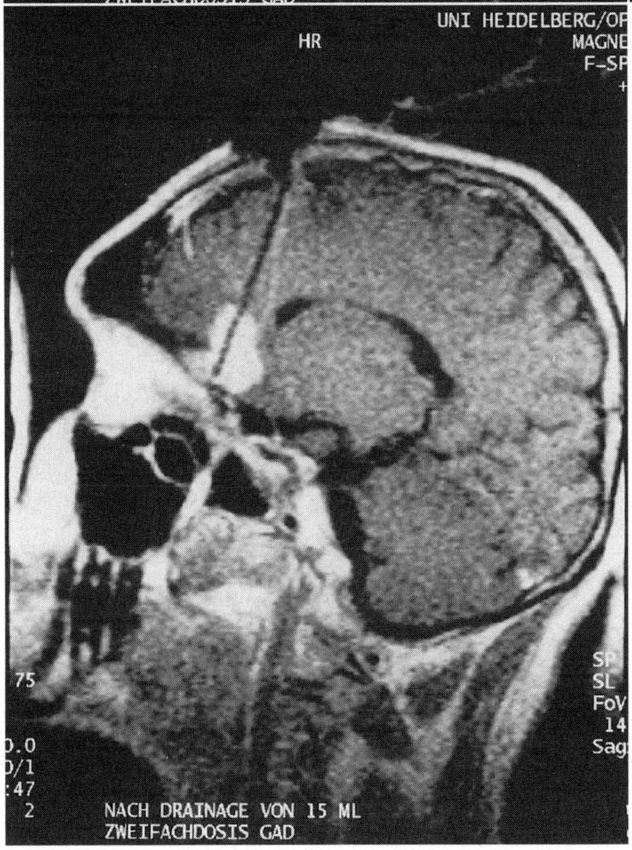

Fig. 28-6. **A,** Subsequent drainage of a frontobasal abscess after aspiration of 5 ml of pus; **B,** after aspiration of 10 ml of pus; and **C,** at the end of the procedure and aspiration of 15 ml of pus.

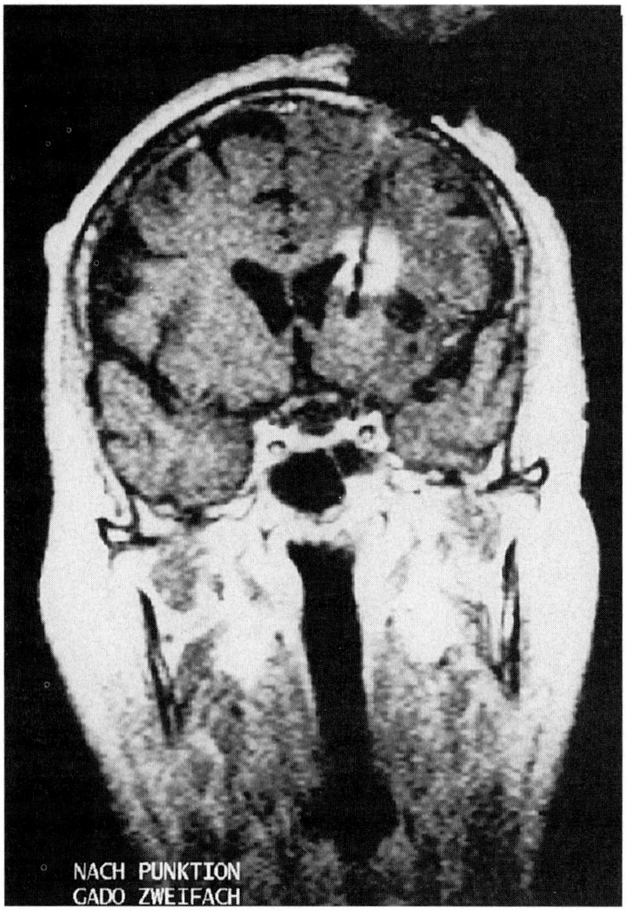

Fig. 28-7. Frontal malignant glioma. Biopsy with the Heidelberg Brain Biopsy cannula (Somatex, Medizintechnische Instrumente GmbH, Berlin, Germany), which has the side window in the center of the lesion.

Table 28-1. MR–guided biopsies performed at the Heidelberg University Hospital

Tumor type	Biopsies *(n)*
Low-grade gliomas	6
High-grade gliomas	9
Lymphomas	4
Metastases	2
Craniopharyngiomas	2
Others (e.g., radiation necrosis, Leigh syndrome, toxoplasmosis)	6

So far, 29 biopsies of different brain lesions (Table 28-1), 4 cyst aspirations, and drainage of 4 abscesses have been performed at the authors' institution using this technique. For brachytherapy applications, patients were placed in the scanner, and general anesthesia was applied. The head was fixed in a ceramic stereotactic frame (Howmedica-Leibinger, Freiburg, Germany). The target for the central catheter was determined with conventional stereotactic methods, and the catheter was applied

A

B

C

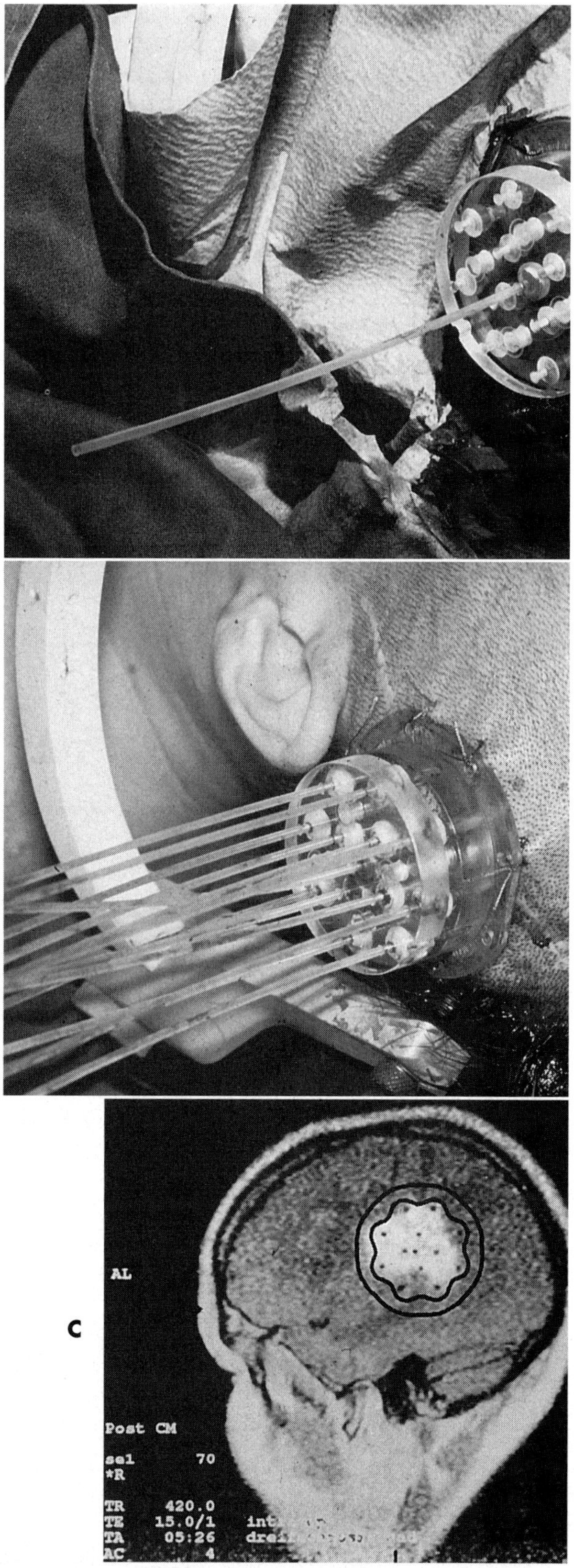

Fig. 28-8. A, Stereotactic placement of a brachytherapy catheter in the center of the target. **B,** At the end of the procedure, 13 parallel catheters were placed in a recurrent glioblastoma. The depth of the catheters was controlled on-line under magnetic resonance guidance. **C,** A sagittal view shows the twist drill burrholes used for radiation planning.

with the help of a stereotactic aiming bow, while the patient couch was moved out of the magnetic field. Additionally, a template with parallel bores was used (Fig. 28-8). The depth of the first catheter was controlled by MRI, and at least 10 other catheters were placed parallel to the first one under MR guidance. The MRI at the end of the procedure was used to plan management by the radiation oncologist.

CONCLUSIONS

MR-guided interventions are safe and reliable procedures with high diagnostic yield. They offer real-time monitoring of needle advancement and targeting. In addition to the advantage of excellent image quality, a sharp frame-based head fixation is not needed in most cases. Intraoperative complications are readily discovered. Another possible major advantage is a shorter operating time when performing the procedure inside the scanner.

REFERENCES

1. Clarke RH, Horsley V: On a method of investigating the deep ganglia and tracts of the central nervous system (cerebellum), *BMJ* 2:1799, 1906.
2. Dittmar C: Uber die Lage des sogenannten Gefässzentrums in der Medulla oblongata, *Ber Sachs Ges Wiss Leipzig* 25:449, 1873.
3. Zernov DN: L'encephalometre, *Proc Gen Clin Ther* 19:302, 1890.
4. Spiegel EA, and others: Stereotaxic apparatus for operations on the human brain, *Science* 106:349, 1947.
5. Drake JM, and others: ISG Viewing Wand, *Neurosurgery* 34:1094, 1994.
6. Leggett WB, and others: The viewing wand: a new system for three-dimensional CT correlated intraoperative localization, *Curr Surg* 48:674, 1991.
7. Olivier A, and others: Frameless stereotaxy for surgery of the epilepsies: preliminary experience, *J Neurosurg* 81:629, 1994.
8. Reinhardt HF, Landolt H: CT-guided "real time" stereotaxy, *Acta Neurochir Suppl (Wien)* 46:107, 1989.
9. Sandeman DR, and others: Advances in image-directed neurosurgery: preliminary experience with the ISG viewing wand compared with the Leksell frame, *Br J Neurosurg* 8:529, 1994.
10. Watanabe E, and others: Three-dimensional digitizer (Neuronavigator): new equipment for CT-guided stereotaxic surgery, *Surg Neurol* 27:543, 1987.
11. Zinreich SJ, and others: Frameless stereotactic integration of CT imaging data: accuracy and initial applications, *Radiology* 188:735, 1993.
12. Heilbrun MP, and others: Stereotactic localization and guidance using a machine vision technique, *Stereotact Funct Neurosurg* 58:94, 1992.
13. Barnett GE, and others: Use of a frameless, armless stereotactic wand for brain tumor localization with two-dimensional and three-dimensional neuroimaging, *Neurosurgery* 33:674, 1993.
14. Koivukangas J, and others: Ultrasound-controlled neuronavigator-guided brain surgery, *J Neurosurg* 79:36, 1993.
15. Roberts DW, and others: A frameless stereotaxic integration of computerized tomographic imaging and the operating microscope, *J Neurosurg* 65:545, 1986.
16. Manwaring KH, Manwaring ML, Moss SD: Magnetic field guided endoscopic dissection through a burrhole may avoid more invasive craniotomies, *Acta Neurochir Suppl (Wien)* 61:34, 1994.
17. Lunsford LD: A dedicated CT-system for the stereotactic operating room, *Appl Neurophysiol* 45:374, 1982.
18. Lunsford LD, Parrish R, Albright L: Intraoperative imaging with a therapeutic computed tomographic scanner, *Neurosurgery* 15:559, 1984.
19. Okudera H, Takemae T, Kobayashi K: Intraoperative computed tomographic scanning during transsphenoidal surgery: technical note, *Neurosurgery* 32:1041, 1993.
20. Schenck JF, and others: Superconductive open-configuration MR imaging system for image-guided therapy, *Radiology* 195:805, 1995.
21. Tronnier VM, and others: Intraoperative diagnostic and interventional magnetic resonance imaging in neurosurgery, *Neurosurgery* 40:891, 1997.
22. Black PM: The development and implementation of intraoperative MRI and its application, *Neurosurgery* 41:831, 1997.
23. Mueller PR, and others: MR-guided aspiration biopsy: needle design and clinical trials, *Radiology* 161:605, 1986.
24. Hayek PC, and others: Localization grid for MR-guided biopsy, *Radiology* 163:825, 1987.
25. Lufkin R, Teresi L, Hanafee W: New needle for MR-guided aspiration cytology of the head and neck, *Am J Roentgenol* 149:380, 1987.
26. Wenokur R, and others: Magnetic resonance imaging-guided fine needle aspiration for the diagnosis of head and neck lesions, *Skull Base Surg* 2:167, 1992.
27. Pitt AM, and others: MRI-guided biopsy in inflammatory myopathy: initial results, *Magn Reson Imaging* 11:1093, 1993.
28. Greenstein SO, and others: MR imaging-guided localization and biopsy of breast lesions: initial experience, *Radiology* 193:97, 1994.
29. Jolesz FA, and others: MR imaging of laser tissue interaction, *Radiology* 168:853, 1988.
30. Masters A, and others: Interstitial laser hyperthermia: a new approach for treating liver metastases, *Br J Cancer* 66:518, 1992.
31. Kahn T, and others: MRI-guide laser-induced interstitial thermotherapy of cerebral neoplasms, *J Comput Assist Tomogr* 18:519, 1994.
32. Vogl T, and others: Recurrent nasopharyngeal tumors: preliminary clinical results with interventional MR-imaging controlled laser-induced thermotherapy, *Radiology* 196:725, 1995.
33. Jolesz FA, Blumenfeld SM: Interventional use of magnetic resonance imaging, *Magn Reson Q* 10:85, 1994.
34. Matsumoto R, and others: Tissue temperature monitoring for thermal interventional therapy: comparison of T1-weighted images, *J Magn Reson Imaging* 4:65, 1994.
35. Young I, and others: Further observations on the measurement of tissue T1 to monitor temperature in vivo by MRI, *Magn Reson Med* 31:342, 1994.
36. Schenck, and others: Carbon fiber biopsy cannulas for MR-compatible neurosurgical procedures, *Proc Third Annual Meeting Int Soc Mag Res Med* 1160, 1995.

Chapter 29

MR-GUIDED LASER ABLATION OF BRAIN TUMORS

Thomas Kahn, Hans-Joachim Schwarzmaier, Frank Ulrich

The experience at Dusseldorf and Krefeld
Magnetic resonance heat monitoring
Magnetic resonance tissue monitoring
Pilot human studies
Clinical follow-up
Conclusions

Laser-induced interstitial thermotherapy (LITT) is a minimally invasive technique of local tumor destruction.[1] The laser energy is directed into the target volume through optical fibers implanted interstitially. The main advantages of LITT are precise delivery of energy to tissue and minimal damage to adjacent structures. Additionally, treatment of deep cerebral lesions usually inaccessible to surgical resection can be performed with preservation of superficial tissue. Optical and thermal diffusion of the absorbed laser energy leads to damage of tissue.[2,3] Several factors are involved in the initial laser light distribution (e.g., laser wavelength, fiber tip characteristics, wavelength-dependent absorption, scattering properties of tissue). The initial heat distribution is then modulated by heat conduction and convection by blood perfusion. Additionally, the optical parameters of tissue are changing during therapy. The optical properties of different tissues, especially tumors, vary significantly.[4]

THE EXPERIENCE AT DUSSELDORF AND KREFELD

Use of a special fiberoptic transmission system, the ITT light guide (Dornier Medizintechnik, Gemering, Germany), which operates with reduced power density at the light guide tip compared with a bare fiber, minimizes the risk of carbonization.[5] Temporal temperature profiles measured *in vitro* in pig brain and *in vivo* in rat brain revealed a steep decrease in temperature within several millimeters from the ITT light guide.[2]

Image guidance of LITT should fulfill several aims: target definition, trajectory selection, laser light guide tracking, and monitoring the localization and volume of the induced lesion indicated by an overlay of the spatial temperature distribution on the anatomic data. Magnetic resonance imaging (MRI) is well-suited to monitor LITT because of its high soft-tissue contrast and sensitivity for temperature changes.[6,7] Experimental studies in phantoms and animal models support the value of MRI in monitoring LITT.[8–11]

MAGNETIC RESONANCE HEAT MONITORING

The most promising approach to thermometry using MRI is based on the temperature-dependent chemical shift. The mean phase in a voxel built up during the specific echo time varies because of small temperature-related frequency shifts. These induced phase shifts can be measured with an appropriate gradient echo sequence. Using an experimental set-up with homogeneous heating of pig brain *in vitro* in a water bath, a linear correlation exists between phase shift and temperature of 20° C to 60° C using a two-dimensional (2D) fast low-angle shot (FLASH) sequence (repetition time, 40 msec; echo time, 14 msec; flip angle, 40°). Until now, the phase method seems to show no tissue dependence (with the exception of fat tissue) and offers a chance to accurately calculate actual temperature *in vivo.*[12–14] Results with laser ablation of pig brain emphasize the capabilities of this method for monitoring LITT. Since 1996, this method has been used for monitoring LITT. The complex raw data of the phase images are automatically transferred to a workstation, unwrapped, and subtracted from a baseline phase image. The resulting temperature values are superimposed on an anatomic image. The temporal resolution is approximately 25 sec. The program is integrated in a user surface that allows an arbitrary scaling of the upper and lower limits of the displayed temperature. Preliminary experience with the application of the phase mapping method *in vivo* indicated its feasibility. To avoid gross motion of the patient's head, tight fixation is required. However, tiny movements and intrinsic pulsations of the brain do not significantly disturb the results.

MAGNETIC RESONANCE TISSUE MONITORING

In addition to direct temperature monitoring, MRI can depict irreversible tissue change caused by coagulation and vacuolization. In an experimental animal study, a typical zonal anatomy of a laser-induced lesion in rat brain with a central and a peripheral zone was found.[2] In the central zone, electron microscopic examination of the acute changes showed generalized damage of cellular and subcellular membranes surrounding the light guide track. Likewise, the intravascular erythrocytes displayed membrane defects and appeared empty. On T1-weighted images, this zone is displayed with high signal intensity and on T2-weighted images with low signal intensity, presumably because of hemoglobin decomposition products.

Fine structural examination of the peripheral zone in experimental animals revealed no membrane disruptions, rather edema with generalized swelling and an empty appearance of nerve cell processes and astrocytic foot processes. The MR appearance with low signal intensity on T1-weighted and high signal intensity on T2-weighted images is in good accordance with the histopathologic findings.

PILOT HUMAN STUDIES

After this detailed neuropathologic study of laser–brain tissue interaction in an animal model was completed, a clinical pilot study was started in 1992 in 31 patients with brain tumors.[15,16] All masses were located supratentorially and had an approximately spherical configuration with an MRI-determined diameter ranging from 18 to 35 mm (mean, 27.9 mm). Neoplasms with intratumoral bleeding and mainly cystic components were excluded. All diagnoses were based on preceding stereotactic biopsy and histologic analysis.

There were 24 astrocytomas (World Health Organization [WHO] grade II), 4 anaplastic gliomas (WHO III–IV), 2 brain metastases of renal adenocarcinomas, and 1 malignant lymphoma. Eighteen neoplasms were located in or close to the sensimotor cortical fields, one tumor was located in the hippocampus, one mass in the anterior corpus callosum, and one tumor in the thalamus.

A neodymium:yttrium-aluminum-garnet (Nd:YAG) laser (Medilas 4060N, 1064 nm, continuous wave, Dornier Medizintechnik, Germering, Germany) was used in combination with an ITT light guide. This device causes a directed circumferential emission profile at the tip because of a special fiber coupler. The length of the flexible light guide is 12 m. The laser unit was installed outside the magnet room. A built-in powermeter was used to control the power output. Additionally, before and after every laser therapy, the system was calibrated with an external powermeter (Model 365 AT, detector head 38001, Scientech, Boulder, Colo). Transmission loss varied between 10% and 15% of the given output power.

All patients underwent detailed neurologic and electroencephalographic examination. The patients with tumors in the sensorimotor cortical fields were additionally examined by neurophysiologic methods (somatosensory evoked potentials, motor evoked potentials, and isometric precision force control). In seven patients, functional MRI using the blood oxygenation level–dependent (BOLD) method was performed in a single section technique with one acquisition using a 2D FLASH sequence (repetition time, 90 msec; echo time, 60 msec; flip angle 40°, 128 × 128 matrix). Five images were acquired during rest and five images during repetitive finger flexion movements of the contralateral hand with respect to the side of the tumor. The procedure was repeated over six cycles, resulting in 60 measurements. The images were postprocessed with a temporal correlation analysis and colorcoding of correlation coefficients.[17] MRI was performed using a 1.5-T Magnetom (Siemens, Erlangen, Germany) with a circularly polarized head coil.

Immediately before LITT, computed tomography (Philips Tomoscan 310, Eindhofen, The Netherlands) of the brain for guidance of stereotactic tumor biopsy was performed in each instance. The stereotactic coordinates were calculated with a Riechert-Mundinger stereotactic frame (Leibinger, Freiburg, Germany). After the biopsy, a 7-F polytef sheath (Cordis, Erkrath, Germany) was implanted based on the stereotactic coordinates, with the tip 5 to 10 mm proximal to the margin of the tumor. The sheath was later used to introduce the light guide. After the sheath was fixed at the skull and the stereotactic frame was removed, the patients were transferred to the MRI unit.

After the patients were placed on the MR table, the sterile light guide was introduced via the sheath into the center of the tumor according to the stereotactic calculations. The light guide was fixed to the sheath and the MR table. The patients were awake and received no anesthesia. Patient contact was continuously maintained throughout the procedure.

For the position of the tip of the light guide and the sheath to be determined, multiplanar reconstructions of a 3D turbo FLASH sequence were used. In 15 of 16 patients, the laser output was adjusted to 4 W (in one case to 5 W). The time of irradiation varied from 10 to 20 min. Phase-sensitive 2D FLASH and echo-shifted turbo FLASH were used in later sequences. In accordance with experimental studies *in vitro* in pig brain, the irreversible damaged zone is outlined by the 60° to 65° isotherm (Figs. 29-1 to 29-3).[18]

During follow-up, in all patients a central high signal intensity and a peripheral low signal intensity zone were displayed on T1-weighted images, which corresponded to the 2D FLASH scans during therapy. Moreover, in all cases, a thin (1 to 3 mm) enhancing rim on T1-weighted images after gadopentetate

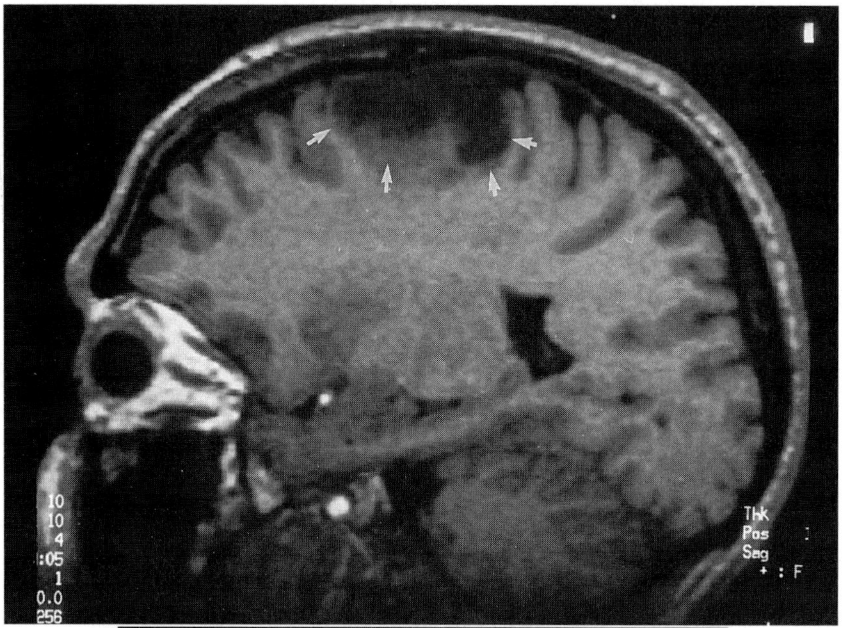

A

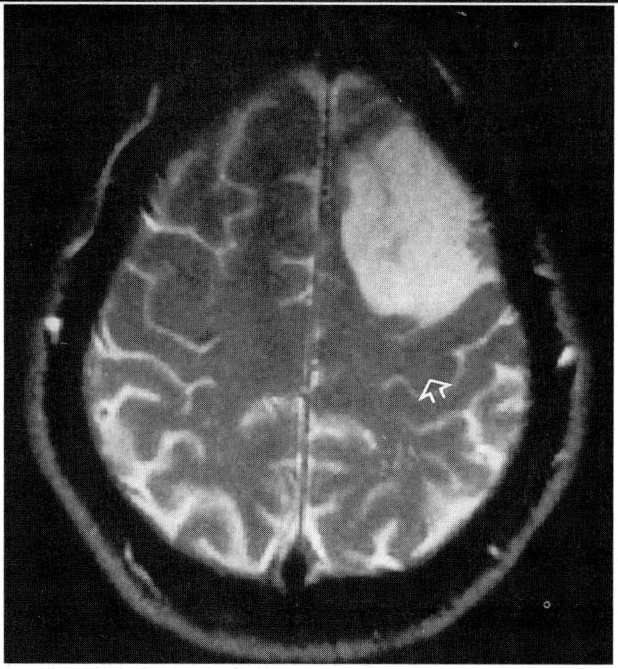

B

Fig. 29-1. Pretherapeutic **A,** sagittal plane T1-weighted three-dimensional turbo fast low-angle shot image and **B,** axial T2-weighted spin-echo image. The mass is located directly adjacent to the precentral gyrus *(arrows).* No distinct perifocal edema is present. No uptake of contrast material occured after intravenous application of Gd:DTPA (not shown). The functional magnetic resonance imaging study located the cortical motor hand area in its typical place in the posterior bank of the precentral gyrus *(open arrow).* (From Kahn TH, and others: In vivo MR thermometry using phase-sensitive sequences: preliminary experience during MRI-guided laser-induced interstitial thermotherapy of brain tumors, *J Magn Reson Imaging* 8:160, 1998.)

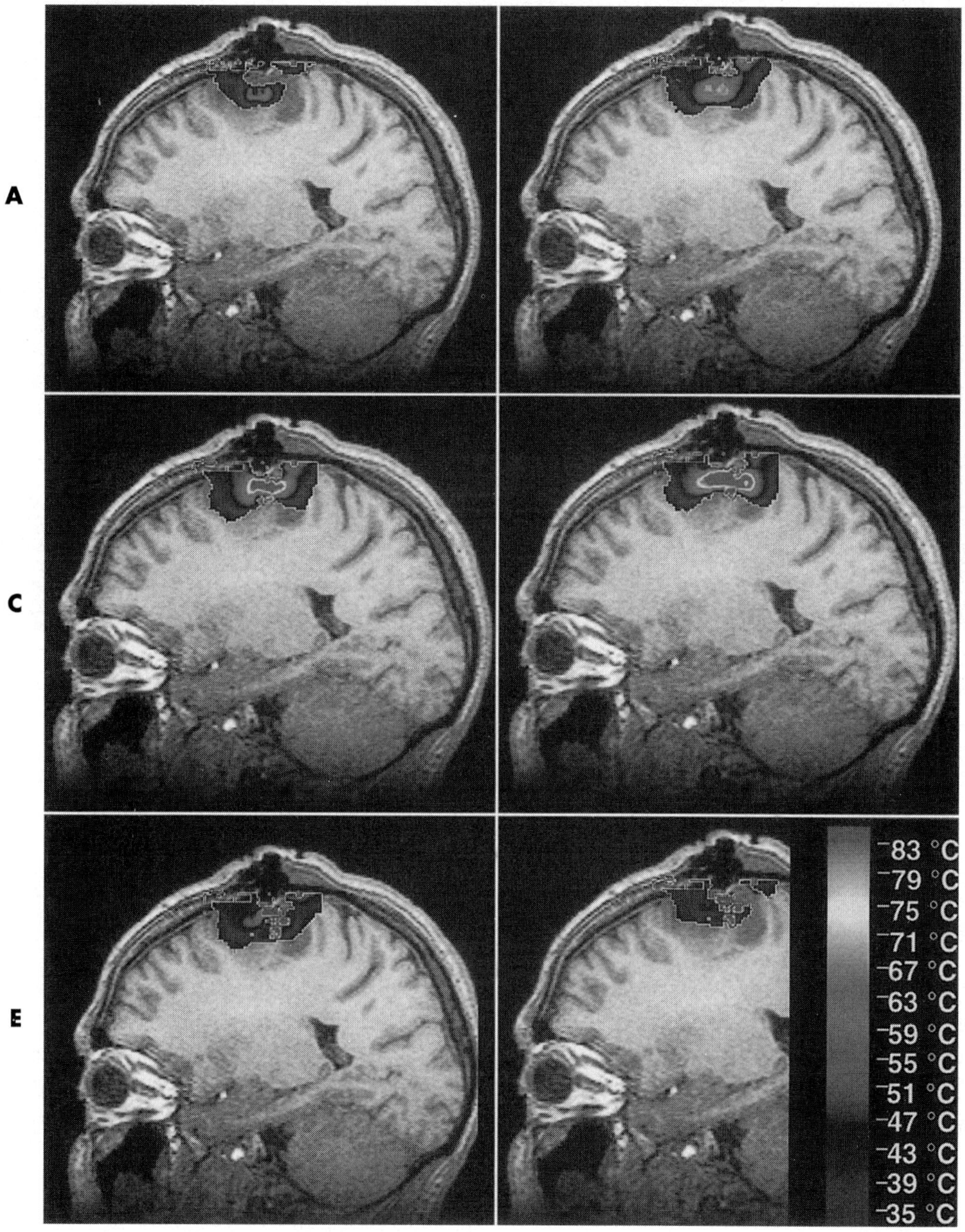

Fig. 29-2. Postprocessed phase-sensitive two-dimensional fast low-angle shot images acquired and displayed during and after laser-induced thermotherapy (LITT). The calculated temperatures are color-coded (bottom right), gradually increasing the heat-affected zone with increasing maximum temperatures. **A** to **D,** Images acquired during LITT 1, 4, 8, and 10 min after starting the laser therapy. **E** and **F,** Temperature distribution 2 and 4 min after switching off the laser. The temperature returned to baseline values. However, some scattered pixels remain unchanged during cooling. See Color Plate 15.

A

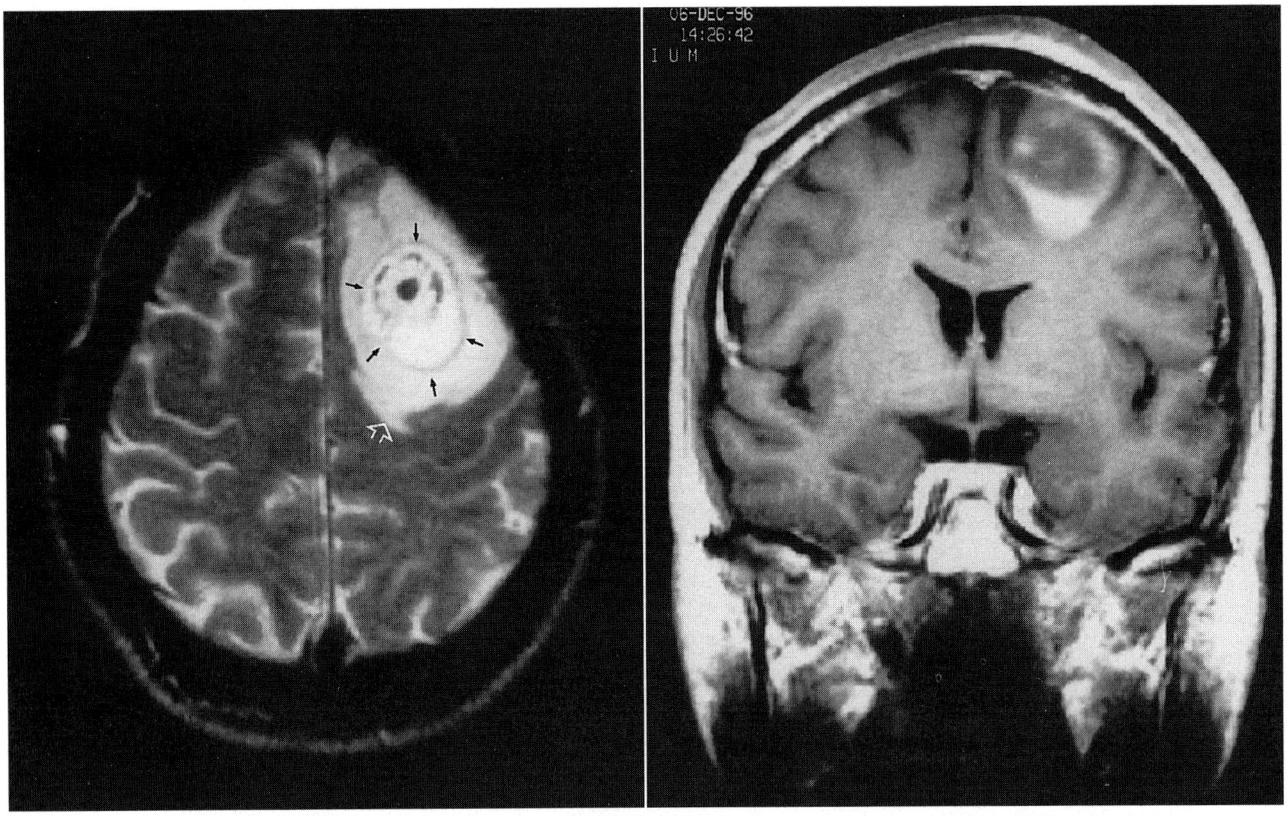

B

Fig. 29-3. A, Axial T2-weighted spin-echo image acquired 1 day after therapy displayed the laser-induced lesion *(arrows)*. Slight increase of the perifocal edema *(open arrow)* is seen. **B,** Coronal T1-weighted contrast-enhanced spin-echo image acquired 1 day after therapy. The enhancing peripheral rim indicates the total lesion size.

(Gd-DTPA) was evident at the border of the peripheral zone.[19] The diameter of these rims was considered the diameter of the total lesion. Lesion size and applied laser energy were not related.

T2-weighted images showed a reverse situation with regard to the signal intensities of the central and peripheral zone. The hyperintense channel of the light guide was surrounded by a central low signal intensity area and a peripheral high signal intensity zone. Follow-up studies revealed a demarcation of the peripheral zone from the surrounding brain by a thin hypointense rim. The diameter of total lesion size determined by T2-weighted images corresponded to the diameter on T1-weighted scans after Gd-DTPA.

CLINICAL FOLLOW-UP

In 28 of 31 patients, follow-up studies showed a slight to severe increase in perifocal edema on T2-weighted images that completely resolved in 2 to 5 wk. There was no association between tumor grade and severity of edema nor between applied laser energy and severity of edema. No patient showed an increase in edema in immediate follow-up studies. Twenty-eight of thirty-one patients received corticosteroids (dexamethasone 12 to 32 mg) perioperatively.

During LITT, two patients had neurologic deterioration. In 29 patients, clinical and neurologic conditions remained unchanged. In the postoperative period, 4 of 31 patients had transient deficits caused by vasogenic edema after LITT. Persistent deficits were only observed in one patient. In this case, the laser-induced lesion exceeded the tumor margin.

Follow-up studies showed neurologic improvement in 18 of 24 patients with astrocytoma WHO II, whereas 6 patients remained unchanged. The outcome of LITT in malignant gliomas was poor. All patients had tumor progression in 3 to 12 months.

CONCLUSIONS

Results show that MRI is well-suited to monitor LITT. A typical laser lesion comprises a central and a peripheral zone that form together the total lesion size. This zone is surrounded by rim enhancement at the border of the peripheral zone after Gd-DTPA. Further follow-up studies with shrinkage of the lesion and accompanying diameter reduction of the enhancing rim after Gd-DTPA support the suggestion that the enhancing rim demarcates the outer border of the irreversible damaged lesion. Tracz and others[20] found similar results in experimental animal studies in cat brain and a good correlation between final histologic lesion size and diameter based on rim enhancement after Gd-DTPA.[20]

The peripheral zone has to be discriminated from the perifocal edema that may show similar signal intensities. The peripheral zone has been labeled as *necrotizing edema* or *delayed liquefaction necrosis,* indicating the irreversible damage within this zone.[2,21] In contrast, the surrounding vasogenic perifocal edema that is not present immediately after therapy is reversible in 15 to 40 days after LITT.

Monitoring LITT could be further improved by introducing phase-sensitive sequences displaying absolute temperature changes.

The advantage of therapeutic control by on-line monitoring of the awake patient makes LITT particularly suitable in brain tumors that are located in areas of functional relevance. In the authors' series, 18 patients had brain tumors located in or close to sensorimotor cortex fields.[22] Because most of these tumors were benign or semibenign, usually slow-growing astrocytomas WHO II, it is particularly critical to avoid post-therapeutic neurologic deficits. Using functional MRI in seven patients, the localization of the cortical motor hand area could be determined, which is important because the localization of the cortical motor hand area may vary especially in the presence of space-occupying lesions nearby or within because of dislocation or reorganization. In these patients, the border of the evolving irreversible lesion facing the motor hand area was monitored; LITT was terminated when the distance was less than 4 to 5 mm.

Currently available light guides for LITT are limited in respect to the maximum lesion size. Newer developments are aimed at increasing inducible lesion size. Besides the enlargement of the fiber tip, this increase can be achieved by cooling of the tissue areas surrounding the optical fiber tips. This additional cooling of the regions also offers in principle the induction of asymmetrical tissue lesions.[23,24]

However, the role of LITT as a therapeutic alternative for brain tumors should be defined. Only a few preliminary reports have been published about the clinical applications of LITT in brain tumors.[25–29] In the authors' series, LITT was of low intraoperative morbidity and no mortality. Only 1 of 31 patients had a persistent deficit. In this case, the laser-induced lesion exceeded the tumor margin. Transient neurologic deficits occurred in the early postoperative period because of vasogenic perifocal edema. In all patients, recovery was obtained in 3 to 5 weeks. These results indicate that LITT is a safe therapy if the laser-induced lesion is confined to the tumor margins. In all patients, a marked tumor reduction could be obtained. Eighteen of twenty-four patients with low-grade gliomas (astrocytoma WHO II) showed a neurologic improvement with decreased severity and frequency of seizures. Although definitive conclusions regarding the value of LITT cannot be drawn based on this study, LITT can be of benefit in patients with low-grade gliomas. However, laser therapy in malignant gliomas—used as a monotherapeutic approach—was unsuccessful. Considering experimental results, a multitherapeutic approach of LITT in combination with radiotherapy or chemotherapy will probably improve the results in malignant brain tumors.[30,31]

REFERENCES

1. Bown SG: Phototherapy of tumors, *World J Surg* 7:700, 1983.
2. Schober R, and others: Fine structure of zonal changes in experimental Nd:YAG laser-induced interstitial hyperthermia, *Lasers Surg Med* 13:234, 1993.
3. Masters A, Bown SG: Interstitial laser hyperthermia in the treatment of tumors, *Lasers Med Sci* 5:129, 1990.
4. Cheong WF, Prahl SA, Welch AJ: A review of the optical properties of biological tissues, *IEEE J Quantum Electronics* 26:2166, 1990.
5. Hessel S, Frank F: Technical prerequisites for the interstitial thermotherapy using the Nd:YAG laser, *Proc SPIE* 1201:233, 1990.
6. Jolecz FA, and others: MR imaging of laser-tissue interactions, *Radiology* 168:249, 1988.
7. Tracz RA, and others: Magnetic resonance imaging of interstitial laser photo coagulation, *Laser Surg Med* 12:165, 1992.
8. Anzai Y, and others: MR imaging guided interstitial Nd-YAG laser phototherapy: dosimetry study of acute tissue damage in an in vivo model, *J Magn Reson Imaging* 1:553, 1991.
9. Anzai Y, and others: MR imaging: histopathologic correlation of thermal injuries induced with interstitial Nd:YAG laser irradiation in the chronic model, *J Magn Reson Imaging* 2:671, 1992.
10. Bleier AR, and others: Real time magnetic resonance imaging of laser heat deposition in tissue, *Magn Reson Med* 21:132, 1991.
11. Matsumoto R, Oshio K, Jolecz FA: Monitoring of laser and freezing-induced ablation in the liver with T1-weighted MR imaging, *J Magn Reson Imaging* 2:555, 1992.
12. Kahn TH, and others: MRI temperature quantification at 1.5 T in vitro: comparison of fast T1-maps and a phase-sensitive sequence, *Fortsch Röntgenstr* 167:187, 1997.
13. Harth T, and others: Determination of laser-induced temperature distributions using echo-shifted turbo-FLASH, *Magn Reson Med* 38:238, 1997.
14. Kahn TH, and others: In vivo MR thermometry using phase-sensitive sequences: preliminary experience during MRI-guided laser-induced interstitial thermotherapy of brain tumors, *J Magn Reson Imaging* 8:160, 1998.
15. Kahn T, and others: MRI-guided laser-induced interstitial thermotherapy of cerebral neoplasms, *J Comput Assist Tomogr* 18:519, 1994.
16. Kahn TH, and others: *MRI-guidance of laser-induced interstitial thermotherapy of brain tumors: three-year experience.* In Müller G, Roggan A, editors: *Laser-induced interstitial thermotherapy,* Bellingham, Wash, 1995, SPIE Press.
17. Kahn TH, and others: Mapping of the cortical motor hand area with functional MR imaging and MR imaging-guided laser-induced interstitial thermotherapy of brain tumors, *Radiology* 200:149, 1996.
18. Kahn TH, and others: Correlation of neuropathological findings and phase-based MRI temperature maps in experimental laser-induced interstitial thermotherapy (LITT): 2nd Interventional MRI Symposium, October 17–18, 1997, Dusseldorf, Germany, *Eur Radiol* 7:1151, 1997.
19. Schwabe B, and others: Laser-induced thermal lesions in the human brain: short- and long-term appearance on MRI, *J Comput Assist Tomogr* 21:818, 1997.
20. Tracz RA and others: Comparison of magnetic resonance images and histopathological findings of lesions induced by interstitial laser photocoagulation in the brain, *Lasers Surg Med* 13:45, 1993.
21. Kiessling M, Herchenhan E, Eggert HR: Cerebrovascular and metabolic effects on the rat brain of focal Nd:YAG laser irradiation, *J Neurosurg* 73:909, 1990.
22. Bettag M, and others: *Neurological and functional changes after laser-induced interstitial thermotherapy (LITT) of brain tumors.* In Müller G, Roggan A, editors: *Laser-induced interstitial thermotherapy,* Bellingham, Wash, 1995, SPIE Press.
23. Schwarzmaier HJ, and others: Improved laser applicators for interstitial thermotherapy of brain structure, *SPIE* 2132:4, 1994.

24. Schwarzmaier HJ, and others: *Applicators for the laser-induced thermotherapy: basic considerations and new developments.* In Müller G, Roggan A, editors: *Laser-induced interstitial thermotherapy,* Bellingham, Wash, 1995, SPIE Press.
25. Roux FX, and others: Laser interstitial thermotherapy in stereotactical neurosurgery, *Lasers Med Sci* 7:121, 1992.
26. Ascher PW: Interstitial thermal therapy of brain tumors with Nd-YAG laser under real time MRI control, *SPIE* 12000:242, 1990.
27. Bettag M, and others: Laser-induced interstitial thermotherapy in malignant gliomas, *Adv Neurosurg* 22:253, 1992.
28. Bettag M, and others: MR-guided laser interventions, *SPIE* 1643:242, 1992.
29. Sakai T, and others: Interstitial laserthermia in neurosurgery, *J Clin Laser Med Surg* 1:37, 1992.
30. Salcman M, Ebert PS: In vitro response of human glioblastoma and canine glioma cells to hyperthermia, radiation, and chemotherapy, *Neurosurgery* 29:526, 1991.
31. Salcman M, Samaras GM: Hyperthermia for brain tumors: biophysical rationale, *Neurosurgery* 9:327, 1981.

Chapter 30

MR–GUIDED RADIOFREQUENCY ABLATION OF BRAIN TUMORS

Gregory J. Rubino, Antonio A. F. DeSalles, Keith L. Black, Robert B. Lufkin

Brain tumors result in significant morbidity and mortality. The prognosis for untreated malignant brain tumors may be 6 to 8 months regardless of histology. Metastatic brain tumors can be seen in approximately 20% of all cancer patients at autopsy. The annual healthcare costs for brain tumor treatment is high.

The treatment options for brain tumors include open craniotomy, radiotherapy, chemotherapy, and radiosurgery. Open craniotomy requires general anesthesia, a long hospital stay, and a long recovery period. Patients with systemic illness (e.g., cardiopulmonary disease, multiorgan failure) may not be appropriate candidates for open craniotomy.

Radiotherapy requires many consecutive hospital visits. The acute adverse effects of radiotherapy include nausea, fatigue, and headache. The risk of radiation necrosis is increased, and some brain tumors may not be radiosensitive. In addition, radiotherapy cannot be repeated beyond the limits of radiation tolerance of healthy brain tissue.

Stereotactic radiosurgery does not involve surgery but more focused external radiation in a single fraction. Because the radiation field can be targeted, radiosurgery can be performed in patients with previous whole-brain radiation. However, because a high dose of radiation is delivered to the tumor in a single fraction, the risks include acute radiation toxicity and radiation necrosis.

Chemotherapy and immunotherapy have been performed in certain brain tumors as a treatment option. Systemic side effects associated with chemotherapy may not be tolerable for some patients.

Magnetic resonance (MR)–guided stereotactic thermal ablation has been developed as an experimental minimally invasive, percutaneous treatment for brain tumors. Conventional hyperthermia raises the local tissue temperature to 42°C to 45°C to augment other treatments. Thermal ablation, however, produces irreversible protein denaturation by increasing the tissue temperature to greater than 60° C. Thermal ablation can be performed with the interstitial use of laser, radiofrequency (RF), or any focal heat source.

RF energy has been successfully used for more than three decades in the neurosurgical field; it proved to be a safe, well-controlled, and reproducible energy source.[1-4] RF transfers rapidly alternating current to tissue, producing heat as a consequence of the resistance of the medium to current. RF has been widely used for management of functional disorders[5-8] but has not extensively been applied to the treatment of brain tumors. With the development of MR-compatible stereotactic frames and other tracking systems, brain tumors can be accurately and safely biopsied.[8,9] Percutaneous focal management of brain tumors using thermal energy can be explored as an extension of the biopsy procedure.

MRI is one of the most powerful soft-tissue diagnostic imaging techniques. The concept of using this advanced imaging technology for diagnosis and guidance of interventional procedures has grown over several years.[10-13] Development of open magnets for improved access to the patient, MR fluoroscopy sequences for real-time needle instrumentation, and MR temperature mapping have facilitated clinical application of interventional MR.

MR-guided stereotactic thermal ablation of brain tumors using RF ablation is reportedly a feasible and promising technique with few immediate complications.[14] This chapter evaluates the efficacy of this technique; examines factors affecting immediate management failure, local control, and recurrence; and reviews the clinical outcome and relationship among several parameters, such as RF dose, size, histology of tumor, and management success.

CLINICAL STUDY DESIGN

Patients with one or more metastatic tumors or a primary brain tumor less than 3 cm in maximal diameter were considered for management. Eighteen brain tumors in 15 patients were treated by MR-guided RF thermal ablation. These patients included 5 men and 10 women aged 20 to 80 years (mean age, 56.7 years). Twelve patients had metastatic brain tumors, and three patients had primary brain tumors. Three patients had two metastatic lesions treated at the same time. Follow-up ranged from 13 to 30 months. Three patients presented with a recurrent brain tumor after whole-brain radiation, surgery, or both.

This protocol was approved by the Human Subject Protection Committee. All patients were informed of possible risks and benefits of the procedure and their management options, including surgical resection, stereotactic radiosurgery, conventional radiation, or chemotherapy. Written informed consent was obtained from all patients. Patients without prior histologic confirmation of their tumor had stereotactic biopsy of the lesion before the thermoablative procedure.

RADIOFREQUENCY ABLATION

All patients were given dexamethasone and anticonvulsants at least 48 hr before the procedure. In the MR suite, an intravenous line was started for antibiotics and light sedation. An MR-compatible Leksell stereotactic frame (Elekta Instruments, Atlanta, Ga) was placed using clean technique. With the frame attached, the patient was placed in the MR scanner where images were obtained. All patients had previous gadolinium-enhanced MR that allowed identification of tumor borders. The stereotactic coordinates of the tumor for placement of the biopsy needle and the RF coagulative lesion were determined in the axial scan. The angles of entrance for the trajectory of the electrode to the tumor were planned on the sagittal and coronal scans.

After the pre-RF MR, the patient was withdrawn from the scanner. Local anesthesia was administered at the location of the electrode entrance. A 5-mm skin incision allowed the placement of a small twist drill hole. Biopsy specimens were obtained from the lesion if necessary. After histopathologic diagnosis was confirmed by frozen section, the biopsy needle was removed. The MR-compatible RF probe was then introduced through the same opening, and RF impedance monitoring was performed as the electrode was advanced (Fig. 30-1).

A modified MR-compatible RF lesion generator system (Radionics, Burlington, Mass), which generated 500-kHz sine wave signals, was used. The RF lesion was generated by raising the probe temperature to 80° C and maintaining it for 1 min. This accepted technique, described in the literature, results in a local area of coagulation necrosis of the tissue.[1-4] This 1-min treatment fraction was repeated at different locations in the tumor until the entire tumor volume was treated. The end point was determined by a combination of known probe position, tumor shape and volume, temperature, duration, and MR appearance. Patients were managed using one insertion of a 5- or

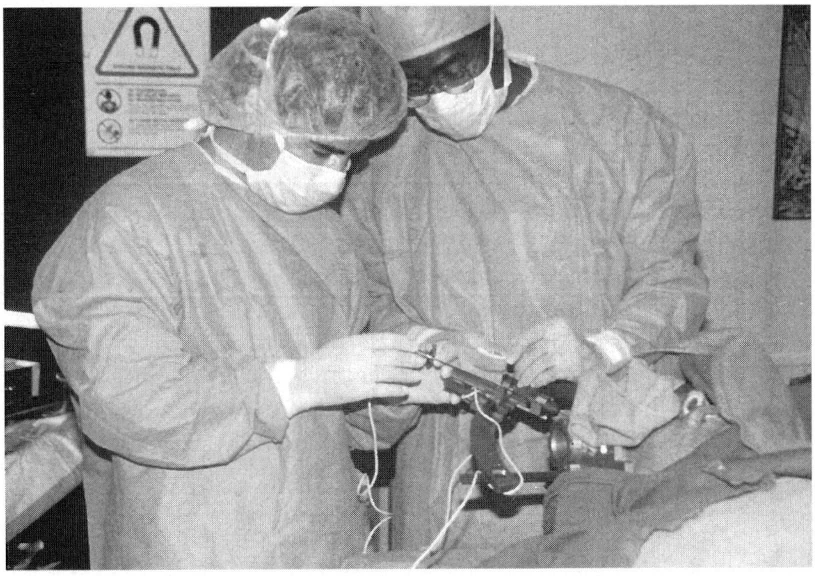

Fig. 30-1. A magnetic resonance (MR)–compatible stereotactic frame in place with a radiofrequency electrode adjacent to the MR scanner.

10-mm exposed tip straight electrode or a side-advance spring that describes a 10-mm diameter semicircle from the tip of the electrode to create a three-dimensional (3D) treatment volume. The goal of the treatment was to cover the entire tumor seen on the pretreatment image plus a small rim of healthy surrounding tissue. The probe was removed and the incision was closed using nylon sutures.

The neurologic status was monitored throughout the procedure in the conscious patient. The procedure took approximately 3 to 4 hr, including pre- and post-MR. Patients were observed for 24 hr before discharge.

MAGNETIC RESONANCE IMAGING AND FINDINGS

Radiofrequency thermal ablation

A 1.5-T superconducting MR unit was modified for improved monitoring of the patient during the procedure. MRI was performed before, during, and immediately after the RF procedure and 1 day, 1 wk, 1 month, 3 months, and every 6 months after RF ablation. The images were reviewed by two neuroradiologists in conjunction with the clinical data.

T2-weighted fast spin-echo imaging (repetition time [TR] 2000-2800 msec; echo time [TE] 80-90 msec) was obtained before treatment in axial, coronal, and sagittal planes, providing localization of the tumor and determination of RF probe trajectory. Fast gradient echo and T2-weighted fast spin-echo were performed during the RF thermal ablation (Fig. 30-2). T1-weighted spin-echo images (TR,500-650 msec; TE, 16-20 msec) were obtained before and after thermal ablation. Gadolinium-enhanced MRI scans were obtained after RF thermal ablation only. MRI before the procedure was performed with a 28-cm field of view (FOV), which is large enough to cover the fiducials of the stereotactic frame to calculate the stereotactic coordinates and angle of trajectory.

The remainder of the MR examination was performed with a 22-cm FOV. A 256 × 192 matrix with two excitations was used for T1-and T2-weighted images. Section thickness was 3 mm with interleaving. In addition, 2D time-of-flight MR angiography (TR, 45 msec; TE, 8 msec) was obtained in some patients using a 60° flip angle and 1.5-mm slice thickness. This technique allowed visualization of vascular structures around the entry point of the RF probe and along its planned trajectory in the brain.

Because the tumor was not removed but coagulated in the brain, the MR signal abnormalities persisted after thermal ablation. The sequential RF lesion volume was calculated to differentiate the healing RF lesion from recurrent or residual tumor. The RF lesion was segmented on gadolinium-enhanced images using a thresholding technique and was reconstructed in a 3D fashion. The sequential RF lesion volume was plotted as a function of time after management.

The MR appearance of the acute RF lesion consisted of four concentric zones A to D: Zone A, an innermost central area of high signal intensity on T1-weighted images, was seen in patients who underwent biopsy immediately before RF ablation (Fig. 30-3). This high signal appearance was not seen in patients who did not receive biopsy immediately before management. Zone B was a second concentric zone isointense to gray matter on T1-weighted images and low signal intensity on T2-weighted images. Zone C was the outermost low signal rim on T1 and T2 sequences. Zone D corresponded to a perilesional high signal area suggestive of edema on T2-weighted images without significant mass effect. On postgadolinium images, peripheral enhancement outside the low signal rim (zone C) was seen. Some small tumors (less than 1 cm in diameter) that required limited RF exposure did not develop zone D after management, and central enhancement after gadolinium administration was noted.

A B C

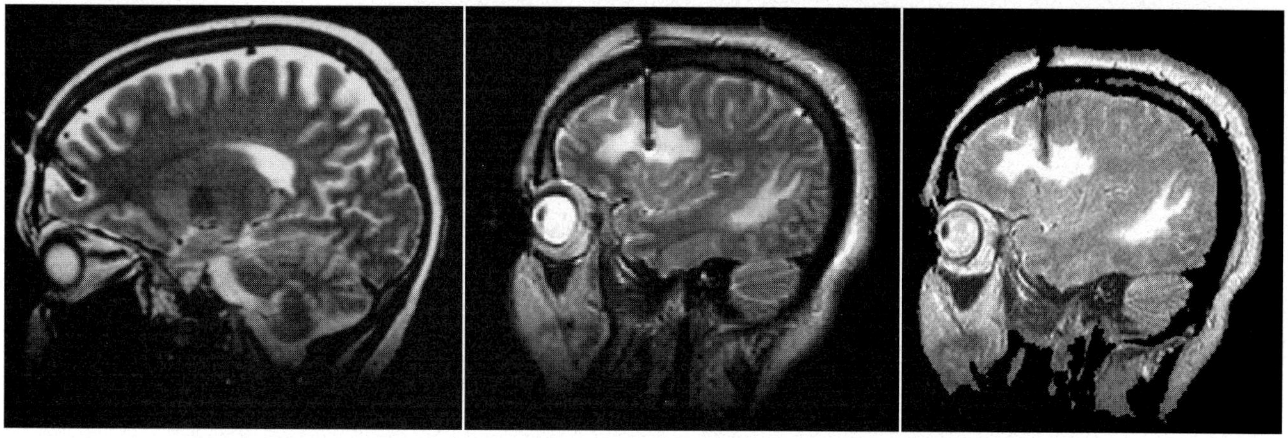

Fig. 30-2. Radiofrequency (RF) electrodes and ablation. **A,** T2-weighted fast spin-echo image of a patient with an anterior RF electrode in place. **B,** T2-weighted fast spin-echo image of another patient with a more posterior RF electrode in place confirms the location of the electrode within the tumor. **C,** T2-weighted fast spin-echo image obtained in the patient in **B** during RF ablation before the appearance of the RF lesion. Noise is slightly increased caused by RF energy delivery inside magnetic resonance unit; however the image quality remains acceptable. (From Anzai Y, and others: *MR-guided radiofrequency ablation of brain tumors.* In Jolesz FA, Young IR, editors: *Interventional MR,* London, 1998, Martin Dunitz Ltd.)

A,B

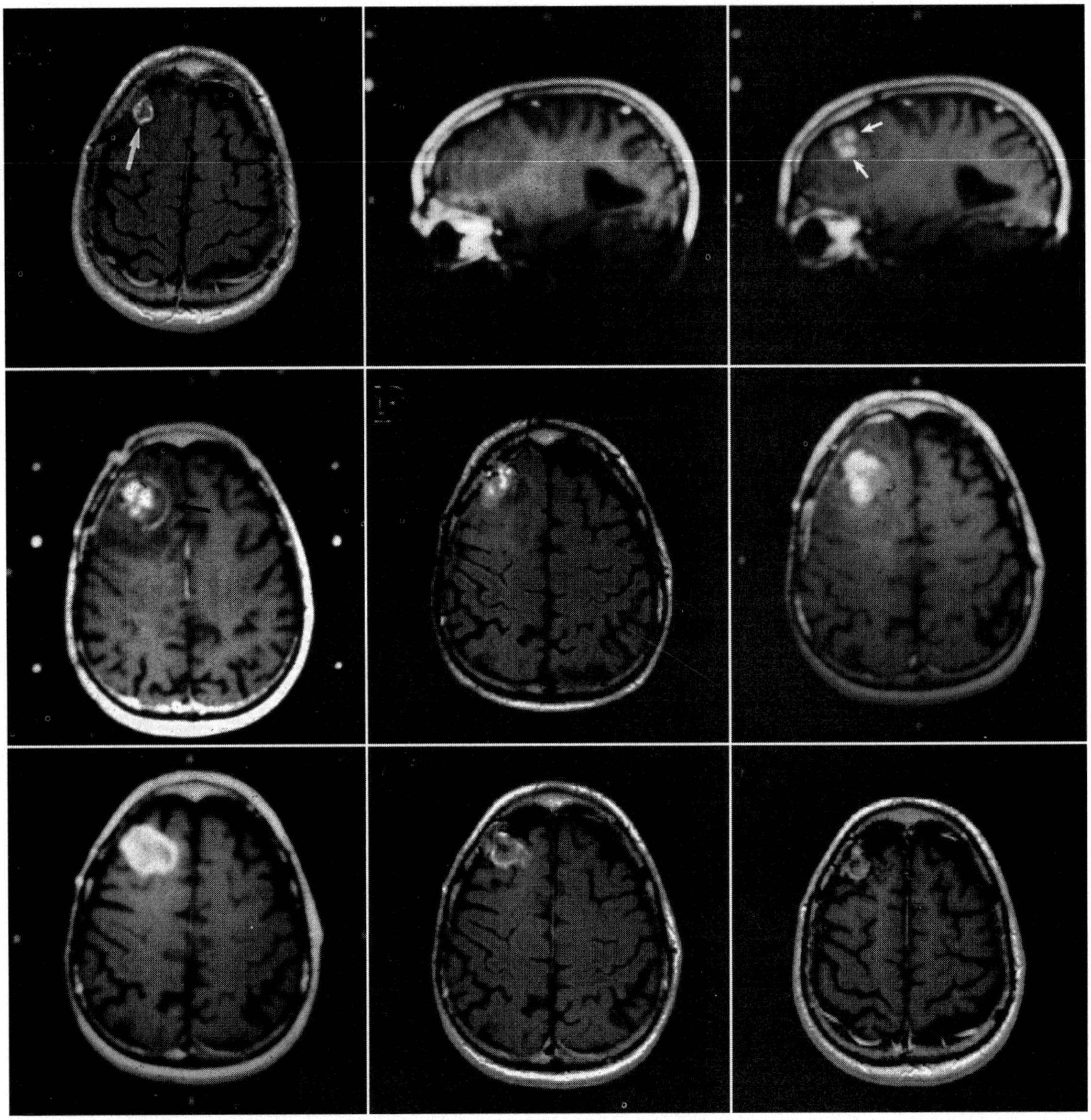

C

D,E

F

G,H

I

Fig. 30-3. A 44-year-old man with metastatic melanoma who had undergone open craniotomy and whole-brain radiation developed another brain metastasis in the right frontal lobe. The patient underwent magnetic resonance (MR)–guided radiofrequency (RF) ablation with no additional treatment. **A,** Outside pretreatment axial T1-weighted MR with enhancement shows a 1.2-cm mass in the right frontal lobe *(arrow)*. **B,** T1-weighted sagittal image before RF treatment shows the large area of edema without evidence of hemorrhage within the tumor. **C,** Non–contrast-enhanced T1-weighted image immediately after RF ablation shows high signal foci in the central portion of the RF lesion *(arrows)*. This finding is often seen in patients who underwent biopsy immediately before thermal ablation and is presumably related to heat-induced methemoglobin formation. **D,** Gadolinium-enhanced axial image immediately after thermal ablation shows well-defined ring enhancement of the RF lesion *(arrow)*. Multiple high signal foci seen outside the head represent fiducials in an MR-compatible stereotactic frame. **E,** Three days after treatment, RF lesion covers the entire initial tumor volume. Contrast-enhanced MR images performed **F,** 1 month; **G,** 3 months; **H,** 6 months; and **I,** 19 months after RF ablation show that the RF lesion gradually decreased in size. No evidence of tumor progression was observed over a 30-month follow-up period. (From Anzai Y, and others: *MR-guided radiofrequency ablation of brain tumors*. In Jolesz FA, Young IR, editors: *Interventional MR,* London, 1998, Martin Dunitz Ltd.)

Sequential changes of the RF lesion on MRI were studied, and several patterns emerged (Figs. 30-3 and 30-4):

- The central high signal on T1-weighted images persisted to 1 to 3 months after the procedure and then gradually resolved.
- The peripheral low signal rim on T2-weighted images became well demarcated and more prominent with time.
- The perilesional high signal area was largest on day 1 to week 1 after therapy, then gradually reduced.

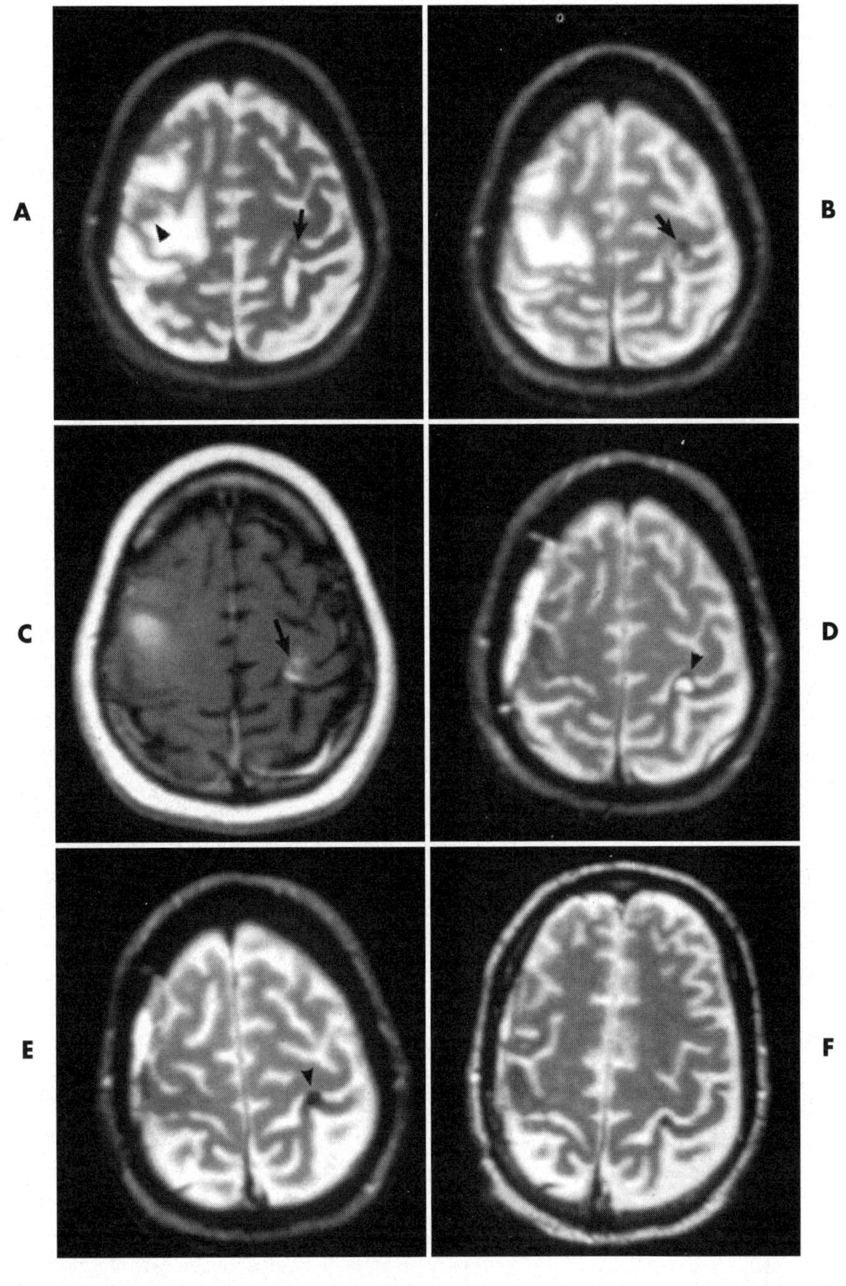

Fig. 30-4. A 56-year-old man with melanoma presented with two metastatic tumors. **A,** A small tumor in the left parietal lobe *(small arrow)* was treated with radiofrequency (RF)-ablation, and the other large tumor *(arrowhead)* in the right parietal lobe was removed by open craniotomy after thermal ablation of the tumor on the left. Biopsy of this small lesion revealed metastatic melanoma. **B,** T2-weighted image immediately after RF ablation shows low signal rim at the boundary *(arrow).* **C,** Gadolinium-enhanced axial image immediately after RF ablation shows enhancement of the RF lesion, representing the area of blood-brain barrier disruption *(arrow).* Sequential T2-weighted images performed **D,** 1 month; **E,** 3 months; and **F,** 6 months after RF ablation show significant volume reduction of the RF lesion. Notice that the peripheral dark rim becomes well demarcated and more prominent 1 month after treatment *(arrowhead)* and the overall lesion size gradually reduces and is barely seen in **F.** (From Anzai Y, and others: *MR-guided radiofrequency ablation of brain tumors.* In Jolesz FA, Young IF, editors: *Interventional MR,* London, 1998, Martin Dunitz Ltd.)

- The overall size of the RF lesions gradually reduced with time.
- Peripheral enhancement was seen up to 6 months after RF ablation.

Radiofrequency lesion volume versus radiofrequency dose

Lesion volumes calculated on gadolinium-enhanced MRI were plotted as a function of the RF dose (time in minutes at 80° C), which reflects tissue heating at the electrode tip (Fig. 30-5). The lesion volume did not correlate well with the RF dose. Furthermore, the lesion size did not increase over a certain volume despite increased RF lesion energy delivery. For example, the volume of the lesion treated for 45 min was similar to that treated for 7 min. The volume of the RF lesion depends on the energy delivered and on the volume over which the energy is applied. Thus, a large RF lesion could be created by advancing or retracting the RF probe and by using the side arm rather than by merely increasing the dose in the same position. The thermal capability of the tissue also varies depending on whether large vessels (acting as heat sinks) nearby can distort the uniform delivery of an RF dose.

Prediction of RF lesion size is helpful for management planning. However, these factors made accurate preoperative dosimetry planning of limited predictive value for lesion volume and underscored the need for imaging feedback during management.

The MR appearance of RF lesions in the brain and interpretation of their signal characteristics has been described[8,13] in two papers describing RF thalamotomy. The signal intensity changes in patients were consistent with those in animal experiments and in previous reports investigating histologic changes after RF ablation in the brain. The innermost high signal on T1-weighted images most likely represents heat-induced methemoglobin conversion from deoxyhemoglobin,[10] which normally takes more than 72 hr in cerebral hematoma without heat induction. These high signal foci were only seen in patients in whom biopsy was performed immediately before RF ablation, which presumably caused a small amount of local bleeding. High signal foci were not observed in three patients who underwent management of five lesions that did not require biopsy. However, the contribution of a highly proteinaceous content fluid collection to the high signal foci on the acute RF lesions cannot be entirely excluded.

The second zone of low signal intensity corresponded to the area of coagulative necrosis, which resulted in loss of cell nuclei seen in the histologic studies. This phenomenon, seen in other examples of RF[10] and interstitial thermal tissue injury caused by neodymium: yttrium-aluminum-garnet (Nd:YAG) laser,[11,12] represents irreversible tissue damage.

The third zone consisting of the low signal rim was well seen, especially in relatively large RF ablations, which required multiple RF applications in different locations in the tumor. This finding most likely represents deoxyhemoglobin in the acute situation and hemosiderin deposition in later follow-up studies.

The outermost zone of peripheral high signal most likely represents edema in the acute lesion and gliosis in the chronic stage.

The hemoglobin products are a potential intrinsic marker to help define resolving RF lesions on follow-up MRI. In small RF lesions, this ring of hemosiderin was not as visible as in the larger lesions. In these cases, gadolinium enhancement may help delineate the RF lesion because peripheral ring enhancement is invariably seen at the boundary of the RF lesion, which presumably corresponds to heat-induced blood-brain barrier disruption.

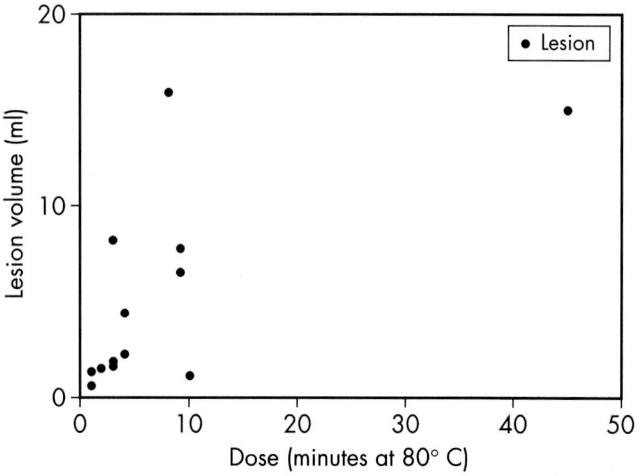

Fig. 30-5. Radiofrequency (RF)-lesion volume versus RF dose. The acute RF lesion volume calculated on the gadolinium-enhanced magnetic resonance (MR)-image was plotted as a function of the RF dose (cumulative times in minutes that the tissue was maintained at 80° C). Lesion size did not increase over a certain volume despite increased RF energy delivery. (From Anzai Y, and others: *MR-guided radiofrequency ablation of brain tumors.* In Jolesz FA, Young IF, editors: *Interventional MR,* London, 1998, Martin Dunitz Ltd.)

CLINICAL OUTCOME ANALYSIS

Treatment success was determined by analyzing sequential RF lesion volume measurement, MRI findings, and clinical findings. Because MR-guided thermal ablation creates focal therapy and has no effect on systemic disease, the focal control of each treated lesion was determined rather than survival or prognosis of patients.

Whether management success was influenced by RF dose was determined by calculating RF dose per tumor volume (or tumor size) using two tailed Student *t*-tests. In addition, a chi-squared test was used for evaluating the gender difference and the effect of combined therapy on management success.

Local control was obtained in 8 of 15 patients (9 of 18 lesions) (Table 30-1). In five tumors in four patients (28%), local control has been obtained for more than 22 months. The longest local control was 2.5 years in a patient with metastatic melanoma. Four patients died from primary cancer or systemic disease within 1 year while metastatic brain tumor was controlled. Three patients who had recurrence after surgery or whole-brain radiation, which usually indicates poor prognosis, were successfully treated by RF ablation. No loss of cognitive function was present in eight patients with local control.

Local recurrence was seen in 7 of 15 patients (9 of 18 lesions) (Table 30-2). Recurrence was noted within 8 months after RF ablation. Three metastatic renal cell carcinomas, three metastatic melanomas, and one glioblastoma multiforme recurred despite relatively large RF lesions. Metastatic adenocarcinoma of the lung, however, was well controlled even with a small RF dose. Although conventional angiography was not performed in this study, hypervascular tumors were assumed to have high tendency for recurrence. Glioblastoma recurred 6 months after RF ablation despite combined treatment with radiosurgery. Acute tissue swelling and marked lesion enlargement were noted in one patient with metastatic melanoma, which was thought to be related to inflammatory reaction after thermal ablation.

Treatment success was not dependent on size of the tumor, RF dose applied, or patient age (Table 30-3). Histology was apparently an important factor affecting success. Hypervascular tumors, such as metastatic renal cell carcinoma and melanoma, tend to recur more frequently than less vascular metastatic adenocarcinomas or squamous cell carcinomas. Occasionally, the firm consistency of these tumor types prohibited placement of the RF probe and prevented treatment. Larger series are needed to achieve statistical significance when analyzing histologic subgroups.

Two patients who had tumors adjacent to the left motor cortex developed Broca's aphasia; one was transient and completely resolved, the other was unresolved motor aphasia. Because of the tumor location, similar deficits would almost certainly have occurred with surgery. One patient developed an acute inflammatory reaction around the RF lesion at 2 weeks that necessitated surgical resection, which did not reveal pathologic evidence of infection.

Table 30-1. Magnetic resonance–guided radiofrequency ablation in locally controlled brain tumors

Age (yr)	Sex	Diagnosis	Location/ size	Radiofrequency dose (min at 80° C)	Pretreatment*	Posttreatment†	Clinical outcome (mo of local control)
44	Male	Melanoma	RF 1.2	45	SG, WRT	None	30, alive
65	Female	Lung adenocarcinoma	RP. 1.0	4	None	None	12, died from lung cancer
71	Female	Lung adenocarcinoma	LF 1.5	9	None	WRT	27, alive
71	Female	Lung adenocarcinoma	RP 1.2	2	WRT	None	22, alive
			LO 0.8	1	WRT	None	22, alive
75	Female	Lung small cell carcinoma	LF 2.6	16	None	WRT	4, died from lung cancer
45	Female	Oligodendroglioma	LF 2.5	9	SG	Ct	25, alive
20	Female	Osteosarcoma	RF 1.0	10	None	Ct	2, died from systemic disease
80	Female	Lung adenocarcinoma	RF 0.8	1	None	None	3, died from lung cancer

Modified from Anzai Y, and others: *MR-guided radiofrequency ablation of brain tumors.* In Jolesz FA, Young IF, editors: *Interventional MR,* London, 1998, Martin Dunitz Ltd.
Ct—chemotherapy; F—frontal; L—left; O—occipital; P—parietal; R—right; SG—surgery; WRT—whole-brain radiation.
*Before radiofrequency ablation.
†After radiofrequency ablation.

Table 30-2. Magnetic resonance–guided radiofrequency ablation in locally recurrent brain tumors

Age (yr)	Sex	Diagnosis	Location/ Size (cm)	Radiofrequency dose (min at 80 °C)	Pretreatment*	Posttreatment	Clinical outcome (mo until recurrence)
56	Male	Melanoma	LP 0.8	3	None	None	8, died at 10 mo from systemic disease
70	Female	Glioblastoma multiforme	LF 2.8	9	None	RS	6, died at 8 mo
40	Female	Adenocarcinoma RCC	RT 1.0	3	None	None	4, surgical resection
			RF 1.0	4	None	None	4, surgical resection
69	Male	Melanoma	LF 1.3	3	None	RS	9, treated by RS
38	Male	Melanoma	LF 1.0	16	None	None	6, treated by WRT
			RF 1.1	1	None	None	0.52 acute inflammatory reaction, resected
71	Male	Adenocarcinoma RCC	LP 2.0	42	None	None	2, surgical resection
36	Female	Astrocytoma	RF 1.2	1	None	None	Treatment failure, surgical resection at 2 mo

Modified from Anzai Y, and others: *MR-guided radiofrequency ablation of brain tumors.* In Jolesz FA, Young IF, editors: *Interventional MR,* London, 1998, Martin Dunitz Ltd.
F—frontal; L—left; P—parietal; RS—radiosurgery; RCC—renal cell carcinoma; R—right; T—temporal; WRT—whole-brain radiation.
*Before radiofrequency ablation.

Table 30-3. Study parameters for radiofrequency (RF) ablation

	Local control	Local recurrence	Significance*
Size, *cm*	1.40	1.36	NS
RF dose, *min*	10.9	9.11	NS
RF dose/volume, *min/cm³*	10.45	7.08	NS
Age, *yr*	58.9	54.3	NS
Sex, M:F	1:7	4:3	NS†
Combined management, % *(n/n)*	44.4 (4/9)	22.2 (2/9)	NS†

Modified from Anzai Y, and others: *MR-guided radiofrequency ablation of brain tumors.* In Jolesz FA, Young IF, editors: *Interventional MR,* London, 1998, Martin Dunitz Ltd.
*Two tailed Student *t*-tests were used to evaluate statistical significance in tumor size, RF dose, and RF dose per tumor volume between local control and recurrence groups.
†Chi-square test was used for gender difference and presence of combined therapy.

A B C D

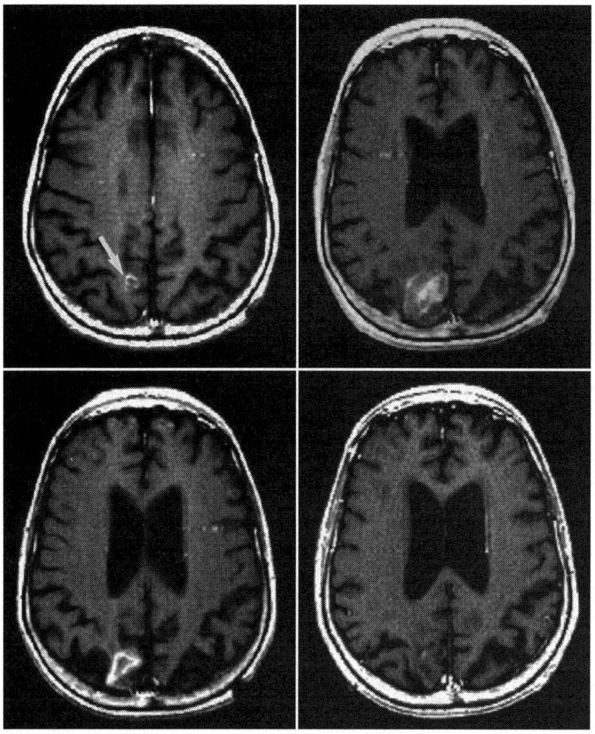

Fig. 30-6. A 65-year-old woman with adenocarcinoma of the lung after left lower lobectomy developed a brain metastasis. **A,** Pretreatment magnetic resonance shows a well-defined small tumor in right occipital lobe (*arrow*). Biopsy confirmed metastatic adenocarcinoma. T2-weighted images **B,** 1 month; **C,** 2 months; and **D,** 10 months after treatment reveal a gradual decrease in RF lesion size. The patient received a 4-min radiofrequency (RF) treatment dose. She died from lung cancer 1 year after RF ablation, and no recurrence was observed in her brain lesion. (From Anzai Y, and others: *MR-guided radiofrequency ablation of brain tumors.* In Jolesz FA, Young IF, editors: *Interventional MR,* London, 1998, Martin Dunitz Ltd.)

A B C D

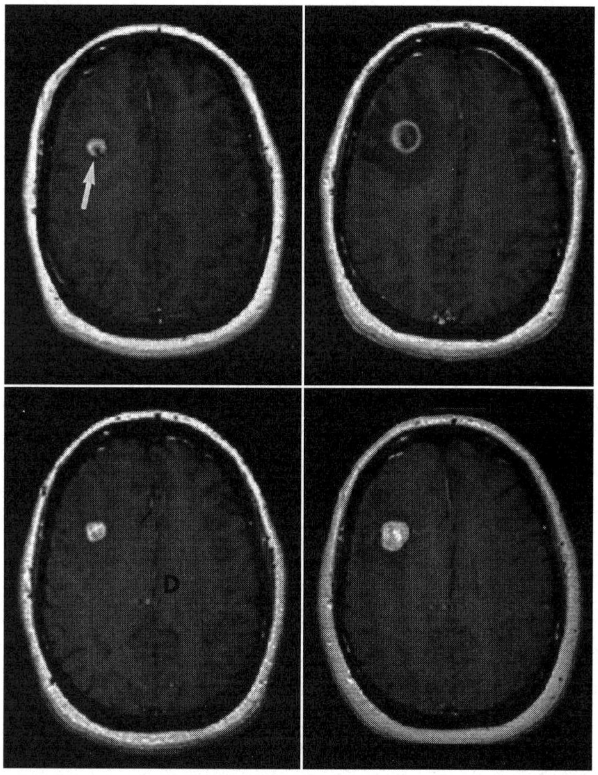

Fig. 30-7. Recurrent disease after radiofrequency (RF)-ablation. A 40-year-old woman with renal cell carcinoma presented with four metastatic tumors; two lesions in the right temporal and frontal lobes were treated by magnetic resonance (MR)–guided RF ablation, and the other two lesions on the left were treated by radiosurgery. All four metastatic tumors recurred 4 months after treatment **A,** Pretreatment gadolinium-enhanced image shows an enhancing tumor in the right frontal lobe *(arrow).* MR images **B,** 1 week; **C,** 1 month; and **D,** 4 months after RF ablation show an increase in RF lesion size and an area of solid enhancement within the previous ablation, suggestive of recurrence. (From Anzai Y, and others: *MR-guided radiofrequency ablation of brain tumors.* In Jolesz FA, Young IF, editors: *Interventional MR,* London, 1998, Martin Dunitz Ltd.)

RADIOLOGIC LONG-TERM FOLLOW-UP EVALUATION

Characteristic MR appearances of thermal-ablated lesions are the presence of high signal foci (heat-induced methemoglobin) and a rim of contrast enhancement (heat-induced blood-brain barrier destruction) (Fig. 30-6).[14] Edema can increase in size up to 1 to 2 wk after thermal ablation but gradually decreases thereafter (see Fig. 30-3).[16] Several imaging findings indicative of recurrence include enlargement of the area of solid enhancement inside the RF lesion on gadolinium-enhanced image (Fig. 30-7), sudden increase in the extent of edema around the RF lesion more than 1 month after treatment, increase in overall lesion size, and new mass effect (effacement of adjacent sulci).

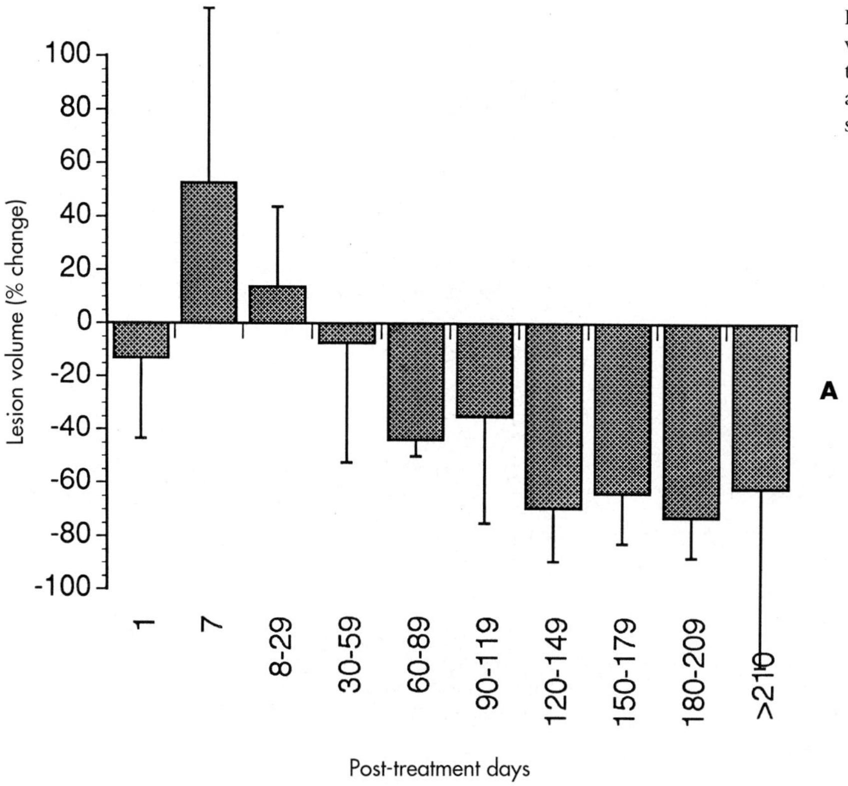

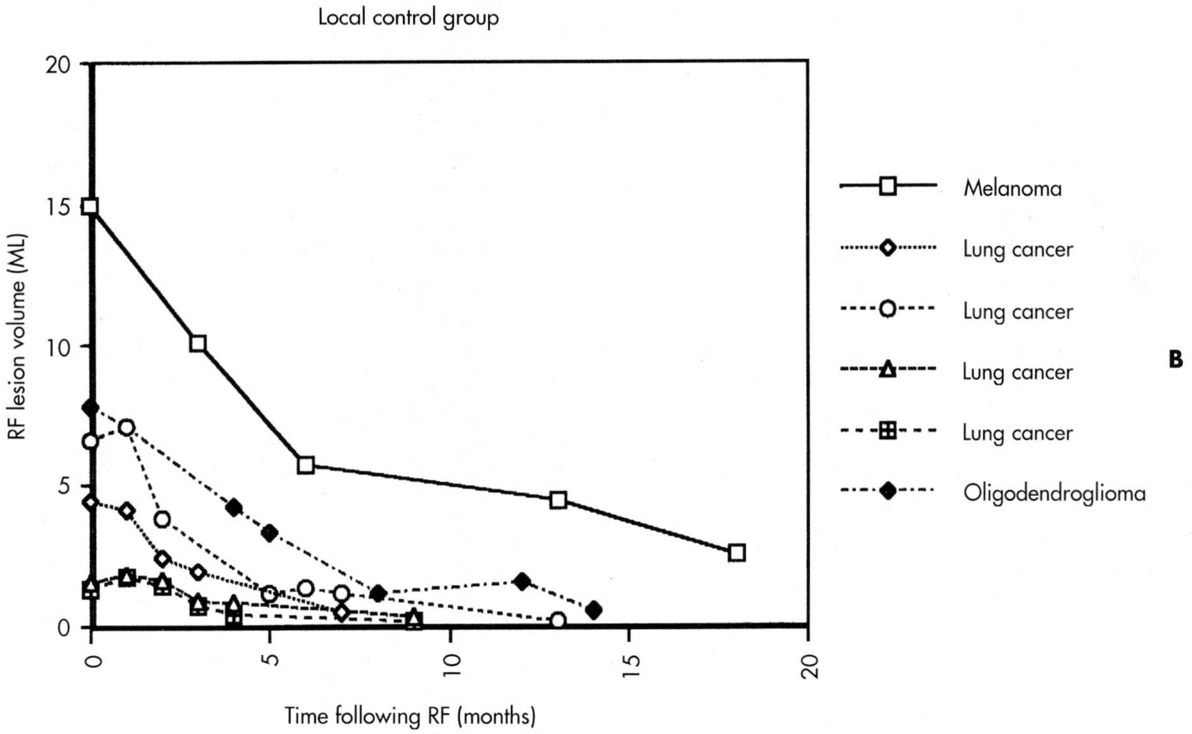

Fig. 30-8. Sequential radiofrequency (RF)-lesion volume measurements as a function of time after treatment. **A,** All lesions were plotted as the percentage of volume change. **B,** The local control group shows gradual decline in the RF lesion volume.

Continued

The sequential RF lesion volumes were calculated based on gadolinium-enhanced 3D reconstruction images. The outer most enhancing portion was segmented as the lesion margin. The sequential RF lesion volumes were plotted as a function of time after treatment in each patient.

The lesion volumes, when averaged over time, showed early expansion of the volume followed by a gradual decline. Some lesions, judged as management failures, continued to expand beyond the first month. Other management failures first expanded, then contracted, and proceeded to re-expand (Fig. 30-8).

C

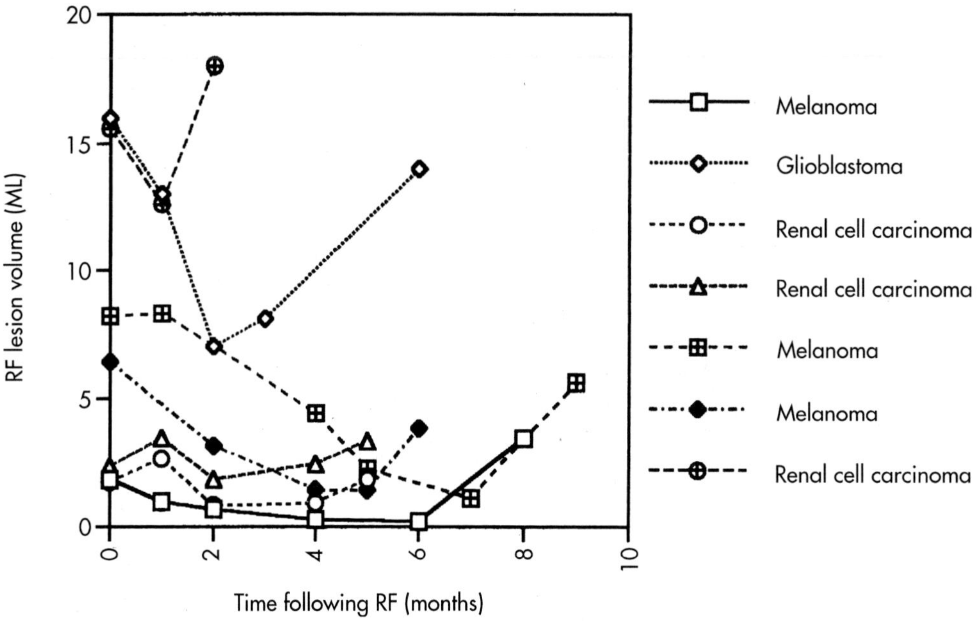

Fig. 30-8, cont'd. C, Sequential RF lesion volume in the recurrence group shows a late increase in RF lesion volume, which suggests tumor growth in the treated area. (From Anzai Y, and others: *MR-guided radiofrequency ablation of brain tumors.* In Jolesz FA, Young IF, editors: *Interventional MR,* London, 1998, Martin Dunitz Ltd.)

RADIOFREQUENCY ABLATION VERSUS SURGERY, RADIOTHERAPY, OR LASER ABLATION

The median survival of 125 metastatic tumors treated by open craniotomy with or without radiotherapy was reported to be 12 months.[17] Another study reviewing patients with solitary metastases revealed longer median survival in a group treatd with surgery and postoperative radiation than in a group managed with surgery alone (20 to 21 months versus 11 to 14 months).[18,19] The study investigated the value of re-irradiation of metastatic brain tumors and revealed that the average survival after second therapy was 5 months.[20] The median survival of recurrent brain metastases managed with re-operation was reported to be 9 months.[21] Stereotactic radiosurgery using a linear accelerator with delivery of high-dose radiation is another management alternative.[22] Stereotactic radiosurgery for 18 patients with brain metastases revealed that radiosurgery was effective for relatively small metastatic brain tumors.[23]

In the RF ablation series, local control was obtained in 8 of 15 patients (53.3%); some patients had previous treatment failure with open craniotomy or radiotherapy. Four patients (27%) treated with RF ablation had no evidence of recurrence for more than 22 months. Another four patients (27%) with metastatic tumor died from primary cancer or systemic disease while the metastatic brain tumor was still controlled. Approximately 50% of patients had recurrence or treatment failure, which necessitated additional treatments. Direct comparison of the treatment effect of thermal ablation and other management modalities, however, was difficult because patient selection and the size of tumors vary significantly among these studies (Fig. 30-9). It is impossible to conclude that this technique is better or worse than other modalities in this noncontrolled study with a small patient sample.

Thermal ablation can be produced with use of interstitial application of laser.[24] Among several widely available lasers, Nd:YAG is most used for interstitial application because of high tissue penetration (see Chapters 10 and 29 for more details). Interstitial laser therapy (ILT) has been applied to eight patients with brain tumors with a follow-up of 1 wk to 13 months.[25] This study showed the feasibility of ILT for brain tumor, however, no clinical outcome data have been reported. Moreover, patients who have been disease-free for 30 months, noted in this series, have never been reported with thermal ablation.

Use of laser and RF for thermal ablation of brain tumors is under investigation. ILT transmits light directly into deep tissue through a fiberoptic cable, resulting in thermal tissue damage. Laser, an extremely powerful light source, produces a steep thermal gradient. The thermal effect of ILT depends on several factors, including laser wavelength, fiber tip design, absorption and scattering properties of tissue, and tissue perfusion. Therefore, how much volume of tumor is destroyed in a given laser parameter is difficult to predict, emphasizing the important role of the imaging modality for monitoring. One advantage of the use of interstitial laser is the lack of interference with MR, causing no artifact. However, RF transfers electrical energy to tissue, producing heat as a consequence of the resistance of the medium to the passage of the rapidly alternating current. RF ablation provides a relatively gradual thermal gradient, which results in better controlled and reproducible thermal ablation. In the use of laser, output power, exposure time, and pulse mode

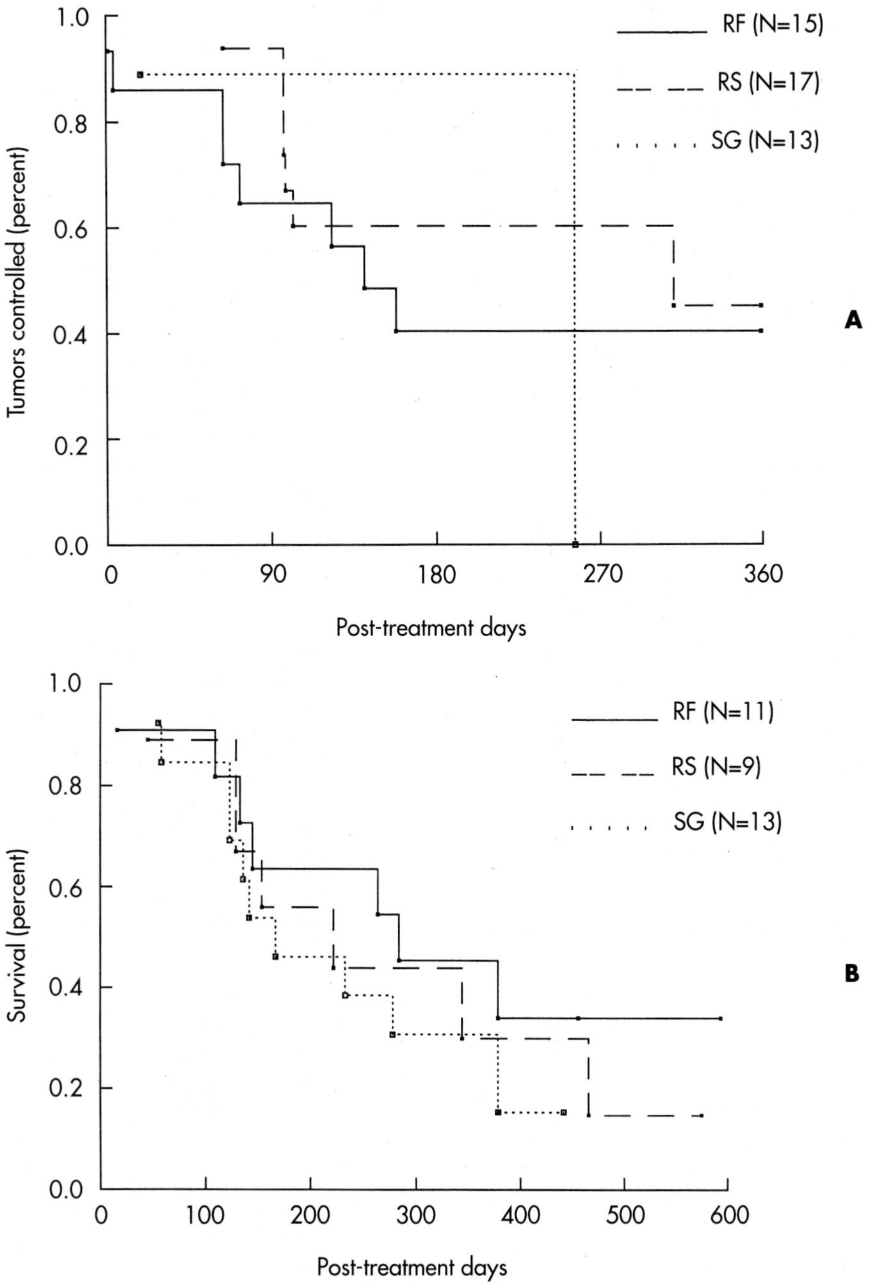

Fig. 30-9. Kaplan-Meier curves comparing age- and histology-matched controls with radiosurgery *(RS)* and conventional surgery *(SG)* and magnetic resonance-guided radiofrequency *(RF)* ablation. **A,** Percentage of tumors controlled versus time. **B,** Survival percentage versus time.

are controlled to obtain desired temperature based on assumption of tissue absorption or scattering. By contrast, a desired temperature can be reliably set up in RF ablation. MR allows visualization of thermal changes induced by laser and RF, and of tissue frozen by cryosurgery.[10-12,15,25,26]

FUTURE ISSUES

The major advantage of this technique for brain tumor management is its minimally invasive nature. The procedure is performed under local anesthesia so that neurologic symptoms can be clinically monitored. RF ablation can be applied to multiple lesions in one setting (requiring a 3-hr procedure and overnight observation). RF ablation may be a powerful alternative for patients who have failed radiation or open craniotomy or for older patients with systemic diseases. Finally, compared with the high patient morbidity and hospitalization costs associated with inpatient surgical procedures, the ultimate cost of medical care may be lower with MR-guided percutaneous interventions. Prospective analysis of cost-effectiveness needs to be conducted to determine this issue.

One limitation of this technique is difficulty controlling hypervascular tumors. Hypervascular tumors failed to respond to RF ablation in one series, likely because of cooling effect by the circulation of blood as seen in the animal model.[27] Numerous vessels in or adjacent to the tumor carry the applied heat away, resulting in insufficient tumor coagulation. Embolization before RF ablation or cryotherapy (freezing) instead of thermal ablation may be beneficial for patients with hypervascular tumors. Because the pathologic extent of malignant glioma extends beyond the areas of gadolinium enhancement or T2 signal abnormalities,[28] focal thermal therapy without any other management should not be considered curative for malignant astrocytoma.

The other limitation of this technique is indirect assessment of tumor recurrence using MR morphology. Clinical use of functional imaging, (e.g., positron emission tomography with ^{18}fluorodeoxyglucose, thallium single photon emission computed tomography, MR spectroscopy) needs to be addressed in conjunction with cost-effective analysis to detect early recurrence. Application of this minimally invasive management for brainstem or deep grey matter lesions will be forthcoming. MR-guided RF ablation may have a strong impact on the management of brain tumor patients.

REFERENCES

1. Sweet WH, Mark VH, Hamlin H: Radiofrequency lesions in the central nervous system of man and cat: including case reports of eight bulbar pain-tract interruptions, *J Neurosurg* 17:213, 1960.
2. Aronow S: The use of radiofrequency power in making lesions in the brain, *J Neurosurg* 17:431, 1960.
3. Zervas NT, Kuwayama A: Pathological characteristics of experimental thermal lesions: comparison of induction heating and radiofrequency electrocoagulation, *J Neurosurg* 37:418, 1972.
4. Organ LW: Electrophysiologic principles of radiofrequency lesion making, *Appl Neurophysiol* 39:69, 1976.
5. Kelly PL, Gillingham FJ: The long term results of stereotaxic surgery and L-dopa therapy in patients with Parkinson's disease: a 10 year follow-up study, *J Neurosurg* 53:322, 1980.
6. Matsumoto K, Shichijo F, Fukami T: Long term follow-up review of cases of Parkinson's disease after unilateral or bilateral thalamotomy, *J Neurosurg* 60:1033, 1984.
7. Hassenbusch SJ, Pillary PK, Barnett GH: Radiofrequency cingulotomy for intractable cancer pain using stereotactic guided by magnetic resonance imaging, *Neurosurgery* 27:220, 1990.
8. Tomlison FH, Jack CR, Kelly PJ: Sequential magnetic resonance imaging following stereotactic radiofrequency ventralis lateralis thalamotomy, *J Neurosurg* 74:579, 1991.
9. Kondziolka D, and others: A comparison between magnetic resonance imaging and computed tomography for stereotactic coordinate determination, *Neurosurgery* 30:402, 1992.
10. Farahani K, and others: Hyperacute thermal lesions: MR imaging evaluation of development in the brain, *Radiology* 196:517, 1995.
11. Anzai Y, and others: MR imaging guided interstitial Nd:YAG laser phototherapy: dosimetry study of acute tissue damage in an in vivo model, *J Magn Reson Imaging* 1:553, 1991.
12. Anzai Y, and others: MR imaging: histopathologic correlation of thermal injuries induced with interstitial Nd:YAG laser irradiation in the chronic model, *J Magn Reson Imaging* 2:671, 1992.
13. Matsumoto S, and others: MR imaging of stereotactic thalamotomy using radiofrequency methods, *Nippon Acta Radiol* 52:1559, 1992.
14. Anzai Y, and others: Preliminary experience with MR-guided thermal ablation of brain tumors, *Am J Neuroradiol* 16:39, 1995.
15. Reference deleted in pages.
16. Farahani K, Black KL, Lufkin RB: Long-term MR imaging study of temperature: controlled lesions in the brain, *Radiology* 197:237, 1995.
17. Sundaresan N, Galicich JH: Surgical treatment of brain metastases: clinical and computerized tomography evaluation of the results of treatment, *Cancer* 55:1382, 1985.
18. Smalley SR, and others: Adjuvant radiation therapy after surgical resection of solitary brain metastasis: association with pattern of failure and survival, *Int J Radiat Oncol Biol Phys* 13:1611, 1987.
19. DeAngelis LM, and others: The roles of postoperative radiotherapy after resection of single brain metastasis, *Neurosurgery* 24:798, 1989.
20. Cooper JS, Steinfeld AD, Lerch IA: Cerebral metastases: value of reirradiation in selected patients, *Radiology* 174:883, 1990.
21. Sundaresan N, and others: Reoperation for brain metastases, *J Clin Oncol* 6:1625, 1988.
22. Larson DA, and others: Stereotactic irradiation of brain tumors, *Cancer* 65:792, 1990.
23. Loeffler JS, and others: The treatment of recurrent brain metastases with stereotactic radiosurgery, *J Clin Oncol* 8:576, 1990.
24. Ascher PW, Justich E, Schrottner O: A new surgical but less invasive treatment of central brain tumors: preliminary report, *Acta Neurochir Suppl (Wien)* 52:78, 1991.
25. Kahn T, and others: MRI-guided laser-induced interstitial thermotherapy of cerebral neoplasms, *J Comput Assist Tomogr* 18:519, 1994.
26. Matsumoto R, Oshio K, Jolesz FA: Monitoring of laser and freezing induced ablation in the liver with T1 weighted MR imaging, *J Magn Reson Imaging* 2:555, 1992.
27. Duchman RA, and others: US guided percutaneous laser ablation of liver tissue in a chronic pig model, *Radiology* 176:129, 1990.
28. Earnest F, and others: Cerebral astrocytomas: histopathologic correlation of MR and CT contrast enhancement with stereotactic biopsy, *Radiology* 166:823, 1988.

Chapter 31

MR–GUIDED MINIMALLY INVASIVE THERAPY OF THE SPINE

Rainer M.M. Seibel, Andreas Melzer, Jürgen Plaßmann, Armin Schmidt, Cornelia Sehnert

Minimally invasive techniques for management of spinal disease can be used for many new indications. Most of these techniques are performed as outpatient procedures with local anesthesia. New methods were developed especially for small free fragments in the spine and will be able to replace open surgery. The combination of computed tomography (CT), x-ray fluoroscopy, and endoscopy or magnetic resonance (MR) tomography with endoscopy is safe and effective to increase outcome for different treatment modalities. Periradicular therapy, percutaneous nucleotomy, sequestrectomy, and dissection of postoperative intraspinal and foraminal scar tissue can be performed with minimally invasive techniques.[1]

With the first open magnet, the first patient with a spinal disorder was treated in 1988.[2] A low-field system with 0.064 T was used. The speed of imaging and the signal-to-noise ratio were not comparable with those of modern machines, but it was the first time that during imaging the patient could be treated with surgical procedures without movement inside the scanner. Previous CT-guided procedures were transformed for use in MR. The major benefit of using MR for guidance in spinal treatment is the ability to generate three-dimensional (3D) views of spinal structures without radiation.

Low back pain and cervical pain caused by herniated disks are very common. In Germany, approximately $33 billion was spent in 1996 for management of spinal diseases. However, the loss of gross national product caused by disability is about three to four times greater. Minimally invasive therapy provides a safe alternative to conventional open surgery of disk herniation.

Normally percutaneous techniques for management of herniated disks had been limited to patients with contained disks.[3] Thus, the disk herniation has to be at the level of the disk, and the posterior longitudinal ligament is not ruptured by a free fragment. In 1990 the authors developed a new technique for micro-endoscopic procedures in the spinal canal for treatment of small free fragments and for dissection of spinal scar tissue after open surgery.[4] CT and MRI allow imaging of small structures in the spine and are therefore ideal imaging guidance instruments.

Guidance of instruments in the body is most accurate with CT. The tip of instruments can be detected with an accuracy of 1 mm^3. Unlike x-ray fluoroscopy, CT and MRI provide accurate localization of nerves, vessels, and herniation in the spine. In soft-tissue characterization, MRI is superior to CT. Bony structures are, however, detected better with CT. The possibility of monitoring of instruments and effects during the procedure shows the potential of both methods. Both imaging modalities have increased speed of data acquisition and reconstruction during the past few years. Today, real-time subsecond scan acquisition and reconstruction are possible. Different methods for management of chronic diseases of the spine are available and can be performed under local anesthesia. They include facet joint denervation, periradicular therapy, percutaneous nucleotomy, micro-endoscopic sequestrectomy, and micro-endoscopic scar dissection.

REQUISITES

Neurologic and clinical examination of the patient is essential and should correlate with the findings on CT and MR. For diagnosis, CT and MRI are very important and should follow 2 weeks of failed conservative management or immediately after the onset of neurologic symptoms. Blood coagulation studies should be normal. Spondylodiscitis should be excluded.

FACET JOINT DENERVATION

Low back pain without sciatica is often caused by degeneration of the facet joints. About 80% of facet syndromes are located in L_4/L_5 and L_5/S_1. Surgical neurolysis of facet joints was introduced in 1971 by Rees[5] and was followed a few years later by electrocoagulation.[6] Facet joint block with local anesthetics or facet joint denervation with 50% to 96% ethanol has been performed under CT and now MRI guidance in the authors' institute since 1986. The neurolysis should be done in both joints of the level. If additional compression of the nerve root is present, treatment should be combined with periradicular therapy. Treatment produces good results in 65% to 75% of patients. CT or MR is used to monitor the spread of ethanol, so errors of injections (into the nerve root or vessels) are prevented.[7,8]

PERIRADICULAR THERAPY

Periradicular therapy was developed for patients with failed back surgery syndromes. Indications for periradicular therapy are listed in Box 31-1.

This technique has been used since 1986 with CT guidance and since 1995 with MRI guidance (Fig. 31-1). Under CT and MRI guidance, a 22- or 23-G coaxial needle system can be advanced step by step to the nerve root. The puncture is made in the lower third of the foramen, and the needle crosses the nerve root from lateral to medial. Local anesthetics and cortisone were applied after test injection of contrast (Fig. 31-2). Four to six times the dose of treatment should be repeated after 3 to 4 weeks. After the first good results of this method (Table 31-1) the authors treated disk herniation as well as spinal stenoses. Periradicular therapy is believed to work by reducing the edema of the nerve root and increasing the blood flow in the nerve. Even in patients who are not surgical candidates, weakness of the leg can often be rescued successfully.[9]

A prospective randomized study with 21 male and 19 female patients was performed in 1990. The study compared periradicular therapy with 10-mg versus 40-mg triamcinolonacetonide. Two independent examiners analyzed the CT images before and after the study and evaluated the results. All patients suffered from chronic pain with disk herniation and radicular symptoms at the treated level. The patients had to answer a questionnaire, including the Visual Analogoue Scale (VAS), before and after treatment. A score of 0 meant no pain, 100 was maximum pain. Additional neuroorthopedic examinations were made by independent physicians. Every 3 to 4 wk, four to eight treatments were performed. Statistical evaluation was carried out with the Mann-Whitney test for comparison of both groups before and after treatment as a double-sided plausibility test.[10]

Statistically, the range of pain according to the VAS was not different in the groups. After therapy, symptoms improved significantly in the 40-mg group but only slightly in the 10-mg group. Neuro-orthopedic examination showed complete improvement of the stretched leg from 30° to 60° in most cases.

Box 31-1. Indications of periradicular therapy

- Disk herniation
- Failed back surgery
- Spinal stenosis
- Stenosis of lateral recess
- Stenosis of vertebral foramen
- Weakness and loss of sensation

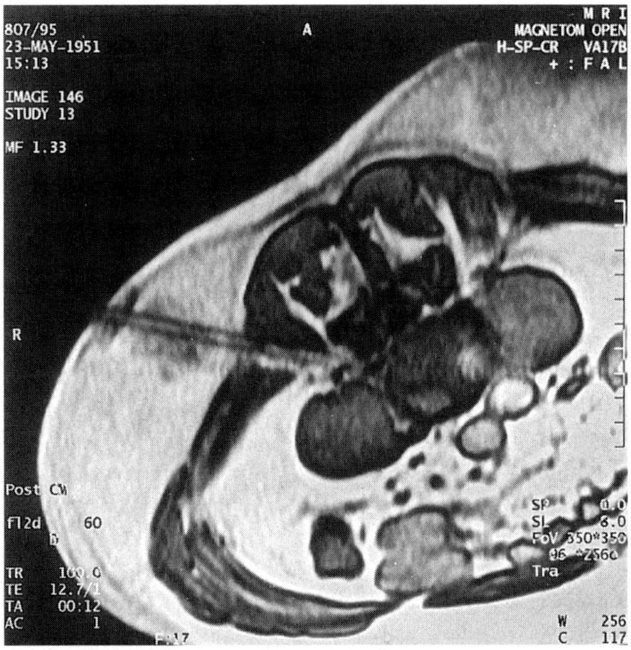

Fig. 31-1. Magnetic resonance–guided periradicular therapy for management of a disk herniation in level L_4/L_5 on the right. The needle tip is advanced directly to the nerve root in the foramen. The double line artifact shows that the center of the needle is in the next plane. If the needle is within the plane, only one black artifact is present.

COMPLICATIONS AND SIDE EFFECTS

Complications and side effects (Table 31-2) are rare after periradicular therapy. One patient with a diastematomyelia had a plegia of the leg immediately after periradicular therapy. The weakness disappeared after a few weeks of conservative treatment. Therefore, patients with spinal cord abnormalities should be excluded for this treatment. Two patients had a spondylodiscitis and a spondylitis after periradicular therapy. No bacterial infection was found at biopsy. These patients were conservatively managed in the hospital.

Patients with acute stomach ulcers should be excluded. Hypertension and diabetes are limitations but not contraindications to therapy. Patients with history of pulmonary embolism should undergo special treatment to prevent thrombosis of the leg. All patients should be given 100 mg/day of aspirin during the treatment period.

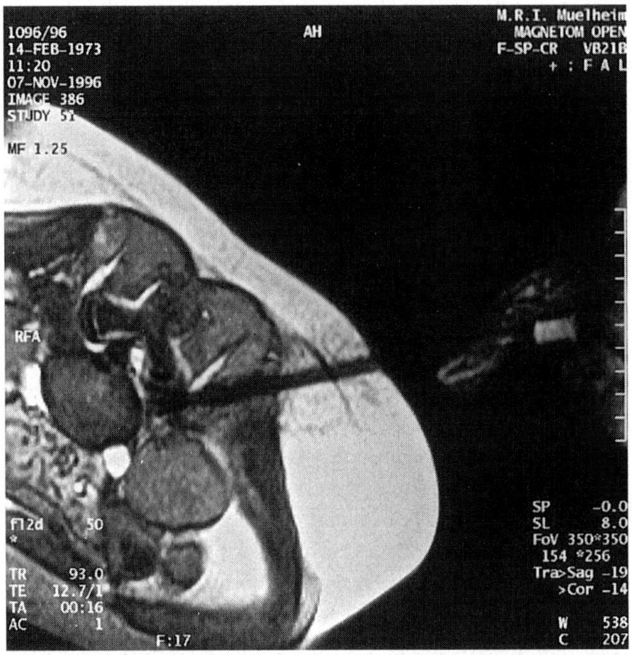

Fig. 31-2. Periradicular therapy in level L_5/S_1 on the left. After contrast injection, the epidural space is highlighted. The dural sac is slightly pushed away by contrast. In the syringe, contrast can be seen. Gadolinium with saline was used. After contrast, local-acting cortisone is injected to the periradicular space.

Table 31-1. Results of periradicular therapy in 370 patients

Finding	Patients (%)
Symptoms improved after first therapy	15
Symptoms improved after fourth therapy	72
No symptoms at the end of treatment	78
No symptoms 3 months after treatment	83
No symptoms 2 years after treatment	68
Disk surgery after periradicular therapy	3

PERCUTANEOUS NUCLEOTOMY

Percutaneous techniques for nucleotomy were first described by Hijikata and others[11] in 1975. Suezawa[12] added discoscopy to fluoroscopy for monitoring the treatment. With the patient under general anesthesia, two trocar systems (diameter 11 mm) were introduced to both foramen intervertebrale. Nucleotomy was performed with conventional instruments. Onik and others[13] invented an automated nucleotomy device with a probe diameter of 2-mm in 1985.

Since 1988 the authors have performed percutaneous nucleotomy with combined CT and fluoroscopy guidance. The authors started with the automated probe of Onik to remove material of the nucleus pulposus. After 1 year, laser nucleotomy was performed using a holmium and neodymium yttrium-aluminum-garnet (Ho:YAG, Nd:YAG) laser (Fig. 31-3). Free fragments in the spinal canal or mass herniation cannot be managed by percutaneous nucleotomy. Small herniation and a contained disk (e.g., the herniation is within the disk level without free fragments) with compression of the nerve root and correlative neurologic symptoms are a good indication for percutaneous nucleotomy or laser nucleotomy.

One hundred ten patients with percutaneous nucleotomy[14] and 116 with laser nucleotomy[15] were treated for herniation. Outcome did not significantly differ in the groups, but laser treatment is technically easier. Both a 20- and 18-guage introducer set were tested for use with the laser. A 23-gauge introducer set is now being tested. The diameter is only 1.2 to 0.65 mm. The study used laser fibers with a 0.4-mm diameter. The risk of nerve root injury in the foramen is very low. Local anesthesia is not used in the nerve root. Patients immediately report any heat effects. For the automated suction device, the introducers had diameters from 2.8 to 4.0 mm.

Patients

Between 1988 and 1991, 110 patients were treated with percutaneous nucleotomy. The mean age was 45 years of age (range, 25 to 66 years). Two patients underwent percutaneous nucleotomy at the level L_3/L_4 (2%), 58 at level L_4/L_5 (53%), and 50 at level L_5/S_1 (45%).

Table 31-2. Side effects of periradicular therapy in a study of 40 patients and a study of 370 patients

Side effect	Patients (*n* (%))	Patients (*n* (%))
Indigestion	1 (2.5)	0 (0)
Edema	1 (2.5)	11 (3)
Acne	1 (2.5)	15 (4)
Tensions and blushing	1 (2.5)	7 (2)
Hair loss	2 (5)	0 (0)
Hormonal disorder	2 (5)	5* (3)
Weight increase	4 (10)	30 (8)
Stomach disorder	5 (12.5)	0 (0)
Calf cramps	15 (37.5)	30 (8)
Petechia	0 (0)	2 (0.5)

*Of 170 female patients.

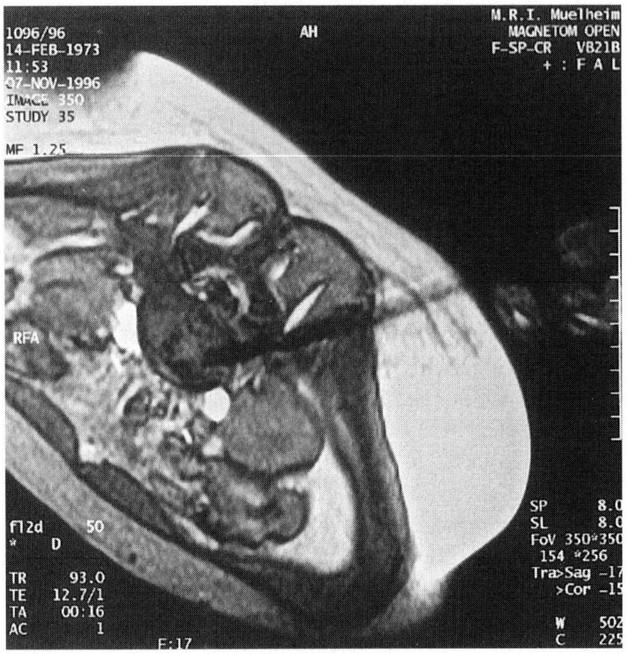

Fig. 31-3. Magnetic resonance (MR)–guided endoscopic laser nucleotomy at level L_5/S_1 on the left. For this level, a double-oblique access is often necessary. In MR, this goal is accomplished by MR fluoroscopy.

Between 1989 and 1991, 116 patients underwent laser nucleotomy. The mean age was 47 years of age, (range, 15 to 81 years). The procedure was performed at the level L_2/L_3 in three patients (2%), at level L_3/L_4 in nine patients (8%), at level L_4/L_5 in 71 patients (62%), and at level L_5/S_1 in 33 patients (28%).

Follow-up

Patients underwent follow-up at 3 weeks, 6 weeks, 3 months, 6 months, and 1 year after percutaneous nucleotomy and laser nucleotomy. The success of both methods was proven by clinical and neurologic examinations at all follow-ups and by CT 3 weeks and 6 months after therapy. MRI of the lumbar spine was routinely done 6 weeks after management to exclude discitis. VAS was used for evaluation of pain.

Results

Of patients, 82% ($n = 110$) experienced complete pain relief after percutaneous nucleotomy. Neurologic findings (e.g., pathologic stretched leg test, weak muscle reflexes) improved immediately after percutaneous nucleotomy in 92%.

Complications and side effects

One percutaneous nucleotomy patient and one laser nucleotomy patient experienced a spondylodiscitis. Of patients, 26% had an irritation of the segmental nerve root for 3 to 5 weeks after percutaneous nucleotomy and 21% after laser nucleotomy.

MINIMALLY INVASIVE THERAPY FOR UNCONTAINED DISK AND SCAR TISSUE

Percutaneous nucleotomy should be used only in a contained disk. Therefore, free fragments in the spinal canal and the foramen, although very common, cannot be treated. The authors developed a new technique with a combination of CT, fluoroscopy, and micro-endoscopy to visualize very small structures inside the foramen and the spinal canal percutaneously. New endoscopes allow this technique using MR inside an open magnet. A new technique for dissection of scar tissue in the spine[16] and for treatment of small free fragments[17] has been performed in the authors' institute for several years under CT guidance.

One study reviewed 20 patients with chronic low back pain. Four patients with free fragment in the spinal canal and eight with lateral herniation and free fragments in the foramen were treated. Under combined endoscopic CT fluoroscopic and micro-endoscopic monitoring, seven patients with prior open surgery with scar tissue in the spinal canal were also treated. One abscess in the foramen was removed. The overall mean age was 51.9 ± 14.8 years. Level L_4/L_5 was treated in 12 patients and L_5/S_1 in 8 patients. Seventeen patients were managed as outpatients. Immediately after therapy, pain relief and improvement of neurologic symptoms were assessed. In follow-up, patients were asked to evaluate treatment success, defined as improvement of pain symptoms estimated on VAS.

Technique

Special introducer sets with diameters from 1.2 to 4 mm were developed for the procedure. The smallest fiberscope with a diameter of 0.29 mm fits into a 22-G coaxial interventional needle set. Good image quality can be achieved with endoscopes having a diameter more than 0.5 mm. Flexible tips allow endoscopes to be introduced transspinally into the foramen or transforaminally into the spinal canal. Micro-instruments having a diameter of 0.9 mm can be used inside the foramen and spinal canal (e.g., forceps, scissors, other instruments). Different laser systems were used for treatment: Nd:YAG and Ho:YAG laser. An interventional CT (Somatom plus 4, Care Vision, Siemens, Erlangen, Germany) is used for tomography. This real-time CT allows two or three surgeons to perform the procedure. For additional fluoroscopy, a digital C arm is used.

Results

Before treatment 20 patients had a pain score between 70 and 100 (VAS). Of patients, 80% ($n = 16$) had neurologic deficits before micro-operation: weakening of the patellar reflex, weakness of the tibialis anterior, and weakness of the extensor brevis and decreased ankle jerk. Immediately after microsurgery, reflexes or weakness improved in 75% of patients. Of patients, 94% showed more than a 50° decreased or a negative stretched leg test. Pain improvement was 50% or greater in all patients at the end of the procedure. The pain score decreased from 88% to 8% on average. Pain relief more than 50% (VAS) was achieved in 90% of patients ($n = 18$) 6 months after treatment.

Complications and side effects

Complications of CT-guided spinal endoscopic procedures did not occur in these few cases. Five patients complained slightly of nerve root irritation at the treated level that lasted several days, sometimes up to 2 weeks. Conservative treatment with periradicular therapy was performed in four patients. Symptoms related to mechanical irritation by pressure to the nerve root during treatment. Of these five patients, three experienced pseudoradicular pain that was managed with blockades of both facet joints (three times in 8 days) by injecting a local anesthetic.

Discussion

Open surgery of the spine is limited because of poor outcome and postnucleotomy syndrome with severe disability after surgery. Therefore, it is important to develop new less-invasive treatments of spinal disease. Periradicular therapy, laser nucleotomy, percutaneous nucleotomy, and micro-endoscopic procedures are successful because of decompression and restoration of the function of the nerve root. Even if complete replacement of open surgery is impossible at this moment, minimally invasive therapy has many indications and offers a new way of treatment for postnucleotomy syndrome with chronic pain.[18]

Free fragments in the spinal canal and in the foramen are a limitation of normal percutaneous nucleotomy. CT-guided micro-endoscopy of the spinal canal make treatment of dislocated herniation possible. Preoperative planning using a 3D technique shows the best access and the right angle to the target volume. CT gives near real-time imaging for monitoring of the procedure and instrument guidance. Micro-endoscopy provides a good view of the surface of the operative field. In combination, these techniques permit the highest safety for minimally invasive therapy in the spine. Under these circumstances, an accuracy of 0.01 mm for handling of instruments may be reached.

Pain therapy and local tumor therapy are the most interesting indications for minimally invasive therapy in oncologic management of the spine. CT and MRI allow precise access to nerves (Fig. 31-4) and tumors (Fig. 31-5). Monitoring of treatment, such as injection of local cytostatic drugs, ethanol injection, application of heat with laser, radiofrequency ablation, focused ultrasound, or cryosurgery, shows the advantages of this technique. Different methods are performed to stabilize metastatic vertebrae. For safety reasons, CT and MRI should be used for local application of toxic materials in tumors of the spine. Injection of local anesthetics into the vertebral artery can cause a convulsion immediately.[19] Negative aspiration is not enough to avoid injury of arterial wall without CT guidance.[20]

With minimally invasive therapy, even primary tumors (e.g., in the liver) can be managed with good results (see Chapters 39 and 40).[21,22] Laser or radiofrequency ablation for metastases of liver and brain seem to be alternatives for open surgery[23–26] and for therapy of head and neck tumors.

New treatments are possible with guidance of recently developed real-time CT and open magnets. The advantage is to

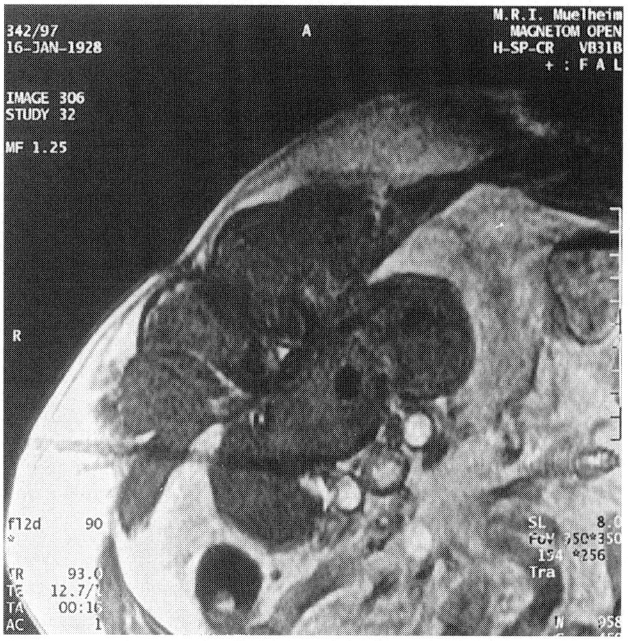

Fig. 31-4. Magnetic resonance–guided lumbar sympathectomy for arterial obstructive disease. The needle tip hit the sympathetic trunk in the "Bermuda triangle" between the psoas muscle, vertebral body, and iliac artery. Contrast is given (white surrounding the needle tip) to prove the correct distribution of ethanol to the trunk. The sympathetic ganglia can be seen black inside the white contrast.

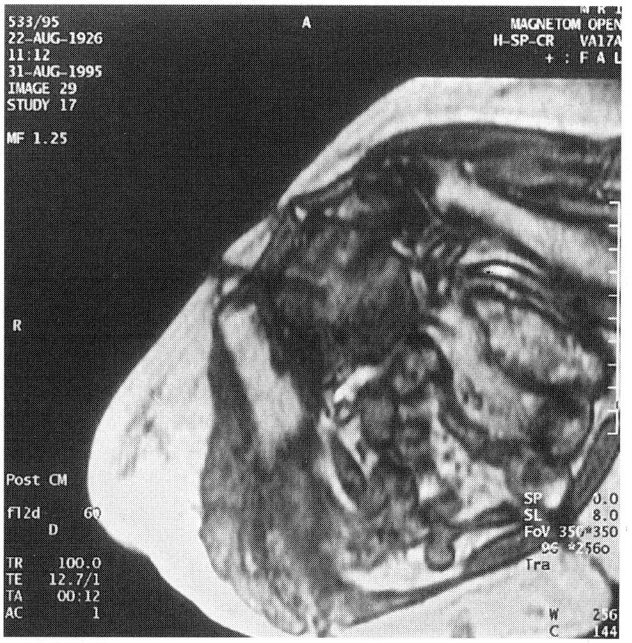

Fig. 31-5. Intratumoral ethanol injection in level S_1. The ethanol injection should be monitored under magnetic resonance fluoroscopy to prevent incorrect spread of the ethanol to the spinal canal. Management is effective for tumor pain reduction and for stabilization of the vertebral body.

perform the procedure while the patient remains in the same position. Both techniques allow free interaction in three planes. Real-time 3D imaging and display may soon be available, especially with the combination of real-time CT and an angiography system. For arterial perfusion of a liver lesion, the same system shows the super selective position of the catheter tip with enhancement of the liver segment.

Open magnets are used in different institutes for surgical procedures.[27] The first tests show a very good ability for use inside the operating room and the possibility to perform image-guided procedures in nearly every region in the body. Additional use of endoscopy is the key to transmit every kind of management modality safely into the body.

The next step in minimally invasive therapy is integration of CT and MR into an operative theater, which will change the face of surgery of the next century. A program to establish and develop a new environment for operating room technology is being developed. The combination of preoperative high-power computer planning, image guidance with capacity of real-time 3D, and CT and MR fluoroscopy with real-time visualization to monitor tissue changes and to network all patient data will be available. In this new operating room, different combinations of CT, MR, angiography, and ultrasound will be integrated. This operating room will be built in a modular fashion, so it can be changed for every special need. The use of microscalpels, microinstruments, radiofrequency, laser, argon plasma coagulation, cryosurgery, hyperenergetic ultrasound, or micromotor-driven remote-control microrobots in the body will be monitored by this combination. Future operative room will include modular systems of imaging machines for minimally invasive surgery.

REFERENCES

1. Seibel RMM, and others: Minimally invasive treatment of spinal diseases, *Min Invas Ther & Allied Technol* 5:226, 1996.
2. Seibel RMM: Image-guided minimally invasive therapy, *Surg Endosc* 11:154, 1997.
3. Onik G, and others: Percutaneous lumbar discetomy using a new aspiration probe: porcine and cadaver model, *Radiology* 155:251, 1985.
4. Seibel RMM, Grönemeyer DHW: Technique for CT guided microendoscopic dissection of the spine, *End Surg* 2:226, 1994.
5. Rees WS: Multiple bilateral subcutaneous rhizolysis of segmental nerves in the treatment of the intervertebral disc syndrome, *Ann Gen Prac* 26:126, 1971.
6. Shealy CN: Percutaneous radiofrequency denervation of spinal facets: treatment of chronic back pain and sciatica, *J Neurosurg* 43:448, 1975.
7. Seibel RMM, Grönemeyer DHW, Grumme TH: *New treatments of the spinal column diseases using interventional radiological techniques.* In Seibel RMM, Grönemeyer DHW: *Interventional computed tomography,* Oxford, 1990, Blackwell.
8. Lora J, Long MD: So called facet denervation in the management of intractable back pain, *Spine* 1:121, 1976.
9. Seibel RMM, Grönemeyer DHW, Grumme TH: *New treatments of the spinal column diseases using interventional radiological techniques.* In Seibel RMM, Grönemeyer DHW: *Interventional computed tomography,* Oxford, 1990, Blackwell.
10. Grönemeyer DHW, and others: Die mikroinvasive CT gesteuerte periradikuläre therapie zur behandlung von chronischen bandscheibenbedingten funktionsstörungen, *Wien Med Wochenschr* 145:129, 1995.
11. Hijikata S, and others: Percutaneous diskectomy: a new treatment method for lumbar disc herniation, *J Toden Hosp* 5:5, 1975.
12. Suezawa Y: Kreuzschmerzen in der orthopädie: heutiger stand ihrer therapie, *Schweiz Rundsch Med Prax* 71:783, 1982.
13. Onik G, and others: Percutaneous lumbar discetomy using a new aspiration probe: porcine and cadaver model, *Radiology* 155:251, 1985.
14. Seibel RMM, Grönemeyer DHW, Sörensen RAL: Percutaneous nucleotomy with CT and fluoroscopic guidance, *J Vasc Interv Radiol* 3:571, 1992.
15. Grönemeyer DHW, and others: Atraumatic CT-controlled percutaneous laser nucleotomy, *Min Inv Ther* 2:247, 1993.
16. Seibel RMM, Grönemeyer DHW: Technique for CT guided microendoscopic dissection of the spine, *End Surg* 2:226, 1994.
17. Seibel RMM: CT guided endoscopy of sequestered disk herniation, *J Vasc Interv Radiol* 1(suppl):222, 1996.
18. Seibel RMM, and others: Minimally invasive treatment of spinal diseases, *Min Inv Ther All Tech* 5:226, 1996.
19. Ariani J, Parmley J, Ochsner A: Facilities and complications after attempts at stellate ganglion, *Surgery* 32:615, 1952.
20. Mastroianni A: The effects of stellate ganglion block. Schmerzdiagnostik und Therapie, Volume 2 Bochum (1986) 80–93.
21. Livraghi T, Vettori C, Lazzaroni S: Liver metastases: results of percutaneous ethanol injection in 14 patients, *Radiology* 179:709, 1991.
22. Vogl TH, and others: MR imaging guided laser induced thermotherapy, *Min Inv Ther All Tech* 5:243, 1996.
23. Fan M, and others: Interstitial 1.06 Nd:YAG laser thermotherapy in malignant gliomas under real time monitoring of MRI: experimental studies and phase I clinical trial, *J Clin Laser Med Surg* 10:355, 1992.
24. Anzai Y, and others: MR imaging guided interstitial NDYAG laser phototherapy: dosimetry study of acute damage in an in vivo model, *J Magn Reson Imaging* 1:553, 1991.
25. Kahn TH, and others: MRI guided laser induced interstitial thermotherapy of cerebral neoplasms, *J Comput Assist Tomogr* 6:519, 1994.
26. Silverman ST: Percutaneous abdominal biopsy: recent advances and future directions, *Sem Int Radiol* 13:3, 1996.
27. Jolecz F, and others: MR imaging of laser tissue interactions, *Radiology* 168:249, 1988.

Chapter 32

MR–GUIDED LUMBAR SYMPATHECTOMY

Andreas Melzer, Rainer M.M. Seibel, Armin Schmidt, Wolfram Triebe

Although lumbar sympathectomy has been an established therapy of peripheral occlusive artery disease for more than 20 years,[1] the appropriate technique is controversial. From the technical standpoint, computed tomography (CT) guidance provides the highest accuracy and the lowest risk of complications.[2,3] This chapter discusses the feasibility of magnetic resonance (MR)–guided lumbar sympathectomy. Temperature and flow sensitivity, arbitrary slice orientation, and excellent soft-tissue contrast make MRI superior to other imaging systems. However, the display of instruments is inferior. The authors have evaluated interventional MR techniques and collaborated in the development of the required MR-compatible instruments.

HISTORICAL REMARKS

The first report of a periarterial sympathectomy by Jaboulay in 1899[4] documented a surgical approach to the sympathetic trunk. In 1913, this technique was improved by Leriche.[5] Adson and Brown[6] reported excision of the lumbar ganglia and communicating branches in 1925. The first paravertebral chemical neurolysis of the sympathetic trunk with 85% ethanol was performed by Swetlow[7] in 1926. In 1949, Haxton[8] presented results from 220 patients treated by lumbar sympathectomy with phenyl alcohol. Today, lumbar sympathectomy has an established place in the treatment of peripheral artery diseases, circulation disorders of the lower limb, and pain therapy for cancer that irritates the lumbar sympathetic trunk. Radiologic and surgical methods are under increasing competition, particularly with the introduction of laparoscopic surgery.[9]

The retroperitoneoscopic approach requires general anesthesia and exposure of the operative field by means of balloon dissection. The ganglia are surgically removed under endoscopic control. The magnification of the endoscope provides a detailed view of the anatomic structures, allowing precise surgical excision.

Until the introduction of CT guidance, chemical sympathectomy was performed under fluoroscopic control or by means of single x-ray images. The major advantage of CT guidance is the preoperative planning and the puncture accuracy of 1 mm[3]. In addition, distribution of a control injection with contrast media can be displayed.

The procedure can be monitored by introducing a micro-endoscope (0.5 mm). CT-guided micro-endoscopic surgical dissection of the sympathetic trunk is being evaluated by Mülheim.[10] For the major disadvantages of CT guidance (exposure to ionizing radiation, limitation to axial scans) to be avoided, lumbar sympathectomy was evaluated with ethanol under MR guidance in a 0.2-T horizontal open magnet.[11] The first clinical MR-guided lumbar sympathectomy with ethanol was performed in 1995. In 1996, Lufkin[12] reported an occasional radiofrequency (RF) ablation of the sympathetic trunk.

ANATOMY

The lumbar sympathetic trunk has three to four ganglia located laterally at both sides of the anterior surface of the vertebral bodies. The communicating branches between the ganglia are relatively long. Grey communicating branches are present in all lumbar ganglia, whereas white communicating branches are found at the upper one or two ganglia. The preganglionic fibers in the lower lumbar sympathetic trunk run into the interganglionic branches. Anatomic variance of communicating branches between two ganglia at one segment nerve or at two segment nerves and one ganglion is found frequently.

After synaptic pre- to postganglionic transition, the postganglionic fibers traverse with the lumbar spinal nerve. These fibers contain the vasomotor nerves and should be interrupted by the lumbar sympathectomy (Figs. 32-1 and 32-2).[13,14]

INDICATIONS

In general, indications of chemical sympathectomy are similar to those of any type of sympathectomy. The major indication is causalgia with continuous and incapacitating pain. Therapy for peripheral artery disease by CT-guided lumbar sympathectomy has produced good results.[15] The main indications for this therapy are occlusions of arteries in the lower leg and foot and simultaneous femoral occlusions. Trophic peripheral ulcers and necrotic areas in the region of the toes can also be successfully treated with lumbar sympathectomy. Lumbar sympathectomy is established as adjuvant treatment after revascularization of the femoral or popliteal arteries. The vascular indications can be determined after clinical examination, including pulse status, Doppler ultrasound, and angiography in accordance with the criteria established by Carstensen (Box 32-1).[16]

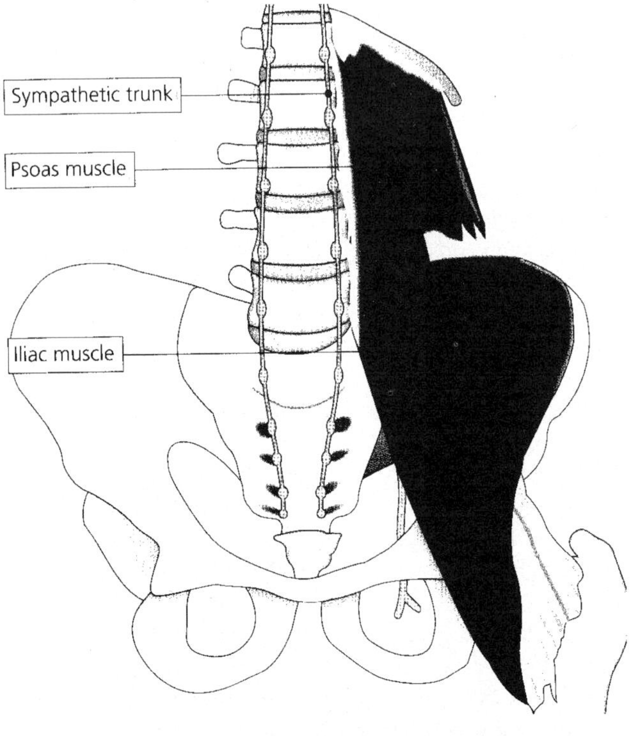

Fig. 32-1. Sectional coronal view of the sympathetic trunk.

CONTRAINDICATIONS

In older patients with generalized arteriosclerosis, the operative lumbar sympathectomy can have contraindications. Most of these often multidiseased patients are classified as New York Heart Association III–IV, so general anesthesia is contraindicated. In patients with isolated aortic occlusions, advanced gangrene, and edema of the lower limb, lumbar sympathectomy should not be performed. If general anesthesia is contraindicated, surgical lumbar sympathectomy is impossible because it is performed only under general anesthesia (Boxes 32-2 and 32-3).[16]

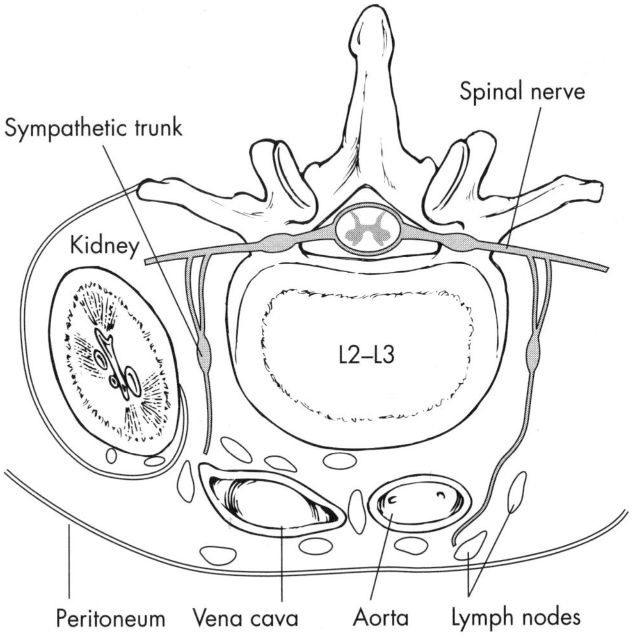

Fig. 32-2. Transverse view of the paravertebral localization of the sympathetic ganglia.

Box 32-1. Indications for lumbar sympathectomy

- Adjuvant treatment to profunda or femoropopliteal bypass or angioplasty
- Causalgia
- Diabetes with peripheral angiopathy*
- Endarteritis obliterans (Winiwarter-Buerger)
- Functional circulation disorders
- Hyperhidrosis
- Peripheral hyperalgesia (burning feet)
- Peripheral necrosis of the toes
- Peripheral occlusive artery disease
- Raynaud's disease
- Trophic ulcers of the lower limb and feet
- Tumor pain

*Only if sympathicus responds to a test blockade.

PATIENTS

Mülheim evaluated treatment with MR-guided lumbar sympathectomies in 15 patients. The patients were 21 to 75 years of age (mean, 57 years). Two patients had diabetes, two had Raynaud's disease, and two had hyperhidrosis. Eleven patients had peripheral artery disease in stage III or IV on the Fontaine scale. In four patients, intervention was performed bilaterally. Bilateral treatment is performed in two sessions; simultaneous treatment is impossible because of the lateroprone position of the patient.

METHODS

Before lumbar sympathectomy, a predictive test using local anesthesia for a temporary sympathetic trunk blockade is useful. The success of lumbar sympathectomy was evaluated by clinical effects, such as warming, increased red skin color, reduced pain, and increased walking distance and pulse intensity. In addition, a thermosensitive liquid crystal display film was used to assess the immediate response of increased blood circulation and warming of the feet (Fig. 32-3).

Box 32-2. Contraindications for lumbar sympathectomy

Isolated aorto-iliac occlusions
Multidiseased patients with extensive arteriosclerosis
Septic gangrene
Treatment-resistant edema of lower limb and feet

Box 32-3. Specific contraindications for magnetic resonance–guided lumbar sympathectomy

Ferromagnetic aneurysm clips
Implanted drug pumps
Major ferromagnetic implants
Pacemaker
Severe ischemic heart disease

Technique of magnetic resonance–guided lumbar sympathectomy

After several tests on phantoms and volunteers and after analysis of conventional axial lumbar spine MR tomography, a preliminary technique of MR lumbar sympathectomy has been defined:

- Exclusion criteria (see indications)
- Informed consent
- Five axial gradient-recalled echo slices (8 mm) of the lumbar spine and fast low-angle shot (Flash) two-dimensional (2D) breathhold
- Evaluation of renal anatomy and paravertebral structures on coronal images (Fig. 32-4)
- Search of respective ureter by FLASH 2D breathhold or rapid acquisition relaxation enhancement (RARE)-like sequence using turbo spin-echo with 60- to 100-mm slices thickness (Fig. 32-5); in doubtful cases, dynamic ureter study with FLASH 2D breathholds every 1 min after intravenous administration of 1 ml/kg gadolinium contrast (Magnevist, Schering, Berlin); if the ureter cannot be localized, diagnosis is completed by CT in level of the planed lumbar sympathectomy after intravenous administration of 50 ml of iodine contrast media (Ultravist, Schering, Berlin)
- Repositioning of the patient to a 45° lateral prone position
- Placement of the interventional 35- or 45-cm coil diagonally to the target around the patient
- Reference scan in the axial direction using FLASH 2D breathhold
- Approval of ureter localization within a reference scan (FLASH 2D breathhold)
- In doubtful cases, referral to CT-guided lumbar sympathectomy
- Displacement of the table to move the target slice into a 0° position

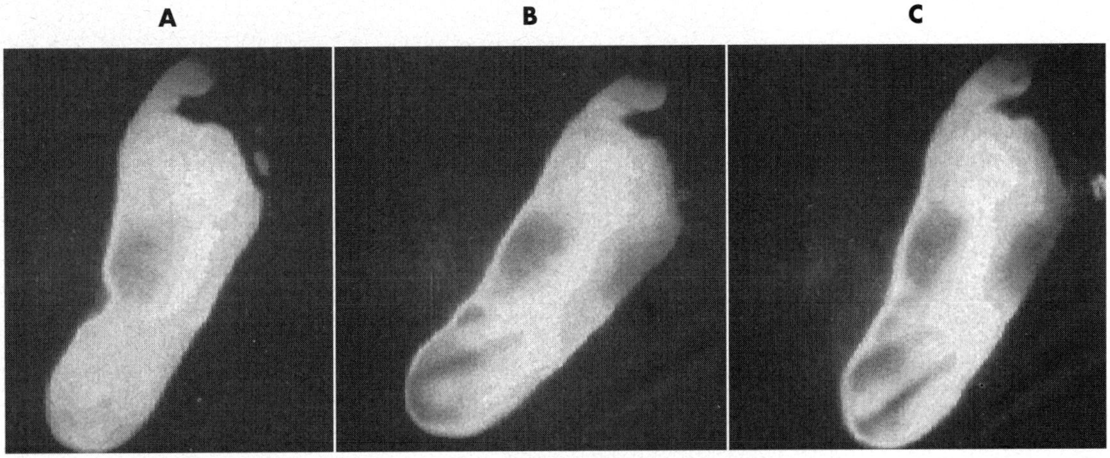

Fig. 32-3. Thermosensitive liquid crystal film allows display of temperature changes of the foot. **A,** before; **B,** 2 min after; and **C,** 5 min after sympathectomy. See Color Plate 16.

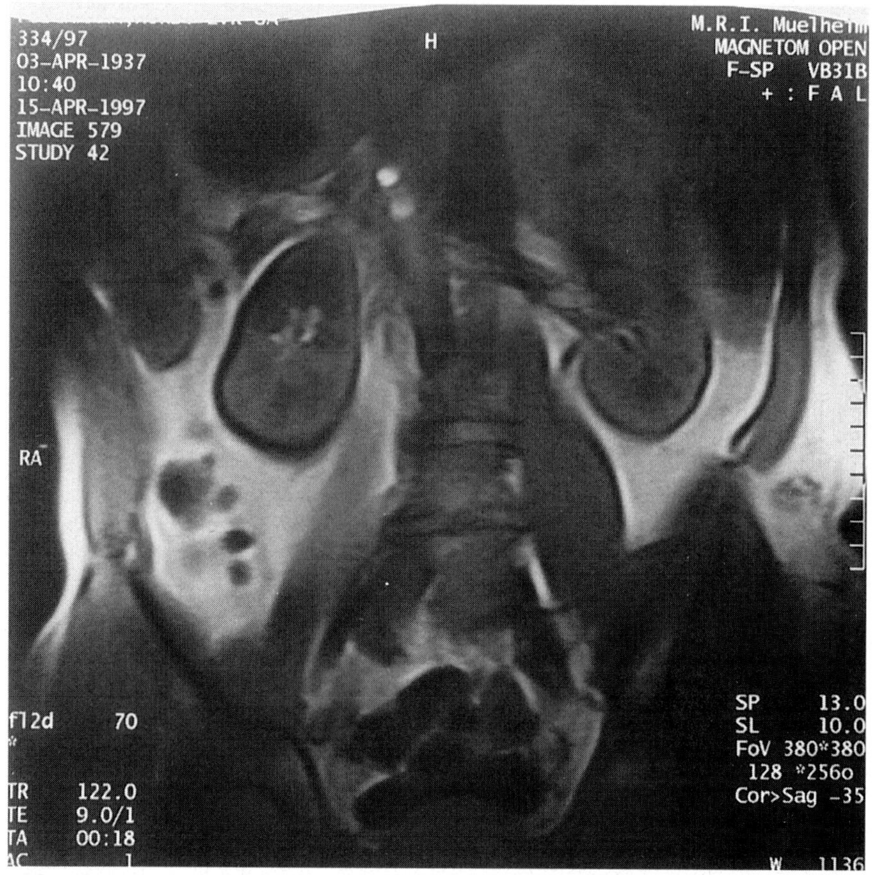

Fig. 32-4. Coronal localization of the ureter with two-dimensional fast low-angle shot (gradient-recalled echo repetition time, 122 msec; echo time, 9 msec; acquisition time, 18 sec; slice, 8 mm).

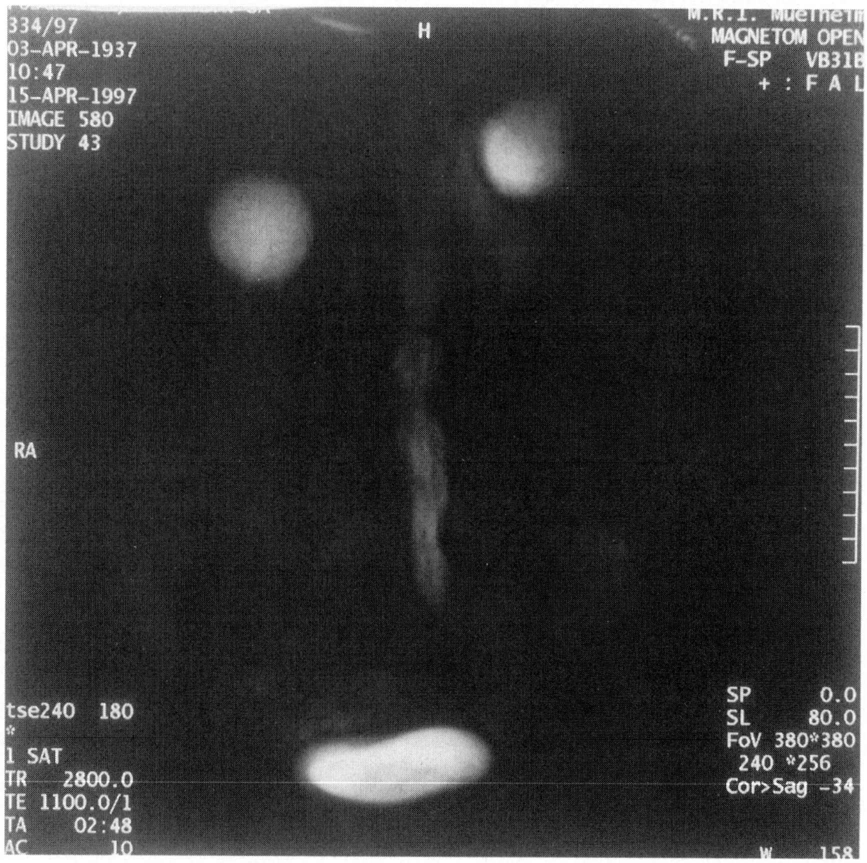

Fig. 32-5. Turbo spin echo (repetition time, 2800 msec; echo time, 1100 msec; acquisition time, 2.48 sec; slice thickness, 80 mm) for localization or exclusion of the ureter in the area of the sympathetic trunk.

- Reference scan and trajectory planning to evaluate distance and angle, using FLASH 2D breathhold
- Referencing of the injection site with the laser pointer by anatomic landmarks (e.g., spinal process) or an MRI grid
- Movement of the table and activation of the laser pointer
- Marking on the skin by means of a black marker (the center of the cross remains free of ink to avoid tattooing)
- Disinfection of skin and sterile draping (Fig. 32-6)
- Local anesthesia and movement of the table to a 0° position in the x-axis (longitudinal)
- Starting of a "fluoro-like sequence" and "digital referencing" with index finger
- If injection site corresponds to the planning, insertion of the needle (150 mm, 22 gauge, Cook, Denmark) and movement forward between the acquisitions to achieve optimal images
- If the needle deteriorates or the patient moves accidentally, the sequence must be stopped. A three-slice breathhold is started, and when the corresponding image of the new needle position is detected, the procedure is finished in breathhold technique or a new "fluoro-like sequence" is started with corrected slice position. In case of significant angulation of the needle trajectory, new planning is required, whereby breathhold slices are acquired in rectangular orientation to the cannula (coronal to sagittal to transversal).
- When the target is reached, contrast solution (2 mmol gadolinium contrast solution, Magnevist, Schering, Berlin) is injected (Fig. 32-7, *A*).
- Three breathhold slices in axial, rectangular coronal, or sagittal orientation sequence confirm the constrast distribution.
- If correct distribution is displayed, ethanol is injected in three 2-ml steps and controlled by fluoro-like sequences or breathhold (Fig. 32-7, *B, C*).
- Final sagittal and axial breathholds and T2 images are obtained to document the procedure and to exclude bleeding (Fig. 32-7,*C*).

RESULTS

Since October 1995, eight women and seven men 21 to 75 years of age, (mean, 57 years) underwent 20 MR-guided lumbar sympathectomies by administration of 6 ml of 80% ethanol.

Two patients could not be treated under MR guidance because one had a major syndesmophytic vertebral bone formation that impeded access to the sympathetic ganglion. A second patient had a large abdominal aortic aneurysm, which was discovered during the initial MR planning scans, and thus was referred to vascular surgery. In both cases, lumbar sympathectomy was performed later using CT guidance. Sympathicolysis had a successful outcome in 12 patients and 16 procedures. Immediately after treatment 14 patients showed flush of the lower limb and toes and subjective heating sensation. Two patients (a 21-year-old female and a 42-year-old male) who had suffered from hyperhidrosis presented after 18 and 12-month follow-ups with significantly reduced sweating to a tolerable level. One patient with severe multiple peripheral stenosis did not improve symptoms and walking distance. In five patients, walking distance notably increased. Eczema at the lower extremities healed completely. In five patients with stage IV occlusive arterial disease (OAD), necrosis healed. Other than pain during needle insertion or during injection of ethanol, no complications occurred. In one patient, bleeding occurred through the needle, but no hematoma was found during follow-up.

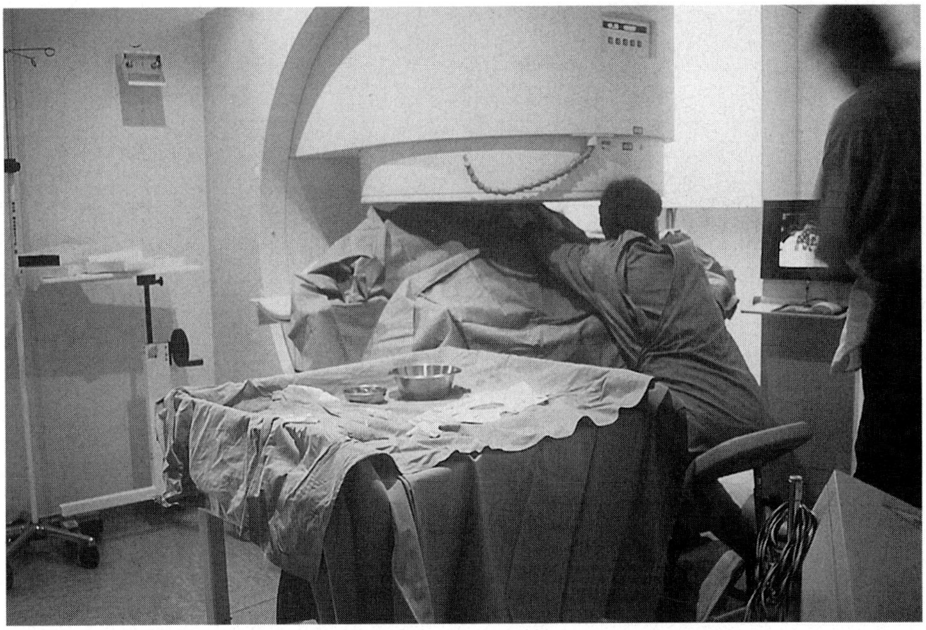

Fig. 32-6. Sterile draping of the patient in the magnetic resonance unit and position of the interventionist.

A

B

C

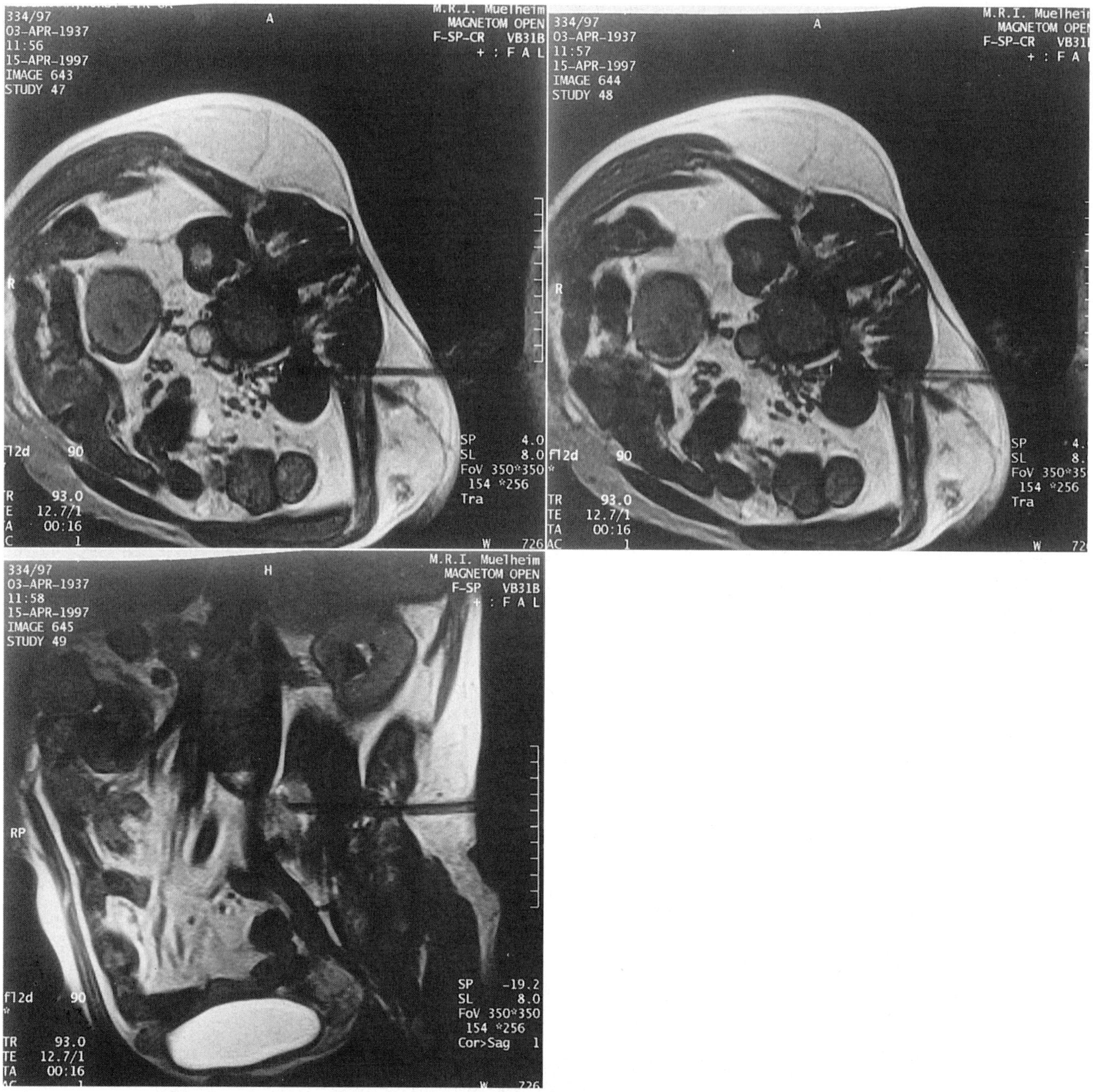

Fig. 32-7. **A,** Magnetic resonance guidance of a 150-mm, 22-gauge cannula (Cook, Denmark) to the sympathetic trunk and injection of 2 mmol/1 contrast solution (Magnevist, Schering, Berlin, Germany). **B,** Injection of 6 ml of 80% ethanol. **C,** Sagittal control image of the ethanol distribution (8-mm gradient-recalled echo two-dimensional fast low-angle shot; repetition time, 93 msec; echo time, 12.7 msec; acquisition time, 16 sec).

DISCUSSION

MR-guided lumbar sympathectomy is possible. In 70% of the authors' patients, there was an improvement after lumbar sympathectomy. MR-guided lumbar sympathectomy can be repeated if sympathetic tone reappears similar to the CT technique.[17] Two questions should be discussed: Is chemical sympathectomy an adequate treatment modality? What are the specific advantages or disadvantages of MR-guided lumbar sympathectomy?

Quantitative appraisal of the success of lumbar sympathectomy has been difficult to evaluate because the effects of therapy and the walking exercise cannot be differentiated with respect to increased walking distance. With intensive walking exercise, patients can improve circulation considerably after

Table 32-1. Complications after lumbar sympathectomy (LS)

	Surgical LS, %	CT-guided LS, %	MR-guided LS, %
Mortality	0.5–7.0	0	0
Hyperesthesia of the genitofemoral nerve	5.0–18.0	2.0	10
Sexual disorders	2.0–9.0	0	0
Paradoxic gangrene	1.0–4.0	0	0
Ureteral damage	1.0	0.01	0
Bleeding			5
Local pain during injection			10

From Seibel RMM, and others: *CT guided lumbar sympathetic trunk neurolysis for the treatment of occlusive arterial disease OAD.* In *Interventional Computed Tomography,* Oxford, 1990, Blackwell Scientific.
CT—computed tomography; MR—magnetic resonance.

lumbar sympathectomy. However, the positive effects of lumbar sympathectomy in Fontaine stage III were proven in a randomized prospective study by Cross and Cotton.[18] In the authors' study on CT-guided lumbar sympathectomy,[15] an improvement from stage III to stage IV (particularly in distally located necroses) was noted. Complete healing of necrosis, preservation of toes,[19] or borderline amputation after a lumbar sympathectomy can be achieved in most cases.

The combination of lumbar sympathectomy, angioplasty, or vascular surgery can be successful if circulation of the lower limb and foot arteries is present.[15]

Two major studies with 150[18] and 830 patients[20] reported postoperative mortality of 0.5% to 7%. Postoperative hyperesthesia in the region of the genitofemoral or lateral cutaneous nerve of the thigh occurred in 5% to 18% of cases and sexual disorders in 2% to 9% of patients. These complications did not occur in the authors' study, but the number of procedures is too low to compare the results (Table 32-1).

Before lumbar sympathectomy, a predictive test using local anesthesia for a temporary sympathetic trunk blockade is useful. Because of the inferior needle visualization under MRI guidance, diagnostic blockade of the lumbar sympathetic trunk with local anesthetic is recommended before ethanol injection. If the localization of the anesthetic drug is correct, warming of the lower limb in the respective dermatome will occur.[21] Also, circulation measurements with an infrared camera can be useful.[22] The authors have used a thermosensitive liquid crystal display film to assess the immediate response of increased blood circulation and warming of the feet (see Fig. 32-3). However, this examination depends on various aspects, such as position of the patient, time, and room temperature. Thus, the examination is helpful only if it compares pre- and postinterventional blood circulation. The most useful methods of assessing the results are clinical: warming of foot and lower limb, skin changes from pale to light red, and improvement in what the patient feels. If the desired effect is achieved, chemical neurolysis can be performed in the same session. However, a dilution of the ethanol should be considered; thus, 5 minutes should pass before the final injection is performed. In cases of hyperhidrosis, a pre- and postinterventional sweating test with iodine-oil-starch emulsion can help check whether sympathectomy was successful.[23] Secondary factors are the healing of ulcers, drying of necrosis, and improved dystrophic skin.

Major concerns are related to the performance of the MR-guided procedures. Although the open magnets represent a significant step toward the feasibility of MR-guided interventions, many technologic drawbacks will impede wide clinical acceptance. For example, slice-orientation planning and handling of the sequence software are difficult and time consuming. If the patient accidentally moves on the table or if the needle (150 mm long) moves out of the image plane, the single-slice fluoroscopic study should be changed to three breathhold slices. For display of the needle in accurate alignment, extensive planning is required to find the respective slice orientation. This procedure is inconvenient for the interventionist and requires excellent assistance at the in-room console, which is not usable under sterile conditions. Regrettably, the procedure steps have been increased with the latest software version. Siemens (Erlangen, Germany) is working on an optoelectronic navigation system that will hopefully improve the situation. The system will trace the position of a cannula holder and automatically transfer the coordinates of the instrument to the MR processor. The sequence can then be reloaded, whereby the slice orientation is aligned to the needle.

Another particular drawback is the impossibility to change sequence parameters quickly, i.e., the sympathectomies are performed in approximation to the vena cava, aorta, and ureter. The blood flow can be signal intensive or low intensive. This feature is important to allow differentiation of vascular structures and the injection fluids. It can simply be gathered by using fast imaging with steady-state precession (FISP) 2D or true FISP 2D sequences or three slice FLASH 2D breathhold. Although MR basically allows display of ureter and urinary flow by using RARE or HASTE sequences, this particular feature is not available with the low-field system. Thus, discrimination of the ureter is difficult if the only available sequence is a turbo spin-echo single-shot sequence. Administration of contrast before search of the ureter is also not very helpful and involves additional time and cost.

Major drawbacks are related to the elaborate use of the sequences of the MR unit. Although refinements of the sequence protocols have led to excellent image quality, their use for interventions is more elaborate because of additional safety features. Sequence handling should be specifically designed for interventional MR. During diagnostic MR, the patient is usually not at risk and does not feel pain, whereas during intervention or surgery, the patient can be endangered and is uncomfortable. Use of general anesthesia during MR-guided surgery should be as short as possible. One crucial aspect is that automatic slice orientation will be solved to some extent by opto-electronic navigation. If sequence change and adaptation of sequence parameters (e.g., repetition time, echo time, matrix, field of view) are simplified and fast, interventional MR can show its real advantages and potential.

REFERENCES

1. Rau G: *Sympathektomie, angiologie,* Stuttgart, 1974, Thieme Verlag.
2. Seibel RMM, Balzer K, Grönemeyer DHW: Erfahrungen mit der CT-gesteuerten Sympathikusausschaltung bei der Behandlung der peripheren AVK, *Angio Arch* 17:75, 1989.
3. Ernst S, and others: Komplikationen der CT-gesteuerten lumbalensympathikolyse: Eigene Erfahrungen und literaturübersicht, *Fortschr Rontgenstr* 168:77, 1998.
4. Jaboulay M: Le traitment de quelques troubles trophiques du pied et de la jambe par la denudation de l'artere femorale et la distension des nerfs vasculaires, *Lyon med* 91:467, 1899.
5. Leriche R: De l'elongation et de la section des nerfs perivasculaires dans certains syndromes douloureux d'origine arterielle et dans quelques troubles trophiques, *Lyon chir* 10:378, 1913.
6. Adson AW, Brown GE: Treatment of Raynaud's disease by lumbar ramisection ganglionectomy and perivascular sympathetic neurectomy of the common iliacs, *JAMA* 84:1908, 1925.
7. Swetlow GI: Alcoholic injections into nerve tissue for the relief of pain, *Am J Med Sci* 171:397, 1926.
8. Haxton HA: Chemical sympathectomy, *BMJ* 68:1026, 1949.
9. Bannenberg JJ: Retroperitoneal endoscopic lumbar sympathectomy: laboratory and clinical experience, *End Surg* 3:16, 1995.
10. Melzer A, and others: Methodology, technological prerequisites and preliminary clinical results of interventions in a horizontal open MRI unit, *Proc Soc Magn Reson* 2:897, 1996.
11. Schmidt A, Melzer A, Seibel R: CT-endoskopische Sympathektomie, *Endoskopie heute* 12:84,M101, 1995.
12. Lufkin RB: RF ablation systems in interventional MRI, *High Care 97 S.* IIIA, Bochum, Germany, 1-2.2.1997.
13. Netter FH: *Autonomes Nervensystem, Nervensystem 1: neuroanatomie und Physiologie,* Stuttgart, 1987, Thieme.
14. Rickenbacher J, Landolt AM, Theiler K: *Rücken, Praktische Anatomie,* Berlin, 1982, Springer Verlag.
15. Seibel RMM, and others: *CT guided lumbar sympathetic trunk neurolysis for the treatment of occlusive arterial disease OAD: interventional computed tomography,* Oxford, 1990, Blackwell Scientific.
16. Carstensen G: *Eingriffe am Sympathikus bei peripheren Durchblutungsstörungen, Spezielle Chirurgie für die Praxis,* Stuttgart, 1975, Thieme.
17. Schild H: *Perkutane Neurolyse des lumbalen Sympathikus, Interventionelle Radiologie,* Stuttgart, 1988, Thieme.
18. Lemmens HAJ: *Sympathikus, intra- und postoperative komplikationen,* Berlin, 1983, Springer Verlag.
19. Lee BY, and others: Lumbar sympathectomy for toe gangrene: longterm follow-up, *Am J Surg* 145:398, 1983.
20. Kruse CA: Thirty years experience with predictive lumbar sympathectomy: method for selection of patients, *Am J Surg* 150:232, 1985.
21. Cross FW, Cotton LT: Chemical lumbar sympathectomy for ischemic rest pain: a randomized, prospective controlled clinical trial, *Am J Surg* 150:341, 1985.
22. McCollum PT, and others: Quantitative assessment of the effectiveness of chemical lumbar sympathectomy, *Br J Anaesth* 57:1146, 1985.
23. Wittmoser R: *Thoracoscopic sympathectomy and vagotomy operative manual of endoscopic surgery I,* Berlin, 1992, Springer-Verlag.

Chapter 33

MR–GUIDED BIOPSY IN THE HEAD AND NECK

Alexandra R. Borges, J. Pablo Villablanca, Joel Sercarz, Elliot Abemayor, Dan J. Castro, John G. Curran, Robert B. Lufkin

In addition to the impact that magnetic resonance imaging (MRI) has made in the depiction of head and neck pathology, interventional techniques with imaging guidance are one of the more exciting and rapidly developing areas in the field of radiology. These techniques include fine-needle aspiration (FNA) of deep-seated lesions previously inaccessible to clinical guidance and minimally invasive management modalities.[1,2] The most striking advantages are lower cost and decreased overall morbidity compared with open surgical procedures. High resolution depiction of lesions and accurate needle placement have revolutionized the management of head and neck pathology.

Although ultrasound is the ideal method for FNA guidance in the infrahyoid neck, the suprahyoid neck remains inaccessible for this imaging modality because of the interposition of bony and airway structures. Computed tomography (CT) and MR have therefore become the preferred modalities for interventional procedures of the deep spaces of the suprahyoid neck.[3,4] The rule for deciding which imaging modality to use is to use the imaging method that best depicts the lesion and its surroundings and the one that is safest in each particular clinical setting.

Image-guided FNAs and core biopsies are widely accepted and commonly used procedures that allow diagnosis of clinically inaccessible lesions in an outpatient basis without the need for open surgery.

DESCRIPTION OF CLINICAL PROBLEM

The head and neck consists of small, closely spaced anatomic structures. Intimate knowledge of normal spatial relationships and anatomic variations is required for safe image-guided procedures. Lesions often lie near vital structures, complicating intervention. Improved visualization during a procedure can therefore provide the physician with critical information, facilitating innovative procedures and enhanced outcomes.

Although CT remains ideal for imaging cortical bone, MRI's superior soft-tissue contrast makes it well-suited for spatial localization and for early and accurate detection of instrument placement during interventions. Unlike CT, the high flow sensitivity of MRI permits delineation of blood vessels without the use of contrast agents. Furthermore, the characteristics of MR that make it a powerful clinical diagnostic imaging tool also make it appealing for use in guiding interventional procedures in the head and neck. The ability to perform oblique and multiplanar imaging and the lack of ionizing radiation are particularly valuable. The sensitivity of the ocular lens to ionizing radiation, a problem in CT studies, also makes MRI the more desirable modality. The absence of beam-hardening artifacts from bone allows unobstructed visualization to guide approaches that may be difficult or impossible with other modalities (e.g., conventional CT). In addition, many experts now consider MR to be the best imaging technique for guiding interventional procedures of an interstitial, rather than an endovascular or endoluminal, natute.

For image-guided procedures, MRI has several shortcomings, which are being solved with advanced MR technology. These shortcomings include slow image acquisition, high cost, and suboptimal patient access. However, with faster imaging techniques, image reconstruction is approaching real-time. Faster scans also lead to decreased costs. Early scanner designs limited access to the patient; new MR instruments feature more open design magnets, which greatly improve patient access.

IMAGE-GUIDED ASPIRATION CYTOLOGY

Description

FNA cytology is a diagnostic tool with a high degree of sensitivity and specificity. In one large series, accuracy rates for FNA in the head and neck ranged from 85% to 98%.[1] Even lymphoma patients can be evaluated using flow cytometry on the aspirated cells. The ability to obtain tissue specimens from deep regions using FNA without surgical intervention has had a dramatic impact in the management of various head and neck lesions.[2-4] Although some lesions may be aspirated under direct palpation, many lesions are deep-seated and are recognized only through tomographic imaging. Image-guided aspiration cytology is particularly useful for such nonpalpable deep lesions.[1,2]

MRI is rapidly replacing CT in this area because MRI permits precise needle placement into comparatively inaccessible areas, such as the skull base and submandibular region, where beam-hardening artifacts limit the effectiveness of CT (Fig. 33-1).

A

B

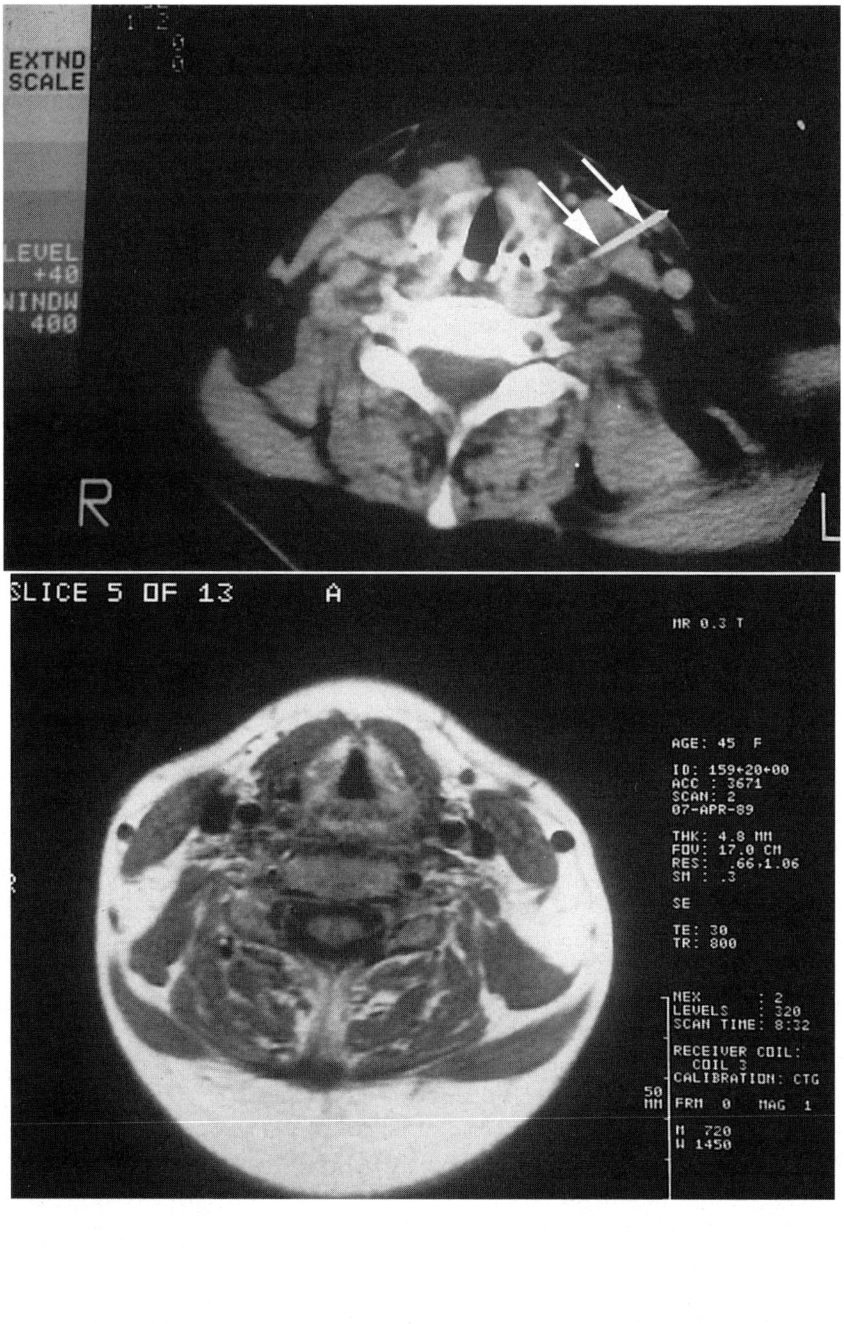

Fig. 33-1. A comparison of computed tomography (CT) and magnetic resonance (MR) axial images from a patient with a suspected neck mass. **A,** CT image from another hospital taken during image-guided needle biopsy. Findings were negative. *Arrows* indicate needle locations. **B,** Follow-up MRI scan reveals normal anatomy. The "mass" was apparently caused by a CT beam-hardening artifact. (From Bittner C, and others: *MR-guided biopsy of the head, neck and brain.* In Jolesz FA, Young IR, editors: *Interventional MR,* London, 1998, Martin Dunitz Ltd.)

Another advantage of MRI over CT is superior tip localization by obtaining an oblique or orthogonal image along the course of the needle without repositioning the patient.[5-13] Finally, the new open MR systems with MR fluoroscopy have greatly simplified these approaches (Fig. 33-2).

Technique

MR-guided FNA or core biopsy begins with a limited scan over the region of interest to precisely localize the lesion and determine the best way to approach it. Usually, the best approach is the one that traverses least important structures, avoids potentially vital structures, and is perpendicular to the scanning plane. After the best course for needle placement is chosen, a marker or the physician's finger is placed on the skin over the region of interest and a single scan is obtained. The distance between the skin and the lesion is measured, as is the angle of the needle when angulation is needed. Patient preparation is identical to that of non–image-guided biopsies and includes informed consent, sterile draping, and local anesthesia. The prebiopsy requirements concerning coagulation parameters are also the same. The procedure can be done free-hand or by using a stereotaxic device.

The needle is introduced into the subcutaneous tissues, and the needle direction is confirmed. If appropriately directed to the lesion, the needle is advanced into the lesion, and scanning is performed to confirm its position. The use of coaxial systems allows multiple samples of different areas of the lesion from a single skin entry site.

During the procedure, commercially available high nickel content needles are used with a coaxial needle system.[6] The system uses a 26-gauge needle of variable length and curvature, which fits through the lumen of a 22-gauge needle. The larger needle is placed into the lesion, and multiple samples are obtained with the smaller needle. This system is especially useful

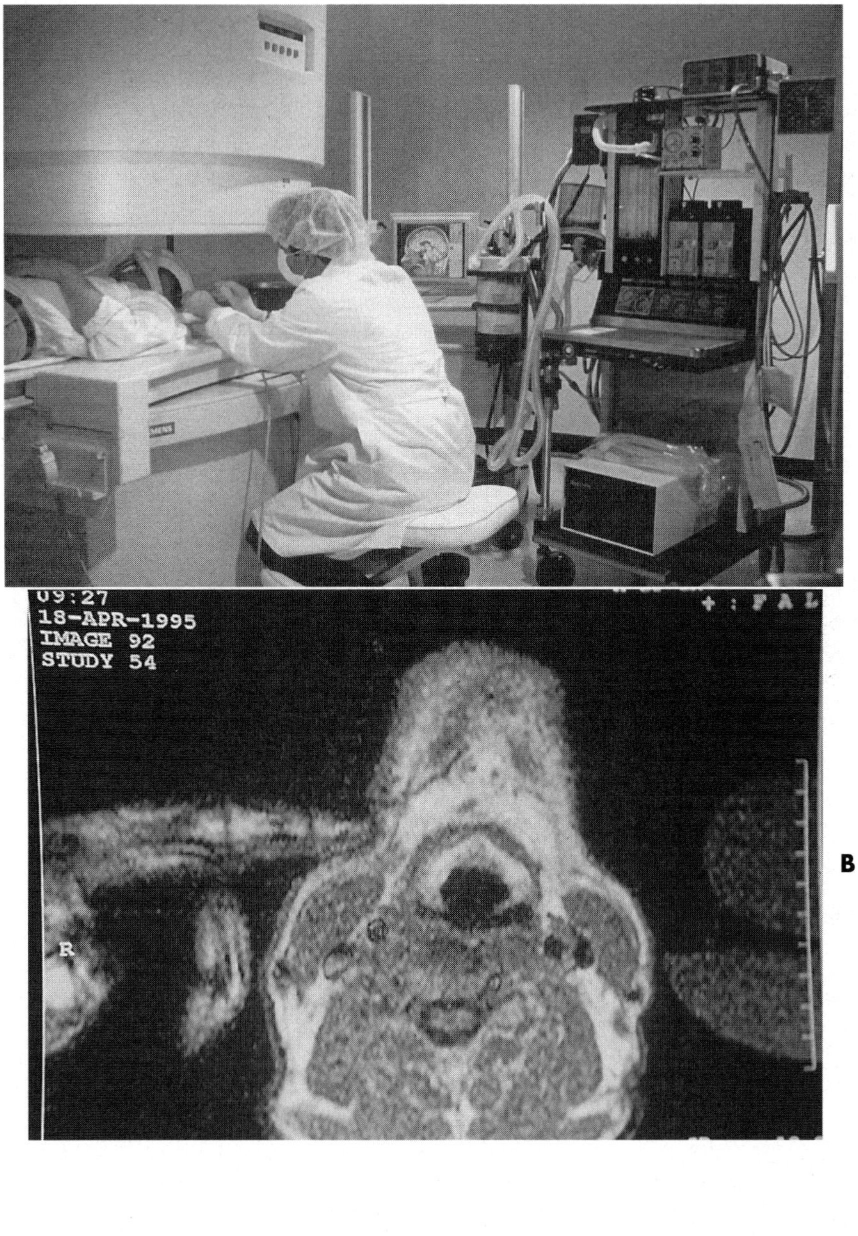

A

B

Fig. 33-2. An open design scanner. **A,** An example of improved patient access with an open design system (Siemens 0.2T Open MR system, Erlangen, Germany). **B,** The position of a lesion can be easily localized with such a system. (**A** from Lufkin RB, Gronemeyer DHW, Seibel RMM: *Interventional magnetic resonance imaging.* In Stark DD, Bradley WG, editors: *Magnetic resonance imaging,* ed 3, St Louis, 1999, Mosby. **B** from Bittner C, and others: *MR-guided biopsy of the head, neck and brain.* In Jolesz FA, Young IR, editors: *Interventional MR,* London, 1998, Martin Dunitz Ltd.)

in the head and neck, where even a small amount of tissue trauma to surrounding neural and vascular structures may be deleterious.

SPECIFIC APPROACHES

The following specific approaches have proven useful for aspiration cytology of head and neck lesions:

Subzygomatic or infratemporal

A subzygomatic or infratemporal approach is valuable for parapharyngeal and infratemporal fossa lesions. The patient's mouth is held open, using a bite block if necessary, and the temporomandibular joint is palpated along the inferior border of the zygoma. The coronoid process can be felt anteriorly. The zygoma, coronoid process, and mandibular condyle form a triangular space through which the needle can be inserted (Fig. 33-3).

Retromandibular

The retromandibular approach is used for parapharyngeal, parotid, and masticator space lesions. The angle of the mandible is palpated, and the needle placed posterior to the angle. For the major proximal branches of the facial nerve beyond the stylomastoid foramen to be avoided, the needle should not be placed higher than 1 cm below the inferior of the tragus. The carotid artery should be palpated below the angle of the mandible and controlled during needle placement (Fig. 33-4).

Submastoid

The submastoid approach is useful for lesions of the skull base. The needle should be placed approximately 1 cm below the mastoid tip, along the anterior aspect of the sternocleidomastoid muscle. Again, the carotid artery should be palpated below the angle of the mandible and controlled during needle placement.

Direct

A direct approach is used for superficial lesions, such as those in the thyroid or parotid glands. It is important to avoid the airway and major vascular structures when approaching these lesions. Other less common paths include the infraorbital canal to reach the infraorbital nerve, the anterior subzygomatic approach to reach anterior lesions, and the transnasal approach for deep nasal cavity lesions (Fig. 33-5).

ERRORS AND MISINTERPRETATIONS

Most errors of image-guided procedures relate to inadequate identification of the lesion or selection of a suboptimal approach. The most important step of image-guided FNA is identification of the lesion. A true lesion may be absent, rather an artifact, a normal variant, or a pseudolesion may be present. Examples of possible artifacts in the head and neck region include beam-hardening artifacts from bone (see Fig. 33-1), dental amalgams, or shoulder girdle. With MR, pulsation artifacts, chemical shift artifacts, and metallic susceptibility artifacts may mimic focal lesions. Masseter muscle hypertrophy, accessory parotid tissue, aberrant carotid artery, prominent and tortuous jugular vein, and muscle asymmetries caused by denervation atrophy are the most common normal variants and pseudolesions confused for pathology. Review of the scans and a limited imaging study to confirm the presence of a lesion in doubtful cases should always be performed before the procedure.

Selection of a suboptimal approach to a lesion is associated with more complications and frequently leads to an inadequate sample. Complications of image-guided FNAs are the same for

A

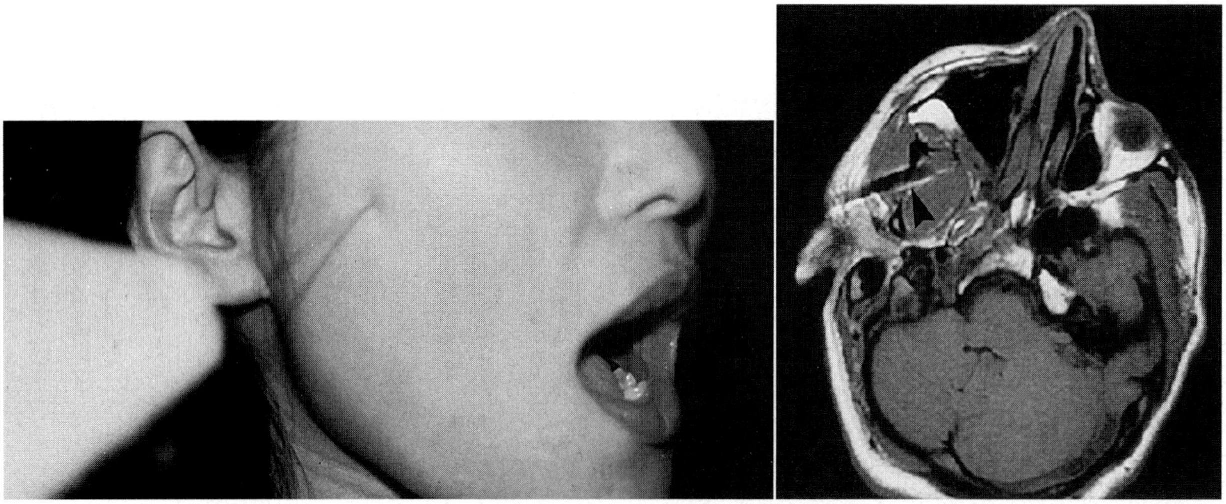

B

Fig. 33-3. In the subzygomatic approach, **A,** The needle is placed between the coronoid and condyle on the open mouth view. **B,** A magnetic resonance image was obtained during biopsy using this approach (*arrowhead* indicates needle position). The patient had a history of treated juvenile angiofibroma. Biopsy was performed to rule out recurrence. The cytology sample was negative. (From Bittner C, and others: *MR-guided biopsy of the head, neck and brain.* In Jolesz FA, Young IR, editors: *Interventional MR,* London, 1998, Martin Dunitz Ltd.)

A

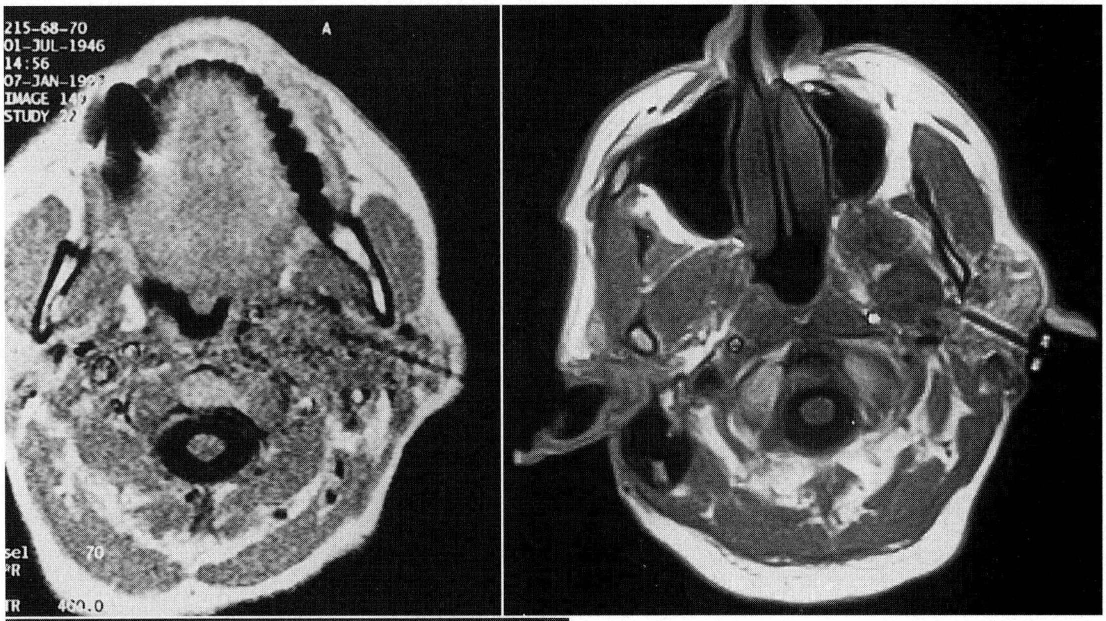

B

C

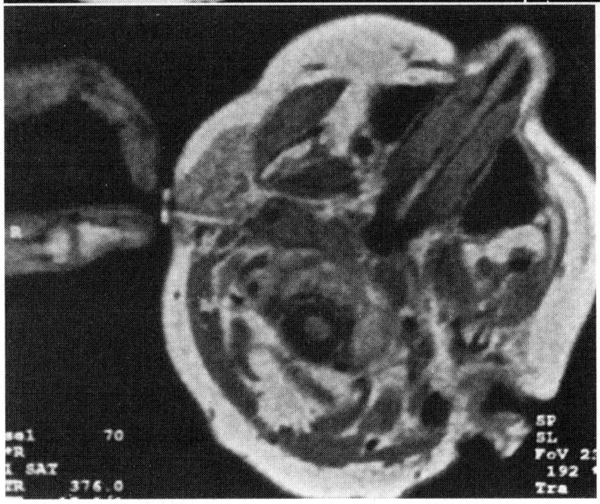

Fig. 33-4. The retromandibular approach was used to diagnose glomus jugulare in **A,** a patient with a poststyloid parapharyngeal space mass. **B,** The needle in a prestyloid parapharyngeal space mass shows pleomorphic adenoma. **C,** The needle is placed in a metastatic squamous cell carcinoma surrounding the carotid artery.

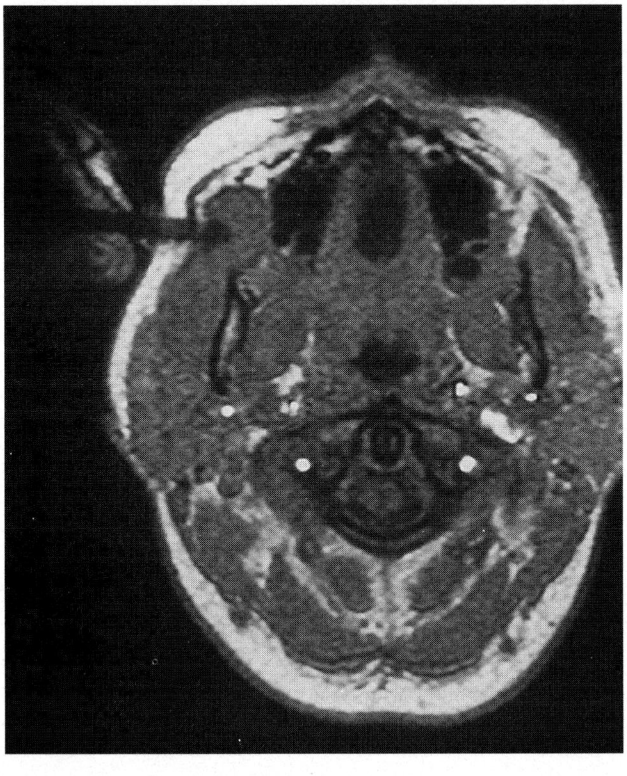

Fig. 33-5. A direct anterior subzygomatic approach to an anterior soft tissue mass was used to diagnose hemangioma.

non–image-guided procedures and include infection, hemorrhage, and rarely nerve damage.

SUMMARY

MR-guided biopsy of the head and neck is an accepted and safe clinical tool and should be considered as the imaging tool of choice in patients with nonpalpable or clinically inaccessible lesions.

REFERENCES

1. Abemayor E, and others: CT-directed aspiration biopsies of masses in the head and neck, *Laryngoscope 95*, 1985.
2. Duckwiler G, and others: Head and neck lesions: MR-guided aspiration biopsy, *Radiology* 170, 1989.
3. Frable M, Frable W: Fine needle aspiration biopsy revisited, *Laryngoscope* 92, 1982.
4. Frable W, Frable M: Thin needle aspiration biopsy in the diagnosis of head and neck tumors, *Laryngoscope* 85, 1974.
5. Lufkin R, and others: Technical note: MR body stereotaxis. An aid for MR guided biopsies, *J Comput Assist Tomogr* 12:6, 1988.
6. Lufkin R, Layfield L: Coaxial needle system for MR and CT guided aspiration cytology, *J Comput Assist Tomogr* 13:6, 1989.
7. Lufkin R, and others: A technique for MR guided needle placement in the head and neck, *Am J Roentgenol* 151, 1988.
8. Lufkin R, Teresi L, Hanafee W: New needle for MR-guided aspiration cytology of the head and neck, *Am J Roentgenol* 149:2, 1987.
9. Mueller PR, and others: MR-guided aspiration biopsy: needle design and clinical trials, *Radiology* 161, 1986.
10. Sinha S, and others: Technical note: pulse sequence optimization for use with a biopsy needle in MRI, *Magn Reson Imaging* 7:5, 1989.
11. To S, Lufkin R, Chiu L: MR compatible winged infusion set, *Comput Med Imaging Graph* 13:6, 1989.
12. Trapp T, and others: MR guided aspiration cytology of the head and neck, *Laryngoscope 99*, 1989.
13. Wenokur R, and others: Magnetic resonance imaging-guided fine needle aspiration for the diagnosis of skull base lesions, *Skull Base Surgery* 2:3, 1992.

Chapter 34

INTERSTITIAL LASER THERAPY OF HEAD AND NECK LESIONS

Martin G. Mack, Thomas J. Vogl

Interstitial laser-induced thermotherapy (LITT) is a recently developed, minimally invasive technique for local tumor destruction in solid organs.

Low-power laser, with delivery of light energy through thin optical fibers, results in a well-defined area of coagulative necrosis. Thus, laser can destroy tumor by direct heating, while greatly limiting damage to surrounding structures.[1–6] Experimental work has shown that a well-defined area of coagulative necrosis is obtained around the fiber tip, with minimal damage to surrounding structures.

The head and neck area includes many small and complex anatomic structures; intimate knowledge of normal spatial relationships and variations is necessary to plan and implement appropriate therapy. Lesions often lie near vital structures, complicating diagnostic and therapeutic procedures. Improved visualization during such procedures can therefore provide the physician with critical information, permitting innovative procedures and improved outcomes.[7–9]

Palliative treatment options for recurrent head and neck cancer are limited by the proximity of vital vascular and neural structures and the aggressive nature of these tumors.

MATERIAL AND METHODS

Laser system and application set

Laser coagulation was performed using a neodymium: yttrium-aluminum-garnet laser (MediLas 5060 and 5100 Germering, Germany; Martin MY 30, Hüttinger Medrzintechnik, Umkirch, Germany) with a specially developed scattering light emitter. Furthermore, an application kit for percutaneous management was developed and optimized.

Laser light with a wavelength of 1046 nm was transmitted to tissue with a diffusing applicator. Laser light of this wavelength penetrates relatively deep into biologic tissue, where photon absorption and heat conduction lead to coagulative and hyperthermic effects. Tissue destruction may be immediate or delayed.

The laser application kit (SOMATEX, Berlin, Germany) consists of a cannulation needle with a tetragonally sharpened tip and guidewire; a sheath system with mandrin (15 cm, 7 F); and a special protective catheter (43 cm, 4 F), which is closed at the distal end. The protective catheter prevents direct contact of the laser applicator with the patient and enables complete removal of the applicator even in the unlikely event of its damage. This device increases patient safety and simplifies the procedure. The catheter is transparent for laser radiation and is heat resistant (up to 400° C). Marks on the sheath and the protective catheter allow exact positioning of both in the lesion.

The system is fully compatible with magnetic resonance imaging (MRI) systems. Magnetite markers on the laser applicator allow easier visualization and positioning.[10] For two applications, a power laser system[11] was used to increase the volume of coagulative necrosis. This application system was developed using a scattering laser applicator introduced into a double-tube protective catheter, which can be cooled by internal flushing with physiologic saline. The glass outer diameter of the diffusing tip applicator (active length, 25 mm) was 0.9 mm to achieve appropriate flushing rates. With this system, the power of the laser could be increased up to 25 W.

The laser is installed outside of the examination unit. The light is transmitted via a 10-m long optical fiber. The complete set-up used for LITT is shown in Figure 34-1.

Procedure monitoring and computer simulation

On-line monitoring of actual temperature distribution is critical in LITT. First, a computer simulation is used to calculate the parameters for laser management (e.g., energy, total application time). The tissue damage can be calculated numerically from the Arrhenius formula, which describes the process of coagulation as:

$$\Omega(T,t) = A\int_{t_1}^{t_f} \exp\left(-\frac{E}{RT(t)}\right)dt$$

where A and E are constants, depending on the specific tissue; R is the universal gas constant (8.31 $Jmol^{-1}$ K^{-1}); and T is the absolute temperature (K) at time t. The integration starts at tr (start of laser radiation) and finishes at t_f (time when temperature equalization takes place after exposure). In the simulation, the integral was solved numerically for each volume element. The damage integral describes the probability for protein denaturation, whereby 1 corresponds to a degree of denaturation of 63%. A value of 0.53 was used for irreversible tissue damage, corresponding to a change of the optical properties from the native to the coagulated values. For the constants A and E, only a few experimentally derived values are available (e.g., A $= 9.4 \times 10^{104}$ sec^{-1}; $E = 6.68 \times 10^5$ $Jmol^{-1}$).

Technique of magnetic resonance–guided laser-induced thermotherapy

All patients undergo computed tomography (CT) and a contrast-enhanced MRI study at least 2 days before LITT; informed consent is obtained from the patient. Immediately before the procedure, patients receive diazepam (if necessary) and meperidine (50 to 100 mg) intravenously. After localization of the tumor with CT, 20 ml of 1% lidocaine is infiltrated. The distance to the lesion and the puncture angle are calculated electronically. For recurrent nasopharyngeal malignant tumors and pleomorphic adenomas, a subzygomatic approach provides optimum access to the lesion. Lesions of the larynx and the floor of the mouth are punctured directly. A 7-F catheter is inserted via a percutaneous approach under CT guidance. A special thermostable plastic catheter is thereafter introduced. In a third step, a software program calculates the parameters for the laser management (e.g., energy, total application time). After the patient is positioned at the MR table, the laser catheter is inserted into the guiding catheter. After the procedure, the cannulation canal is closed with fibrin glue (Tissucol, Immuno GmbH, Heidelberg, Germany).

Magnetic resonance thermometry

MR thermometry is performed via a turbo fast low-angle shot (FLASH) sequence (repetition time, 7 msec; echo time,

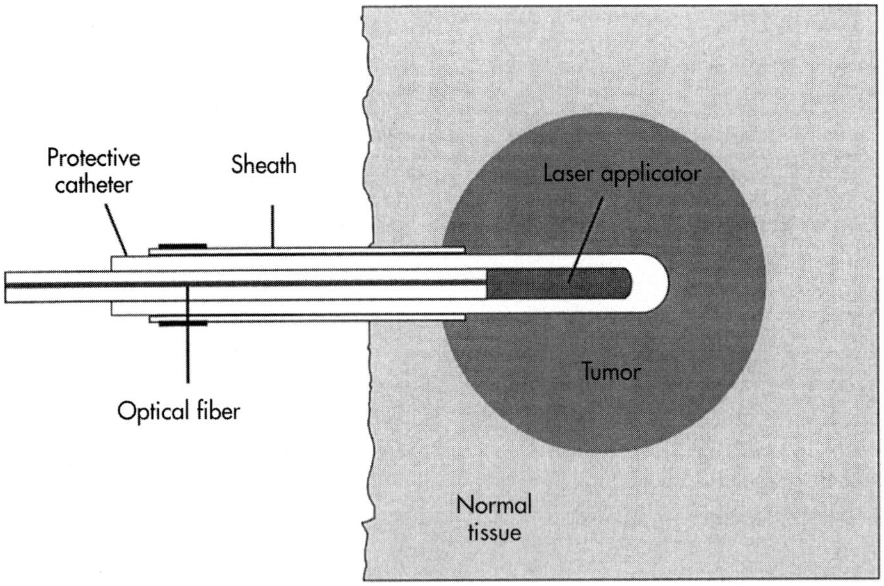

Fig. 34-1. The set-up for laser-induced thermotherapy. (From Mach MG, Vogl TJ: *Interstitial laser therapy of head and neck lesions.* In Debatin JF, Adam G, editors: *Interventional magnetic resonance imaging,* Heidelberg, 1998, Springer-Verlag.)

3 msec; inversion time, 400 msec) and a thermo FLASH two-dimensional (2D) sequence (repetition time, 102 msec; echo time, 8 msec; flip angle, 5°), which is more sensitive for the detection of thermal-induced changes in signal and morphology.[1–3,12–16]

Before and after LITT, T1-weighted spin-echo, gradient echo and T2-weighted spin-echo images are obtained on the 1.5-T magnet. Of special importance is a dynamic turbo FLASH sequence protocol, which is started before contrast and with a short delay (6 sec) after contrast over 180 sec. Nonenhanced and contrast-enhanced imaging studies are also performed 1 wk, 3 months, and 6 months after therapy. Qualitative and quantitative parameters are evaluated, including size, morphology, and contrast enhancement pattern, at early and late follow-up.

PATIENT MATERIAL

Fourteen patients (mean age, 64.2 years) with recurrent head and neck tumors were managed using MR-controlled LITT. Sixteen lesions were treated with 24 laser applications. Two laser applications were performed using the power laser application system described. All patients had primary head and neck tumors (histologically undifferentiated squamous cell carcinoma, $n = 12$; pleomorphic adenoma, $n = 2$). The primary management modalities were surgical resection, postoperative radiation, radiochemotherapy, or a combination of these techniques. Clinical examinations and MRI follow-up provided evidence for tumor recurrence 1 to 16 months after primary therapy. Nine patients presented with clinical signs of tumor recurrence, such as malfunction of the eustachian tube ($n = 6$), pain ($n = 7$), dysphagia ($n = 7$), hoarseness ($n = 3$), and symptoms of intracranial nerve involvement (e.g., diplopia).

RESULTS

In vitro magnetic resonance thermometry

An *in vitro* study using muscle tissue showed reproducible loss of signal intensity corresponding to increasing tissue temperatures. Using an energy of 5 W and an application time of 12 min, the maximum diameter of the region with signal loss was 25 mm. This effect was best monitored using the thermo-turbo FLASH sequence at inversion times of 300 to 400 msec, providing a nearly linear inverse correlation between signal intensity and temperature. By comparison, this correlation was somewhat less linear using the FLASH 2D sequence; which, however, provided higher spatial resolution and clearer delineation of topographic structures.

Laser-induced thermotherapy and *in vivo* magnetic resonance thermometry

Under CT guidance, optimal positioning of the cannula and mandrin was achieved in all patients. All tolerated the puncture well with a moderate amount of systemic analgetics and local infiltrative anesthesia. After the protective catheter was positioned and the laser tip inserted, the energy of the laser and the duration of the management were calculated individually, depending on the position of the laser tip in relation to the tumor borders, the homogeneity of the tumor, and its relationship to neighboring vascular structures, in particular the internal carotid artery and major branches of the external carotid artery, including the maxillary, lingual, and ascending pharyngeal arteries. The results of *in vivo* MR thermometry were similar to *in vitro* results, regardless of the location of the recurrent tumor. Preinterventional scans were optimized individually to show the tumor as tissue having signal intensity lower than that of fat and higher than that of muscle tissue. For each patient, these images were used as baseline for visualizing changes in signal loss during LITT.

MR thermometry enabled on-line display of hyperthermic effects, seen in all patients as an area with progressively decreasing signal intensity surrounding the laser-emitter tip. This feature enabled accurate monitoring of the progress of LITT and abortion of the laser procedure if vital structures were threatened by coagulative necrosis. In this regard, the most important feature of MR thermometry using the thermo-turbo FLASH and FLASH 2D sequences for tumors of these types was the possibility to monitor the perfusion of the internal carotid artery by analyzing the high signal intensity of this vessel.

The regions of necrosis were defined as areas with increased signal intensity on T2-weighted images, low signal intensity on T1-weighted noncontrast images, and lack of contrast enhancement on T1-weighted contrast-enhanced images.

In vivo study

In a prospective study, 14 patients underwent LITT of the head and neck under MRI guidance using an interventional subzygomatic approach for recurrent tumors of the nasopharynx and parapharyngeal space. Lesions of the floor of the mouth and the larynx were directly punctured. Pretherapeutic MR scans revealed tumor recurrence in all patients. All patients had surgery or chemotherapy before LITT intervention.

Thirteen patients tolerated the procedure well. The mean laser power for the standard applications was 5.1 W and for the power laser applications 23.2 W. One patient with a recurrent squamous cell carcinoma and infiltration of the sublingual gland developed pain 5 min after starting the laser with 5.3 W; the laser treatment was stopped before delivering the full dose. No long-term side effects related to treatment were observed. The follow-up MR study 2 years and 9 months after treatment in one patient with a pleomorphic adenoma showed no recurrent tumor.

MR thermometry enabled on-line display of the hyperthermic effects, seen as progressively decreased signal from the tissue surrounding tumor (Fig. 34-2). The criteria for evaluating success of management included clinical data, such as pain or other local symptoms, and pre- and posttherapeutic changes in signal and tumor morphology. Coagulative necrosis was induced in all patients (Figs. 34-3 and 34-4).

DISCUSSION

Palliative management options for recurrent head and neck cancer are limited by the proximity of vital vascular and neural

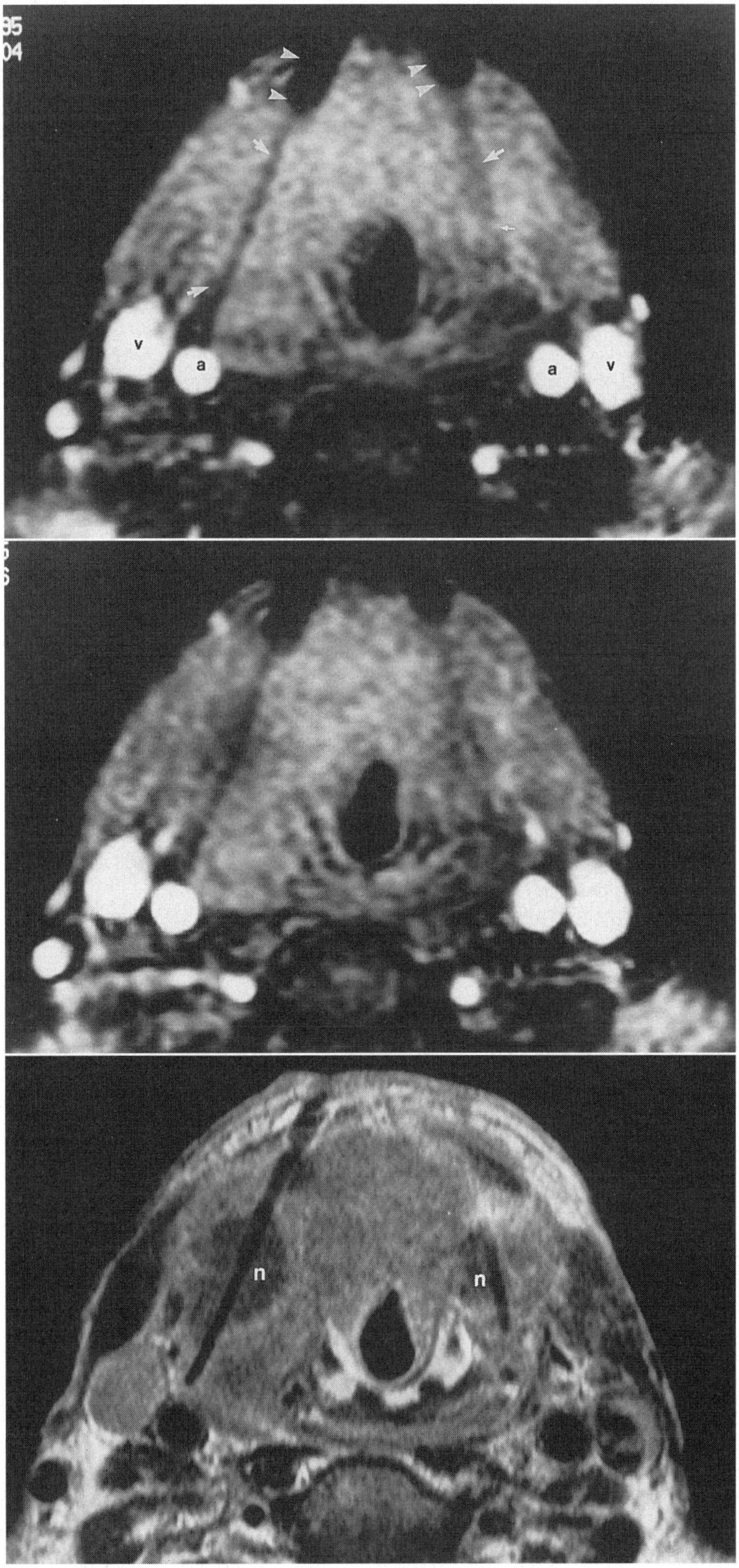

A

B

C

Fig. 34-2. Recurrent squamous cell carcinoma of the larynx after laryngectomy. **A,** Magnetic resonance (MR) turbo fast low-angle shot (FLASH) image shows the positioned laser applicators with the magnetite markers *(arrowheads)* in the lesions and the active zone *(between arrows)*. Note the flow signal in the carotid artery *(2)* and jugular vein *(v)*. **B,** MR turbo FLASH image 6 min after starting the laser shows the area of signal decrease around the active laser zone, representing obtained coagulative necrosis caused by the increase in tissue temperature and T1 relaxation time. **C,** T1-weighted image immediately after laser management shows the induced coagulative necrosis *(n)*.

A

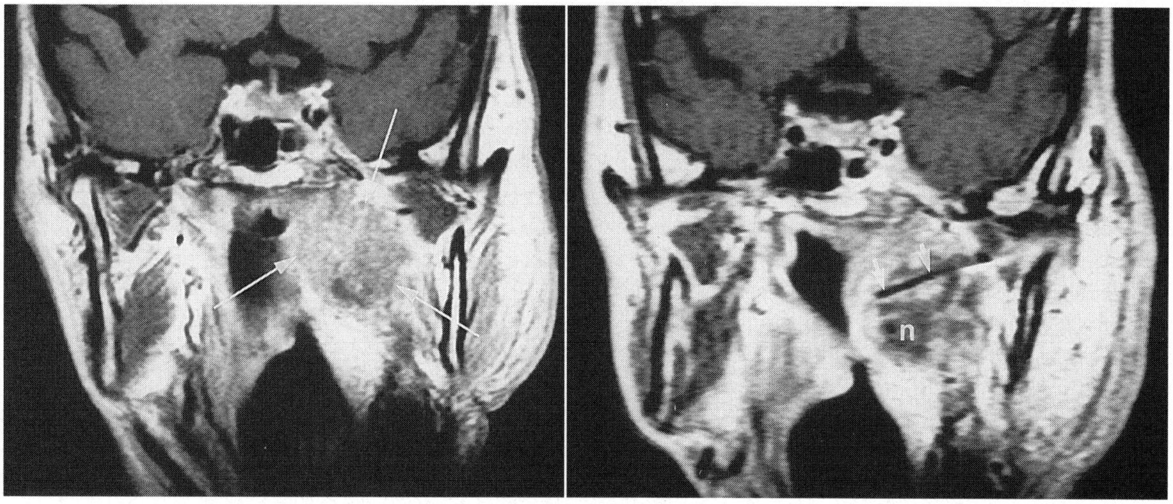

B

Fig. 34-3. Recurrent nasopharyngeal carcinoma 1 year after radiotherapy (70 Gy) is seen with T1-weighted spin-echo sequence in coronal slice orientation (repetition time, 700 msec; echo time 14 msec) before and after laser-induced thermotherapy (LITT). **A,** Preinterventional T1-weighted image (repetition time, 700 msec; echo time 15 msec) in coronal slice orientation shows the recurrent nasopharyngeal carcinoma *(arrows)* as a homogenous mass with skull base and parapharyngeal space involvement. **B,** Contrast-enhanced T1-weighted sequence after LITT (15 min, 4.5 W) shows a significant amount of necrosis *(n)* in the middle and inferior compartments of the tumor. Note the active zone *(arrows)* of the laser applicator.

A

B

C

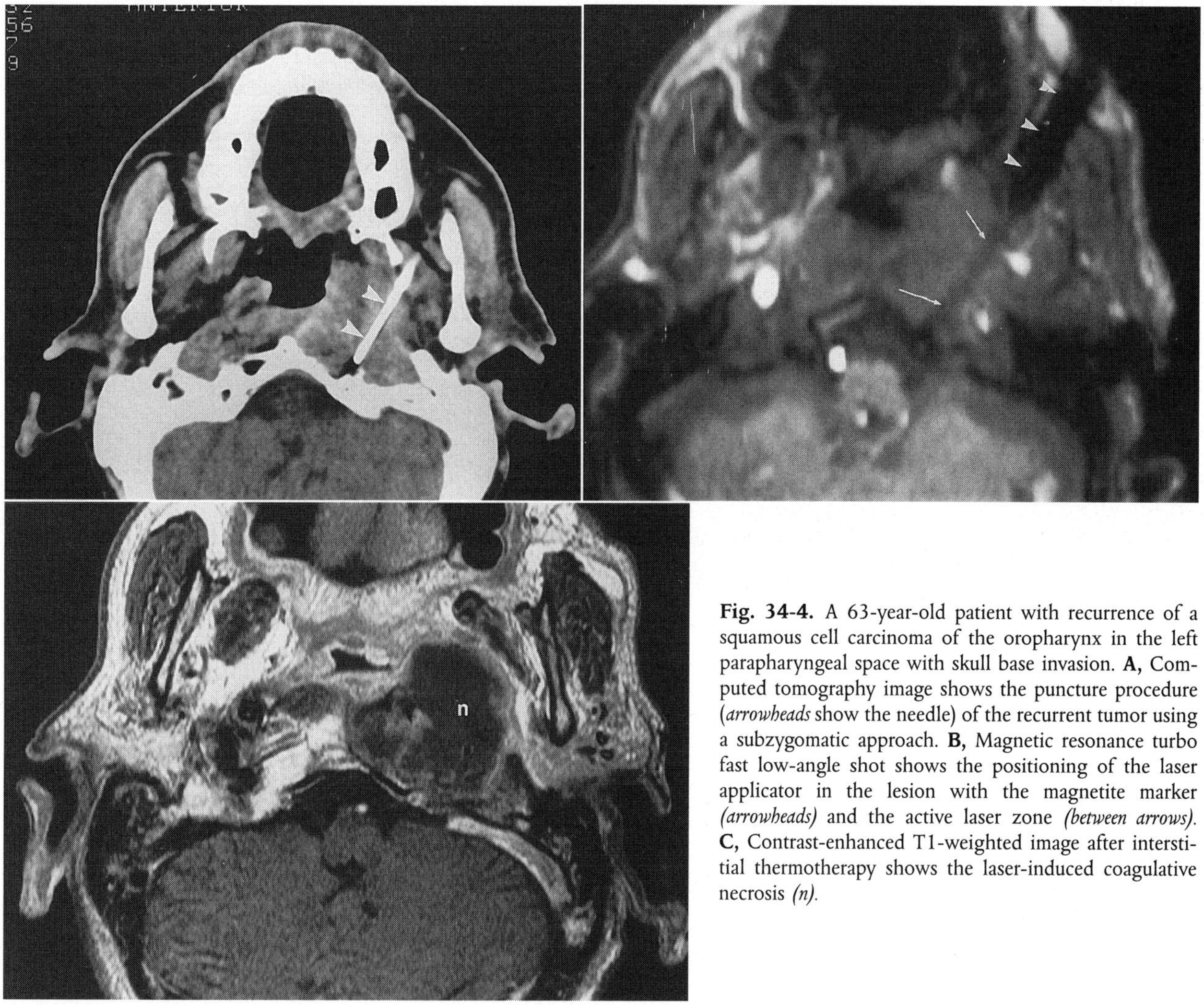

Fig. 34-4. A 63-year-old patient with recurrence of a squamous cell carcinoma of the oropharynx in the left parapharyngeal space with skull base invasion. **A,** Computed tomography image shows the puncture procedure (*arrowheads* show the needle) of the recurrent tumor using a subzygomatic approach. **B,** Magnetic resonance turbo fast low-angle shot shows the positioning of the laser applicator in the lesion with the magnetite marker *(arrowheads)* and the active laser zone *(between arrows).* **C,** Contrast-enhanced T1-weighted image after interstitial thermotherapy shows the laser-induced coagulative necrosis *(n).*

structures and the aggressive nature of these tumors. A minimally invasive management modality, such as interventional MR-guided laser-induced thermotherapy, offers several potential management benefits.

First, MRI provides unparalleled topographic accuracy because of its excellent soft-tissue contrast and high spatial resolution. Second, the temperature sensitivity of the thermo-turbo FLASH and FLASH 2D sequences can be used to monitor the temperature elevation in the tumor and surrounding healthy tissues, thus increasing safety. On-line MRI during LITT therefore allows early detection of local complications and management effects, such as bleeding, hemorrhage, or necrosis. Third, recovery times, lengths of hospital stay, and the risk of infection and other complications can be reduced compared with conventional palliative surgery. Finally, successful implementation of such minimally invasive procedures would significantly reduce costs in comparison with surgical procedures. A further, indirect advantage is the psychological effect caused by avoidance of cosmetic deformities that can result from major reconstructive surgery.

Although few interventions have been performed, several interesting results have occurred: treatment induced a great amount of necrosis. No clinically relevant anesthetic problems occurred; in all patients, diazepam (10 to 15 mg) and meperidine (50 to 100 mg) and local anesthetic infiltration were sufficient.

The major limitation of these data is that all patients had previously treated lesions, so information as to how primary tumors of the head and neck might respond to LITT cannot be provided.

The results should be discussed in the context of possible complications arising from this special form of therapy. The risk of bleeding is rather low because of the protective effect of the laser and closure of the puncture channel after therapy with Tissucol R fibrin glue. A major risk is the possibility of arterial injury during LITT. MR monitoring of the flow in the major branches of the external and internal carotid artery can prevent such injury by allowing abortion of the procedure when the area of necrosis approached the vessels. Another important complication could be perforation of the mucosa with subsequent fistulation, inflammatory infiltration, and edema. Under appropriate monitoring conditions with MRI, such complications can occur at a very low rate. However, no clinical relevant complication was observed.

CONCLUSIONS

MR-guided LITT allows accurate on-line thermometry during the interventional procedure. Dynamic gadolinium-enhanced MRI is suitable for early and late follow-up studies for lesions managed with LITT. Follow-up studies indicate that the laser-induced effects lead to reliable palliation in recurrent head and neck tumors.

REFERENCES

1. Batnar R, and others: Absolute temperature quantification in near real-time with an open 0.5 Tesla interventional MR-scanner, *Proc Int Soc Magn Reson Med* 3:1957, 1997.
2. Bleier AR, and others: Real-time magnetic resonance imaging of laser heat deposition in tissue, *Magn Reson Med* 21:132, 1991.
3. Delannoy J, and others: Noninvasive temperature imaging using diffusion MRI, *Magn Reson Med* 19:333, 1991.
4. Dickinson RJ, and others: Measurement of changes in tissue temperature using MR imaging, *J Comput Assist Tomogr* 10:468, 1986.
5. Jolesz FA, and others: MR imaging of laser-tissue interactions, *Radiology* 168:249, 1988.
6. Vogl TJ, and others: In-vitro evaluation of MR-thermometry for laser-induced thermotherapy, *Fortschr Röntgenstr* 167:638, 1997.
7. Vogl TJ, and others: Recurrent nasopharyngeal tumors: preliminary clinical results with interventional MR imaging–controlled laser-induced thermotherapy, *Radiology* 196:725, 1995.
8. Castro DJ, and others: Metastatic head and neck malignancy treated using MRI guided interstitial laser phototherapy: an initial case report, *Laryngoscope* 102:26, 1992.
9. Castro DJ, Saxton RE, Lufkin RB: Interstitial photoablative laser therapy guided by magnetic resonance imaging for the treatment of deep tumors, *Semin Surg Oncol* 8:233, 1992.
10. Mack MG, and others: Design of a percutaneous application set for MR-controlled laser induced thermotherapy, *ISMRM Abstracts* 1951, 1997.
11. Vogl TJ, and others: Internally cooled laser applicator system for MR-guided laser induced thermotherapy, *Radiology* 205:177, 1997.
12. Castren Persons M, and others: Laser-induced hyperthermia: comparison of two different methods, *Lasers Surg Med* 12:665, 1992.
13. Castro DJ, and others: Interstitial laser phototherapy assisted by magnetic resonance imaging: a new technique for monitoring laser-tissue interaction, *Laryngoscope* 100:541, 1990.
14. Cline HE, and others: MR temperature mapping of focused ultrasound surgery, *Magn Reson Med* 31:628, 1994.
15. Matsumoto R, Oshio K, Jolesz FA: Monitoring of laser and freezing-induced ablation in the liver with T1-weighted MR imaging, *J Magn Reson Imaging* 2:555, 1992.
16. Panych LP, and others: Effects related to temperature changes during MR imaging, *J Magn Reson Imaging* 2:69, 1992.

Chapter 35

MR–GUIDED BREAST BIOPSY

Mitchell D. Schnall

Magnetic resonance imaging (MRI) of the breast represents a promising modality for the detection and diagnosis of breast cancer.[1–3] The most exciting aspect of breast MRI is its potential to show cancer occult to traditional mammographic imaging and clinical examination. MRI has great potential in the detection of occult multifocal disease in patients with breast cancer and in screening patients at extremely high risk for breast cancer.[3–5]

Although the presence of contrast enhancement on a breast MRI examination is extremely sensitive for breast cancer, it is not specific. The finding of contrast enhancement alone is approximately 40% specific for breast cancer.[3] Intense research has focused on improving the specificity of breast MRI through the use of enhancement kinetics and architectural features.[1,2,6,7] This intense research has led to significant improvement in the specificity of breast MRI to approximately 70%. Although the improved specificity from improved interpretation criteria is important, it is not sufficient to obviate the need for pathologic diagnosis of MR-detected lesions through biopsy.

Abnormalities that are detected primarily on MRI may be visualized by more traditional imaging modalities (ultrasound, mammography) in retrospect. If so, more traditional modalities can easily be used to guide biopsy. Confirming that a finding on the more traditional imaging modality and the finding on MRI represent the same structure is imperative. However, in many cases, lesions detected initially with MRI cannot be detected with other imaging modalities even in retrospect. Therefore, breast biopsy should be guided directly through MRI. At a recent meeting of the Federal Multi-Agency Consortium on Imaging Technologies to Improve Women's Health on May 1, 1997, the lack of MR-guided biopsy was cited as the major technical barrier to the clinical dissemination of breast MRI.

DESIGN CONSIDERATIONS FOR MAGNETIC RESONANCE IMAGING–GUIDED BIOPSY

Several major design issues should be considered when planning a system for MR-guided breast biopsy. Most successful breast MRI is performed at high magnetic field strength. Therefore, biopsies will typically be performed in high-field superconducting magnets. Patients should be removed from the magnet for needle placement. Access to the breast should be made available when the patient is withdrawn from the magnet. Most prototype breast imaging and biopsy systems maintain the patient in the prone position.[8–10] The patient lies on a platform elevated off of the scanner table while the breast extends away from the patient's chest below the support platform. Maintaining an open architecture to the space below the patient platform allows access to the breast for needle placement. An alternative approach would be to image the patient supine, maintaining access to the breast through an anterior approach.[11]

A second major design issue for MR-guided breast biopsy is stabilization. The breast should be stabilized so a needle can be passed into the breast without causing major perturbations of the existing anatomy. The traditional way to stabilize a breast for needle placement remains compression (Figs. 35-1 and 35-2). With the patient lying prone on the MRI platform and the breast extending below the imaging platform, the breast can be easily compressed in the craniocaudal, mediolateral, or other oblique views to allow for needle placement. The most obvious configuration is to compress the breast mediolaterally, allowing

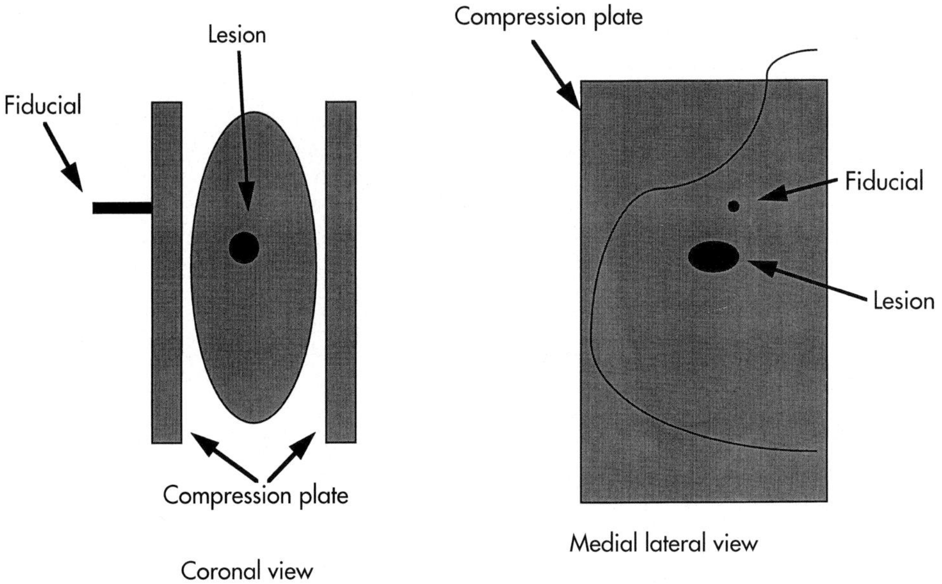

Fig. 35-1. Coronal and mediolateral views of a breast under compression prepared for biopsy. A fiducial is placed on one of the imaging plates. The mediolateral projection of the fiducial onto the imaging slice that contains the lesion provides the information for calculating the appropriate position for needle placement.

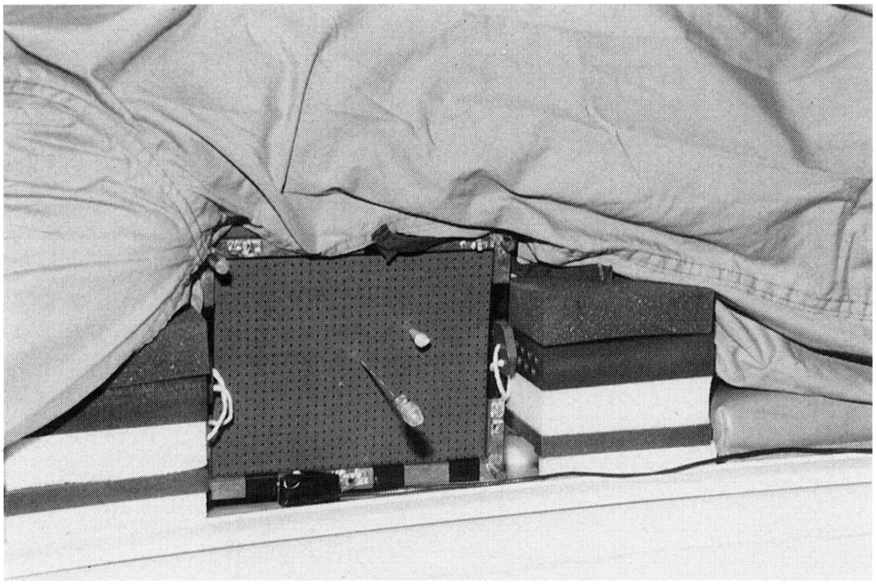

Fig. 35-2. A lateral compression plate shows a fiducial and a needle placed in the grid holes.

easy access to the breast from the medial or lateral approach. There have been reports of compressing the breast against the chest wall with the patient lying supine as a means of stabilizing the breast and gaining access during needle placement.[11] Although this approach is successful, the risk of puncturing the chest wall is greater.

A third major consideration in designing an MR-guided breast biopsy is needle guidance. For the needle to be appropriately guided into the desired location in the breast, it is necessary to relate the position of the needle to the coordinate system of the MRI. This placement is typically accomplished by fiducial markers on the compression plate through which the needle is placed. The location of the fiducial markers can be seen in the MRI scan and on the plate (see Fig. 35-1). Thus, the location of the lesion in the plane parallel to the compressing plate can be established by measuring the lesion location relative to the fiducials. This measurement will provide the distances that the needle is offset from the fiducial when placing it into the breast. The depth of the needle can then be calculated by measuring the distance from the plate to the plane that con-

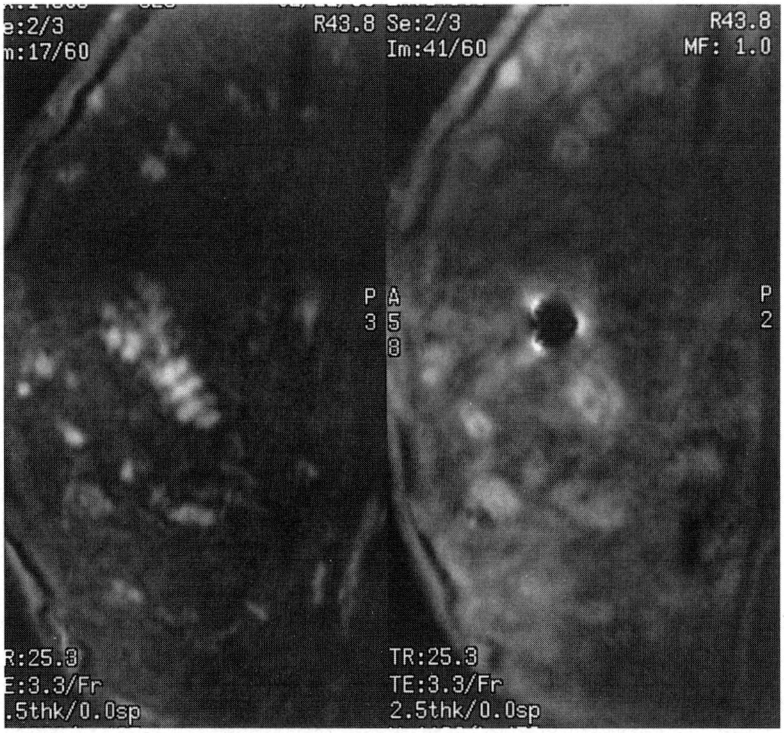

Fig. 35-3. Left, Sagittal slice from a postcontrast three-dimensional examination of the breast shows an enhancing lesion. **Right,** The black susceptibility artifact from the needle depicts the needle passing through a portion of the enhancing lesion.

tains the lesion in the direction perpendicular to the plate. For the needle to be passed into the breast, an opening in the compression plate is necessary. A large single opening in the compression plate can provide access to the breast. The needle may be guided by hand into the correct position or by an external needle guide that can locate the correct position by use of a mechanical positioner. Alternatively, the plate can be perforated with multiple small holes at fixed intervals. The needle can be passed into the hole closest to the exact coordinates that are calculated for needle placement. The use of a grid of holes on the compression plate is particularly convenient because it reduces the deflection of the needle as it passes into the breast.

Another technical consideration for MR-guided breast biopsy is that of available needles. MR-compatible needles are available from multiple manufacturers. Several manufacturers also have MR-compatible localization wires. Prototype, spring-loaded, core biopsy guns are being tested by multiple manufacturers. Although the MR-guided needles are adequate for placement of localization wires, core biopsy guns have difficulty in reliably obtaining core samples from the breast. The current evolution in MR-compatible core biopsy guns will hopefully provide reliable core samples in the future.

BIOPSY PROCEDURE

The procedure for performing MR-guided breast biopsy is similar to that used in standard mammographically or ultrasound-guided procedures. Initially, an intravenous line is placed for gadolinium injection, preferably before the patient gets on the scanner so there is no need to manipulate or move the patient during the procedure itself. The patient is then placed on the MR table. In most systems, the patient is placed prone. The breast is then sterilized, and compression is applied. As discussed, compression is most easily applied mediolaterally. The fiducial markers are not intrinsic to the coil apparatus itself; they should be placed so that localization can be achieved. The patient is then placed in the magnet, and localizing scan is performed. This approach is used to set up the postcontrast images and to ensure that the fiducial markers are visualized. Pre- and postgadolinium images are performed to localize the enhancing lesion. Although the images do not need to be the same quality of those obtained during diagnostic MRI, they should be of sufficient quality to ensure that the area to be biopsied can be easily identified. Once the postgadolinium scan is obtained, the patient is removed from the magnet. The location of the lesion may be calculated relative to the fiducial markers. This calculation can be done manually or via an automated system. Once the relative position of the lesion to the fiducial marker is established, the position for the needle pass can be calculated. The needle is then passed into the desired location (Fig. 35-3). With standard Lufkin needles (E-Z-EM, Glenn Falls, NY), it is necessary to remove the stylet before performing gradient echo images to confirm lesion position. The size of the artifact is greatly reduced, and a more accurate depiction of the needle location can be established. When the needle is in proper position, the patient may be removed from the scanner, and a localization wire may be passed through the needle. If necessary, the needle may be repositioned and its location may be rechecked.

One nuance of the MR-guided breast biopsy is that the contrast within the image changes as a function of time after contrast injection. Therefore, a lesion with very crisp borders that may be easily detectable on the initial postgadolinium image may be very difficult to see on the scan done to check lesion position (Fig. 35-4). Often, enough breast architecture is visible to establish that the needle is positioned in the appropriate location. However, the patient should remain still during the procedure so that the appearance of the breast does not dramatically change from the postgadolinium to the post–needle pass scan.

Another nuance of the MRI-guided localization procedure is that it is impossible to perform specimen MRI scans in a fashion similar to the specimen mammograms to confirm excision. In the case of focal masses detected by MRI, specimen mammograms are useful. Although a mammogram of the entire breast may not reveal the lesion, a specimen mammogram of a small segment of the breast often will depict the abnormality. The only way to ensure that the lesion has been excised is by follow-up MR several weeks after excision. Very detailed MR pathologic correlation is important to confirm that the suspicious area has been excised. If doubt exists as to whether the lesion has truly been excised, the patient is reimaged 2 weeks after biopsy.

INDICATIONS FOR MAGNETIC RESONANCE–GUIDED BREAST BIOPSY

MRI is a new breast imaging modality without established clinical indications. The indications for biopsy under MR guidance are even less established. In general terms, an MR-guided biopsy procedure should be entertained anytime a suspicious enhancing lesion seen on MR is occult on clinical examination and conventional imaging. Many MR-detected lesions that are

A
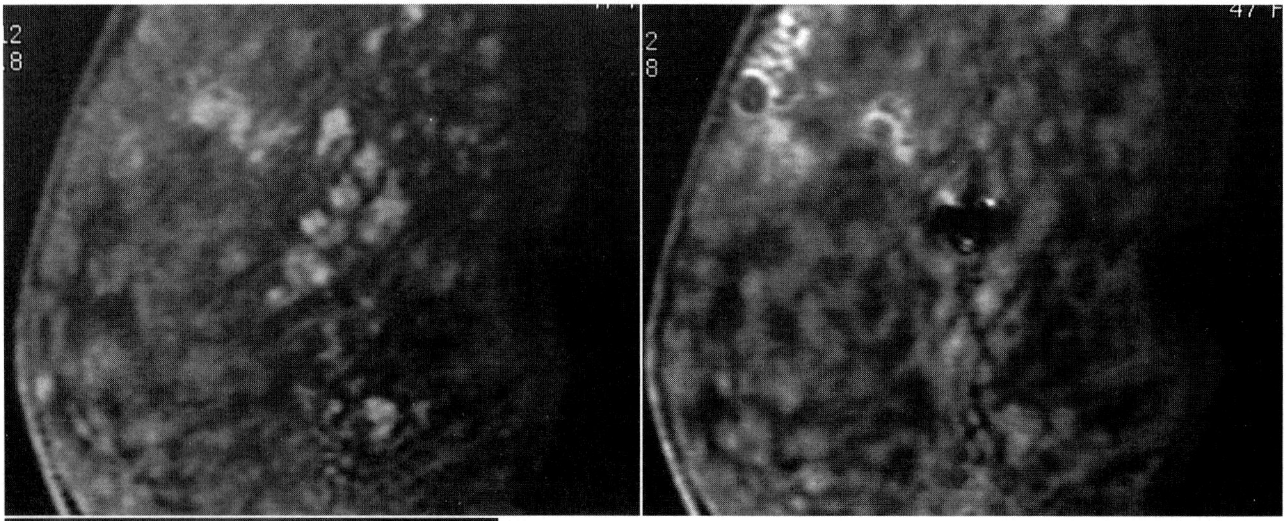
B

C
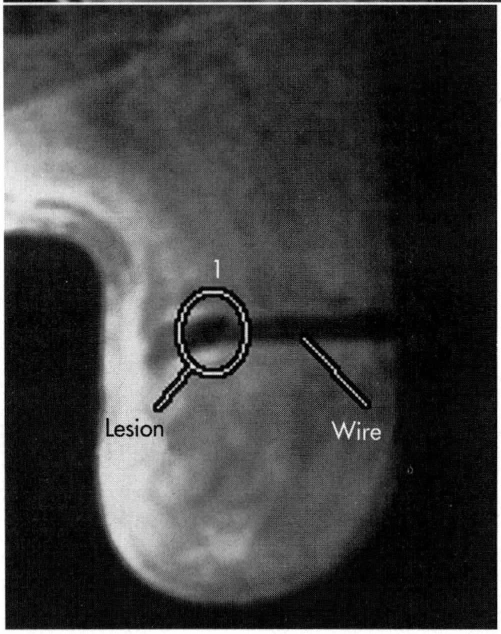

Fig. 35-4. A, Sagittal slice from a postcontrast acquisition shows multiple small enhancing lesions in the breast. **B,** Delayed postcontrast image after needle placement shows the needle position. On the delayed image, the enhancing portion of the lesion is difficult to visualize. **C,** A delayed axial view shows the trajectory of the needle. Although no lesion can be detected, lesion location can be superimposed on the needle to document accurate needle position. This approach assumes that the lesion has not moved during the biopsy and follow-up imaging procedure.

initially occult to other imaging modalities may be detected in retrospect. However, proceeding in this way would require an additional diagnostic examination to determine if these lesions could be detected, and the risk exists that the findings seen on different modalities represent different anatomic structures. Therefore, if MRI-guided breast biopsy is available, occult lesions detected by MR should be biopsied under MR guidance. The most common clinical scenario that leads to MR-guided breast biopsy is the detection of additional enhancing lesions on breast MRI performed for local staging of breast cancer.[4] In this setting, MRI localization wires may be placed so that these additional lesions can be excised during excision of the primary lesions. This technique may also be used to clearly define the margins of abnormal enhancement so that a lesion with its surrounding intraductal component may be excised in one setting. An additional application of MR-guided biopsy is the identification of occult lesions in patients with maxillary node presentation. Eighteen patients who presented with a positive axillary node biopsy and normal conventional imaging studies were studied. In 15 of 18 patients, MRI correctly detected an abnormality that on excision under MR guidance was shown to be cancer. Other settings in which MR can detect carcinoma include evaluation of patients with nipple discharge or high-risk patients. Occasionally, lesions that are visualized on only a single view of a mammogram may be easily localized and biopsied by MRI.

Eighty-six MR-guided procedures have been performed at the author's institution for the various indications discussed, including 1 cyst aspiration, 8 core biopsies, and 77 wire placements. Of these procedures, 31 yielded cancer. All procedures were considered technical successes. Five required repositioning of the needle after initial needle placement. Repositioning was necessary because of patient motion or miscalculation of the guidance hole. The average distance from desired needle position tip to actual needle position tip was 3 mm.

Results from prototype MR breast biopsy systems worldwide clearly show the feasibility and usefulness of performing this procedure with diagnostic breast MRI. For breast MRI to reach its potential as a valuable tool in the detection, diagnosis, and staging of breast cancer, commercial breast MRI biopsy systems should be available. Commercial suppliers will soon have prototypes available.

REFERENCES

1. Kaiser WA, Zeitler E: MR imaging of the breast: fast imaging sequences with and without Gd-DTPA, *Radiology* 170:681, 1989.
2. Heywang SH, and others: MR imaging of the breast with GD-DTPA: use and limitations, *Radiology* 171:95, 1989.
3. Harms SE, and others: MR imaging of the breast with rotating delivery of excitation off resonance: clinical experience with pathologic correlation, *Radiology* 171:493, 1993.
4. Orel SG, and others: Staging of suspected breast cancer: effect of MR imaging and MR-guided biopsy, *Radiology* 196:115, 1995.
5. Morris EA, and others: MR imaging of the breast in patients with occult primary breast carcinoma, *Radiology* 205:437, 1997.
6. Nunes LW, and others: Breast MR imaging: interpretation model, *Radiology* 202:833, 1997.
7. Boetes C, and others: MR characterization of suspicious breast lesions with a gadolinium-enhanced turbo FLASH subtraction technique, *Radiology* 193:777, 1994.
8. Heywang-Kobrunner SH, and others: Prototype breast coil for MR guided needle localization, *J Comput Assist Tomogr* 18:876, 1994.
9. Orel SG, and others: MR-imaging-guided localization and biopsy of breast lesions: initial experience, *Radiology* 193:97, 1994.
10. Kuhl CK, and others: Interventional breast MR imaging: clinical use of a stereotactic localization and biopsy device, *Radiology* 204:667, 1997.
11. Fischer U, and others: MR-guided biopsy of suspect breast lesions with a stereotaxic add-on device for surface coils, *Radiology* 192:272, 1994.

Chapter 36

MR–GUIDED LASER BREAST TREATMENT

Lee Min Lai, Margaret A. Hall-Craggs

In recent years, management of breast cancer has moved toward breast conservation. The aim of breast conservation is to maximize cosmesis without compromising overall survival. Several prospective trials have shown that, in patients with early-stage breast cancer, breast-conserving surgery (e.g., lumpectomy, wide local excision) with adjuvant radiotherapy is safe and achieves rates of overall survival comparable with those for radical mastectomy.[1-6] Nevertheless, surgery has risks of hematoma formation and infection, and the cosmetic outcome may be less than satisfactory because of deformity and scarring. Therefore, minimally invasive methods of destroying breast tumors *in situ* have been explored in an attempt to improve the cosmetic outcome of treatment. Several techniques have been investigated for the treatment of tumors in solid organs, including interstitial laser photocoagulation (ILP),[7-9] radiofrequency interstitial thermal ablation,[10,11] high-intensity focused ultrasound (US),[12,13] cryotherapy, and photodynamic therapy.[14,15]

Studies have concentrated mainly on developing ILP as a minimally invasive therapy for breast tumors. In this simple procedure, low-power laser energy is delivered directly into the tumor substance via thin optical fibers inserted percutaneously.[16] ILP has the potential to replace lumpectomy in treating selected cases of breast cancer and thus fits into the schema of breast conservation. However, all minimally invasive techniques are dependent on imaging for visualizing the target lesion, guiding the placement of fibers, and monitoring and assessing management effect. Various imaging modalities including US, computed tomography (CT), and magnetic resonance imaging (MRI) have been investigated for use in conjunction with ILP in the breast; the most promising appears to be MRI.

LASER ASPECTS

Laser light has three defining characteristics: it is monochromatic (of a single wavelength), coherent (light waves are in-phase), and collimated (waves are exactly parallel). These properties enable precise delivery of laser light to a very small area in a predictable manner. During ILP, laser light is delivered interstitially into tumor tissue via thin optical fibers, which can range from 0.1 to 1 mm in diameter. The fibers are made of a fused silica core surrounded by a cladding (made of plastic, hard polymer, or silica), which has a smaller refractive index than the core does. Consequently, light is transmitted by total internal reflection along the fiber with minimal power loss. ILP induces tissue necrosis by thermal coagulation, which occurs when laser light is absorbed by tissue surrounding the fiber. The laser light

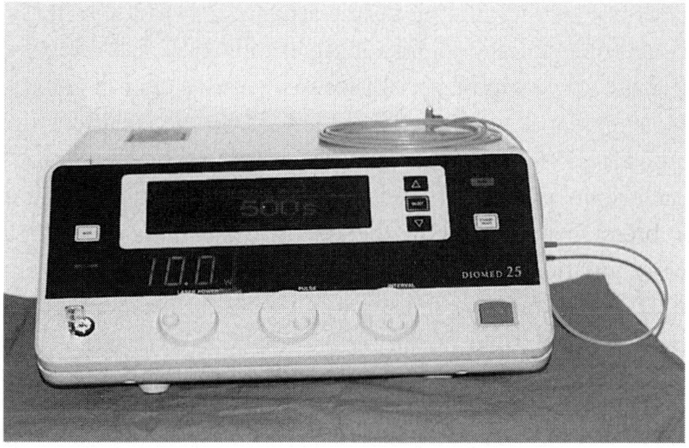

Fig. 36-1. A Diomed-25 semiconductor diode laser (Diomed, Cambridge, UK).

is transformed into heat, resulting in charring, which acts as a point heat source.[17,18] Coagulation necrosis of the tissue occurs as a result of thermal conduction rather than light penetration; the extent of thermal damage is related to the temperature gradient achieved.

Fibers with modified (diffuser) tips that allow tissue heating over a larger surface area were considered for use in ILP in an attempt to achieve larger thermal lesions, but early studies showed that these fibers were not better than bare fiber tips in generating thermal lesions (Personal communications). Moreover, diffuser tips cost considerably more than bare fibers and are not reusable. Nevertheless, diffuser tips continue to be developed and their use reviewed.

Several lasers have been evaluated for use in ILP: the neodymium: yttrium-aluminum-garnet (Nd:YAG) laser (1064 and 1320 nm), the semiconductor diode laser (805 nm), and the argon ion laser (488 and 514 nm). Of these lasers, the 805-nm diode laser has been used extensively for ILP because it is portable (the size of a typewriter), operates with a standard electrical supply, and has a wavelength that is effectively absorbed by most biologic tissues (Fig. 36-1).

INTERSTITIAL LASER PHOTOCOAGULATION EXPERIMENTS

Preclinical experiments to determine the optimal laser parameters for ILP were conducted in liver tissue. *In vivo* studies of ILP have been performed in healthy rat, rabbit, and pig livers.[19-21] The earliest and most comprehensive study was performed in a rat liver using a 400-mm bare-tipped optical fiber with the 1064-nm Nd:YAG laser.[19] Well-defined necrotic lesions of up to 16 mm were consistently generated with single-fiber ILP; the sizes could be increased by increasing the power and energy used. A plateau effect was observed above a power of 1 W and energy of 600 J, and charring around the fiber tip occurred above 0.75-W even for exposure durations as short as 200 sec.

Matsumoto, and others[21] showed that similar necrotic lesions could be induced by ILP in rabbit liver and noted that the longitudinal diameter (along the fiber track) of necrosis was greater than the transverse diameter (perpendicular to the fiber track), thus forming an ellipsoid lesion. The diameters of the lesions could be increased by increasing the power or the energy of the laser.

Amin and others[17] investigated the significance of charring in ILP using the 1320-nm Nd:YAG, the 1064-nm Nd:YAG, and the 805-nm diode in rat livers *in vivo.* Charring occurred relatively quickly and at low power (1 to 2 W) with the 1320-nm and 805-nm lasers but not with the 1064-nm laser. The thermal lesions generated were significantly larger when charring was present. At low power, precharring the bare fiber (by dipping it in a drop of rat's blood and firing at 4 to 5 W) produced consistently larger necrotic lesions than use of a clean fiber did. The authors concluded that charring induced larger lesions by preventing light penetration and therefore caused higher local temperatures. Precharring the fiber allows this process to begin much earlier during ILP. In a later study, Harries, and others[8] noted that areas of necrosis measuring 10 to 14 mm in diameter can be produced consistently in human breast when the bare fiber tip is charred before ILP.

For larger lesions to be generated with a single energy source, fiber-coupling systems or beam splitters have been used to enable simultaneous activation of more than one fiber.[22] Early beam splitters were relatively inefficient in conserving energy. Initial tests of one system (1 × 4 Starcoupler-Canstar, Canada) showed that although it achieved equal splitting ratios from a single-output fiber, up to 40% of input power was lost at fiber junctions. More efficient systems are now available; the 1 × 2 × 4 optical splitter designed by Diomed (Cambridge, UK) reliably splits the laser beam with a 30% energy loss (Fig. 36-2). Another way of increasing the laser burn size is to use a pull-back technique, in which fibers are withdrawn about 10 mm after the first dose and the laser is then reapplied.

ROLE OF IMAGING

Imaging is an integral part of minimally invasive procedures when access is limited and the view of the operative field is restricted. It is essential for the accurate planning, guiding, and follow-up of management in interventional procedures. The key roles of imaging in these procedures are to assess disease extent (locoregional staging), to visualize and guide tools to the target lesion, and to assess the efficacy of treatment during and after therapy. The ideal imaging modality should produce good tissue resolution, scan, and process images in real-time with minimal risks to the patient.

Breast tumors are conventionally diagnosed using triple assessment, which refers to the combination of clinical examination, tissue diagnosis (by fine-needle aspiration cytology or core biopsy histology), and imaging. Current available imaging techniques for evaluating breast disease include conventional x-ray mammography, US, CT, and MRI.

Locoregional staging of disease

Accurate locoregional staging of disease is essential in breast cancer management to select appropriate therapy. For patients undergoing surgery, staging and completeness of excision can be confirmed by histopathologic examination of the excised specimen and exploration of the axilla. With minimally invasive therapies in which tumors are destroyed *in situ,* these parameters are not available; consequently, the most accurate imaging modality for pretreatment tumor staging should be used.

X-ray mammography is the most widely used imaging modality in the diagnosis and follow-up of breast cancer and is the only imaging modality with proven efficacy for breast cancer screening. Although x-ray mammography is relatively sensitive for detecting early-stage cancers, its accuracy in assessing locoregional disease is low. Moreover, in a review of 10 studies, Fentiman[23] found that the sensitivity of mammography in detecting breast cancer varied from 61% to 87%. Sensitivity was lower in women younger than 50 years of age (56%) than in women older than 51 years of age (78%).

US is a valuable adjunct to clinical examination and mammography in diagnosing breast lumps, especially in younger women with dense breasts on mammography and in women who have undergone breast augmentation. Although US is extremely accurate for diagnosing cystic lesions if all criteria for diagnosing a simple cyst are met (96% to 100%), its accuracy for differentiating between benign and malignant solid lumps is lower because of a significant overlap in the US features of benign and malignant tumors. Moreover, the quality of information of US examination is highly dependent on the type of equipment used and the experience of the examiner.

In a recent study by Hagay, and others,[24] contrast-enhanced CT was found to be useful for the diagnosis of local recurrence after breast-conservation surgery. The sensitivity and specificity for diagnosing recurrent cancer in the conserved breast in this study were 91% and 85%, respectively. However, despite encouraging results, breast CT has not been used routinely because of the radiation hazard to both breasts and thorax and the relatively large dose of contrast medium required. The effectiveness of CT compared with mammography in diagnosing breast lesions has not been adequately evaluated.

MRI of the breast has been intensively studied over the past decade. MRI provides excellent soft-tissue resolution, which is further enhanced by the use of intravenous gadopentetate (Gd-DTPA). Kaiser[25] and Harms, and others[26] showed that a sensitivity of more than 90% for detecting cancer in the breast can be achieved with contrast-enhanced MRI. Furthermore, MR appears to be more sensitive than mammography for detecting tumor recurrence after surgery[27] and for staging locoregional disease.[28-30] However, the specificity of breast MR is less impressive, ranging from 53% to 97%.[31-35]

Targeting and tool guidance

Until recently, interventional use of x-ray mammography was largely limited to stereotactic localization and biopsy procedures. It has also been used for guiding the newly developed technique of mammotomy for large-core percutaneous breast biopsy.[36] However, it has not been used for guiding or monitoring thermal therapies.

US is useful in guiding needle aspiration or biopsy of breast lesions for cytologic or histologic examination.[37] It is also an excellent image-guiding tool because real-time US can facilitate needle guidance into the target lesion for therapeutic procedures. However, not all breast tumors are clearly defined on US, which limits the effectiveness of US in therapeutic procedures for breast cancer because the treatment margins need to be clearly identified.

CT-guided biopsy procedures in the thoracic and abdominal viscera continue to be invaluable in these cases. CT's use in guiding procedures in the breast has been mainly limited to needle localization of impalpable breast lesions, which are difficult to image on conventional two-view x-ray mammography.[38]

MR guidance has been used successfully in stereotactic biopsies and for preoperative localization of impalpable breast lesions.[39-42] Development of newer open-access MR scanners and MR fluoroscopy has made MR amenable for use in guiding placement of interventional tools (Figs. 36-2 and 36-3, *A, B*).

Imaging of treatment effects

Imaging provides a noninvasive way of monitoring tissue changes during and after therapy. There are two conceptual methods of image guidance: on-line imaging, which requires near real-time imaging, and stereotactic guidance, which is based on previously acquired images.[43] The advantage of accurate real-time imaging is that adequacy of treatment can be determined and necessary adjustments made in the same session. US, CT, and MRI have been evaluated for defining tumor extent and monitoring ILP. Early attempts at monitoring thermal treatments were conducted in the liver using CT and US.[7] US was excellent in measuring tumor size but could not accurately show laser-induced changes during or after treatment. During ILP, US showed a hyperechoeic region gradually developing around the fiber tip, but the size of this region did not correlate with the size of the burn on histology.[7] Dynamic contrast-enhanced CT scans accurately depicted laser-induced necrosis in the liver[7,44] but were less reliable in showing the extent of laser damage after ILP of breast cancers.[8]

MR has some thermally dependent effects that may facilitate the imaging of thermal treatments during therapy. T1 relaxation times and other temperature-dependent parameters have been investigated for use in monitoring thermal therapies. These parameters include diffusion coefficients,[45-47] chemical shift, magnetization transfer coefficient,[48] and susceptibility changes occurring with tissue and hemoglobin degradation.[49] The laser light and optical fibers do not degrade MRI providing that the laser source remains outside the Faraday cage. MRI also does not interfere with the delivery of laser light. Clinical studies of ILP involving MR guidance mainly looked at its role in palliation of inoperable hepatic metastases and brain tumors.[50-53] Only Fried, and others[52] and Roberts, and others,[53] in their experimental studies, attempted to correlate changes in MR signals with histologic analysis.

No imaging modality fulfils all the requisite criteria for staging and monitoring of treatment in minimally invasive therapy

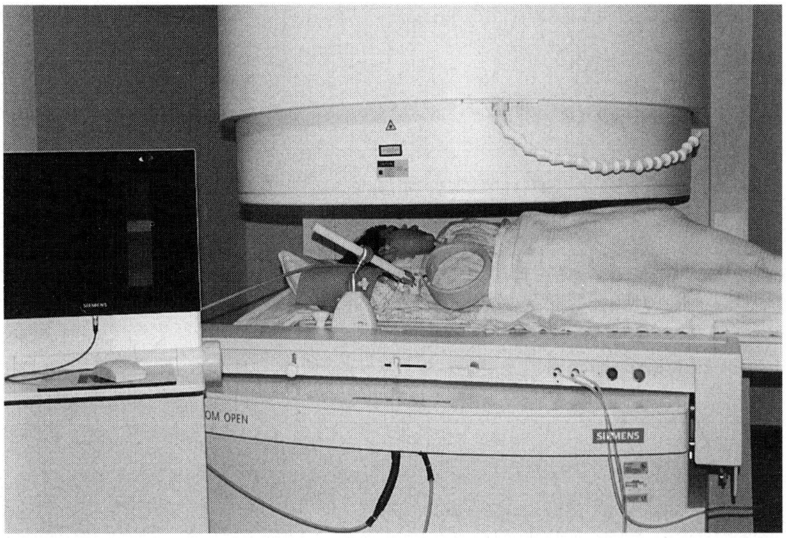

Fig. 36-2. Breast imaging in an open-access scanner (0.2T Magnetom Open, Siemens, Erlangen, Germany). A 21-cm flexicoil is positioned around the breast leaving sufficient access to guide and manipulate needles and fibers.

A

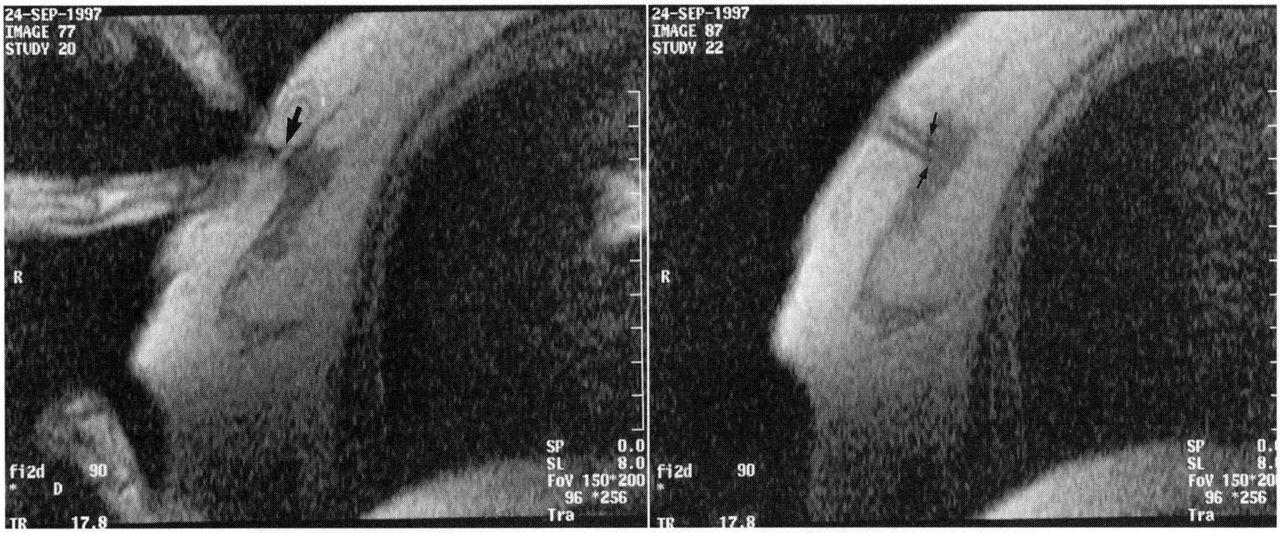

B

Fig. 36-3. A, Needle localization in an open-access magnet. The needle tip *(arrow)* is guided into the breast tumor using magnetic resonance (MR) fluoroscopy (two-dimensional fast low-angle shot; repetition time, 17.8 sec; echo time, 8.1 sec; flip angle, 90°; acquisition time, 11 sec). **B,** After insertion of two MR-compatible needles, the needle tip positions can be clearly visualized *(small arrows)*.

to the breast. However, MRI offers the highest sensitivity to staging tumors, has the potential to monitor treatment effects, and does not involve the use of ionizing radiation. It has been primarily used in the application of ILP to the breast.

INTERSTITIAL LASER PHOTOCOAGULATION TECHNIQUE IN THE BREAST

In some studies, the Diomed-25 semiconductor diode laser (Diomed, Cambridge, UK) is used at a wavelength of 805 nm. Although this laser is low power (maximum output, 25 W), ILP should be performed in a room with full laser safety precautions, which include interlockable doors, suitably blinded windows, coverage of reflective surfaces, and goggles (suited to the wavelength of the laser) worn by all personnel and the patient. The laser source is sited in the scanning console room, and long optical fibers (up to 10 m) are passed through a wave guide into the scanning room.

The optical fibers used for breast ILP are 400 μm in diameter and are prepared: the distal ends of the fibers are stripped to remove the cladding, the bare fiber tips are cleaved, and the entire length of the fibers are sterilized in ethylene dioxide. The sterilized fibers are then precharred by applying a flame to the bare tips (Fig. 36-4) and are loaded into 18-gauge needles until the fiber protorudes 4 mm from the needle tip (Fig. 36-5). A marker is placed on the fiber to indicate the proximal end of the needle (Fig. 36-5). If the procedure is to be carried out in an MR scanner, MR-compatible needles (William Cook Europe, A/S) should be used to minimize the susceptibility artifacts.

Breast ILP is performed aseptically and under imaging guidance (US or MRI). Local anesthetic (lidocaine 1%) is infiltrated into the skin and peritumoral region before insertion of needles. Eighteen-gauge needles are inserted under US or MR guidance followed by the precharred optical fibers, which are loaded singly into each needle. Once the needle is in position, the fiber is advanced through the needle until its tip extends a few mm distal to the needle tip as indicated by the Steristrip® flag (Fig. 36-6). The laser is set to deliver a power of 2.5 W per fiber for 500 sec.

The procedure is well tolerated using local anesthetic and intravenous sedation. Patients' vital signs are monitored throughout the procedure, and resuscitation equipment is kept on hand.

Because ILP has the potential to destroy tumor totally, all material necessary for adequate cytologic or histologic examination is obtained before treatment. In breast lesions, this takes

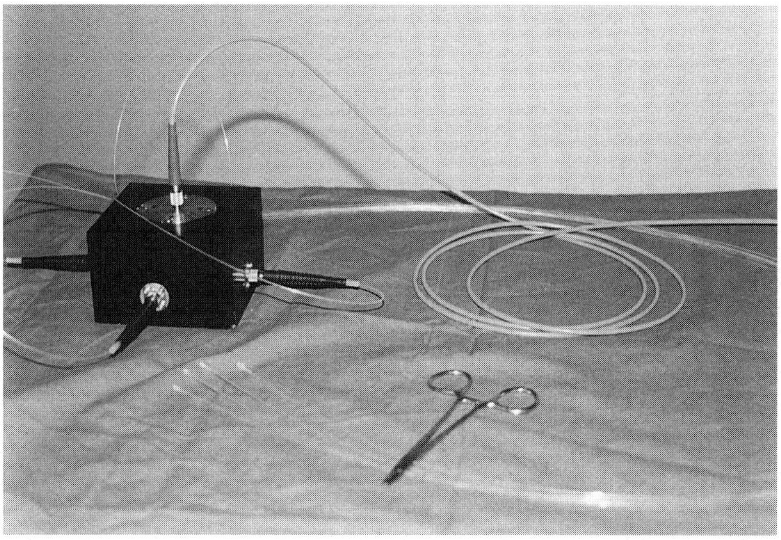

Fig. 36-4. A beam splitter is attached to four sterilized and cleaved optical fibers.

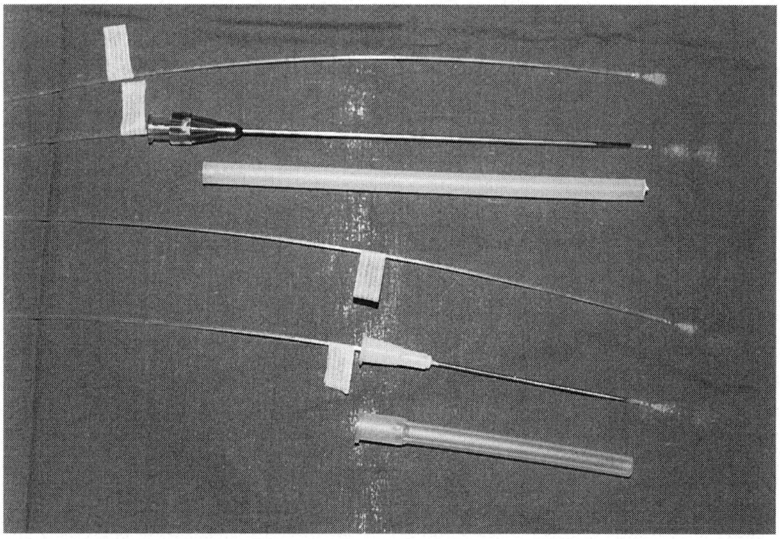

Fig. 36-5. A flagged and preloaded 18-gauge magnetic resonance–compatible needle **(top)** with a similarly prepared standard hypodermic needle **(bottom).**

the form of fine-needle aspiration cytology or core biopsy of the tumor.

INTERSTITIAL LASER PHOTOCOAGULATION IN BREAST CANCER

The aim of ILP in breast cancer treatment is to achieve ablation of the tumor and a margin of healthy tissue equivalent to surgical excision. A minimally invasive procedure, ILP should ideally be carried out as a daycase procedure, and the extent of laser damage should be ascertained at the time of treatment, so any modifications to treatment can be performed in the same session.

The most extensive studies of ILP in breast cancer treatment were performed using a single bare-tipped fiber with the 805-nm semiconductor diode laser in a treat-and-excise protocol.[8,9] The procedure was safe and well tolerated. Minor complications occurred, including pain and sensation of heat, which stopped immediately when treatment was terminated. One patient had prolonged bleeding after withdrawal of the needle that stopped when a pressure dressing was applied. One patient had a pectoralis muscle burn, and one other patient a small skin burn, both of which were excised at surgery.

With one precharred fiber, the size of laser burn is small (median diameter, 11 mm)[9] and therefore inadequate for ablating most tumors. Development of beam splitters has enabled ILP treatments with multiple fibers; early treatments in hepatic metastases yielded larger volumes of necrosis.[7] The size of thermal lesions can be increased by a pull-back technique, as described. Preliminary treatments in breast tumors with multiple-fiber ILP has produced lesions up to 40 mm in diameter (Unpublished data), which is theoretically sufficient to treat small tumors with a margin of clearance.

HISTOPATHOLOGY OF BREAST TUMORS AFTER INTERSTITIAL LASER PHOTOCOAGULATION

Macroscopically, the ILP-induced lesion consists of a central charred cavity surrounded by a broad area of pale tissue and a peripheral hemorrhagic rim beyond which is viable tumor. Microscopically, the pale zone of tissue shows *in situ* heat fixation characterized by cells that are morphologically normal but have hyperchromatic smeared nuclei and hypereosinophilic cytoplasm consistent with the presence of coagulated proteins. The extent of *in situ* fixation varies depending on the site of laser fiber in the tumor and its relationship to healthy breast tissue and fat. The hemorrhagic rim contains cells that are less damaged; their nuclei are only slightly hyperchromatic and retain their chromatin pattern and nucleoli. These cells were surrounded by proliferating fibroblasts, blood vessels, and extravasated erythrocytes. Immunocytochemical staining in specimens from two patients confirmed the nonviability of cells in all three zones.

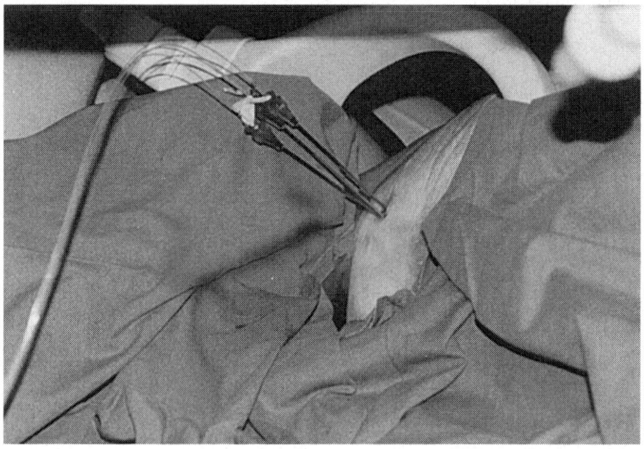

Fig. 36-6. Four-fiber interstitial laser coagulation treatment to breast tumor.

IMAGING OF INTERSTITIAL LASER PHOTOCOAGULATION IN THE BREAST

Patients who underwent early ILP in the breast using real-time US to monitor treatment effects showed similar results to those when ILP was used in the liver. Hyperechoeic regions appeared around the laser fiber, probably because of microbubble formation. The area of hyperechogenicity did not correlate with the extent of laser-induced necrosis.[8]

Most breast ILP treatments were imaged in a 1-T magnet (42 SP, Siemens, Erlangen, Germany). A double breast, receive-only coil was used for diagnostic imaging and locoregional staging. Mumtaz and others[9] showed that contrast-enhanced MR with T1-weighted, three-dimensional (3D) fast low-angle shot (FLASH) sequence performed 24 to 96 hr after single-fiber ILP accurately depicted the extent of laser damage as areas of nonenhancement (Fig. 36-7). The areas of nonenhancement correlated closely to the histopathologic size of laser-induced necrosis ($r = 0.86$). Furthermore, MR measurements of residual viable tumor, seen as residual enhancing zones on the posttreatment scan, correlate well with histopathologic measurements of viable residual disease (Fig. 36-7, *A* to *E*). Contrast-enhanced MR scans performed immediately or a few hours after ILP were unreliable for predicting the extent of laser-induced damage.

The results of imaging multiple fiber treatments have been less clear. With more extensive damage to the tumor margins, an inflammatory reaction appears around the area of necrosis, which enhances with Gd-DTPA. Consequently, measurement of residual viable disease becomes unreliable in the short-term. Delayed MR studies may predict the extent of residual disease more accurately when the inflammatory response subsides.

In a recent study, dynamic imaging of ILP was evaluated in 14 women who had biopsy-proven diagnosis of breast cancer using 2D FLASH sequence (repetition time, 111 msec; echo time, 10 msec; flip angle, 60°; slice thickness, 10 mm; three slices/30 sec). An expanding zone of signal loss around the optical fiber tip was observed during ILP.[54] This zone first appeared at approximately 30 sec into treatment and reached maximum size at 270 to 400 sec. Close correlation between the maximum size of signal loss and histopathologic dimensions of the laser burn was found ($r = 0.85$). The correlation was marginally better for single fibers than for multiple fibers. However, use of a

A B C D

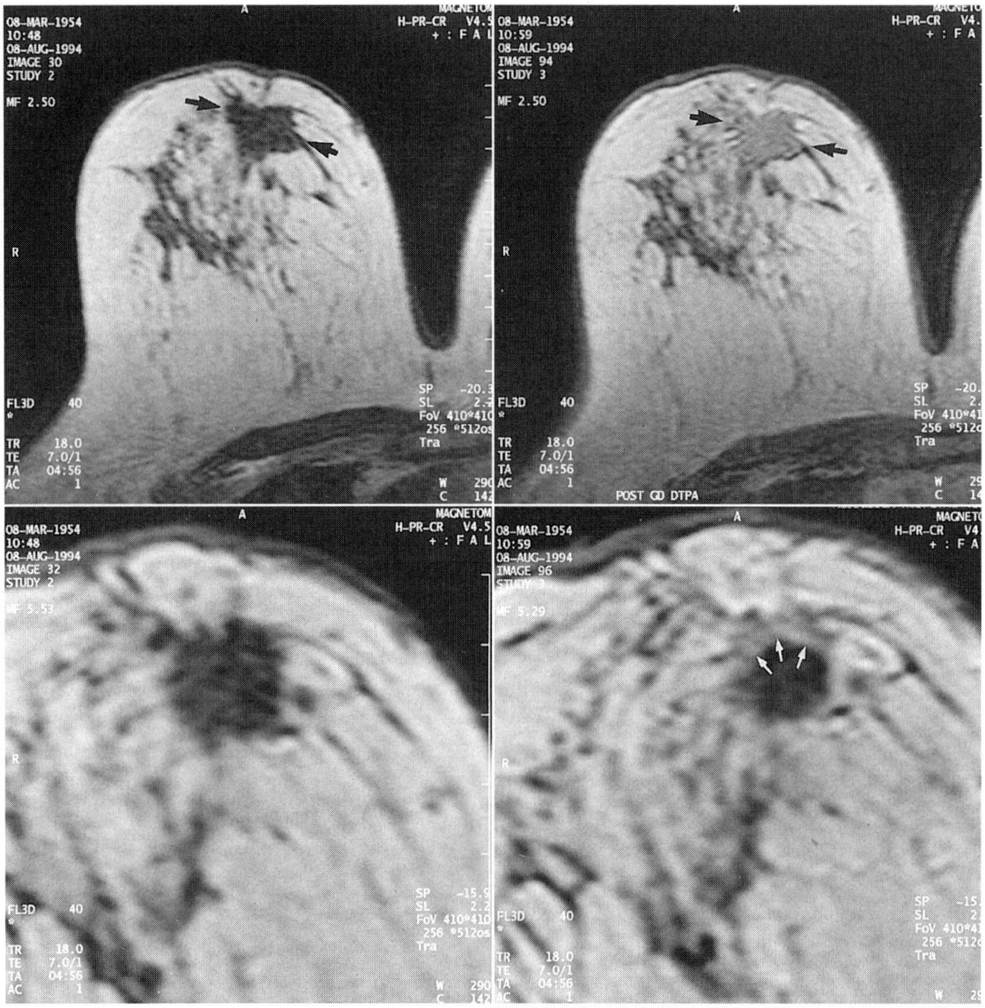

E

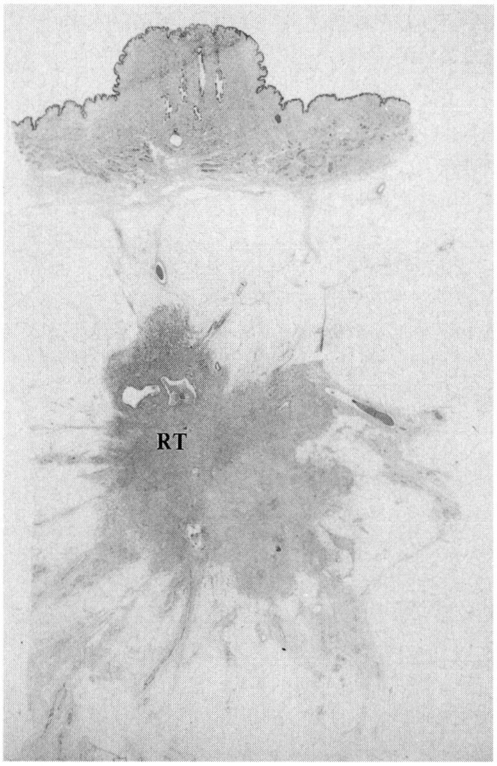

Fig. 36-7. Magnetic resonance (MR) images of pretreated breast cancer *(arrow)* **A**, before and **B**, after contrast enhancement with gadopentetate. MR images obtained after interstitial laser photocoagulation (ILP) of the same lesion **C**, before and **D**, after contrast enhancement. **E**, Histopathology of the excised tumor. **A** and **B** show an intensely enhancing breast cancer. **C** and **D** show images after single-fiber ILP. In **D**, an 11-mm zone of nonenhancement is seen in the tumor with an eccentric enhancing rim *(white arrows)*. In **E**, the area of the enhancing rim correlates well with the dimensions of residual viable tumor *(RT)* found on histopathology. See Color Plate 17.

conventional scanner and only a side-access breast coil (MRI Devices) did not achieve accurate targeting of the lesions, largely because of restricted access to the patient.

Further studies to evaluate spatial and temporal changes of MR signal intensity with ILP are being conducted using a scanner with a more open configuration and operating at a lower field strength. Ideally, thermal changes will be imaged in or close to real-time, and measurements can be made of the areas showing signal loss for comparison with histopathologic findings.

INTERSTITIAL LASER PHOTOCOAGULATION TREATMENT OF BREAST FIBROADENOMAS

Fibroadenomas are common benign tumors in young women; the peak incidence occurs at age 21 to 25 years. These tumors can be accurately diagnosed by clinical examination, US, and fine-needle aspiration cytology. The natural history of fibroadenomas is unpredictable; the spontaneous resolution rate is approximately 16% to 37% over 1 to 3 years. Of these lumps, one third will become smaller and one third will increase in size.

Conventionally, treatment of these lesions is surgical excision, usually under general anesthesia. The main disadvantages of surgery are the risks of general anesthesia, wound infection, hemorrhage, and scarring, which may be cosmetically unacceptable. Moreover, some women develop multiple fibroadenomas, and surgical excision means multiple operations and multiple scars. Studies have more recently validated the safety of using a conservative approach in managing breast fibroadenomas.[55,56] Consequently, women diagnosed with breast fibroadenomas have two treatment options: surgical excision or no treatment with limited follow-up. The main problem with the no treatment option is that a persistent lump in the breast can be a source of constant anxiety to the patient. In such cases, a treatment such as ILP is an attractive alternative because it may destroy the tumor without leaving a scar.

In a pilot study, 15 women aged 19 to 24 years with confirmed breast fibroadenomas (on triple assessment) were treated with ILP. All patients were awaiting surgery. ILP was performed using two to four fibers (depending on the size of the fibroadenoma). Immediately after ILP, treated lumps swelled 4 to 5 mm as evident on US, probably because of tumoral and peritumoral edema. Treatment was associated with localized bruising and redness of the breast, particularly with the four fiber treatments; these complications resolved within 1 wk in all patients. The procedure was otherwise well tolerated with the use of a local anesthetic, intravenous analgesia, and sedation.

All the treated fibroadenomas were smaller on serial US measurements. The reduction in lesion size was approximately 45% at 8 weeks and 70% at 6 months. In three patients, the treated fibroadenomas were clinically and US undetectable at 6 months follow-up. Furthermore, 10 of 15 patients declined surgery after their initial favorable response to ILP. In this series, the only complication was a skin burn at one of the needle entry points in a patient with superficial fibroadenoma treated with four fibers. This healed with regular dry dressings, leaving a faint scar measuring 5 mm in diameter. No prophylactic antibiotics were used, and no patient developed any infection.

PROBLEMS AND COMPLICATIONS

The problems encountered in MRI of breast ILP treatments are partly attributable to the restricted access to the patient in a conventional scanner. As a result, needle localization of tumors was difficult to perform. These problems may be overcome by newer open-access MR scanners and MR fluoroscopy. Imaging difficulties were also experienced at 1 T with the present generation of MR-compatible needles, which cause sufficient artifact to obscure small targets.

The only significant complications in treated patients were skin and pectoralis muscle burns arising from misplaced fibers, mainly because optical fibers are MR invisible unless specially coated.[57] These burns can be prevented with real-time imaging during therapy, which would detect the thermal effect of the laser on healthy and tumor tissue. The skin can be cooled with cold swabs and cold water irrigation during and after ILP to limit inadvertent thermal damage. No infection occurred in the ILP-treated sites in any patient. One patient with a fibroadenoma recently treated with four-fiber ILP had a persistent sterile discharge for 3 wks. The discharge was not infected on microbiologic examination and was probably related to the large volume of coagulative necrosis induced. With more aggressive ILP treatment using multiple fibers, this complication will likely occur more often.

SUMMARY AND THERAPEUTIC CONSIDERATIONS

Several issues should be addressed before ILP can replace lumpectomy in conservative treatment of breast cancer. One reservation is the loss of material for histopathologic examination when the whole tumor is ablated because useful information can be gained to prognosticate and help plan further treatment, such as radiotherapy and chemotherapy. New biopsy techniques[31] that allow larger blocks of tissue to be sampled may have a significant role in addressing this issue.

Another major issue is validation of clearance margins after ILP of these tumors. As discussed, studies have shown that residual enhancing material seen in MRI 48 to 72 hr after treatment can be caused by an inflammatory response or the presence of persistent tumor. Therefore, the characteristics of the enhancing rim should be further evaluated. Much work is needed to develop dynamic monitoring of ILP in real-time. Even then, multiple biopsies of the treated margins with MR or US guidance may be necessary to ensure that no residual tumor is present.

MR-guided ILP of breast tumors is safe and feasible. Small cancers (<2 cm) would appear to be more suitable for ILP because the chances of complete ablation are greater. ILP will require stringent clinical trials before it can be considered for routine clinical use as a treatment option for breast cancer in carefully selected patients. Strict patient selection criteria will need to be established to avoid possible complications from incomplete tumor ablation. Likewise, in the treatment of breast fibroadenomas in young women, further studies of ILP (randomized if possible) with more patients are necessary to validate the efficacy of this treatment.

REFERENCES

1. Fisher B, and others: Eight year results of a randomized clinical trial comparing total mastectomy and lumpectomy with or without irradiation in the treatment of breast cancer, *N Engl J Med* 320:822, 1989.
2. Sarrazin D, and others: Ten year results of a randomised trial comparing conservative treatment to mastectomy in early breast cancer, *Radiother Oncol* 14:177, 1989.
3. Veronesi U, and others: Breast conservation is the treatment of choice in small breast cancer: long term results of a randomised clinical trial, *Eur J Cancer* 26:668, 1990.
4. Veronesi U, and others: Conservative treatment of early breast cancer. Long term results of 1232 cases treated with quadrantectomy, axillary dissection and radiotherapy, *Ann Surg* 211:250, 1990.
5. Veronesi U, and others: Conservative approaches for the management of stage I/II carcinoma of the breast: Milan Cancer Institute trials, *World J Surg* 18:70, 1994.
6. Jacobsen JA, and others: Ten year results of a comparison of conservation with mastectomy in the treatment of stage I and II breast cancer, *N Engl J Med* 332:907, 1995.
7. Amin Z, and others: Hepatic metastases: interstitial laser photocoagulation with real-time US monitoring and dynamic CT evaluation of treatment, *Radiology* 187:339, 1993.
8. Harries SA, and others: Interstitial laser photocoagulation as a treatment for breast cancer, *Br J Surg* 81:1617, 1994.
9. Mumtaz H, and others: Laser therapy for breast cancer: magnetic resonance imaging and histopathological correlation, *Radiology* 200:651, 1996.
10. McGahan JP, and others: Hepatic ablation using radiofrequency electrocautery, *Invest Radiol* 25:267, 1990.
11. Rossi S, and others: Percutaneous RF interstitial thermal ablation in the treatment of hepatic cancer, *Am J Roentgenol* 167:759, 1996.
12. Hill CR, ter-Haar GR: Review article: high intensity focused ultrasound-potential for cancer treatment, *Br J Radiol* 68:1296, 1995.
13. Cline HE, and others: Focused ultrasound system for MR imaging-guided tumour ablation, *Radiology* 194:731, 1995.
14. Lowdell CP, and others: Interstitial photodynamic therapy: clinical experience with diffusing fibres in the treatment of cutaneous and subcutaneous tumours, *Br J Cancer* 67:1398, 1993.
15. Koechli OR, and others: Assessment of effect of photosensitisers on cytotoxicity of photodynamic therapy in human breast cancer cell cultures, *Arch Gynecol Obstet* 256:167, 1995.
16. Bown SG: Phototherapy of tumours, *World J Surg* 7:700, 1983.
17. Amin Z, and others: Interstitial laser photocoagulation: evaluation of a 1320nm Nd:YAG and an 805nm diode laser. The significance of charring and the value of precharring the fibre tip, *Lasers Med SCI* 8:113, 1993.
18. Wyman D, Whelan W, Wilson BC: Interstitial laser photocoagulation: NdYAG 1064nm optical fibre source compared to point heat source, *Lasers Surg Med* 12:659, 1992.
19. Mathewson K, and others: Biological effects of intrahepatic neodymium: yttrium-aluminium-garnet laser photocoagulation in rats, *Gastroenterology* 93:550, 1987.
20. Dachman AH, and others: US-guided percutaneous laser ablation of liver tissue in a chronic pig model, *Radiology* 176:129, 1990.
21. Matsumoto R, and others: Interstitial Nd:YAG laser ablation in normal rabbit liver: trial to maximise the size of laser induced lesions, *Lasers Surg Med* 12:650, 1992.
22. Steger AC, and others: Multiple-fibre low-power interstitial laser hyperthermia: studies in the normal liver, *Br J Surg* 79:139, 1992.
23. Fentiman I: *Detection and treatment of early breast cancer,* London, 1990, Martin Dunitz.
24. Hagay C, and others: Contrast-enhanced CT: value for diagnosing local breast cancer recurrence after conservative treatment, *Radiology* 200:631, 1996.
25. Kaiser WA: *MR Mammography (MRM),* 1993, Springer-Verlag.
26. Harms SE, and others: MR imaging of the breast with rotating delivery of excitation off resonance: clinical experience with pathologic correlation, *Radiology* 187:485, 1993.
27. Mumtaz H, and others: Comparison of magnetic resonance imaging and conventional triple assessment in locally recurrent breast cancer, *Br J Surg* 84:1147, 1997.
28. Boetes C, and others: Breast tumours: comparative accuracy of MR imaging relative to mammography and ultrasound for demonstrating extent, *Radiology* 197:743, 1995.
29. Orel SG, and others: Staging of suspected breast cancer: effect of MR imaging and MR-guided biopsy, *Radiology* 196:115, 1995.
30. Mumtaz H, and others: Staging of symptomatic primary breast cancer with MR imaging, *Am J Roentgenol* 169:417, 1997.
31. Flickinger FW, and others: Differentiation of benign from malignant breast masses by time-intensity evaluation of contrast-enhanced MRI, *Magn Reson Imaging* 11:617, 1993.
32. Orel SG, and others: Suspicious breast lesions: MR imaging with radiopathologic correlation, *Radiology* 190:485, 1994.
33. Kerslake RW, and others: Dynamic gradient-echo and fat suppressed spin-echo contrast enhanced MRI of the breast, *Clin Radiol* 50:440, 1995.
34. Stomper PC, and others: Suspicious breast lesions: findings at dynamic gadolinium enhanced MR imaging correlated with mammographic and pathologic features, *Radiology* 197:387, 1995.
35. Bone B, and others: Sensitivity and specificity of MR mammography with histopathological correlation in 250 breasts, *Acta Radiol* 32:208, 1996.
36. Parker SH, Burbank F: A practical approach to minimally invasive breast biopsy, *Radiology* 200:11, 1996.
37. Bruneton JN, and others: Axillary lymph nodes metastases in breast cancer: preoperative detection with US, *Radiology* 158:325, 1986.
38. Spillane RM, and others: Computed tomography-guided needle localisation of nonpalpable breast lesions: review of 24 cases, *Acad Radiol* 3:115, 1996.
39. Doler W, and others: Stereotaxic add-on device for MR-guided biopsy of breast lesions, *Radiology* 200:863, 1996.
40. Fischer U, and others: MR imaging guided breast intervention: experience with two systems, *Radiology* 195:533, 1995.
41. Adam G, and others: Interventional magnetic resonance: initial clinical experience with 1.5-tesla magnetic resonance system combined with c-arm fluoroscopy, *Invest Radiol* 32:191, 1997.
42. deSouza NM, and others: Magnetic resonance imaging guided breast biopsy using a frameless stereotactic technique, *Clin Radiol* 51:425, 1996.
43. Jolesz FA, Blumenfeld SM: Interventional use of magnetic resonance imaging, *Magn Reson Q* 10:85, 1994.
44. Steger A, and others: Ultrasound features of interstitial laser hyperthermia, *Clin Radiol* 46:88, 1992.
45. Dickinson RJ, and others: Measurement of changes in tissue temperature using MR imaging, *J Comput Assist Tomogr* 10:468, 1986.
46. Le Bihan D, Delannoy J, Levin RI: Temperature mapping with MR imaging of molecular diffusion: application to hyperthermia, *Radiology* 171: 853, 1989.
47. Bleier AR, and others: Real-time magnetic resonance imaging of laser heat deposition in tissue, *Magn Reson Med* 21:132, 1991.
48. Young IR, and others: Further observations on the measurement on tissue T1 to monitor temperature in vivo by MRI, *Magn Reson Med* 31:342, 1994.
49. Farahani K, and others: Methaemoglobin formation and T1 shortening in thermal coagulation (abstract). Proceedings of the Society of Magnetic Resonance. Berkeley, CA:1576.
50. Kahn D, and others: MRI-guided laser-induced interstitial thermotherapy of cerebral neoplasms, *J Comput Assist Tomogr* 18:519, 1994.

51. Vogl TJ, and others: Malignant liver tumours treated with MR imaging guided laser induced thermotherapy: technique and prospective results, *Radiology* 196:257, 1995.
52. Fried MP, and others: Dynamic T1-weighted magnetic resonance imaging of interstitial laser photocoagulation in the liver, *Lasers Surg Med* 18:410, 1996.
53. Roberts HRS, and others: Magnetic resonance imaging of interstitial laser photocoagulation of normal rat liver: imaging-histopathological correlation, *Min Invas Ther* 6:41, 1997.
54. Hall-Craggs MA, and others: Dynamic MR guidance of laser therapy to breast cancer, *Radiology* 201:177, 1996.
55. Carty NJ, and others: Management of fibroadenoma of the breast, *Ann R Coll Surg Engl* 77:127, 1995.
56. Cant PJ, and others: Case for conservative management of selected fibroadenomas of the breast, *Br J Surg* 74:857, 1987.
57. Paley M, and others: High magnetic susceptibility coatings for visualization of optical fibres on a specialised interventional MRI system, *Eur Radiol* 7:1341, 1997.

Chapter 37

INTERVENTIONAL MRI OF THE THORAX

Jonathan G. Goldin

Magnetic resonance imaging (MRI) has become an established technique for evaluation of the chest[1-4] and is considered superior to other imaging modalities in the evaluation of specific mediastinal,[5-7] hilar,[8,9] and chest wall[10-13] abnormalities. MRI should be the perfect technique for imaging the thorax because of the exquisite soft-tissue contrast, multiplanar capability, intrinsic flow sensitivity, and lack of ionizing radiation. Its use in the assessment of the lung has been limited by the signal loss caused by magnetic susceptibility artifacts (caused by the many air and soft-tissue interfaces), respiratory and cardiac motion artifacts, and poor signal-to-noise ratios (SNRs). Low-field MR systems offer the advantage of significantly less susceptibility artifact and the potential for better visualization of the lung parenchyma.

Interventional MR is receiving great interest as minimally invasive surgical procedures become the preferred method of management.[14-16] Developments in computed tomography (CT) and three-dimensional (3D) visualization software have allowed sophisticated biopsy and surgical procedures to be performed under image guidance. The ability to perform these procedures with a nonionizing imaging source is of great interest. Currently, interventional MR is being developed using several magnet configurations. Early procedures in the thorax have been closely modeled on biopsy and surgical techniques performed under CT or videoscopic guidance. Interventional MR can use previously prepared image data from various different modalities and provide cross-section imaging in near real-time. In addition, the use of new treatment methods specifically targeted by localization offers the potential for the ablation or size reduction of tumors, giving rise to a new spectrum of interventional MR capabilities.[14,16]

The rational use of low-field MRI in chest disease requires an understanding of the basic MR physics particular to chest imaging and a familiarity with pulse sequences, techniques of interventional MR, and the clinical conditions in which thoracic MRI has shown to be of benefit. This chapter reviews these topics and discusses potential uses of interventional MR in the management of pathology in the mediastinum, lung parenchyma, and chest wall.

PHYSICS PRINCIPLES

Traditional spin-echo sequences remain the most commonly used pulse sequences in imaging the chest. Both 90° and 180° radiofrequency (RF) pulses are used in spin-echo sequences. These RF pulses rotate the magnetic vector aligned along the z axis into the x-y plane, where it produces a detectable signal. By varying the interval between the RF pulses, images of different characteristics can be obtained primarily by determining the T1 and T2 relaxation times of the tissues encountered.

The T1 relaxation time is a measure of the rate of recovery of the longitudinal or z magnetic vector in a patient and is caused by the transfer of energy from the hydrogen proton to the surrounding lattice. T1 varies, with magnetic field strength being longer in higher magnetic fields; it tends to be longer in water and shorter in fat. Any process that increases tissue water content (e.g., edema) will thus lengthen the T1 relaxation time. The interval between successive 90° pulses, known as the repetition time (TR), determines the ability to differentiate the relaxation times of different tissues. This differentiation is best achieved with short TRs because tissue relaxation during long TRs makes differentiation impossible. Using a 1.5-T magnet, the usual TR is approximately 600 msec for T1-weighted sequences, which corresponds to one R-R interval in cardiac-gated scans.

The T2 relaxation time is a measure of the time protons take to go out of phase after the end of an RF pulse. It has primarily two causes: inhomogeneities of the external magnetic field and inhomogeneities of local magnetic fields, from neighboring nuclei, in the tissues. In general, T2 is longer in homogeneous environments (e.g., water, in which differences in magnetic field strength are relatively small) and shorter in inhomogeneous environments (e.g., soft tissue, in which variations in the local magnetic fields are great and molecules cannot move around fast, resulting in protons getting out of phase faster). Therefore, an increase in tissue water (e.g., edema) tends to prolong the T2 relaxation time. An echo time (TE) of less than 30 msec is considered short.

The failure to visualize lung on conventional spin-echo sequences, even with relatively short TEs of 20 to 30 msec, is caused by the innumerable magnetic field gradients caused by the large differences in magnetic susceptibility between air and soft tissue at each alveolar interface.[17,18] This susceptibility artifact is related to the degree of lung inflation, being 7 msec at full inflation and 80 msec in deflated gasless lungs.[19] In pathologic states in which inflammation or tumor replaces air, these conventional sequences yield abundant signal.[20]

A sequence with a long TR and a short TE is often used, in which the effects of T1 and T2 are minimized, and the contrast results from differences in water or proton density. The resultant images have relatively high signal strength and the lowest SNR. However, the degree of contrast is limited because of the elimination of the positive features of T1 and T2 relaxation.

Conventional MR scanners use gradient magnetic fields and 2D Fourier transformation to obtain spatial localization.[21] The 2D Fourier transformation is very sensitive to motion. Motion results in phase changes that result in signal misregistration because signals are incorrectly ascribed to the phase-encoding gradient. This artifact is visible on the images as a band of signal along the phase-encoding direction originating from the moving structure. In the chest, such phase-encoding motion artifacts most often arise from the major blood vessels or the heart. It is therefore advantageous to choose a phase-encoding direction that avoids obscuring the region of interest by considering the direction of the expected artifact. A more complex technique to minimize the effect of this phase-encoding motion artifact can sometimes be used with discretion in thoracic MRI. The result of these complex gradient profiles is that the SNR on T1-weighted and proton density–weighted scans is decreased. The signal arising from flowing blood is also increased, which further reduces the contrast between blood and the vessel wall.

Respiratory motion results in a series of ghost images that extend through the image, being most visible in the subcutaneous fat of the anterior chest wall, oriented along the phase-encoding direction. This artifact can be reduced by altering the sequence in which the phase-encoding views or steps are obtained.[22,23] This technique in which the respiratory cycle is monitored and the level of phase encoding is chosen according to the level of inspiration is known as *respiratory compensation.* In the reconstruction process, the phase-encoding steps can be reordered to shorten the apparent respiratory cycle (high-order sort) or to make it appear as if only very long inspiration has occurred (low-order sort). Either technique minimizes the respiratory motion artifact without lengthening the scan time or decreasing the signal strength. Respiratory compensation should be used in most thoracic imaging sequences. A flow artifact arises from blood flowing into the plane at imaging during a scan sequence. The region adjacent to the image volume in conventional multisliced imaging does not receive RF pulses. As a consequence, the spin momentum of the tissues is completely relaxed. When these relaxed spins enter the image plane, they are of relatively high signal intensity. Furthermore, the consequence of flow during the pulse sequence is that the molecules acquire a random phase, which results in a large phase-encoding motion artifact. This artifact can be decreased by presaturating and dephasing the inflowing spins with 90° pulses,[24] reducing the signal produced by the inflowing blood. This reduction, however, results in increased slice acquisition time and increased power deposition. Spatial presaturation should nevertheless be used in all MR thoracic scans.

OVERVIEW

Open-configuration MR systems use various magnet types and allow easy access to the patient. They allow the patient table to be placed along the axis of the magnet, allowing easy access to the patient from either side. If necessary, the table can be placed perpendicular to the axis of the magnet, allowing easy access for an operator at the head of the table.

Conventional spin-echo T1, T2, and other image sequences are easily obtained on the magnet. These images are used as a baseline to localize the area of interest and to compare with cross-section or other image data acquired in the previous work-up of the patient. Once the area of interest is localized, care is taken to ensure that the region is included in the central 30 cm of the field; this approach has the most homogeneous flux and defines the region in which electronic spatial coordinate guidance is possible.[25]

For precise placement of a biopsy needle or RF ablation, many systems use a hand-held probe, which allows the operator to select and control image orientation and location. Close communication between the operator and technologist at the MR console is important. Current systems allow sequential and simultaneous image data collection, processing, and display, so new images may be visualized as fast as every 2 sec. Images can be displayed on various consoles, including those located in the magnet room, to allow the operator real-time feedback.

The ability to advance the RF probe or the tip of an instrument to the exact target region is of great interest in the development of interventional MR systems. Optical digitizer systems that allow 3D localization of a probe are available. These systems allow localization and spatial relationship of the probe to be known at all times. Similar techniques are being used to assist with tip localization of various instruments. These techniques include diagnostic bronchoscopy, laryngoscopy, interventional biopsy, and RF ablation.[26]

DIAGNOSTIC APPLICATIONS

Lung parenchyma

MR is more sensitive than CT for detecting lung nodules that are difficult to differentiate from adjacent vessels on CT.[27] MR is as least as sensitive as CT for the detection of pulmonary metastatic nodules larger than 5 mm in diameter.[27,28] The detection rate of small nodules is improved by using short time inversion recovery (STIR) sequences[29] and may also be improved by the use of low-field strength magnets (0.2 T) rather than the usual high-field strength magnets (1.5 T). The low-field strengths reduce the induced susceptibility gradients in aerated lung compared with high-field strengths. MRI can help better characterize cystic lesions as a result of the higher signal strength[30,31] or fluid levels[32] seen on T2-weighted sequences. This differentiation can sometimes be difficult on CT because the high protein content results in soft-tissue attenuation in some lesions.[33]

MRI of the lung parenchyma has been of little clinical value.[1,4,32,34] Conventional spin-echo sequences yield little signal intensity from inflated lung parenchyma because of low proton density. The presence of innumerable air or soft-tissue (alveolar wall) interfaces (which result in large susceptibility-induced magnetic field gradients caused by internal magnetic field inhomogeneities and intravoxel phase dispersion) and cardiac and respiratory motion, (which results in significant signal loss and image degradation).[35,36] Healthy or subtle lung infiltration cannot be adequately assessed with MRI.[37] Additionally, the inability to reliably detect calcification further results in MR being inferior to CT in the detection and characterization of solitary lung nodules.[38] MR can, however, differentiate one pulmonary nodule from end-on vessels, especially in the perihilar region.[27,38]

Ultrashort TE gradient echo sequences[10] and short TE spin-echo sequences[39,40] have been developed as a potential solution to some of the problems encountered when imaging the lung parenchyma. Use of an alternate projection reconstruction algorithm, similar to that used in CT, allows the production of proton density–weighted images. This technique improves visualization of aerated lung parenchyma in peripheral vessels, but the effect of physiologic motion in the chest is accentuated, and the images show little tissue contrast. Moreover, the projection reconstruction algorithm is highly susceptible to magnetic field inhomogeneity, which leads to further blurring in the reconstructed images.[35]

Short echo delay (TE, 7 msec) has been used to compensate for the very short T2 relaxation time in inflated lung parenchyma when using conventional spin-echo sequences. This technique uses a standard 2D Fourier transformation reconstruction algorithm and can be easily performed with only minimal modifications on most commercial scanners. This technique leads to a 3.5-fold increase in the SNR from aerated lung.[39]

MR has been used to quantitate lung water content and to differentiate cardiogenic from noncardiogenic causes.[3,41–44] Several animal models using small bore magnets have shown that MRI techniques can be used to quantitate absolute lung water content,[45] to reliably detect changes in lung water content, and to show its distribution in various types of experimental edema.[9,46] Recent work in healthy volunteers suggests that MRI measurements of relative lung water changes in clinical pulmonary edema should be feasible. In healthy volunteers, measurements of average lung density, lung density gradient, and pleural pressure gradients obtained with MR were similar to those obtained with more invasive techniques.[19] Disease processes decrease the elastic properties of the lung and thus affect lung density, suggesting that MRI determination of lung water content and lung density should prove useful in the assessment of parenchymal lung disease. Different MRI characteristics for types of experimental pulmonary edema have been found in some studies[42] but not in others.[47,48] Although high-resolution CT remains superior to MRI for assessing parenchymal disease,[49,50] MRI may have a role in assessing the activity of the disease process.[20,48,51,52] The ability of MRI to differentiate relaxation times of different tissues based on their differences in free and bound water fractions may be of value. MRI may be able to differentiate acute and chronic alveolar tissue from chronic fibrosis. In well-established animal models involving radiation pneumonitis in rats[52] and bleomycin-induced toxicity in mice,[41] the T2 values measured in the parenchyma lengthened with the development of acute edema and inflammatory cell infiltrate, whereas T1 shortening occurred with the onset of fibrosis. In clinical studies, MRI was equivalent to high-resolution CT in its ability to show abnormalities correlating with active disease, although high-resolution CT was superior overall.[53] MR signal intensity correlates with clinical severity of disease and potential response to treatment, with a decrease in signal intensity in patients who show clinical improvement after treatment.[52]

MR has a potential role in differentiating various causes of alveolar opacification[20,50,54] and is comparable with high-resolution CT in the assessment of alveolar opacification.[53] The pathologic appearances are comparable to those on the simultaneously acquired MRI scans.[54] The presence of alveolar opacification, reticulation, nodules, and interlobular septal thickening is reflected best by proton density– and T1-weighted MRI scans. T2-weighted images add no further diagnostic information because of a marked decrease in signal intensity.

Fibrosis is often a result of treatment in patients with thoracic malignancies. Because of different relaxation characteristics, MR should allow differentiation of active inflammatory or neoplastic disease from fibrotic disease. Several reports using T2-weighted MRI[55] or T1-weighted gadopentetate-enhanced sequences[56] have shown that fibrosis can be differentiated from recurrent tumor. Because of the inflation-dependent T2 shortening caused by susceptibility artifact, this use of signal differences is not clinically useful. Further differentiation of tumor and associated inflammatory disease is difficult because of overlapping in the influence on T2 and T1 relaxation curves.[55,57]

The ability to guide biopsy procedures to specific locations of abnormal signal using interventional MR offers the potential for improved diagnostic yield not possible with conventional CT. This capability may be of particular benefit for differentiating neoplastic disease from inflammatory tissue or surgical fibrosis in the initial staging and follow-up of patients with lymphoma, lung cancer, and metastatic disease.

The mediastinum and hila

MRI is the modality of choice for diagnosing mediastinal or hilar lesions in patients who cannot tolerate iodinated contrast agents and for imaging posterior mediastinal or prevertebral masses.[32,58] Accurate delineation of the spinal cord and spinal canal on MR, together with the ability to perform multiplanar reconstructions, affords MR an advantage over CT in the evaluation of lesions adjacent to the spine.[32] MRI may also be used in the evaluation of the mediastinum and hila after conventional CT examination when further clarification is required. MRI has better inherent soft-tissue contrast; the streak artifacts that occur from edges of pulsatile vascular structures, especially in contrast-enhanced CT, are not seen. Although MRI is not superior to CT in the differentiation of benign from malignant lesions (and should not be performed for this purpose),[37,59–61] it can occasionally characterize fluid-filled or necrotic lesions better than CT. The proteinaceous content of these lesions may result in soft-tissue attenuation on CT,[33] whereas prolongation of the T1 and T2 values in these lesions is well-shown on MRI.[61]

MRI is more accurate than CT in diagnosing mediastinal invasion[62] and vascular invasion by lung cancer.[7,56,63,64] MRI is therefore recommended as a secondary imaging modality in the evaluation of lung cancer staging, particularly when mediastinal, vascular, or cardiac invasion is suspected. Despite early optimism, MRI is not better than CT in its ability to detect and define mediastinal lymph nodes.[29,62,63,65–70] Although some studies have reported that MRI shows nodes in the aortic-pulmonary window and subcarinal regions[37,46,64,71,72] because mf the ability to image in multiaxial planes, it is not more accurate. However, MRI is more accurate than CT in the diagnosis of tracheobronchial lymphadenopathy in patients with lung cancer,[7–9,29,63] but this accuracy may not offer any advantage with respect to clinical management and outcome. MRI is no more sensitive than CT in the differentiation of benign hyperplasia from malignant involvement.[73,73a] The MR appearances of a healthy thymus and thymic abnormalities are well-described;[1,74,75] although MR is excellent for the diagnosis and evaluation of thymic lesions, it does not have a significant advantage over conventional CT.[76,77]

Heavily T2-weighted MR sequences may help differentiate nonobstructive passive lobar atelectasis from atelectasis caused by a hilar-obstructing lesion if CT evaluation has been inconclusive.[29,56,78,79] On T2-weighted images, lung consolidation has a higher signal than the hilar mass, whereas the nonobstructive collapse has a lower signal intensity.[79] It has been reported that by using gadopentetate-enhanced T1-weighted imaging, this differentiation can be improved further.[64] MR is also useful in identifying underlying mass lesions in the completely opacified hemithorax.[80]

Radiation-induced fibrosis and recurrent tumor in the mediastinum can sometimes be differentiated. Because of the similar signal from acute inflammatory tissue and tumor, differentiation between the two is impossible.[55,57] MRI has a significant role in the follow-up of patients with treated mediastinal Hodgkin's lymphoma.[32,81] After radiation treatment, the residual mediastinal masses on T2-weighted images showed significantly decreased intensity in most patients.[81] Detection of a high-intensity residual mass is not specific for tumor but has been used as an indication for the need for biopsy or close follow-up.[82] The MR appearances of untreated mediastinal masses associated with fibrosis have also been reported in patients with lymphomas[83] and fibrosing mediastinitis.[84]

MRI should be ideal for performing image-guided procedures of the mediastinum and hilum because of the exquisite soft-tissue contrast, multiplanar capability, intrinsic flow sensitivity, and lack of ionizing radiation. However, respiratory and cardiac motion artifacts are an increased problem with real-time continuous imaging than with the conventional breathhold imaging techniques. The detection of lesions is improved by using STIR sequences[29] and, possibly by the use of low-field magnets. Better characterization of lesions is also a result of the higher signal strength of tumor-containing tissue or fluid levels (seen on T2-weighted sequences).[30,31] This differentiation can sometimes be difficult on CT because the high protein content results in the same tissue attenuation in some lesions.[33] Thus, low-field MR is a useful technique for identifying the nature of the lesion, which influences the nature of the therapeutic or interventional diagnostic procedure being planned.

Chest wall and pleural lesions

MR is excellent for the assessment of the chest wall. T1-weighted sequences are best for evaluation of tumor invasion of intramuscular fat and for assessment of the extent of chest wall involvement. T2-weighted sequences are optimal for differentiation of tumor and edema (which produce high signal) from the surrounding muscle (which has low signal intensity). Although the destruction of cortical bone is better seen with CT, marrow involvement by tumor is better identified by signal changes with MR. As a result of the superior contrast and multiple imaging planes, MR allows better presurgical delineation of the extent of chest wall disease than obtained by CT. MR reliably assesses primary chest wall tumors[64] and chest wall extension of bronchogenic carcinoma[8,78,82] and lymphoma.[63] This tissue characterization and spatial resolution allow localization for both biopsy procedures and RF ablation therapy on an open low-field system.

MR appearances of lymph nodes and arteriovenous malformation are characteristic, and these problems can be easily diagnosed on thoracic MR evaluation. In general, however, considerable overlap exists between the MR signal characteristics of benign and malignant lesions, and MR offers no benefit over CT in the differentiation between these two pathologies. It has been suggested that homogeneous signal intensity and smooth margins are more common in benign tumors, whereas malignant lesions are more likely to have heterogeneous signal and irregular margins.[64]

Pleural fluid collections can be easily identified, as can associated pleural thickening or nodularity. Drainage of a pleural fluid (with an interactive feedback as to how much fluid is being drained) and the effect of lung reexpansion can easily be achieved using open MR techniques. This capability can improve overall outcome in the drainage and installation of sclerosing agents for recurrent symptomatic effusions in the setting of malignancy. In addition, direct installation of antibiotic therapy using visualization of the site of deposition may improve the outcome for treatment of infective pleural collections in immunocompromised patients.

Brachial-plexopathy

MRI provides superior delineation of healthy anatomy of the brachial-plexus,[85,86] mainly because of its multiplanar capabilities and superior soft-tissue contrast.[87–89] The lack of beam attenuation artifacts from bone and the accurate identification of adjacent vasculature are further advantages of thoracic MR over CT.[90] Although few experiences have been published, MR is superior to other imaging techniques for evaluating brachial plexus trauma,[87,91] differentiating fibrosis from tumor,[91] and documenting or excluding brachial plexus involvement by malignancy.[12,88,89,91]

The suggested MR technique for suspected peripheral brachial-plexopathy is as follows: the anatomy is first mapped with T1-weighted images in at least two planes, and the study is completed with selective use of other pulse sequences in the appropriate anatomic plane to delineate lesions and associated (e.g., vascular) pathologic abnormalities. Limitations in MR evaluations of brachial-plexopathy include limited experience with appropriate use of gadolinium; limited data concerning differentiation between tumor, fibrosis, and radiation injury, specifically in this region; and limited experience with subgross trauma[91] and idiopathic neuritis.

CONCLUSIONS

The potential for open low-field interventional MR techniques seems great. Many minimally invasive procedures, ranging from biopsies to RF ablation, and minimally invasive surgical resections seem possible. With the advent of increasingly aggressive treatment of severe obstructive pulmonary disease in the form of lung reduction surgery, the potential to perform such procedures using a minimally invasive technique is attractive. Interventional MR techniques may allow these complicated procedures to be performed in patients who are highly susceptible to cardiac or respiratory instability without major changes in the thoracic chest wall function resulting in decreasing morbidity and overall health care costs. RF ablation may allow tumors to be reduced in size before surgical resection. Interventional therapeutic techniques using 3D imaging modalities with good visualization are likely to become an important part of medical practice. Techniques that allow excellent characterization without exposing patients to radiation will likely dominate this exciting area.

REFERENCES

1. Gamsu G, Sostman D: Magnetic resonance imaging of the thorax, *Am Rev Respir Dis* 139:254, 1989.
2. Webb WR: The role of magnetic resonance imaging in the assessment of patients with lung cancer: a comparison with computed tomography, *J Thorac Imaging* 4:65, 1989.
3. Webb WR, Sostman HD: MR imaging of thoracic disease: clinical uses, *Radiology* 182:621, 1992.
4. Fisher MR: Magnetic resonance for the evaluation of the thorax, *Chest* 95:166, 1989.
5. Webb WR: *Mediastinum and hila.* In Partain CL and others, editors: *Magnetic resonance imaging,* ed 2, Philadelphia, 1988, WB Saunders.
6. Brown LR, Aughenbaugh GL: Masses of the anterior mediastinum: CT and MR imaging, *Am J Roentgenol* 157:1171, 1991.
7. Webb WR: Magnetic resonance imaging of the hila and mediastinum, *Cardiovasc Intervent Radiol* 8:306, 1986.
8. Glazer GM, and others: Imaging of the pulmonary hilum: a prospective comparative study in patients with lung cancer, *Am J Roentgenol* 145:245, 1985.
9. Webb WR, and others: Magnetic resonance imaging of the normal and abnormal pulmonary hila, *Radiology* 152:89, 1984.
10. Bergin CJ, and others: MR evaluation of chest wall involvement in malignant lymphoma, *J Comput Assist Tomogr* 14:928, 1990.
11. Haggar AM, and others: Chest-wall invasion by carcinoma of the lung: detection by MR imaging, *Am J Roentgenol* 148:1075, 1987.
12. Heelan RT, and others: Superior sulcus tumors: CT and MR imaging, *Radiology* 170:637, 1989.
13. McLoud TC, and others: MR imaging of superior sulcus carcinoma, *J Comput Assist Tomogr* 12:233, 1989.
14. Jolesz FA, Shtern F: The operating room of the future: report of the National Cancer Institutes workshop. Imaging-guided stereotactic tumor diagnosis and treatment, *Invest Radiol* 27:326, 1992.
15. Jolesz FA, Blumenfield SM: Interventional use of magnetic resonance imaging, *Magn Reson Q* 10:85, 1994.
16. Silverman SG, and others: Interactive MR-guided biopsy in an open configuration MR imaging system, *Radiology* 197:175, 1995.
17. Durney CH, and others: Calculation and interpretation of inhomogeneous line broadening in models of lungs and other heterogeneous structures, *J Magn Reson* 85:554, 1989.
18. Morris AH, and others: A new nuclear magnetic resonance property of lung, *J Appl Physiol* 58:759, 1985.
19. Mayo JR, McKay A, Müller NL: T2 relaxation time in MR imaging of normal and abnormal lung parenchyma, *Radiology* 177:313, 1990 (abstract).
20. Moore EH, and others: MRI of pulmonary airspace disease: experimental model and preliminary clinical results, *Am J Roentgenol* 146:1123, 1986.
21. Edelstein WA, and others: Spin warp NMR imaging and applications to human whole-body imaging, *Phys Med Biol* 25:751, 1980 (letter).
22. Bailes DR, and others: Respiratory ordered phase encoding (ROPE): a method for reducing respiratory motion artifacts in MR imaging, *J Comput Assist Tomogr* 9:835, 1985.

23. Wood ML, Henkelman RM: Suppression of respiratory motion artifacts in magnetic resonance imaging, *Med Phys* 13:794, 1986.
24. Felmlee JP, Ehmann RL: Spatial presaturation: a method for suppressing flow artifacts and improving depiction of vascular anatomy in MR imaging, *Radiology* 164:559, 1987.
25. Sinha S, and others: Pulse sequence optimization for use with a biopsy needle in MRI, *Magn Reson Imaging* 7:575, 1989.
26. vanSonnenberg E, and others: A wire-sheath system for MR-guided biopsy and drainage: laboratory studies and experience in 10 patients, *Am J Roentgenol* 151:1088, 1988.
27. Doppman JL, and others: Detection of ACTH-producing bronchial carcinoid tumors: MR imaging vs. CT, *Am J Roentgenol* 156:39, 1991.
28. Feuerstein IM, and others: Pulmonary metastases: MR imaging with surgical correlation-a prospective study, *Radiology* 192:123, 1992.
29. Webb WR, and others: Bronchogenic carcinoma: staging with MR compared with staging with CT and surgery, *Radiology* 156:117, 1985.
30. Barakos JA, and others: High signal intensity lesions of the chest in MR imaging, *J Comput Assist Tomogr* 13:797, 1989.
31. Naidich DP, and others: Congenital anomalies of the lungs in adults: MR diagnosis, *Am J Roentgenol* 151:13, 1988.
32. Weinreb JC, Naidich DP: Thoracic magnetic resonance imaging, *Clin Chest Med* 12:33, 1991.
33. Mendelson DS, and others: Bronchogenic cysts with high CT numbers, *Am J Roentgenol* 140:463, 1983.
34. Gefter W: Chest applications of magnetic resonance imaging: an update, *Radiol Clin North Am* 26:573, 1988.
35. Bergin CJ, Glover GH, Pauly JM: Lung parenchyma: magnetic susceptibility in MR imaging, *Radiology* 180:845, 1991.
36. Naidich DP, Weinreb JC, Schinella R: MR imaging of pulmonary parenchyma: comparison with CT in evaluating cadaveric lung specimens, *J Comput Assist Tomogr* 14:595, 1990.
37. de Geer G, and others: MR characteristics of benign lymph node enlargement in sarcoidosis and Castleman's disease, *Eur J Radiol* 6:145, 1986.
38. Muller NL, Gamsu G, Webb WR: Pulmonary nodules: detection using magnetic resonance and computed tomography, *Radiology* 155:687, 1985.
39. Mayo JR, McKay A, Müller NL: MR imaging of the lungs: value of short TE spin-echo pulse sequences, *Am J Roentgenol* 159:951, 1992.
40. Bergin CJ, Pauly JM, Macovski MA: Lung parenchyma: projection reconstruction MR imaging, *Radiology* 179:777, 1991.
41. Taylor CR, and others: Proton relaxation times in bleomycin-induced lung injury, *Invest Radiol* 22:621, 1987.
42. Schmidt HC, Daw-Guey T, Higgins CB: Pulmonary edema: an MR study of permeability and hydrostatic types in animals, *Radiology* 158:297, 1986.
43. Cutillo AG, and others: Determination of lung water content and distribution by nuclear magnetic resonance, *J Appl Physiol* 57:583, 1984.
44. Cutillo AG, and others: Determination of lung water content and distribution by nuclear magnetic resonance imaging, *J Thorac Imaging* 1:39, 1986.
45. Levitt RG, and others: Magnetic resonance imaging of mediastinal and hilar masses: comparison with CT, *Am J Roentgenol* 145:9, 1985.
46. Webb WR, and others: Sagittal MR imaging of the chest: normal and abnormal, *J Comput Assist Tomogr* 9:471, 1985.
47. Vinitski S, and others: Assessment of lung water by magnetic resonance in three types of pulmonary edema, *Heart Vessels* 4:88, 1988.
48. Cutillo AG, and others: Clinical implications of nuclear magnetic resonance lung research, *Chest* 96:643, 1989.
49. Kinsella D, and others: The role of magnetic resonance imaging in cystic fibrosis, *Clin Radiol* 44:23, 1991.
50. Müller NL, Mayo JR, Lentle BC: Imaging of diffuse lung diseases: past, present, and future, *Radiol Clin North Am* 29:1115, 1991.
51. Craig DA, and others: MRI findings in pulmonary sarcoidosis, *Magn Reson Imaging* 6:567, 1988.
52. McFadden RG, Carr TJ, Wood TE: Proton magnetic resonance imaging to stage activity of interstitial lung disease, *Chest* 92:31, 1987.
53. Müller NL, Mayo JR, Zwirewich CV: Value of MR imaging in the evaluation of chronic infiltrative lung diseases: comparison with CT, *Am J Roentgenol* 158:1205, 1992.
54. Primack SL, and others: MR imaging of infiltrative lung disease: comparison with pathologic findings in 22 patients, *J Comput Assist Tomogr* 18:233, 1994.
55. Glazer HS, and others: Radiation fibrosis: differentiation from recurrent tumor by MR imaging, *Radiology* 156:721, 1985.
56. Kameda K, Adachi S, Kono M: Detection of T-factor in lung cancer using magnetic resonance imaging and computed tomography, *J Thorac Imaging* 3:73, 1988.
57. Lee JKT, Glazer HS: Controversy in the MR imaging appearance of fibrosis, *Radiology* 177:21, 1990.
58. Burk DJ, and others: Spinal and paraspinal neurofibromatosis: surface coils MR imaging at 1.5 T, *Radiology* 156:721, 1987.
59. Glazer GM, and others: Mediastinal lymph nodes: relaxation time/pathologic correlation and implications in staging of lung cancer with MR imaging, *Radiology* 168:429, 1988.
60. Ross JS, and others: Magnetic resonance of the chest: initial experience with imaging and in vivo T1 and T2 calculations, *Radiology* 152:95, 1984.
61. Gamsu G, and others: Magnetic resonance imaging of benign mediastinal masses, *Radiology* 151:709, 1984.
62. Laurent F, and others: Bronchogenic carcinoma staging: CT vs. MR imaging; assessment with surgery, *Eur J Cardiothorac Surg* 2:31, 1988.
63. Webb WR, and others: CT and MR imaging in staging non-small cell bronchogenic carcinoma: report of the Radiologic Diagnostic Oncology Group, *Radiology* 178:705, 1991.
64. Kono M, and others: MR imaging in the assessment of lung cancer patients: primary lung cancer staging, evaluation of therapeutic effect and diagnosis of recurrent tumor, *Nippon Igaku Hoshasen Gakkai Zasshi* 49:831, 1989.
65. Musset D, and others: Primary lung cancer staging: prospective comparative study of MR imaging with CT, *Radiology* 160:607, 1986.
66. Batra P, and others: Evaluation of intrathoracic extent of lung cancer by plain chest radiography, computed tomography, and magnetic resonance imaging, *Am Rev Respir Dis* 137:1456, 1988.
67. Poon PY, and others: Mediastinal lymph node metastases from bronchogenic carcinoma: detection with MNR imaging and CT, *Radiology* 162:651, 1987.
68. Grenier P, and others: Preoperative thoracic staging of lung cancer: CT and MR evaluation, *Diagn Intervent Radiol* 1:23, 1989.
69. Patterson GA, and others: A prospective evaluation of magnetic resonance imaging, computed tomography, and mediastinoscopy in the preoperative assessment of mediastinal node status in bronchogenic carcinoma, *J Thorac Cardiovasc Surg* 94:679, 1987.
70. Platt JF, and others: Radiologic evaluation of the subcarinal lymph nodes: a comparative study, *Am J Roentgenol* 151:279, 1988.
71. Batra P, and others: MR imaging of the thorax: a comparison of axial, coronal, and sagittal imaging planes, *J Comput Assist Tomogr* 12:75, 1988.
72. Webb WR, and others: Coronal magnetic resonance imaging of the chest: normal and abnormal, *Radiology* 153:729, 1984.
73. Glazer HS, and others: The thoracic aorta studies by MR imaging, *Radiology* 157:149, 1985.

73a. Panicek DM: MR imaging for pulmonary metastases? *Radiology* 182:10, 1992.

74. de Geer G, Webb WR, Gamsu G: Normal thymus: assessment with MR and CT, *Radiology* 158:313, 1986.
75. Molina PL, Siegel MJ, Glazer HS: Thymic masses on MR imaging, *Am J Roentgenol* 155:495, 1990.
76. Batra P, Herrmann C, Mulder D: Mediastinal imaging in myasthenia gravis: correlation of chest radiography, CT, MR, and surgical findings, *Am J Roentgenol* 148:515, 1987.
77. Emskotter T, Trampe H, Lachenmayer L: Magnetic resonance imaging in myasthenia gravis: an alternative to mediastinal computerized tomography? *Dtsch Med Wochenschr* 113:1508, 1988.
78. Tobler J, and others: Differentiation of proximal bronchogenic carcinoma from postobstructive lobar collapse by magnetic resonance imaging: comparison with computed tomography, *Invest Radiol* 22:538, 1987.

79. Herold CJ, Kuhlman JE, Zerhouni EA: Pulmonary atelectasis: signal patterns with MR imaging, *Radiology* 178:715, 1991.
80. Laissey JP, and others: Post-pneumonectomy evaluation of the chest: a prospective comparative study of MRI with CT, *Magn Reson Imaging* 7:55, 1989.
81. Nyman RS, and others: Residual mediastinal masses in Hodgkin disease: prediction of size with MR imaging, *Radiology* 170:435, 1989.
82. Webb WR: MR imaging of treated mediastinal Hodgkin disease, *Radiology* 170:315, 1989 (editorial).
83. Negendank WG, and others: Lymphomas: MR imaging contrast characteristics with clinical-pathologic correlations, *Radiology* 177:209, 1990.
84. Rholl KS, Levitt RG, Glazer HS: Magnetic resonance imaging of fibrosing mediastinitis, *Am J Roentgenol* 145:255, 1985.
85. Blair DN, and others: Normal brachial plexus: MR imaging, *Radiology* 165:763, 1987.
86. Kellman GM, and others: MR imaging of the supraclavicular region: normal anatomy, *Am J Roentgenol* 148:77, 1987.
87. Gupta RK, and others: MR evaluation of brachial plexus injuries, *Neuroradiology* 31:377, 1989.
88. Castagno AA, Shuman WP: MR imaging in clinically suspected brachial plexus tumor, *Am J Roentgenol* 149:1219, 1987.
89. Kneeland JB, and others: Diagnosis of diseases of the supraclavicular region by use of MR imaging, *Am J Roentgenol* 148:1149, 1987.
90. Armington WG, and others: Radiographic evaluation of brachial plexopathy, *Am J Neuroradiol* 8:361, 1987.
91. Rapoport S, and others: Brachial plexus: correlation of MR imaging with CT and pathologic findings, *Radiology* 167:161, 1988.

Chapter 38

MR–GUIDED BIOPSY IN THE ABDOMEN

David S. K. Lu, Stuart G. Silverman

With the advent of magnetic resonance (MR)–compatible instruments, monitoring devices, and open-configuration MR scanners, almost all of the major limitations of MR guidance for interventional procedures have been overcome. Although many forms of MRI-guided therapy are being envisioned, the ability to perform an MR-guided biopsy is basic to all MR-guided therapy. The development of a robust and practical system for MRI-guided biopsy is therefore of major importance. The need to perform abdominal biopsies under MRI guidance is increasing because improving MR technology is enabling detection of some lesions, especially hepatic lesions, not otherwise visible by ultrasound (US) or computed tomography (CT).[1]

MRI-guided biopsy for the liver was first described by Mueller, and others[2,3] using closed magnets and prototype nonferromagnetic needles. In these early reports, needle placement was first performed under US guidance, and the MRI scans confirmed needle placement in the lesion. These initial studies were the first to show the use of an MR-compatible needle. Other early works included the use of a wire-sheath system for biopsy in a closed magnet system.[4] In these closed magnet systems, conventional spin-echo pulse sequences were initially used. These sequences are being replaced with much faster gradient echo sequences.[5] However, despite faster imaging times, a fundamental problem of closed MR systems for abdominal biopsy remained: the radiologist does not have direct access to the patient, and multiple needle advancement steps are usually necessary to ensure proper needle advancement toward a target lesion. Also, the procedure is cumbersome and time consuming, with the patient having to move out of the magnet bore each time the needle is advanced.[6]

The recent development of open-configuration MRI systems solved the problem of patient access. Silverman and others first reported MRI-guided biopsies of the abdomen using an open-configuration MR system.[7] In this report, a 0.5-T vertically open MRI system specifically designed to guide interventions and surgery (Signa SP, General Electric Medical Systems, Milwaukee, Wis)[8] was used. The interventional scanner system included an integrated optical localizer and tracker, which allowed interactive control of the biopsy needle such that the biopsy could be guided by MRI alone. Other open-configuration MR systems have been successfully used for abdominal biopsies, including magnets that permit a horizontally open field for patient access (Magnetom Open, Siemens Medical Systems, Erlangen, Germany).[9,10] A complete discussion of the different open-configuration MRI systems is beyond the scope of this chapter and is discussed elsewhere.[11] Some open MR scanners were originally designed for claustrophobic patients and have limited guidance equipment. However, optional methods of localization (e.g., optical tracking, mechanical sensors, radiofrequency [RF] localizers, tip tracking[12,13]) are available as add-on equipment. Also, open systems can be used alone without an integrated guidance system or with a simple adjacent needle localizer to guide the entire biopsy procedure with MRI. This guidance can be accomplished as long as simultaneous imaging during needle manipulations and near immediate image feedback onto an in-room display monitor are available so that biopsy needles can be easily repositioned.

Basic localization techniques used in CT can be used for MR guidance. For example, skin markers can be used to locate the skin entry site relative to the target. The skin entrance site can also be localized with laser light or with a special grid designed for MRI taped to the skin surface.[14] Even the radiologist's finger can be used as a skin marker,[10] which can simultaneously approximate the needle angulation needed. Once the skin entrance site and needle angulation have been selected, the needle is advanced stepwise toward the lesion. Because upper abdominal structures move substantially during respiration, the true needle trajectory may not correspond to the original planned needle trajectory, therefore necessitating stepwise angulation adjustments. Thus, interactive, real-time (or near real-time) image updating is critical. On the 0.2-T horizontally open system and the 0.5-T vertically open system, an in-room display monitor shows rapidly updated images.

BIOPSY ON THE 0.5-T VERTICALLY OPEN-CONFIGURATION MAGNETIC RESONANCE IMAGING SYSTEM

At the Brigham & Women's Hospital, the first Signa SP vertically open MR system (General Electric Medical Systems, Milwaukee, Wis) was installed in 1994 (Fig. 38-1) with a fully equipped interventional MRI suite.[15] In this suite, all equipment is MRI compatible, including a noninvasive blood pressure monitor, an anesthesia delivery system (XL10 MRI Compatible Anesthesia Station, Ohmeda, Madison, Wis), a patient monitoring system with a pulse oximeter, an airway carbon dioxide monitor, electrocardiography (MagLife ODAM, Bruker, Wissembourg, France), and two-way audiovisual communication devices. Additional custom-made devices include an MR-compatible stethoscope, a laryngoscope containing lithium batteries, an intravenous pole, and an aluminum oxygen tank. Connections are also provided for vacuum, air, and anesthetic gases and for electrocautery, laser, and cryotherapy devices. Adjacent rooms were set up for the scanner console and for computer hardware. The suite also contains decontamination and clean rooms for handling and assembling instruments and a three-bed holding area for pre- and postoperative care.

Images are obtained from the center of the magnet where the homogeneous part of the field is located (12 ppm over 30 cm). Specially designed flexible surface coils operate as RF transmitters and receivers. These coils are applied to the surface of the patient overlying the anatomic region of interest. Imaging can be performed in a standard mode (as in a conventional scanner) or an interactive mode; the latter was designed specifically for interventional procedures. The two-way audio system facilitates the interactive mode by allowing communication be-

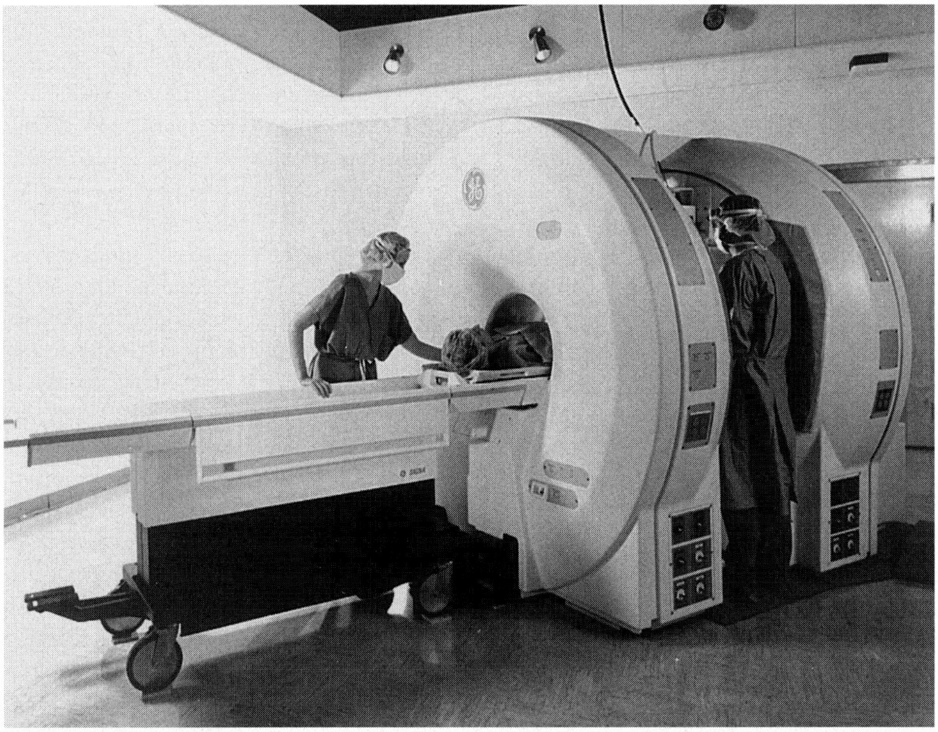

Fig. 38-1. Interventional magnetic resonance imaging (MRI) system (Signa SP, General Electric Medical Systems, Milwaukee, Wis) used at Brigham & Women's Hospital, Boston. The magnet is constructed using two interconnected cryostats with an opening to permit access to the patient. MRI is possible over a spherical volume about the center of the gap. An optical tracking system with sensors embedded above the interventional field determines the spatial location of a hand-held probe, which in turn determines the scan plane then displayed on the monitor. (From Lufkin RB, Gronemeyer DHW, Seibel RMM: *Interventional magnetic resonance imaging.* In Stark DD, Bradley WG: *Magnetic resonance imaging,* ed 3, St Louis, 1999, Mosby.)

tween the interventionalist in the suite and the technologist in the control room. The radiologist verbally communicates the imaging plane to the technologist in reference to a hand-held probe over the region of interest. Once scanning has been completed, the radiologist then views the images displayed on a video screen in the suite.

In the interactive mode, an optical tracking system is used to constantly identify the position of the probe. A three-dimensional (3D) optical digitizer (Pixsys 5000 Flashpoint Position Encoder, Image-guided Technologies, Boulder, Colo) uses three video sensors (built into the system on a rail above the interventional field), which localize the spatial position of two infrared light-emitting diodes (LEDs) mounted on a hand-held biopsy probe. The spatial information provided by the probe's LEDs is used to generate a normal axis along the handle of the probe and a position located at a specified offset from the probe. This spatial information is transmitted to a workstation (Sun Sparc 20, Sun Microsystems, Mountain View, Calif), which uses menu-driven applications to define the scan plane obtained by the MRI scanner. Thus, the position of the biopsy probe determines the scan plane.

The radiologist verbally communicates a desired plane to the technologist in the control room. Any plane may be selected. For example, standard axial, sagittal, and coronal planes can be obtained at the needle tip. Image planes relative to the instrument may be selected. Virtually any oblique or orthogonal plane relative to the long axis of the probe may be used. For abdominal biopsy, only the three orthogonal image planes are selected (Fig. 38-2). When the in-plane mode is selected, the image is in the plane of the long axis of the probe attached to the needle. When a perpendicular plane is selected, the image is in a plane perpendicular to the probe's long axis. The nomenclature *in-plane 90°* results in an image that is in the plane of the probe's long axis and is perpendicular to the floor. The nomenclature *in-plane 0°* results in an image that is in the plane of the needle's long axis and in a plane that is 90° or perpendicular to the in-plane 90° image. The perpendicular plane mode results in an image that is perpendicular to the long axis of the needle and can be positioned at the level of the needle tip. The displayed plane is relevant only to the probe position and not to the patient or the magnet. For a biopsy using an approach from the patient's lateral aspect with the long axis of the probe parallel to the floor, an in-plane 90° image is axial-like. However, when the probe is held in a vertical position perpendicular to the floor, an in-plane 90° image is sagittal-like.

The fundamental mechanism for this form of instrument tracking is that spatial information derived from the location of the LEDs is used to predict the path of the needle and the position of the needle tip. However, predicting the path of the needle and displaying it on the image require that the needle be straight. When the biopsy needle is attached to the end of the probe and an in-plane image is selected, the image will be in the long axis of the probe and will contain a straight needle. If the needle bends, however, the entire shaft (including the tip) may not be on the displayed image. When in the perpendicular mode, the system should know the exact length of the needle.

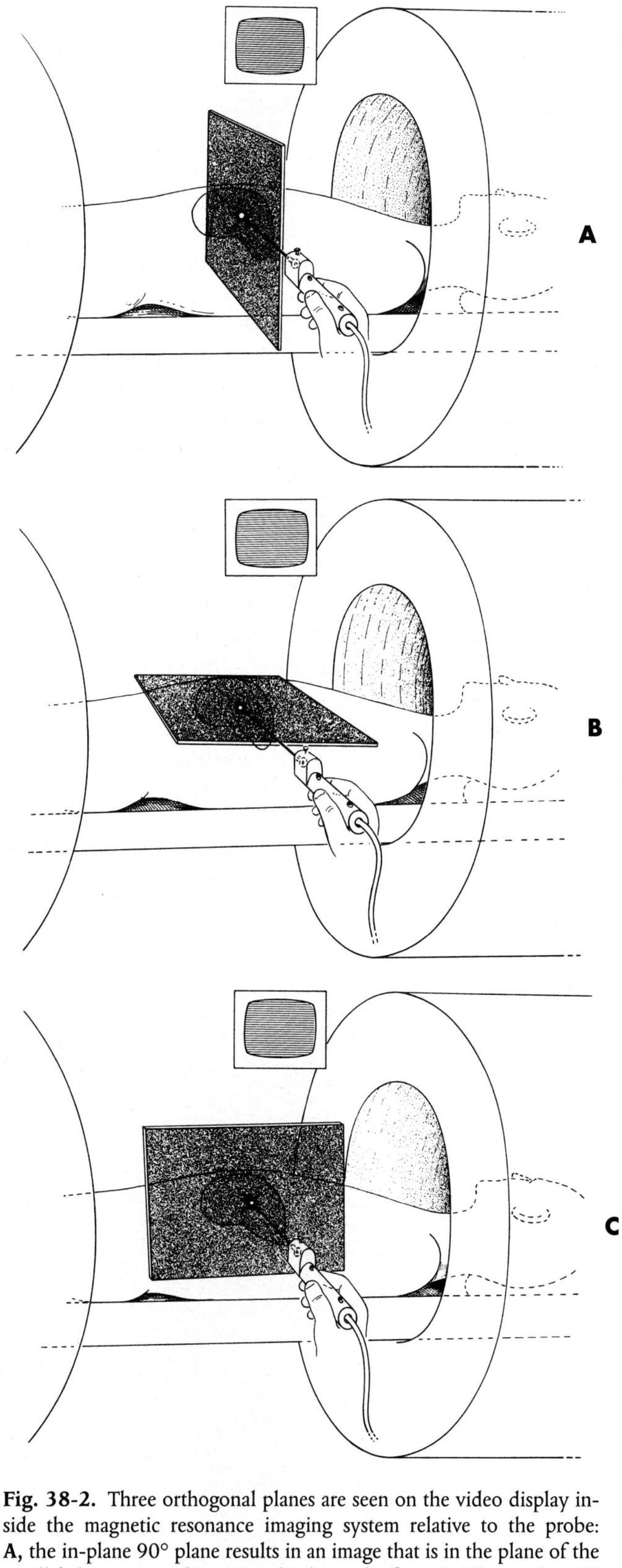

Fig. 38-2. Three orthogonal planes are seen on the video display inside the magnetic resonance imaging system relative to the probe: **A,** the in-plane 90° plane results in an image that is in the plane of the needle's long axis and is perpendicular to the floor. **B,** The in-plane 0° plane results in an image that is in the plane of the needle's long axis and in a plane that is 90° to the in-plane 90° view. **C,** The perpendicular plane results in an image that is perpendicular to the long axis of the needle at the level of the needle tip.

Then, a perpendicular image obtained at the same distance from the probe will accurately predict the position of the needle tip. If the precise needle length is unknown, the tip may not be displayed. Needle tip localization in MRI is a problem relative to CT because the appearance of the tip is not always discernible from the shaft. When the radiologist holds the probe attached to a biopsy needle for targeting, the expected trajectory of the needle is displayed as an icon or "virtual needle." This predicted trajectory is superimposed on the video screen image in the magnet bore as a white vertical contiguous line followed by a dashed line. The end of the contiguous line represents the predicted position of the needle tip. The dashed line displays the path the needle would take if it were advanced further. During the procedure, as the needle is advanced, the display shows the radiologist the position of the needle tip and the transgressed structures, the predicted path of the needle, the structures in the region of the path should the needle be advanced, and, when in-plane, the distance the needle should be advanced for the needle tip to reach the target.

The procedure for performing a biopsy using this system is as follows: using a prior MRI or CT scan, a flexible surface coil is positioned on the abdomen such that the entry point and lesion are within the imaging volume and such that the probe is within the field-of-view of the optical tracking system's videosensors (Fig. 38-3). Standard noninteractive scanning using a gradient echo sequence is used to check the surface coil placement. T1- and T2-weighted spin-echo pulse sequences may be needed to optimize lesion visualization. The region is scanned in the interactive mode using a nonsterile biopsy probe without an attached needle. For more rapid scanning, a fast gradient echo sequence (repetition time, 15.7 msec; echo time, 7.5 msec; flip angle, 30°, 10-mm thick sections) is used such that images are updated every 1.5 sec. The optimal entry point and angle to the lesion are determined by showing the needle icon projecting in the lesion on all three orthogonal planes. The skin site is then marked. A sterile interventional field is prepared along with a specially designed MRI-compatible procedure tray, which includes a ceramic MRI-compatible blade (Micro-Surgical Techniques, Fort Collins, Colo). All biopsy needles are MRI compatible (E-Z-EM, Westbury, NY; Cook, Bloomington, Ind). A needle of sufficient length to reach the lesion is chosen based on the depth of the lesion determined at the time of the initial interactive scanning. The biopsy needle is attached to the probe and the needle advanced (and viewed in the three orthogonal planes) along the planned path. Once the needle tip reaches the target lesion, it can be viewed in the lesion in all three planes (Fig. 38-4). The depth of needle insertion is determined by the images not by the depth estimate.

Preliminary biopsy data suggest that MRI-guided biopsy using this system is safe and accurate.[7] Test characteristics are similar to those reported with US- and CT-guided techniques. MRI can be used to biopsy lesions visible with MRI alone or seen best with MRI. However, although rare, equipment failure, claustrophobia, and lesion visibility may prevent the use of this system. Patients with cardiac pacemakers, cerebral aneurysm clips, or other MRI-incompatible devices and implants have not undergone MRI-guided biopsy. Also, patients with a history of active ischemic heart disease (ischemia on electrocardiography or re-

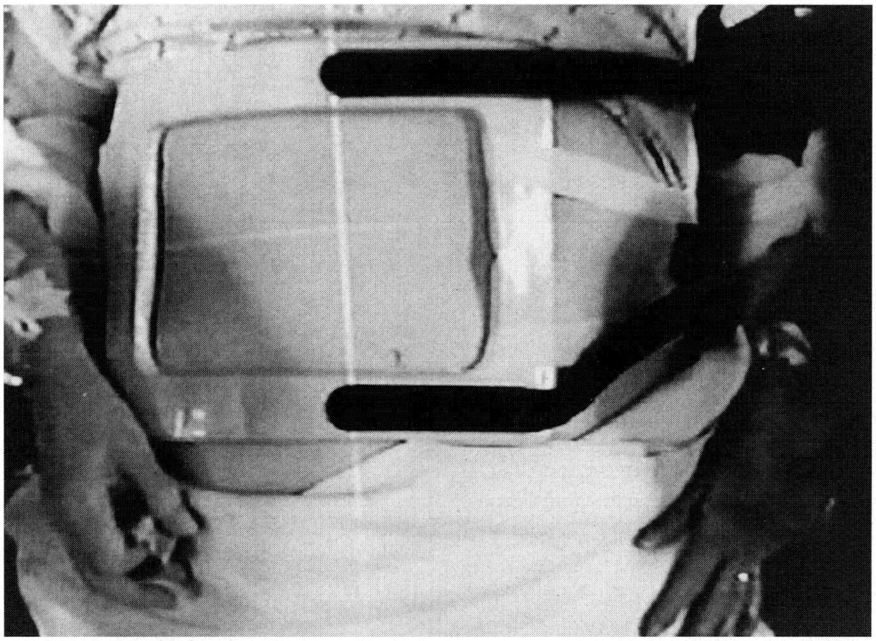

Fig. 38-3. The transmit and receive flexible surface coil used in the Signa SP system (General Electric Medical Systems, Milwaukee, Wis) shown in position from an overhead view during a magnetic resonance imaging–guided abdominal biopsy. The rectangular region is the surface area in which the cutaneous entry route is chosen.

cent symptoms of angina) have not been biopsied because ST and T wave electrocardiographic changes are distorted; therefore, intraprocedural silent ischemia could occur undetected.[16]

BIOPSY ON THE 0.2-T HORIZONTALLY OPEN-CONFIGURATION MAGNETIC RESONANCE IMAGING SYSTEM

The 0.2-T horizontally open-configuration MRI system consists of a C-shaped iron-core resistive magnet (Magnetom Open, Siemens Medical Systems, Erlangen, Germany) whose two magnet poles are 42 cm apart, allowing for a horizontally oriented open field for patient access (Fig. 38-5). Multiple MR-compatible accessories are also built into the suite, including a specially designed MR-compatible chair that facilitates access by the interventionalist to the patient, an adjustable optical light source specifically designed to illuminate the interventional field, and a mobile console with MR-compatible active matrix liquid crystal display monitor (1024 lines and 1280 pixels/line resolution). The height and angle of the liquid crystal display screen can be adjusted for optimal viewing by the physician. The console is also equipped with an RF-shielded mouse by which menu-driven functions of the scanner can be

A B C

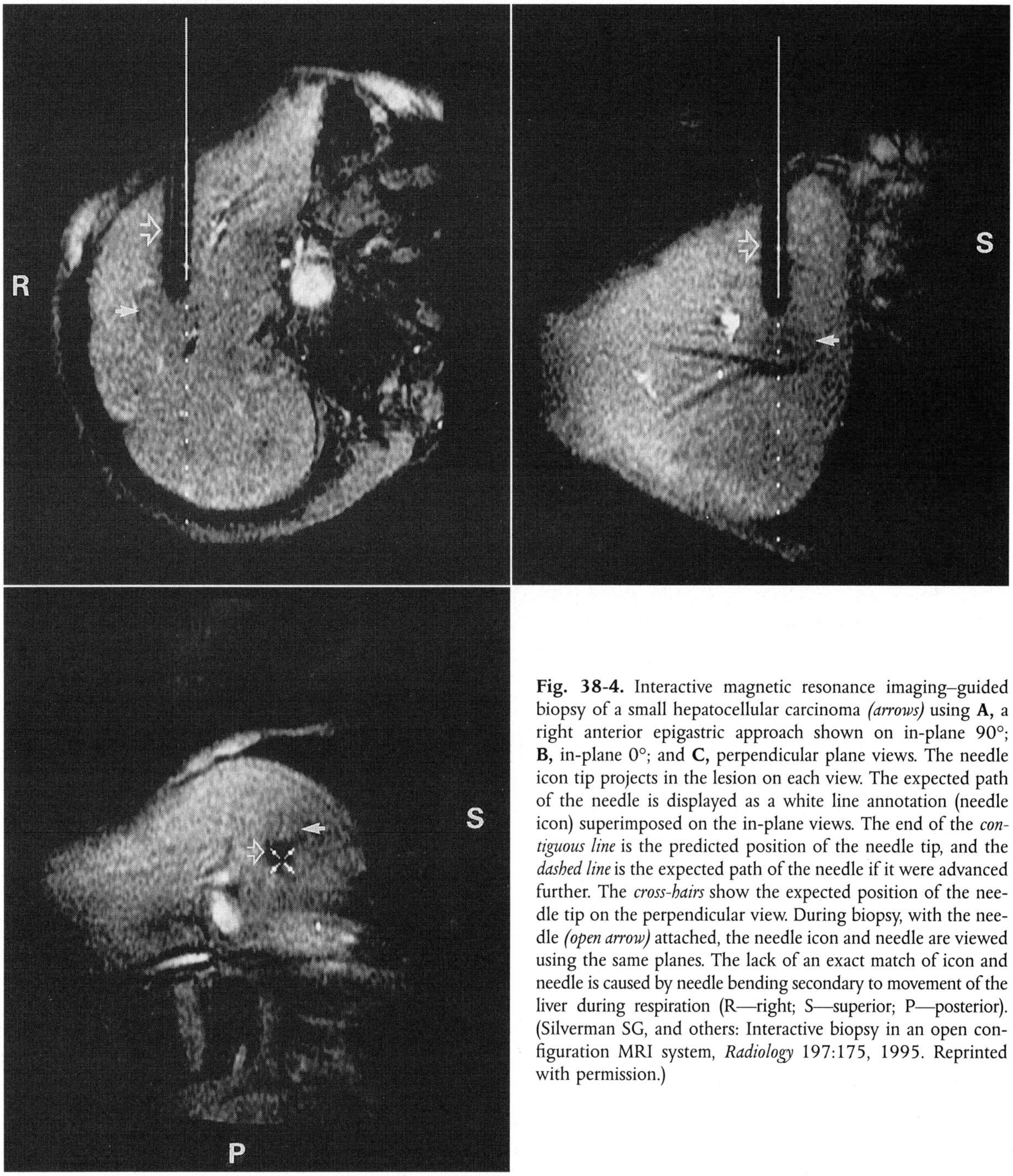

Fig. 38-4. Interactive magnetic resonance imaging–guided biopsy of a small hepatocellular carcinoma *(arrows)* using **A,** a right anterior epigastric approach shown on in-plane 90°; **B,** in-plane 0°; and **C,** perpendicular plane views. The needle icon tip projects in the lesion on each view. The expected path of the needle is displayed as a white line annotation (needle icon) superimposed on the in-plane views. The end of the *contiguous line* is the predicted position of the needle tip, and the *dashed line* is the expected path of the needle if it were advanced further. The *cross-hairs* show the expected position of the needle tip on the perpendicular view. During biopsy, with the needle *(open arrow)* attached, the needle icon and needle are viewed using the same planes. The lack of an exact match of icon and needle is caused by needle bending secondary to movement of the liver during respiration (R—right; S—superior; P—posterior). (Silverman SG, and others: Interactive biopsy in an open configuration MRI system, *Radiology* 197:175, 1995. Reprinted with permission.)

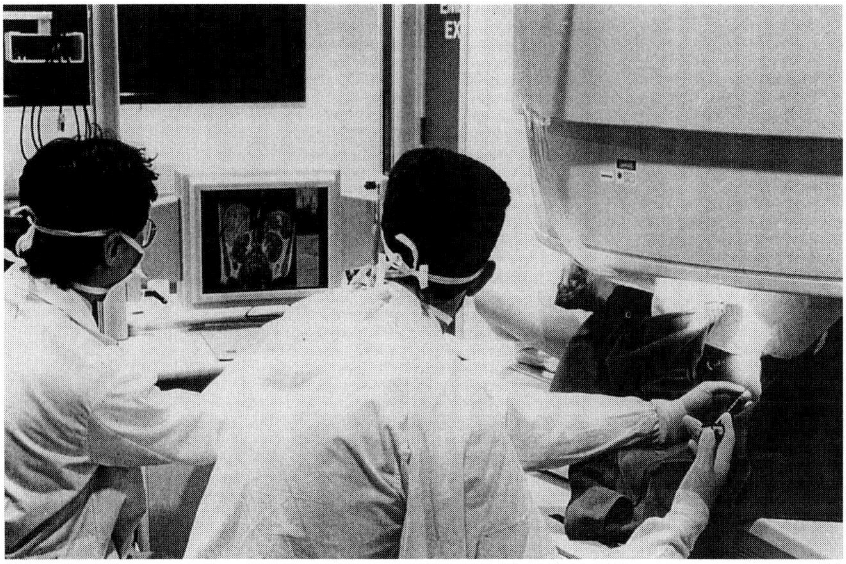

Fig. 38-5. A liver biopsy in the 0.2-T Magnetom open scanner system (Siemens Medical Systems, Erlangen, Germany). The patient is lying inside the scanner between vertically oriented magnet poles *(far right)*. Note the horizontally open access to the patient by the treating radiologist, who is continually holding the biopsy needle as it is advanced into the liver. At the same time, the radiologist is actively viewing the latest image updates on the liquid crystal display monitor (which shows the needle halfway toward the lesion) so that rapid interactive needle adjustments can be made. The technologist *(far left)* may control the scanner from inside the room next to the radiologist by using menu-driven functions through a mouse attached to the monitor.

operated from within the interventional suite, including selection of pulse sequences. Therefore, scanning can be controlled from within the room if desired. This option allows the MR technologist to work in the interventional suite, a useful feature if the technologist is also assisting with the biopsy procedure.

One of the first systems is installed at the University of California at Los Angeles Medical Center. Researchers have developed an abdominal biopsy technique using a free-hand technique with no need for additional stereotactic devices.[10] In this technique, first reported for liver biopsies, a conventional axial diagnostic sequence (T1 spin-echo, T2 fast spin-echo, or gradient echo sequence) is first used to find the plane containing the target lesion. Usually a T1-weighted gradient echo fast low-angle shot (FLASH) sequence is preferred because of the imaging speed and the possibility of breath-hold scanning. Once the lesion is identified, the radiologist decides on the approximate skin entrance site. The path from the skin entrance site to the target lesion defines the imaging plane. Because of the presence of the pleural reflection, many hepatic lesions tend to be located superior to where the ideal skin entrance site would be; therefore, a coronal or off-coronal plane may be desirable to image the needle path. A 10-sec breathhold, three-section, T1-weighted gradient echo sequence (FLASH) is then performed centered on the lesion, based on the reference axial image and in the chosen plane, with the radiologist's finger marking the skin entrance site. This approach can be repeated by adjusting the finger until it is seen with the lesion in the center slice. The fingertip marks the precise skin entrance site. At the same time, the radiologist's finger may also be used to give an approximation of the degree of cranial angulation needed to target the lesion.

Once the skin entrance site is marked and sterilely prepared, the MR-compatible biopsy needle is used to puncture the skin and is advanced toward the lesion. Fine needle angulation adjustments are made stepwise based on repeated image updating using the same coronal three-section gradient echo sequence. Departures of the actual needle course from the planned needle path can be identified in-plane and off-plane, the latter by seeing the needle in the adjacent sections. Because it takes 10 sec for each image acquisition and 3 sec for image display, a minimum of 13 seconds is needed for each needle adjustment. However, usually only several adjustment and advancement steps are necessary for the needle tip to reach the target lesion. The average time it requires, therefore, from initial skin puncture to accurate positioning of the needle tip in the lesion is approximately 2 to 3 min (Fig. 38-6).

Frahm, Gehl, and Robberg[9] reported successful MRI-guided biopsies of adrenal and pelvic masses using the Magnetom open scanner (Siemens Medical Systems, Erlangen, Germany).[9] Techniques similar to the liver biopsy technique could be applied in any open-configuration MR scanner and to other anatomic regions in the abdomen. For upper abdominal structures, because of respiratory motion, fast gradient echo sequences with adequate contrast resolution to reliably delineate the lesion and the needle trajectory would be preferred.

A significant limitation of the horizontally open magnet design is that some regions of the abdomen that require an ante-

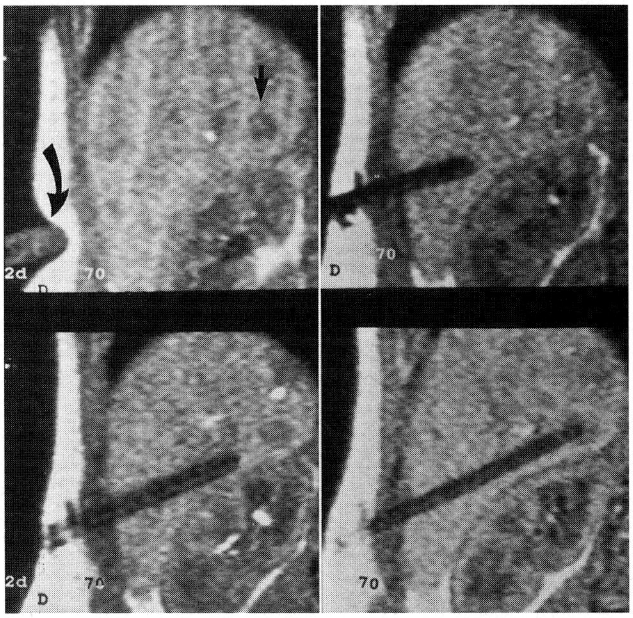

Fig. 38-6. Magnetic resonance–guided biopsy of focal liver mass using sequential coronal fast low-angle shot images (repetition time, 66 sec; echo time, 9 sec; flip angle, 70°) shows intermittent image updates during a biopsy. Note the radiologist's finger marking the skin entrance site *(curved arrow)* and approximate angulation toward the lesion *(black arrow),* with subsequent advancements of the needle.

rior percutaneous approach (e.g., left lobe of liver, pancreatic body, or omentum) cannot be easily performed. Some small adults and children may be able to be lie inside the scanner in the lateral decubitus position so that the anterior abdomen can be accessed. However, because most patients are not small enough for this position, patients with anterior masses that require an anterior approach are not candidates for biopsy in this type of scanner.

MRI-guided abdominal biopsy is used clinically in some centers. Although experience with MRI-guided abdominal biopsies using the 0.2-T open configuration scanner is still early and limited, the initial results are encouraging. Since US-guided abdominal biopsies are so efficient and accurate, MRI is rarely preferred if a lesion is easily visualized by US (particularly when cost is considered). However, some patients have lesions that are not seen well by US but that are seen by CT and MRI. In choosing between CT and MRI guidance, it should be noted that MRI provides continuous patient access and multiplanar imaging, which do not exist with current CT guidance techniques. Examples of lesions for which MR guidance would be preferable to CT guidance include hepatic masses located in the dome of the liver and adrenal gland masses. MR guidance avoids the pleural space and lung, and near real-time image feedback facilitates targeting a moving target.

Therefore, MRI-guided abdominal biopsy will likely be reserved for the following special circumstances:

1. Lesions not seen by US, seen equally well by CT and MRI, and requiring an angled or oblique approach to target will benefit.
2. Some lesions are viewed best (or only) with MRI. The interventional guidance modality should be the modality that visualizes the lesion the best. Many lesions may be clearly delineated by contrast-enhanced CT but not by precontrast CT, and most such lesions would be better depicted by MRI. Also, as diagnostic MRI techniques improve, more liver, pancreas, and other abdominal lesions are being detected only with MRI.[1]
3. Lesions that may also need MRI-guided therapy or have been treated with MRI-guided therapy (e.g., RF, laser, percutaneous ethanol ablation) may benefit. If MRI-guided therapy is planned, MRI can be used to biopsy the lesion before and after treatment.

Despite the significant progress in MR guidance of biopsy procedures, MRI-guided biopsy has some limitations. For example, some lesions may be well-visualized using a conventional closed (often 1.5-T) MRI system but may not be visualized with an interventional MRI system of lower field strength. Some lesions may be seen with US and CT and not with MRI. In these cases, MRI may not be able to be used to guide biopsy or treatment. Also, as stated, limitations specific to an MRI environment (e.g., inability to detect silent cardiac ischemia) may prevent the use of MRI for guiding invasive procedures in some patients. Nevertheless, the field of interventional MRI is relatively new, and some of these limitations are likely to be overcome.

CONCLUSIONS

Much progress has been made in the ability to biopsy masses under MR guidance. As technology improves, indications for this modality as the primary image guidance tool may expand. Already, this technique has formed the basis for various MR-guided therapeutic procedures, all of which are natural extensions of the biopsy technique.

REFERENCES

1. Ferrucci JT: Liver tumor imaging: current concepts, *Am J Roentgenol* 155:473, 1990.
2. Mueller PR, and others: MR-guided aspiration biopsy: needle design and clinical trials, *Radiology* 161:605, 1986.
3. Mueller PR, and others: Clinical use of a nonferromagnetic needle for magnetic resonance-guided biopsy, *Gastrointest Radiol* 14:61, 1989.
4. van Sonnenberg E, and others: A wire-sheath system for MR-guided biopsy and drainage: laboratory studies and experience in 10 patients, *Am J Roentgenol* 151:815, 1988.
5. Mahfouz AE, and others: MR-guided biopsy using ultrafast T1- and T2-weighted reordered turbo fast low-angle shot sequences: feasibility and preliminary clinical applications, *Am J Roentgenol* 167:167, 1996.
6. Silverman SG, and others: Needle-tip localization during CT-guided abdominal biopsy: comparison of conventional and spiral CT, *Am J Roentgenol* 159:1095, 1992.
7. Silverman SG, and others: Interactive biopsy in an open configuration MRI system, *Radiology* 197:175, 1995.
8. Schenck JF, and others: Superconducting open configuration MRI system for image-guided therapy, *Radiology* 195:805, 1995.
9. Frahm VC, Gehl HB, Robberg WA: Technique of MR-guided core biopsy of abdominal masses using an open low-field scanner: feasibility and first clinical results, *Fortschrgeb Rontgenstr Nuklearmed Erganzungsbd* 164:62, 1996.

10. Lu DSK, and others: Biopsy of hepatic dome lesions: semi-real-time coronal MR guidance technique.
11. Lu DSK: *Am J Roentgenol* 168:737, 1997.
12. Gronemeyer DH, and others: New possibilities and aspects of low-field magnetic resonance tomography, *Radiol Diagn (Berlin)* 30:519, 1989.
13. Leung DA, and others: Real-time biplanar needle tracking for interventional MR imaging procedures, *Radiology* 197:485, 1995.
14. Dumoulin CL, Souza SP, Darrow D: Real-time position monitoring of invasive devices using magnetic resonance, *Magn Reson Med* 29:411, 1993.
15. Hajek PC, and others: Localization grid for MR-guided biopsy, *Radiology* 163:825, 1987.
16. Silverman SG, and others: Design and implementation of an interventional MR imaging suite, *Am J Roentgenol* 168:1465, 1997.
17. Hughes CW, Bell C: *Anesthesia equipment in remote hospital locations.* In Rogers MC and others, editors: *Principles and practice of anesthesiology,* St Louis, 1993, Mosby.

Chapter 39

MR–GUIDED RADIOFREQUENCY ABLATION OF THE LIVER

Travis L. Boaz, Jonathan S. Lewin

Until recently, the long imaging times and the difficulty in directly accessing the patient in a cylindrical imaging system rendered magnetic resonance (MR) an unlikely guidance modality for "hands on" procedures. These problems have been overcome over the past several years with the advent of system hardware and pulse sequence improvements, which have allowed the development of rapid imaging on open-imaging systems.[1-6] The feasibility of MR as a guidance modality has been dependent on the development of needles and probes that are undeflected by the magnetic field and that create little or no field distortions or image degradation.[7-9] Other innovations that have made MR an attractive guidance alternative include in-room liquid crystal display monitors and frameless stereotactic localization systems, which allow interactive scan plane manipulation analogous to real-time ultrasound (US) imaging.[10] These advances have stimulated the development of MR-guided interventional techniques.

The main focus of therapeutic interventional MR has been in the minimally invasive treatment of cancer and cancer metastases. Regional metastasis may be the only life-threatening component of disease in many patients. For example, of the 160,000 patients newly diagnosed with colorectal carcinoma each year, approximately 24,000 have metastatic disease at the time of diagnosis, 30,000 to 50,000 will subsequently develop metastases, and at least half of these patients will die of their metastatic disease.[11,12] For many, progressive involvement of the liver will be a major or sole determinant of survival.[13,14] For patients who are surgical candidates, resection of hepatic metastases alters the natural history of the disease, increasing survival from a median of 6 months to a median of 29 to 30 months, with up to a 40% 5-year survival.[11,15] A major motivation and working model supporting the development of methods for local therapy is the demonstration that effective local therapy can significantly improve outcome in these patients.

With growing experience in interventional MR, investigators have used MR as an effective means of guidance for the percutaneous destruction of neoplastic tissue. The use of chemotherapeutic or chemoablative substances and thermal energy tissue destruction have been investigated. Previously studied chemoactive agents include absolute alcohol and various chemotherapeutic agents.[16] More recently, attention has focused on the delivery of thermal energy creating thermoablative lesions. Current thermoablative modalities include laser interstitial therapy, radiofrequency (RF) thermal ablation, focused US, and cryotherapy.[17-20] The thermoablative modalities are perhaps most exciting because of the inherent capability of MR to monitor temperature fluctuations.[21,22] The combination of MRI monitoring of tumor destruction and minimally invasive methods for tumor destruction has the potential to interactively visualize and direct the ablative procedure to ensure complete tumor destruction with an adequate margin. This aspect is a major difference compared with other ablative techniques and could markedly alter the options available to patients who are not surgical candidates.

The addition of MR temperature monitoring and necrosis confirmation to interstitial thermal ablation was initially performed in brain tumors, using laser and RF generators as sources of heat.[23,24] Preliminary clinical data have been very encouraging. Temperature-sensitive MR sequences have also been developed to enable accurate on-line monitoring of heat deposition.[25] The relationship of MRI signal intensity change to tissue temperature is complex, and precise MR measurement of temperature is difficult. However, the phase transition from viable to necrotic tissue can also be imaged using changes in the tissue relaxation parameters, T1 and T2, which occur in the process of necrosis.[26,27] The accuracy of MR findings in defining thermal lesion size has been repeatedly shown using several different energy sources.[20,28,29]

RADIOFREQUENCY THERMOTHERAPY

Interstitial RF thermal ablation depends on the transfer of electrical energy to tissue with the deposition of heat secondary to the increased resistivity of the intervening tissue to the passage of rapidly alternating current.[30] This transfer is achieved by passing RF energy from an RF generator through a shielded electrode with an exposed tip of varying length, which has been placed within a focus of abnormal tissue. Tissue heated to 60° C or greater undergoes coagulative necrosis and can be considered adequately treated in thermal ablative techniques, such as interstitial RF thermotherapy. RF therapy is not a new therapeutic modality; it has been used with great success for more than 3 decades in the neurosurgical community.[24] The placement of RF electrodes into pathologic tissue has typically been performed under direct visualization or stereotactic guidance based on preoperative computed tomography (CT) data. Indications for this form of therapy have historically included cordotomy, pallidotomy, leukotomy, and thalamotomy for the treatment of intractable pain and involuntary movement disorders.[31-37] More recently, investigators have used RF ablative therapy in the abdomen using US to direct therapy in the treatment of primary and secondary hepatic tumors.[38-40] However, assessment of treatment success or failure in this setting has been dependent on follow-up imaging, typically performed with contrast-enhanced CT.

Interstitial RF thermotherapy is an attractive treatment option for several reasons. As described, this modality has a long history of use. Also, complications resulting from RF ablation are unlikely, with the coagulation effect of the heating process contributing to a very low incidence of hemorrhage in the central nervous system[41,42] and abdomen, based on preliminary data.[38,43] The generating equipment necessary to create RF lesions is typically readily accessible because it is well-established in the neurosurgical community and is relatively inexpensive compared with laser light sources. Reproducible tissue destruction has been observed in various tissues. Furthermore, studies in humans and animals have shown that thermal lesion shape and size can be controlled through the electrode design and the duration and magnitude of the energy delivered.[30,41,42,44,45] Energy deposition is easy to control with RF ablation and allows gradual heating.[41] The presence of a thermister in the electrode tip gives continuous temperature feedback, and impedance measurements are another parameter related to tissue changes at the ablation site. These features are of particular importance when destroying tumors adjacent to neurovascular structures. Unlike radiotherapy, interstitial RF thermal ablation, similar to other thermal ablative therapies, can be repeated *ad infinitum* without concern for cumulative dose.

INTERSTITIAL RADIOFREQUENCY THERMOTHERAPY WITH MAGNETIC RESONANCE GUIDANCE

The use of interstitial RF thermotherapy under MR guidance is based on the direct destruction of tissue through the application of RF energy. The methodology differs significantly from the empirical (blind) approach typically used in neurosurgical applications of RF ablation technology. Variations in lesion size and shape caused by unanticipated thermal conduction during treatment cannot be predicted and are not usually recognized until follow-up imaging studies are performed. The major contribution of MRI is its outstanding ability to monitor the zone of thermal tissue destruction during the procedure and to provide real-time guidance for deposition of the RF energy. Through MR monitoring, thermal lesion size and configuration can be directly controlled by the operator and adjusted during the procedure to compensate for deviations from preoperative predictions. MR is exceptionally well-suited for this purpose because of its lack of ionizing radiation, excellent soft-tissue discrimination, spatial resolution, and sensitivity to temperature and blood flow.[2,19,46] This technique permits accurate destruction of the tumor, including margins, and extends the application of RF ablation to the safe destruction of tumor within visceral organs and adjacent to vital neurovascular structures. Furthermore, MR is not hampered by difficulties caused by changes in tissue imaging characteristics brought about by RF ablation as has been described by some authors using US guidance.[38]

Until recently, MR-guided RF therapy has been limited by its inability to actively monitor the lesion as it is created. This feature is secondary to the inherent imaging interference caused by the RF source. New software and hardware modifications have recently been developed that allow RF energy to be deposited during imaging between the brief sampling periods of temperature-sensitive sequences, thereby maintaining tissue temperature while making interference-free real-time monitoring possible.[47]

Other recent improvements include the development of a water-cooled RF electrode designed by Goldberg and others,[48] in which the electrode is cooled by constant infusion of iced saline. Although lesion length depends on exposed tip length, lesion diameter was previously limited to approximately 2 cm.[40] This drawback was thought to be caused by charring at the electrode and tissue interface, which in turn impaired energy transfer. With the new water-cooled electrode, charring at the interface is prevented, allowing energy to be further transmitted. With this form of energy deposition, a second application of RF energy may be necessary without cooling once the desired margins are achieved to destroy the area adjacent to the cooled electrode. Lesions can be created with this electrode design that would have required multiple ablations with intervening electrode repositioning with a standard RF electrode.

INTERVENTIONAL TECHNIQUES

Interstitial RF thermotherapy monitored by MR has been performed in patients with RF electrode placement outside of the scanner in a neurosurgical stereotactic frame or with the RF electrode interactively placed under MR guidance in an open interventional system.[24,43] Technical requirements differ primarily with regard to the MR imager and interventional accessories. Once the electrode is placed, energy deposition and treatment monitoring are performed in a similar manner.

The primary focus has been minimally invasive interstitial RF thermotherapy of tumors of the liver and retroperitoneum with electrode placement performed under direct MR guidance in the MR imager. MR-guided electrode placement and monitoring of therapy are performed using a commercially available c-arm MR system (Siemens MAGNETOM OPEN, Erlangen, Germany) supplemented with (1) an in-room 1024 × 1280 liquid crystal display monitor; (2) in-room imager controls; (3) an optically linked frameless stereotaxy system (developed in collaboration with Radionics, Inc., Burlington, Mass, and Siemens Medical Systems, Erlangen, Germany) to interactively drive image acquisition; (4) a 50- to 120-W RF generator (Radionics, Inc.); (5) and an MR-compatible 17 cm × 2 mm shielded electrode with a 2- to 3-cm exposed tip with or without water cooling (Fig. 39-1).

Electrodes are placed in the liver or retroperitoneum under continuous imaging with automated acquisition, reconstruction, and display using 1 to 2 sec per frame using short repetition time, short echo time gradient-echo sequences. Fast imaging with steady-state precision (FISP) or true FISP sequence designs are applied, depending on the tissue contrast necessary for tumor visualization. With a standard RF electrode, interstitial thermal ablation is performed at an electrode tip temperature of 85° C to 90° C for 6 to 20 min at each electrode location before repositioning for larger tumors. The ablation time at each location and electrode repositioning are based on MRI during ablation to achieve maximal ablation tissue necrosis for the MR-compatible electrode in use. Electrode repositioning is performed in the scanner in an interactive manner under continuous MRI guidance similar to that used for initial electrode placement. Larger thermo-ablative lesions can be formed when using the water-cooled electrode, thus requiring fewer electrode repositionings in large tumors.

Multiplanar short tau inversion recovery (STIR) and T2-weighted images are performed before the procedure. These sequences are repeated intermittently during ablation to monitor thermal lesion size and configuration. After ablation, they are repeated with the addition of gadopentetate-enhanced T1-weighted images to confirm the final zone of tissue destruction.

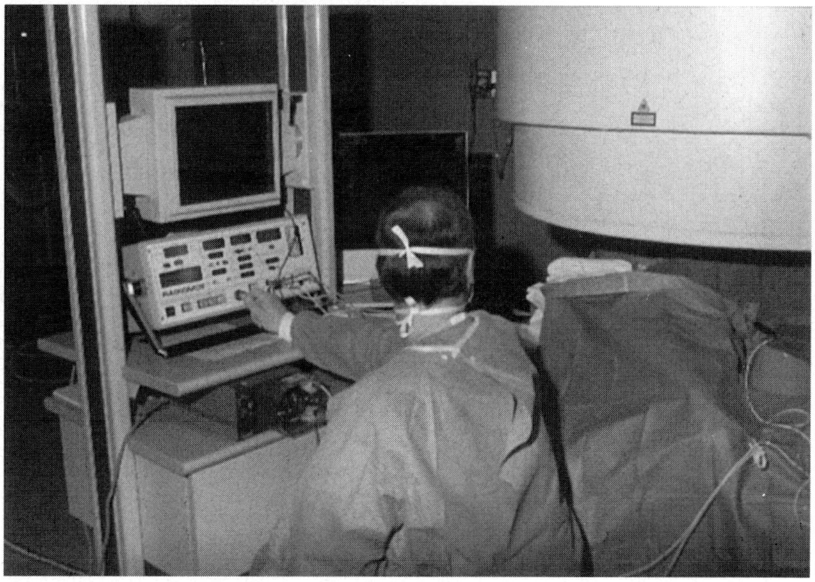

Fig. 39-1. An open magnetic resonance imaging (MRI) system with an in-room physician image monitor, a radiofrequency ablation system, and an MR-compatible mouse to control the system. The open bore allows access for interactive electrode manipulation, viewed on the monitor at 1 to 2 sec per frame in a fluoroscopic mode. The MR-compatible Radionics RFG-3C (Radionics, Inc, Burlington, Mass) RF thermal lesion generator can be seen underneath the image monitor, connected to an electrode in the patient's liver. (Reprinted with permission from Lewin JS, and others: Interactive MR-guided radiofrequency interstitial thermal ablation of abdominal tumors: clinical trial for evaluation of safety and feasibility, *J Magn Reson Imaging* 8:40, 1998.)

CURRENT EXPERIENCE

Animal model

Animal experiments were performed to evaluate the detection and temporal evolution of heat deposition and *in vivo* tissue destruction during RF ablation under direct MR monitoring. Liver RF ablation thermal lesions were produced with a custom-designed MR-compatible electrode on a clinical 0.2-T scanner in a rabbit model under direct MR guidance. Heat deposition and thermal lesion extent were monitored with MRI during and for 20 to 40 min after treatment using phase maps, T2-weighted, and contrast-enhanced T1-weighted images (Figs. 39-2 and 39-3). Animals were killed immediately after thermal lesion creation and pathologic correlation was performed. Hepatic thermal lesions approaching 2×2 to 4 cm were produced, and it was possible to tailor thermal lesion size and shape under MR guidance. Tissue necrosis was delineated by a ring of hyperintensity surrounding central hypointensity on T2-weighted and postcontrast T1-weighted images, similar to the findings reported in the brain by Farahani and others.[42] Correlation of MRI findings of tissue destruct with gross and histologic analysis suggested that MR accurately guided electrode placement and predicted the size and shape of the region of tissue necrosis (Fig. 39-4).[49,50]

Lesion size using the nonperfused electrode was limited to approximately 17 mm in diameter. Lesion length varied depending on the exposed tip length. This exposed tip length can be predefined at the time of manufacture. By having various exposed tip length electrodes, the operator can use the electrode that would make the most appropriate lesion size and shape to the tumor to be ablated. This advantage makes this approach better than chemoablative modalities, which are often limited to spherical lesion formation. Lesion diameter is thought to be limited by charring of the tissue adjacent to the exposed electrode tip. This tissue charring impairs the transmission and distribution of RF thermal energy. Goldberg and others realized that this drawback could be potentially overcome by preventing charring at the electrode and tissue interface. Prevention is achieved by cooling the electrode tip by the passage of ice-chilled water through internal water channels. This water is circulated using a perfusion pump. Cooling the tip of the electrode allows more RF energy to be deposited and a larger lesion size. Lesion size depends largely on the total amount of thermal energy deposited. Once the lesion of the desired size is created, a second ablation is performed without perfusion to coagulate any tissue adjacent to the electrode that may have been sufficiently protected by the chilled electrode to remain viable.

A second series of hepatic thermal ablations were performed in NZW rabbits using the water-perfused RF electrode. Preprocedural imaging and electrode placement were identical to those used for the nonperfused electrode. Electrode placement was confirmed using axial T2-weighted images. Thermal ablation was then performed. The electrode tip was heated to ap-

A

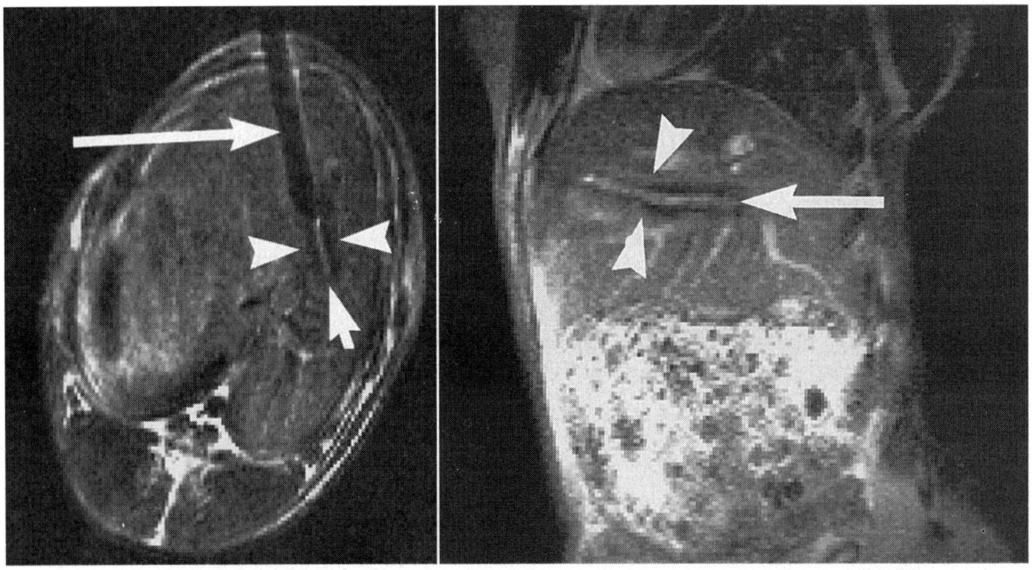

B

Fig. 39-2. A rabbit model of hepatic ablation. **A,** A T2-weighted axial image through the upper abdomen of a rabbit after hepatic radiofrequency (RF) thermal ablation. The thermal lesion shows decreased signal intensity on this T2-weighted image, with its margins clearly demarcated *(arrowheads).* The 2-mm diameter RF electrode after repositioning in preparation for the creation of a second lesion (*straight arrow*) is clearly separate from the remainder of the lesion. The electrode has minimal associated signal distortion and need not be removed to ascertain lesion size. A linear hyperintensity is present in the lesion representing the electrode tract *(short arrow).* **B,** A T2-weighted coronal image through the upper abdomen of a rabbit after hepatic RF thermal ablation. The electrode tract is again identified centrally *(straight arrow).* A sharp lesion margin is present *(arrowheads).*

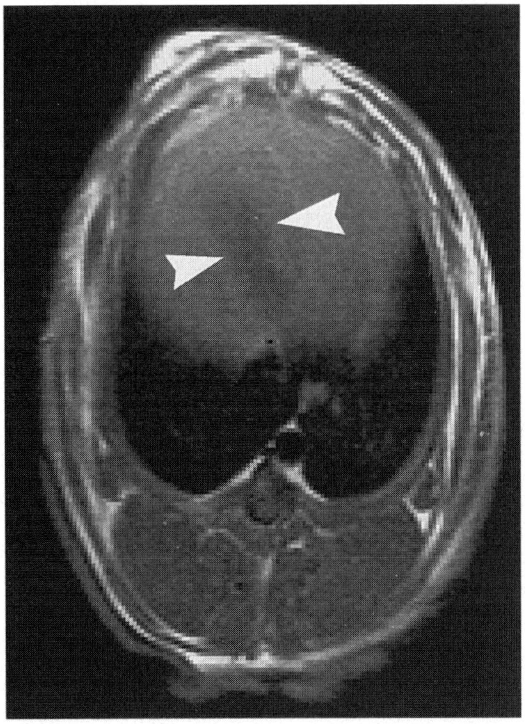

Fig. 39-3. A T1-weighted contrast-enhanced axial image through the upper abdomen of a rabbit after hepatic radiofrequency ablation. There is a central zone of decreased signal corresponding to a zone of coagulative necrosis. Around this area is a zone of enhancement representing the known hyperemia (*arrowheads*).

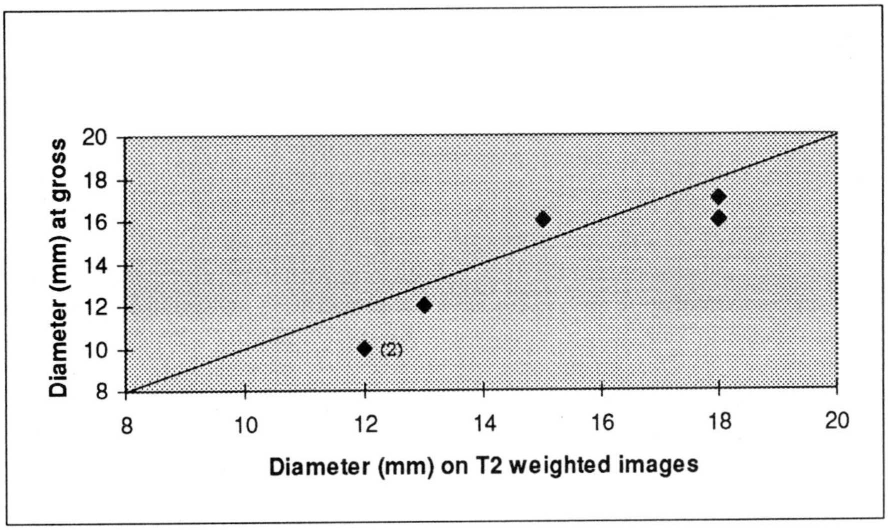

Fig. 39-4. A comparative plot of lesion size (in millimeters) as determined at gross examination compared with dimensions determined during a procedure using T2-weighted images. Imaging diameter correlated well with actual diameter determined at gross examination. Estimated size was always within 2 mm. Imaging tends to slightly overestimate actual lesion size. *(2)* refers to lesions in two rabbit livers with the same dimensions. (Modified with permission from Boaz TL, and others: A rabbit model for MR-monitoring of tissue destruction in MR-guided radiofrequency hepatic thermal ablation, Proceedings of the International Society for Magnetic Resonance in Medicine. 5th Scientific Meeting and Exhibition, Vancouver, 1997.)

proximately 80° C without water perfusion. The impedence and milliamperage at that temperature were noted. The milliamperage was then increased to approximately 150% of the nonperfused value. Chilled saline was circulated through the electrode during RF energy deposition; the rate of saline perfusion was increased to maintain a temperature of 20° C at the electrode tip. This approach was performed for 20 min in each animal. Although this ablation time length was constant in the animal study, the thermal lesion size could be altered by varying the duration of ablation. Imaging was then repeated using T2- and STIR-weighted axial imaging through the lesion. Thermo-ablation was then performed without water cooling using the same electrode for 3 min to ensure thermocoagulation of tissue adjacent to the exposed tip. Postprocedural imaging identical to that performed in the previous trial was then performed, followed by animal sacrifice and postmortem evaluation.

This series using the perfused electrode showed that thermal lesions had similar imaging characteristics to those seen with the nonperfused electrode. The thermal lesions seen on contrast-enhanced T1-weighted images tended to be less distinct than lesions created with the nonperfused electrode. Lesion size varied and depended entirely on the amount of current deposited and the length of time the tissue was exposed to the RF energy (i.e., total ablation time). Lesions ranged from approximately 1 cm in diameter to a lesion involving nearly the entirety of the rabbit liver. Intermediate imaging performed between the ablation with water perfusion and the ablation performed without water perfusion did not show a demarcation between the near zone (zone of tissue adjacent to the perfused electrode, which remained potentially viable secondary to the thermoprotective effects of water cooling) and the far zone (tissue distant from the perfused electrode, which receives full RF energy).

Clinical experience

Eleven tumors in seven patients were treated during 13 ablations using MR-guided RF ablation during 1996 and 1997 as part of a phase I clinical trial. Six of the 11 tumors treated were renal cell carcinoma metastases or local recurrence, three were metastatic leiomyosarcoma, one was an adenocarcinoma of unknown primary and one was a metastatic colon carcinoma. All tumors were refractory to conventional modes of cancer therapy and were not considered appropriate for surgical resection. Treated sites include the liver ($n = 6$), retroperitoneum ($n = 3$), diaphragmatic crus or abdominal wall ($n = 1$), and pelvis ($n = 1$). The last four procedures were performed using the water-perfused RF electrode.

No technical failures or patient complications occurred. Two patients have shown disease progression, and the remaining four have shown stable disease or decreased tumor size during an average follow-up of 152 days.

In each tumor, the region of tissue destruction could be accurately guided through sequential rapid T2-weighted and STIR images obtained during ablation and could be confirmed as an avascular zone on contrast-enhanced MRI scans obtained at the end of ablation (Figs. 39-5 to 39-7).[49,51,52] The maximal ablation size for each electrode position was an oblate spheroid approximately 2.4 cm long and 2 cm in diameter.

Two weeks after ablation, tumors with greater than 50% volume ablation showed a slight enlargement of the region of edema surrounding the central core of tissue necrosis, with subsequent reduction in tumor volume. In the patient with the longest follow-up (18 months), the tumor is absent on CT, with only minimal soft-tissue distortion at the site of electrode placement on MRI. Four tumors were incompletely ablated because of marked hypervascularity, size, or insufficient time to complete the procedure.[43,52]

No morbidity or toxicity has been encountered, although MRI scans obtained immediately after ablation have shown a small amount of fluid adjacent to the liver in two patients after liver ablation, without associated symptoms, change in vital signs, or significant drop in hematocrit level.

Ultrasound-guided radiofrequency experience

Because the follow-up for MR-guided RF therapy is relatively short, comparison with the more established regimen of US-guided RF therapy may be helpful to better understand the natural history of liver metastases treated with RF thermal ablation. Rossi, and others[38] treated 50 patients with 41 hepatocellular carcinoma nodules and 13 metastatic hepatic nodules using a similar protocol of RF interstitial thermal ablation, with a mean follow-up of 22 months. Only 2 of the 50 patients showed local recurrence at the treated site, although additional tumor nodules developed in other patients. Treatment appeared very well tolerated, without significant morbidity.[38]

TECHNICAL CONSIDERATIONS

Recent developments have made the use of MR as an interventional guidance even more attractive. Intraprocedural MR monitoring has recently been made possible by development of a switching mechanism that briefly interrupts RF deposition during the sampling period of imaging pulse sequences, reducing the duty cycle of RF deposition from 100% without imaging to approximately 50% to 60% during imaging, depending on the repetition time and sampling time of the sequence used.[47] Sequences are also being developed that could potentially give more accurate tissue temperature information. At present, tissue temperature is measured only by the thermistor located at the RF electrode tip. The temperature distribution extending from the electrode tip can vary widely depending on the local vascular anatomy because of the heat sink properties of blood flow. This temperature information could help the interventionalist alter the procedure to ensure that the entire target abnormality is ablated.

Another consideration is the heat sink effect of blood flow. Hypervascular tumors, including some hepatomas and renal cell carcinoma metastases, can be very difficult to destroy using

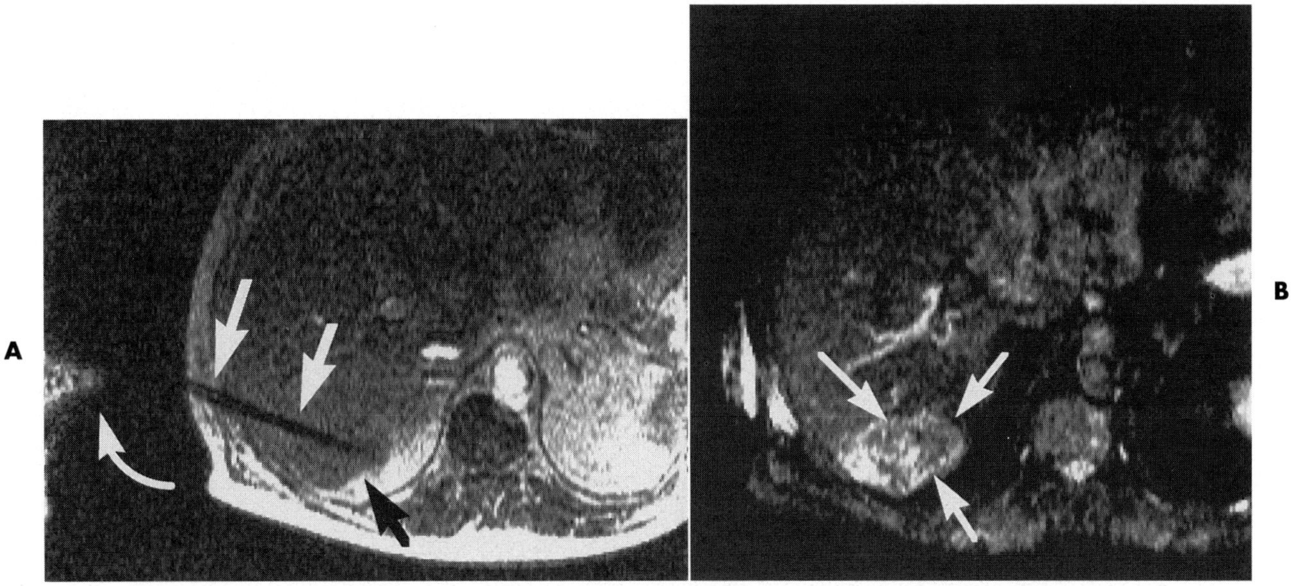

Fig. 39-5. A 73-year-old with colon carcinoma metastatic to the liver. **A,** Fast imaging in steady-state precision (FISP) (repetition time, 17 msec; echo time, 8 msec; flip angle, 90°) sequence used during interactive radiofrequency (RF) electrode insertion and manipulation. One image from a series obtained during breathhold at a frame rate of 2 sec per image shows a magnetic resonance-compatible electrode *(white arrows)* being inserted into an exophytic mass in the posterior aspect of the right lobe of the liver *(black arrow).* The radiologist's hand can be seen advancing the electrode at the edge of the image *(curved arrow).* The lesion was delineated with T2-weighted images before RF electrode insertion. A true FISP sequence with T2 weighting is used for electrode insertion, with a frame rate of 1.5 sec per frame for equivalent 128 ×256 resolution. The frame rate is often increased by using a rectangular field of view. **B,** A short tau inversion recovery axial image through the liver (repetition time, 4470 msec; echo time, 48 msec; inversion time, 110 msec) shows a central area of thermally induced necrosis, which is decreased in signal intensity *(white arrows)* and is surrounded by increased signal consistent with edema. This pattern of signal changes correlates well with the experimental data in healthy rabbit liver. A periportal metastasis seen on the image was not treated during this RF thermal ablation session. (From Lewin JS, Boaz TL: *MR-guided RF treatment.* In Debatin JF, Adam G, editors: *Interventional magnetic resonance imaging,* Heidelberg, 1998, Springer-Verlag.)

thermal ablation techniques because of the rapid flow of blood, which carries away applied heat, preventing cumulative thermal injury. These hypervascular tumors frequently require significantly greater total RF energy deposition and may require repositioning of the electrode multiple times. Even with these maneuvers designed to overcome the difficulties of heat deposition in these hypervascular tumors, complete ablation may be impossible. To a lesser degree, this heat sink effect of blood flow can be a problem in the treatment of tumors immediately adjacent to large vascular structures. This phenomena of decreased efficacy of RF ablation in tissues adjacent to large blood vessels can be seen in thermoablations performed near central branches of the portal vein (Fig. 39-8).

CONCLUSIONS

The excellent soft-tissue contrast, multiplanar capabilities, vascular conspicuity, and temperature sensitivity of MRI are very well-suited for use in guidance and monitoring of interventional procedures, both for diagnostic purposes and for treatment; the use of these interventional techniques continues to increase as MR systems developed or modified for procedure guidance proliferate. Beyond the advantages of diagnostic intervention, successful application of these technologic advances to minimally invasive treatment of cancer has the potential to profoundly reduce the morbidity and cost associated with local cancer therapy and may significantly affect the treatment options and prognosis for patients with regional tumor spread.

RF therapy specifically has many intrinsic benefits, including ease of use, availability, a low complication rate, and the ability to create thermal lesions of variable morphology.[45] Recent advances in MR and RF technology are beginning to overcome previous shortcomings in this therapy and monitoring combination. Preliminary results suggest that this emerging modality has a promising future for the treatment of abdominal tumors. With the ability to immediately assess the results of treatment and to use this information to interactively vary the thermal lesion size and shape, the addition of MR monitoring to interstitial RF thermotherapy has significant potential to provide a much-needed therapeutic modality for the treatment of regional metastatic disease.

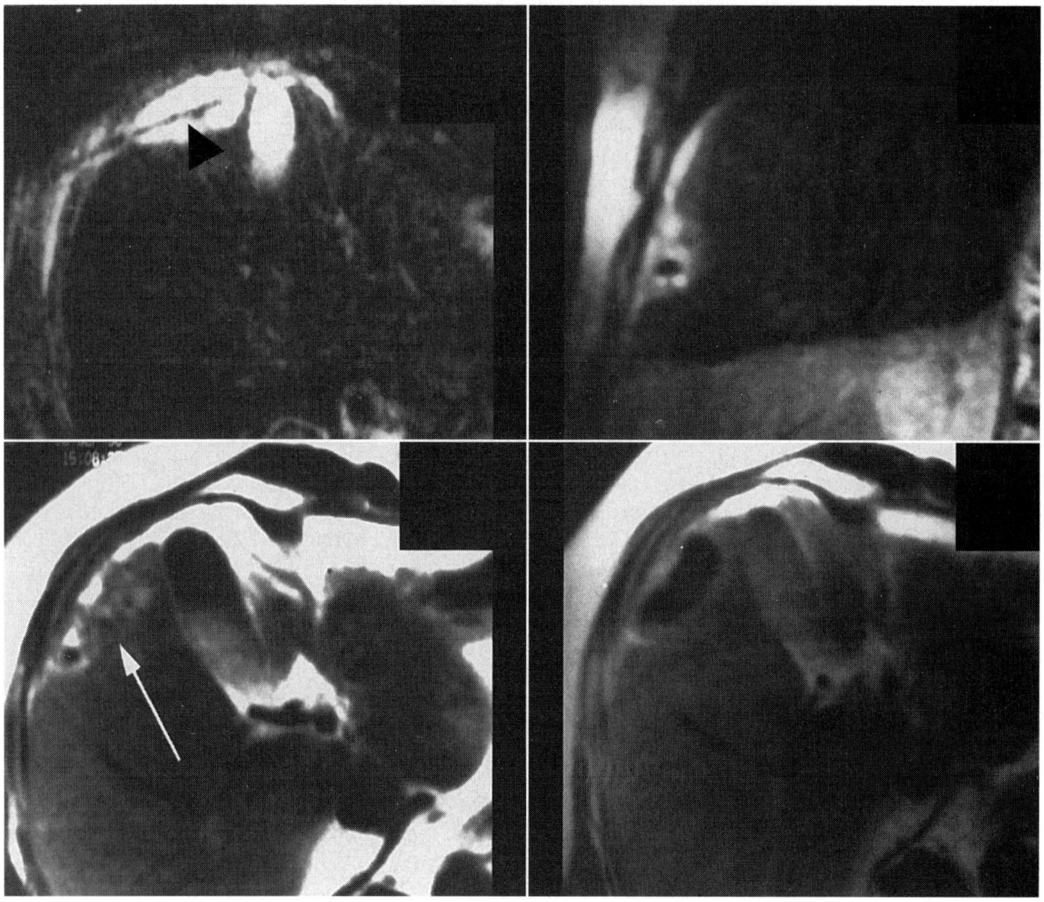

Fig. 39-6. A 74-year-old with three known metastases from a previously resected leiomyosarcoma of the stomach. **A,** A short tau inversion recovery axial image during the ablation procedure shows a very bright 5×3 cm tumor bisected by the dark line of the titanium electrode in its center *(arrowhead)*. The gallbladder is seen as another bright structure medial to the mass. **B,** A T2-weighted oblique image perpendicular to the titanium electrode shows the electrode as a dark dot in the lower third of the lesion. Two longitudinal electrode passes through the lesion were performed to ablate the lower and upper halves of this larger tumor. **C,** A contrast-enhanced T1-weighted axial image obtained before ablation, at the same level as in **A,** shows irregular enhancement in the region of the tumor *(arrow)*. The gallbladder, seen medial to the tumor, is partially filled with contrast. **D,** Immediately after ablation, a contrast-enhanced T1-weighted axial image, at the same level as in **C,** shows a markedly hypointense lesion completely replacing the enhancing mass, with a slight rim of marginal enhancement. This pattern of loss of vascularity with slight reactive marginal enhancement has been seen in all patients treated to date and has shown a very high correlation with pathologic evidence of tissue necrosis in an animal model. This loss of vascularity can be seen on contrast-enhanced computed tomography and persists for several months as the treated tumor is resorbed. (Reprinted with permission from Lewin JS, and others: Interactive MR-guided radiofrequency interstitial thermal ablation of abdominal tumors: clinical trial for evaluation of safety and feasibility, *J Magn Reson Imaging* 8:40, 1998.)

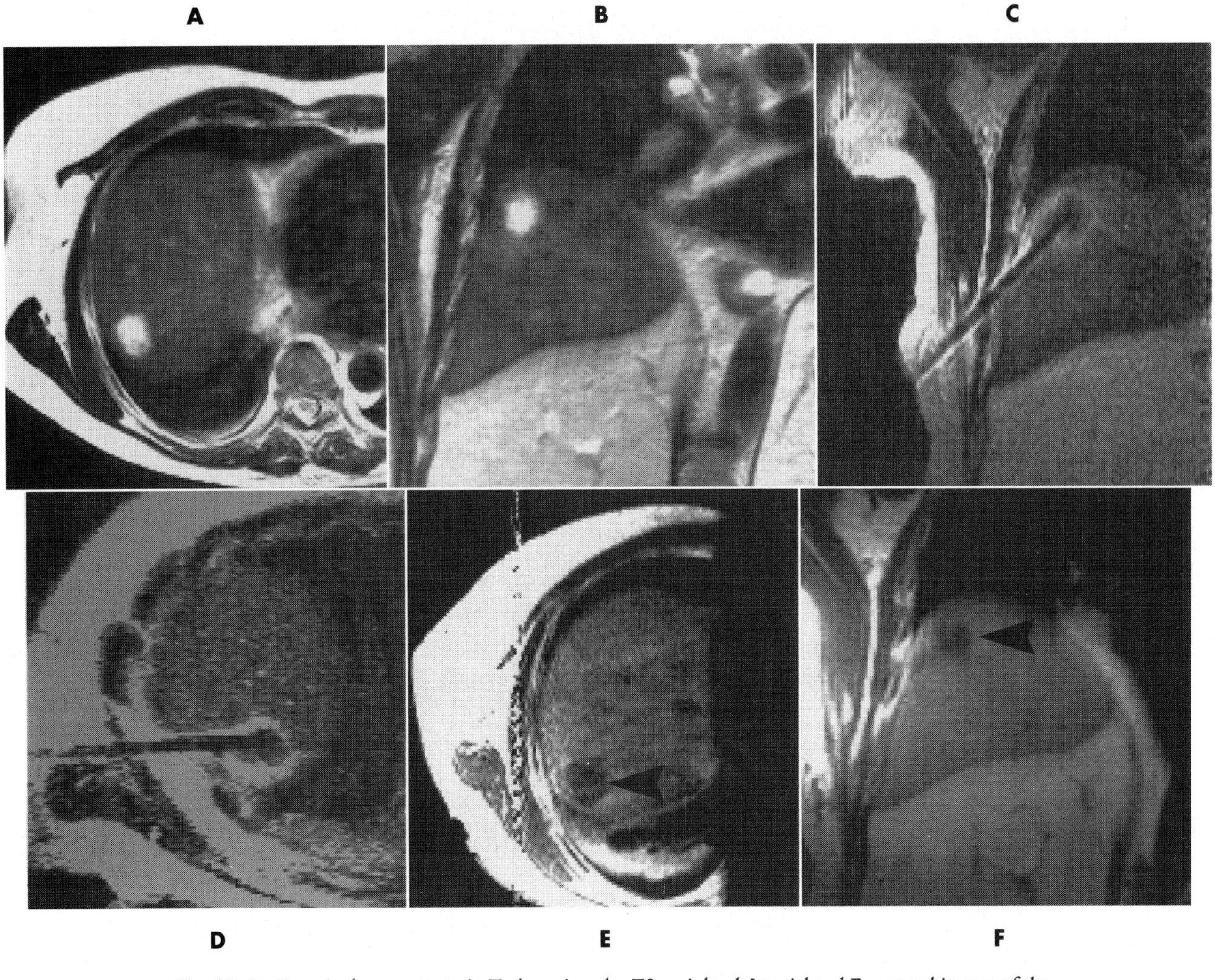

Fig. 39-7. Hepatic dome metastasis. Turbo spin-echo T2-weighted **A,** axial and **B,** coronal images of the abdomen show hyperintense metastasis in the posterior dome of the right lobe of the liver. Turbo spin-echo T2-weighted **C,** coronal and **D,** oblique axial-sagittal images with similar parameters along the course of the magnetic resonance-compatible radiofrequency (RF) electrode show the electrode positioned within the tumor. The effects of RF-interstitial thermal ablation are seen as marked hypointensity developing around the active distal 3 cm of the electrode, surrounded by a rim of hyperintensity reflecting edema and hyperemia. After RF-ITA, contrast-enhanced T1-weighted **E**, axial and **F**, coronal images show hypointensity *(arrowhead)* corresponding to the avascular area of tumor necrosis. This hypointensity approximates the volume of the originally identified tumor, along with a small margin of surrounding healthy parenchyma. (Reprinted with permission from Lewin JS, and others: Interactive MR-guided radiofrequency interstitial thermal ablation of abdominal tumors: clinical trial for evaluation of safety and feasibility, *J Magn Reson Imaging,* 8:40, 1998.)

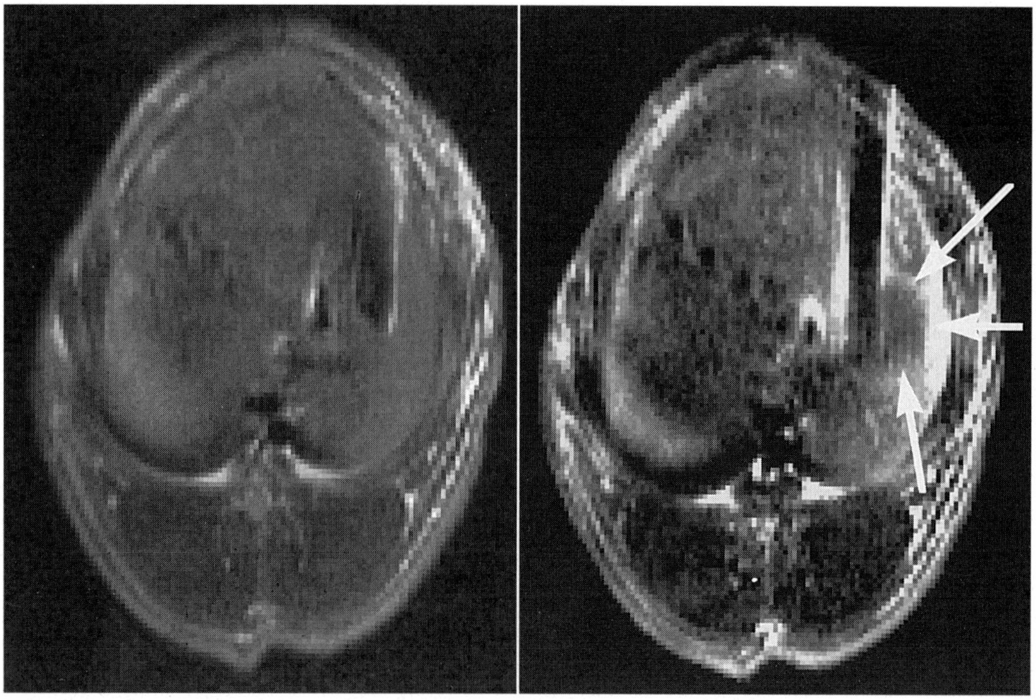

Fig. 39-8. T2-weighted images through rabbit liver show the electrode placement positioned adjacent to a large portal vein. **A** shows electrode placement to the portal vein prior to radiofrequency application. **B** shows an asymmetric lesion following ablation secondary to heat-sinking effects of adjacent vessels. *Arrows* mark the margin of the radiofrequency-induced thermal ablation.

REFERENCES

1. Jolesz FA, Blumenfeld SM: Interventional use of magnetic resonance imaging, *Magn Reson Q* 10:85, 1994.
2. Schenck JF, and others: Superconducting open-configuration MR imaging system for image-guided therapy, *Radiology* 195:805, 1995.
3. Silverman SG, and others: Interactive MR-guided biopsy in an open-configuration MR imaging system, *Radiology* 197:175, 1995.
4. Kaufman L, and others: Accessible magnetic resonance imaging, *Magn Reson Q* 5:283, 1989.
5. Gronemeyer DHW, and others: Neumoglichkeiten und gesichtspunkte der low-field-kernspintomographie, *Radiol Diagn* 30:519, 1989.
6. Duerk JL, Lewin JS, Wu DH: Application of keyhole imaging to interventional MRI: a simulation study to assess sequence requirements, *J Magn Reson Imaging* 6:918, 1996.
7. Lufkin R, Teresi L, Hanafee W: New needle for MR-guided aspiration cytology of the head and neck, *Am J Roentgenol* 149:380, 1987.
8. Lufkin R, and others: A technique for MR-guided needle placement, *Am J Roentgenol* 151:193, 1988.
9. Wenokur R, and others: Magnetic resonance imaging-guided fine needle aspiration for the diagnosis of skull base lesions, *Skull Base Surgery* 2:167, 1992.
10. Lewin JS, and others: *Interactive MRI of procedure guidance on a clinical C-arm system: a pilot biopsy study,* New York, 1996, Proceedings of the International Society for Magnetic Resonance in Medicine 2, 4th Scientific Meeting and Exhibition.
11. Niederhuber JE, Ensminger WD: *Treatment of metastatic cancer to the liver.* In DeVita VT Jr, Hellman S, Rosenberg SA, editors: *Cancer: principles and practice of oncology,* ed 4, Philadelphia, 1993, Lippincott.
12. Alexander HR, and others: Regional treatment strategies for unresectable primary or metastatic cancer confined to the liver, *Principles and Practice of Oncology Update* 10:1, 1996.
13. NIH Consensus Conference: Adjuvant therapy for patients with colon and rectal cancer, *JAMA* 264:1444, 1990.
14. Wood CB, Gillis CR, Blumgart LH: A retrospective study of patients with liver metastases from colorectal cancer, *Clin Oncol* 2:285, 1976.
15. August DA, Sugarbaker PH, Ottow RT: Hepatic resection of colorectal metastases, *Ann Surg* 201:210, 1985.
16. Lewin JS, and others: *MR-monitoring of tissue necrosis following percutaneous ethanol injection in implanted rat hepatoma: evaluation of temporal signal changes at 0.2T,* New York, 1996, Proceedings of the International Society for Magnetic Resonance in Medicine 2, 4th Scientific Meeting and Exhibition.
17. Anzai Y, and others: MR imaging-guided interstitial Nd:YAG laser phototherapy: dosimetry study of acute tissue damage in an in vivo model, *J Magn Reson Imaging* 1:553, 1991.
18. Goldberg SN, and others: Tissue ablation with radiofrequency: effect of probe size, gauge, duration, and temperature on lesion volume, *Acad Radiol* 2:399, 1995.
19. Cline HE, and others: Focused US system for MR imaging-guided tumor ablation, *Radiology* 194:731, 1995.
20. Matsumoto R, and others: MR monitoring during cryotherapy in the liver: predictability of histologic outcome, *J Magn Reson Imaging* 73:770, 1993.
21. Hall AS, and others: Observation by MR imaging of in vivo temperature changes induced by radiofrequency hyperthermia, *J Comput Assist Tomogr* 14:430, 1990.
22. Le Bihan D, Delannoy J, Levin RL: Temperature mapping with MR imaging of molecular diffusion: application to hyperthermia, *Radiology* 171:853, 1989.
23. Tomlinson FH, and others: Sequential magnetic resonance imaging following sterotactic radiofrequency ventralis lateralis thalamotomy, *J Neurosurg* 74:579, 1991.
24. Anzai Y, and others: Preliminary experience with MR-guided thermal ablation of brain tumors, *Am J Neuroradiol* 16:39, 1995.
25. Vogl TJ, and others: Malignant liver tumors treated with MR imaging-guided laser-induced thermotherapy: technique and prospective results, *Radiology* 196:257, 1995.

26. Matsumoto R, Oshio K, Jolesz FA: Monitoring of laser and freezing-induced ablation in the liver with T1-weighted MR imaging, *J Magn Reson Imaging* 2:555, 1992.
27. Bleier AR, and others: Real-time magnetic resonance imaging of laser heat deposition in tissue, *Magn Reson Med* 21:132, 1991.
28. Anzai Y, and others: MR-imaging histopathologic correlation of thermal injuries induced with intersitital Nd:YAG laser irradiation in the chronic model, *J Magn Reson Imaging* 2:671, 1992.
29. Tracz RA, and others: Comparison of magnetic resonance images and the histopathological findings of lesions induced by interstitial laser photocoagulation in the brain, *Lasers Surg Med* 13:45, 1993.
30. Aronow S: The use of radio-frequency power in making lesions in the brain, *J Neurosurg* 17:431, 1960.
31. Sweet WH, Mark VH, Hamlin H: Radiofrequency lesions in the central nervous system of man and cat: including case reports of eight bulbar pain-tract interruptions, *J Neurosurg* 17:213, 1960.
32. Tew JM, Keller JT: *The treatment of trigeminal neuralgia by percutaneous radiofrequency technique.* In Keener EB, editor: *Clinical neurosurgery,* Baltimore, 1977, Williams & Wilkins.
33. Siegfried J: 500 percutaneous thermocoagulation of Gasserian ganglion for trigeminal pain, *Surg Neurol* 8:126, 1977.
34. Hitchcock ER, Teixeira MJ: A comparison of results from center-median and basal thalamotomies for pain, *Surg Neurol* 15:341, 1981.
35. Broggi G, and others: Radiofrequency percutaneous trigeminal rhizotomy: considerations in 1000 consecutive cases of essential trigeminal neuralgia, *J Neurosurg Sci* 29:165, 1985.
36. Rosomoff HL, and others: Percutaneous radiofrequency cervical cordotomy: technique, *J Neurosurg* 23:639, 1965.
37. Nashold BS, Ostdahl RH: Dorsal root entry zone lesions for pain relief, *J Neurosurg* 51:59, 1979.
38. Rossi S, and others: Percutaneous RF interstitial thermal ablation in the treatment of liver cancer, *Am J Roentgenol* 167:759, 1996.
39. McGahan JP, and others: Hepatic ablation using radiofrequency electrocautery, *Invest Radiol* 25:267, 1990.
40. McGahan JP, and others: Treatment of liver tumors by percutaneous radiofrequency electrocautery, *Semin Interven Radiol* 10:143, 1993.
41. Zervas NT, Kuwayama A: Pathological characteristics of experimental thermal lesions: comparison of induction heating and radiofrequency electrocoagulation, *J Neurosurg* 37:418, 1972.
42. Farahani K, and others: Hyperacute thermal lesions: MR imaging evaluation of development in the brain, *Radiology* 1996:517, 1995.
43. Lewin JS: *Interactive MR-guided radiofrequency interstitial thermal ablation of abdominal tumors: a phase I clinical trial,* Vancouver, 1997, Proceedings of the International Society for Magnetic Resonance in Medicine, 5th Scientific Meeting and Exhibition.
44. Zervas NT: Eccentric radio-frequency lesions, *Confin Neurol* 26:143, 1965.
45. Chung YC, Duerk JL, Lewin JS: *Generation and observation of radiofrequency thermal lesion ablation for interventional magnetic resonance imaging,* New York, 1996, Proceedings of the International Society for Magnetic Resonance in Medicine, 4th Scientific Meeting and Exhibition.
46. Cline HE, and others: Magnetic resonance-guided thermal surgery, *Magn Reson Med* 30:98, 1993.
47. Zhang Q, and others: A method for simultaneous RF ablation and MR imaging, *J Magn Reson Imaging* 8:110, 1997.
48. Goldberg SN, and others: Radiofrequency tissue ablation: increased lesion diameter with a perfusion electrode, *Acad Radiol* 3:636, 1996.
49. Boaz TL, and others: Imaging of the temporal evolution of hepatic tissue destruction during MR-guided radiofrequency thermal ablation in a rabbit model, *Radiology* 201:389, 1996 (abstract).
50. Boaz TL, and others: *A rabbit model for MR-monitoring of tissue destruction in MR-guided radiofrequency hepatic thermal ablation,* Vancouver, 1997, Proceedings of the International Society for Magnetic Resonance in Medicine, 5th Scientific Meeting and Exhibition.
51. Lewin JS: Magnetic resonance image guided therapy: clinical applications and future directions, *Med Phys* 23:1146, 1996.
52. Lewin JS, and others: Interactive MR-guided radiofrequency interstitial thermal ablation of abdominal tumors: clinical trial for evaluation of safety and feasibility, *J Magn Reson Imaging* 8:40, 1998.

Chapter 40

CLINICAL USES OF MR–GUIDED LASER ABLATION OF THE LIVER

Thomas J. Vogl, Martin G. Mack

The liver is the most common site of metastatic disease resulting from colorectal carcinoma; metastases are rarely present at other sites if the liver and lung are free of tumor.[1] In 1994 in the United States approximately 149,000 persons developed colorectal carcinoma, and approximately 56,000 died of this neoplasm. Weiss and others[1] estimated that at least 20% of patients with this disease will die with metastases exclusively in the liver. In many patients, the degree of hepatic involvement is the main determinant of survival.[2-4] The median survival for patients with liver metastases resulting from colorectal carcinoma is 4 to 12 months from the time of diagnosis of metastatic disease. Among patients with one metastasis, 45% are alive at 2 years, whereas only 12% are alive at 3 years.

In patients who are not candidates for hepatectomy, palliative management of hepatic metastases is unsatisfactory. An efficient, minimally invasive technique is needed to slow, or halt, growth of metastases. This rationale is valid for management of other primary neoplasms with isolated hepatic metastases (e.g., breast carcinoma, carcinoid, others) and for management of localized hepatocellular neoplams (e.g., hepatocellular carcinoma, well-circumscribed cholangiocarcinomas).

Laser-induced interstitial thermotherapy (LITT) is a minimally invasive technique suitable for local tumor destruction in solid organs. It uses optical fibers to deliver high-energy laser radiation to the target lesion. Because of light absorption, temperatures up to 150° C are reached in the tumor, leading to a substantial thermocoagulation. Magnetic resonance imaging (MRI) is used for placing the laser applicator in the tumor and for monitoring progress of thermocoagulation. The thermosensitivity of certain MR sequences is key to real-time monitoring, allowing accurate estimation of the extent of thermal damage. This chapter discusses the technique of MR-guided minimally invasive laser-induced thermotherapy and the results of local lesion control and survival data.

MATERIAL AND METHODS

LITT protocol and inclusion criteria were approved by the local ethics committee, and written informed consent was obtained from all patients. The study included 61 patients who developed metastases in the remaining liver after hepatectomy, 47 patients who presented with metastases in both liver lobes, 14 patients who had contraindications for surgery, and 3 patients who refused hepatic surgery. Patients with more than five metastases, metastases larger than 4 cm in the greatest diameter, or with extrahepatic tumor spread were excluded. Patients who developed additional liver metastases during follow-up were also treated. Therefore, a maximum of nine lesions were treated per patient.

PATIENTS TREATED WITH LASER-INDUCED INTERSTITIAL THERMOTHERAPY

Between June 1993 and January 1997, 125 consecutive patients with liver metastases, 28 to 84 years of age (mean, 59.2 years), were treated with MR-guided LITT under local anesthesia. The primary tumor was a colorectal carcinoma in 85 patients, breast cancer in 16 patients, and hepatocellular carcinoma in 5 patients. In the remaining 19 patients, the primary tumors were thyroid carcinoma, urothelial carcinoma, esophageal carcinoma, hypernephroid carcinoma, bronchial carcinoma, and melanoma. A total of 355 lesions (mean per patient, 2.8; range; 1 to 9 lesions) were treated in these 125 patients using 998 laser applications (mean per patient, 8; range, 1 to 36 applications). The first 20 patients were included in a phase I study, whereas the remainder were included in a phase II study using improved multi-applicator laser technology.

All patients with colorectal carcinoma underwent chemotherapy with various protocols, usually fluorouracil and leukovorin, after surgical resection of the primary tumor. In all patients, the metastases developed during chemotherapy.

The mean duration between detection of liver metastases (i.e., the time of the LITT decision) and the initial laser procedure was 1.9 months.

LASER SYSTEM AND APPLICATION SET

Laser coagulation was performed using a neodymium: yttrium-aluminum-garnet (Nd:YAG) laser (Dornier MediLas 5060, Martin MY 30, Munich) with a specially developed scattering dome light emitter. For effective LITT, a special diffusing applicator and an application kit for percutaneous treatment were developed and optimized.

Laser light with a wavelength of 1046 nm was transmitted to tissue with a diffusing applicator. A protective glass dome with a diameter of 1.4 mm was mounted on a 400-μm silica fiber core. It was frosted on its inner surface, which emitted laser light 12 to 15 mm. Laser light of this wavelength penetrates deeply into biologic tissue, where photon absorption and heat conduction lead to coagulative and hyperthermic effects. Tissue destruction may be immediate or delayed.

The laser application kit (SOMATEX, Berlin, Germany) consists of a cannulation needle with a tetragonally sharpened tip, the guidewire, a sheath system with mandrin (15 cm, 7), and a special protective catheter (43 cm, 4) that is closed at the distal end (Fig. 40-1). The protective cathether prevents direct contact of the laser applicator with the patient and enables complete removal of the applicator, even in the unlikely event of damage to the fiber during treatment. This device increases patient safety and simplifies the procedure. The catheter is transparent to laser radiation and resistant to heat up to 400° C. Marks on the sheath and the protective catheter allow exact positioning of both in the lesion.

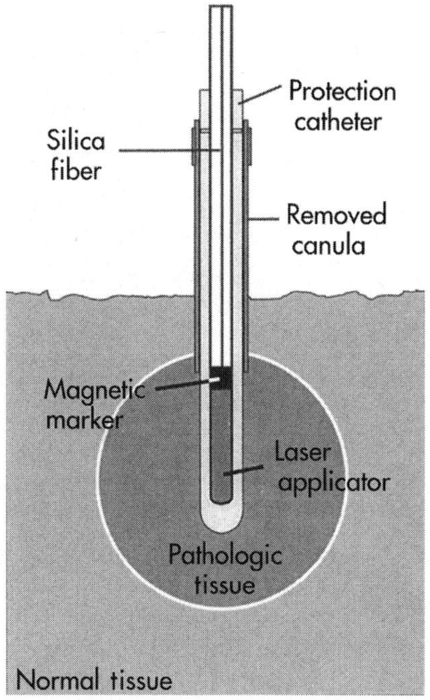

Fig. 40-1. Set-up of magnetic resonance–guided laser-induced thermotherapy. (From Vogl TJ, Mack MG: *Interstitial laser therapy of liver lesions.* In Debatin JF, Adam G: *Interventional magnetic resonance imaging,* Heidelberg, 1998, Springer-Verlag.)

The system is fully compatible with MRI systems. Magnetite markers on the laser applicator facilitate visualization and positioning. The laser is installed outside of the examination unit, and the light is transmitted via a 10-m optical fiber. The complete set-up for LITT is shown in Figure 40-1.

PROTOCOL DURING LASER-INDUCED INTERSTITIAL THERMOTHERAPY

Informed consent was obtained from all patients enrolled in the study. The success of LITT depends on accurate delivery of the optical fibers to the target area, real-time monitoring of the treatment effects, and subsequent evaluation of the extent of thermal damage. Achievement of these objectives depends on the imaging methods used.

Before LITT, all patients undergo contrast-enhanced MRI. After localization of the tumor via computed tomography (CT), 20 ml of 1% lidocaine is infiltrated locally, and pethidine (25 to 50 mg) is administered intravenously.

A 7-F sheath is subsequently inserted via a percutaneous approach under CT guidance (Fig. 40-2, *A* to *C*). A special heat-resistant protective catheter is thereafter introduced. After the patient is positioned on the MRI table, the laser catheter is inserted into the protective catheter.

MR thermometry is performed using specially designed turbo fast low-angle shot (FLASH) (repetition time [TR], 7 msec; echo time [TE], 3 msec; inversion time, 400 msec) and two-dimensional FLASH (TR, 102 msec; TE, 8 msec; flip angle, 15°) sequences, which have been optimized for the detection of thermal changes (Fig. 40-2 *D, E*).

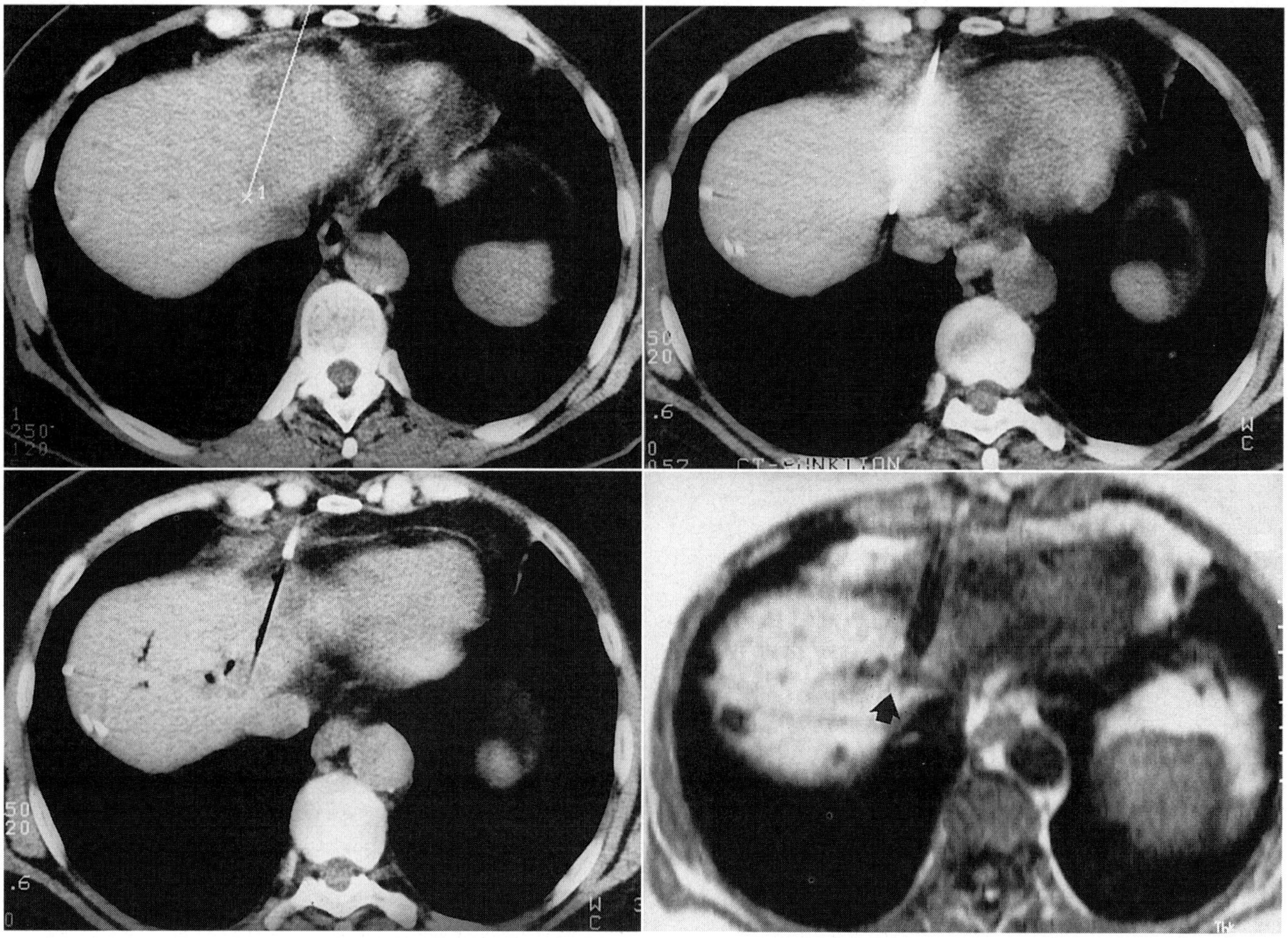

Fig. 40-2. Computed tomography (CT) guidance, magnetic resonance (MR) thermometry, and MR therapy control of metastatic colon cancer in liver segment 4. **A,** Transverse CT scan reveals the position of the two lesions and the marked puncture direction. **B,** The needle enters the lesion in a space anterior to the inferior vena cava. **C,** An inserted laser applicator system is seen, revealing the thermocatheter and the sheath with higher density. **D,** A plain two-dimensional (2D) fast low-angle shot (FLASH) image (repetition time [TR], 154 msec; echo time [TE], 6 msec; flip angle, 70°) in axial slice orientation shows the metastases before laser-induced interstitial thermotherapy (LITT) in liver segment 4 *(arrow),* the active zone of the laser, and the position of the magnetite marker. *Continued*

Before and after LITT, T1-weighted (spin-echo, gradient echo) and T2-weighted (spin-echo) images are obtained (Fig. 40-2, *F, G*). A conventional 1.5-T magnet (Siemens SP 4000, Erlangen, Germany) is used for MRI. Follow-up examinations using the plain and contrast-enhanced (gadopentetate 0.1 ml/kg body weight) sequences are carried out 2 days, 1 month, 3 months, and every 6 months after LITT. Qualitative and quantitative parameters are evaluated, including size, morphology, and contrast-enhancement pattern at early and late follow-up.

DEFINITION OF PATIENTS FOR MAGNETIC RESONANCE–GUIDED LASER-INDUCED INTERSTITIAL THERMOTHERAPY

Patients chosen for LITT should have less than five lesions, and none measuring more than 40 mm in diameter. They are generally nonsurgical candidates because of lesion distribution or localization or because they refuse operative resection. Patients with recurrent disease after partial resection of one hepatic lobe are also suitable for this therapy. All patients are hospitalized for 24 hours after the procedure. Survival was estimated with the Kaplan-Meier method, and statistical analysis was performed for different subgroups (e.g., male versus female, metastases from colorectal carcinoma versus metastases from other primary tumors, phase I versus phase II) using the Breslow test and the Tarone-Ware test.

RESULTS

Complications

All patients tolerated the procedure well under local anesthesia without severe complications. Three patients experienced mild nausea after LITT; in one patient, an asymptomatic right subphrenic hemorrhage developed (visualized on MRI). No deaths, infections, or liver or bile duct injury occurred.

E F G

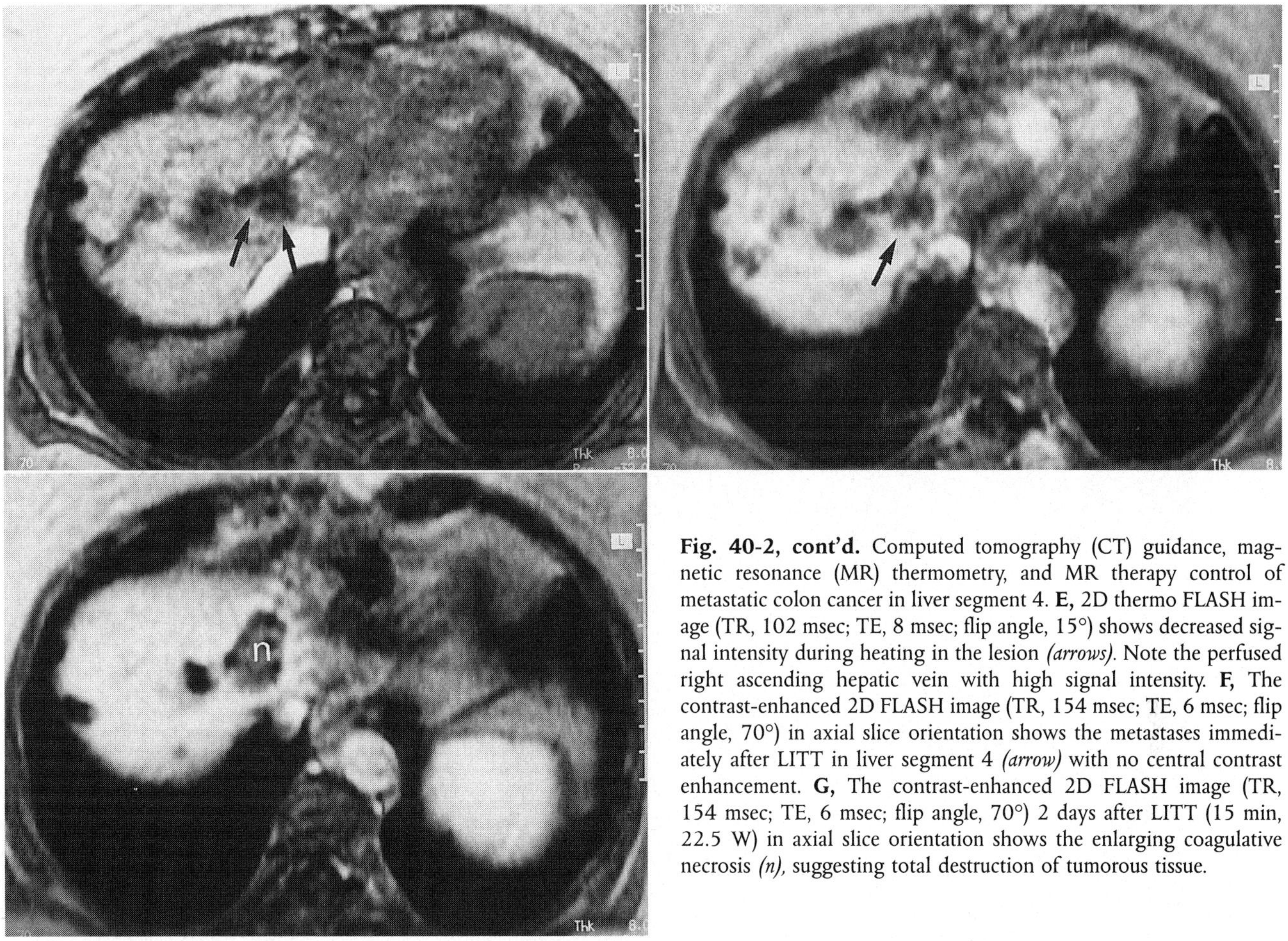

Fig. 40-2, cont'd. Computed tomography (CT) guidance, magnetic resonance (MR) thermometry, and MR therapy control of metastatic colon cancer in liver segment 4. **E,** 2D thermo FLASH image (TR, 102 msec; TE, 8 msec; flip angle, 15°) shows decreased signal intensity during heating in the lesion *(arrows).* Note the perfused right ascending hepatic vein with high signal intensity. **F,** The contrast-enhanced 2D FLASH image (TR, 154 msec; TE, 6 msec; flip angle, 70°) in axial slice orientation shows the metastases immediately after LITT in liver segment 4 *(arrow)* with no central contrast enhancement. **G,** The contrast-enhanced 2D FLASH image (TR, 154 msec; TE, 6 msec; flip angle, 70°) 2 days after LITT (15 min, 22.5 W) in axial slice orientation shows the enlarging coagulative necrosis *(n),* suggesting total destruction of tumorous tissue.

Magnetic resonance response of liver metastases and healthy liver tissue to laser-induced interstitial thermotherapy

In the phase I study, 20 patients with 49 lesions were candidates for LITT. The lesions ranged from 10 to 40 mm in diameter and were treated with one LITT applicator under MRI control. The mean laser power was 5.2 W (range, 2.8 to 8.6 W), and the duration of application was 10 to 35 min (mean, 19.2 min).

The phase II study was carried out between July 1994 and January 1997; 105 patients with 306 lesions were treated with an advanced MR-controlled LITT protocol. Depending on tumor volume, up to eight applicator systems were positioned in the central and peripheral parts of the metastases. This approach resulted in an increased volume of thermal tumor necrosis. The mean laser power was 5.3 W (range, 4.7 to 8.5 W), and the duration of application was 16 to 23 min (mean, 20.8 min).

Local tumor control

Short-term follow-up MRI verified the size and location of the treated lesion and assessed laser-induced tumor necrosis and resultant changes in size and morphology of the lesion (Figs. 40-3 and 40-4).

No statistically significant differences occurred ($P > 0.05$) between the local control rates of the various histopathologic tumor types and between the various positions of the lesions with regard to the segmental topography of the liver.

Of 306 lesions treated in the phase II study, 84% remained constant in size as determined in follow-up studies over at least 3 months. All lesions that were larger (16%) at follow-up had been larger than 10 ml at the time of the initial procedure. In 76%, 100% necrosis of the lesion was obtained; in 19.5%, the volume of necrosis comprised 75% to 99% of the lesion's volume; and in 4%, necrosis was unsatisfactory at 30% to 74% of the lesion's volume. One lesion (0.5%) showed no response to treatment.

Survival rate

During follow-up, 23 of 125 treated patients died of myocardial infarction ($n = 1$), apoplexia ($n = 1$), or tumor progression in the liver ($n = 13$) or in other locations ($n = 8$). The overall cumulative survival rate was 0.86 after 12 months and 0.63 after 28 months. The mean survival time, calculated with the Kaplan-Meier method, was 35 months (limited to 45 months;

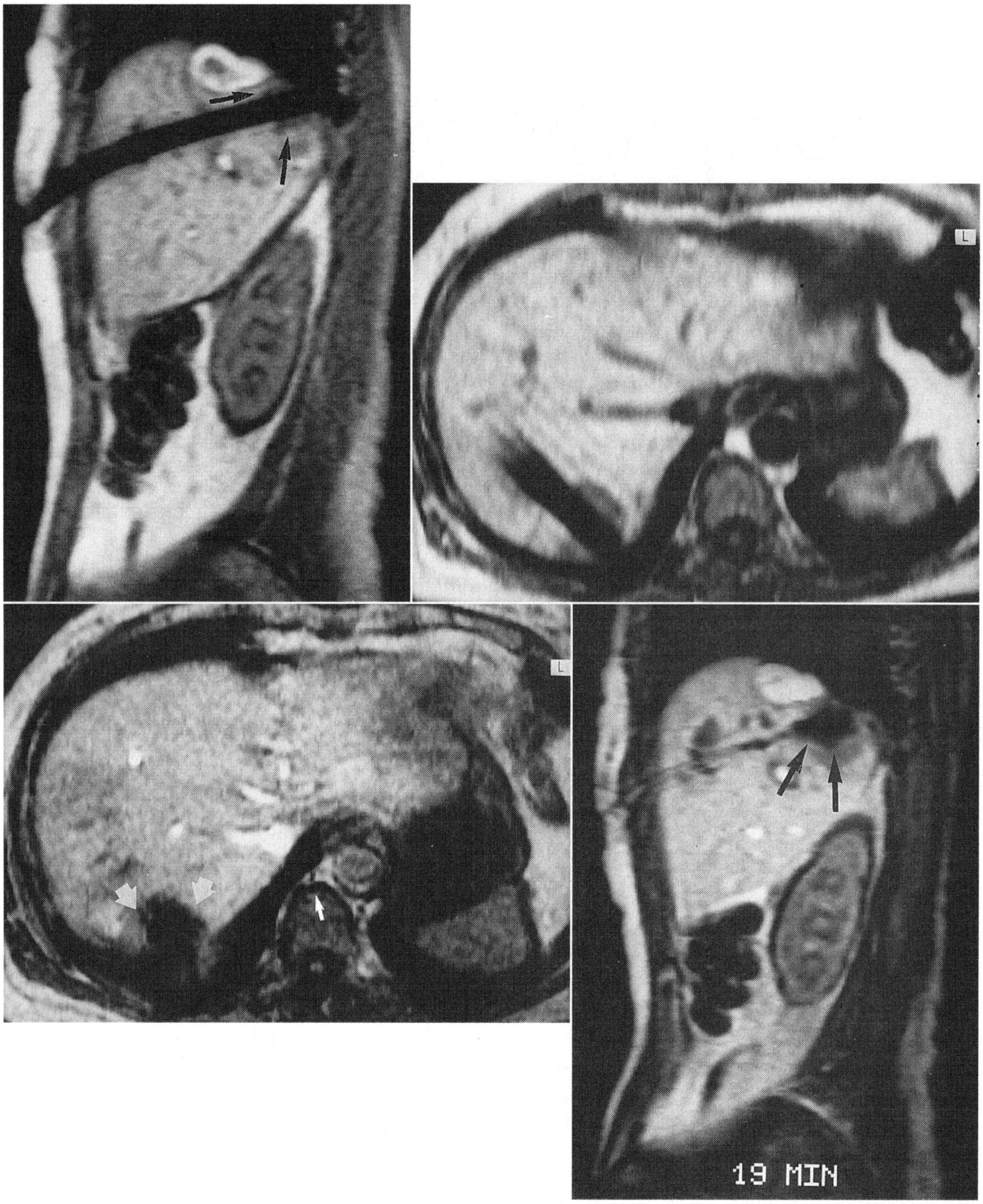

Fig. 40-3. Laser-induced interstitial thermotherapy (LITT) of recurrent metastases of a colorectal carcinoma after partial liver resection. **A,** The plain sagittal two-dimensional (2D) fast low-angle shot (FLASH) image (repetition time [TR], 154 msec; echo time [TE], 6 msec) before LITT shows the liver metastases *(arrows)* of the colorectal carcinoma with the transhepatic inserted applicator system and the introduced magnetite marker. Some bleeding is present in the upper portion of the tumor. **B,** The plain axial 2D FLASH image before LITT shows superiorly the metastases and the position of the application system. **C,** The axial 2D thermo FLASH image (TR, 102 msec; TE, 8 msec; flip angle, 15°) shows decreased signal intensity during heating in the lesion *(arrows)*. Note the perfused right ascending hepatic vein with high signal intensity *(small arrow)*. **D,** The sagittal 2D thermo FLASH image (TR, 102 msec; TE, 8 msec; flip angle, 15°) shows the decrease of signal intensity during heating in the lesion *(arrows)*.

Continued

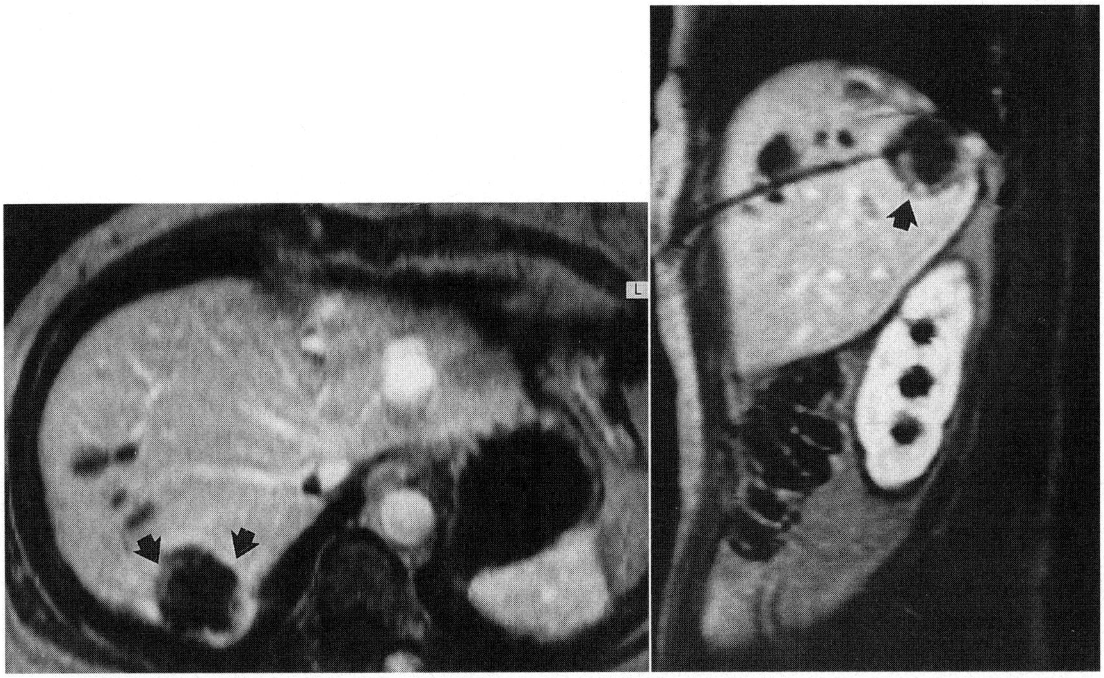

Fig. 40-3, cont'd. Laser-induced interstitial thermotherapy (LITT) of recurrent metastases of a colorectal carcinoma after partial liver resection. **E,** The contrast-enhanced 2D FLASH image obtained 2 days after laser intervention (22 min, 5.8 W) shows the induced coagulative necrosis (*arrows*). A viable tumor cannot be documented. **F,** The sagittal contrast-enhanced 2D FLASH image obtained 2 days after the laser intervention (22 min, 5.8 W) shows the induced coagulative necrosis *(arrow).*

Fig. 40-5). Survival did not differ significantly ($P > 0.05$) between male and female patients, nor between patients with colorectal metastases and those with metastases of other primary tumors. The improved multi-applicator technique gave rise to a statistically significant improvement in survival as determined by comparing the phase I and phase II studies (log-rank test, 0.032; Breslow test, 0.029; Tarone-Ware test, 0.031; Fig. 40-6). Survival was significantly longer ($P < 0.05$) in patients who had recurrent metastases after hemihepatectomy before laser treatment versus patients who had metastases in both liver lobes or who had contraindications to surgery (log-rank test, 0.032; Breslow test, 0.029; Tarone-Ware test, 0.031; Fig. 40-7).

Factors predicting optimal local tumor control

Total inactivation of the lesions (i. e., constant or regressive volume and avascularity as determined by follow-up with MRI) was achieved significantly ($P < 0.05$) more often in patients in whom the initial size of metastases was smaller than 2.5 cm maximum diameter. The location of the hepatic metastases did not result in significant differences in inactivation of the lesion.

DISCUSSION

The liver is one of the most common sites of metastasis in cancer patients. Survival of patients with metastatic liver disease depends on the extent of liver involvement and the presence of metastatic tumor elsewhere.

Two general means exist for managing metastatic liver tumors: systemic and locoregional treatment, including surgical resection. In at least 50% of patients with metastases resulting from colorectal cancer, the liver is the sole or predominant site of metastatic disease. For these patients, the question is whether systemic or locoregional therapy is more beneficial. One trial, performed by the Mayo Clinic and North Central Cancer Treatment Group, showed a survival advantage for patients receiving fluorouracil and leucovorin.[5] Even if such regimens produce a survival advantage, the study showed that remissions are short-term only.

Hepatic resection is the only potentially curative therapy for patients with colorectal cancer metastatic to the liver. Many uncontrolled studies have reported 5-year survival rates of 20% to 40% for patients who underwent resection of metastases.[6-8] Even in highly selected patients, this result is remarkable because 5-year survival in patients with medical treatment of metastatic colorectal cancer is very low.

Palmer, Petrelli, and Herrera[9] followed up 30 patients with unresectable liver metastases who refused to undergo further treatment. In 24 patients (80%), less than 25% of the liver was involved. Fourteen had synchronous metastases, whereas 16 had metachronous tumors. The mean interval from diagnosis of

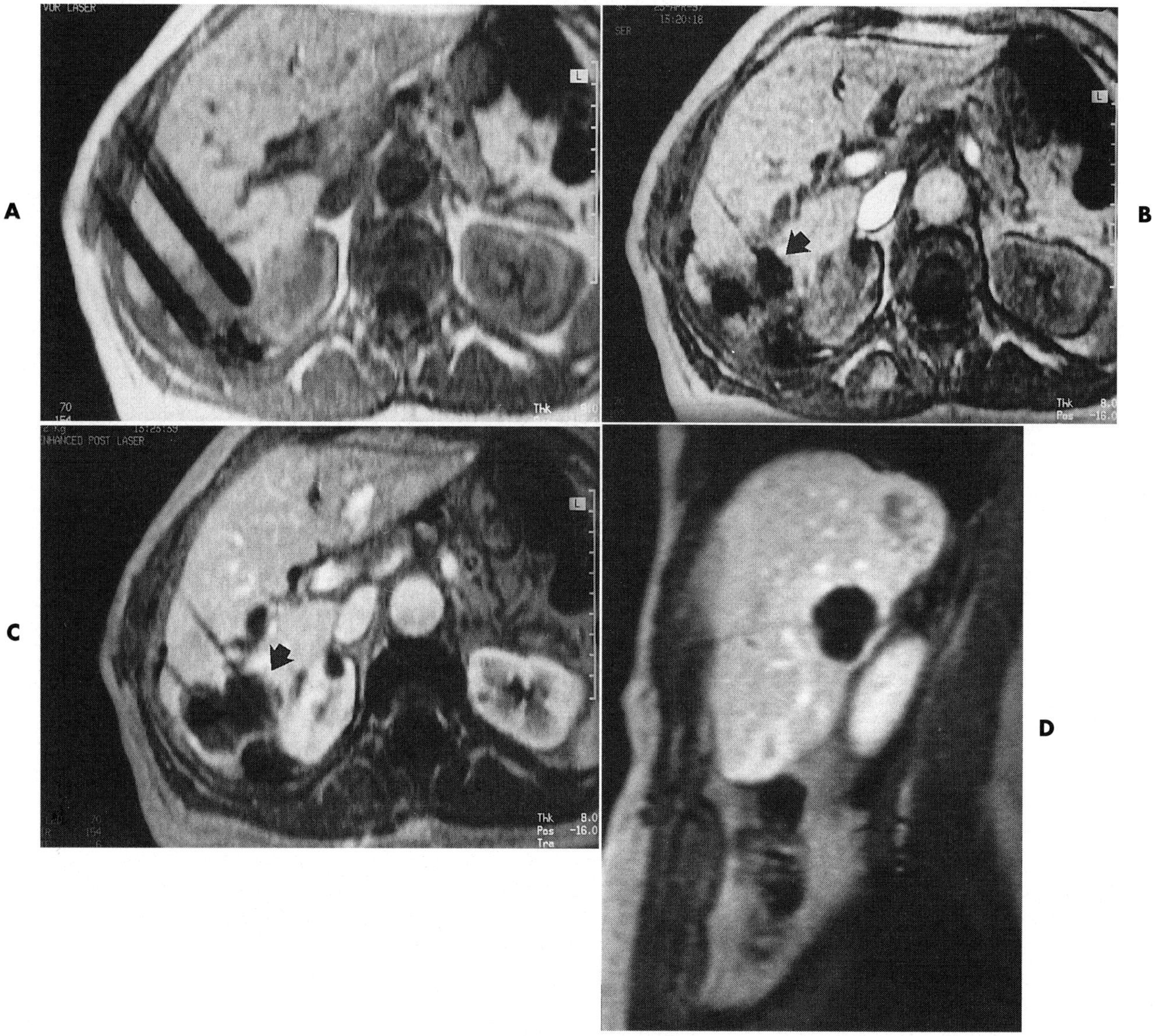

Fig. 40-4. Double-power maneuver in a large metastasis in liver segment 6. **A,** The plain axial two-dimensional (2D) fast low-angle shot (FLASH) image before laser-induced interstitial thermotherapy (LITT) shows superiorly the metastases and the position of the application systems, which have been placed in a parallel fashion. **B,** The axial 2D thermo FLASH image (repetition time, 102 msec; echo time, 8 msec; flip angle, 15°) shows decreased signal intensity during heating in the lesions *(arrow)* 15 min after LITT. **C,** The contrast-enhanced 2D FLASH image obtained 2 days after laser intervention (21 min, 5.8 W) shows the induced coagulative necrosis *(arrow)*. A viable tumor cannot be documented. **D,** Control in sagittal orientation after 2 days shows the confluent amount of laser-induced necrosis.

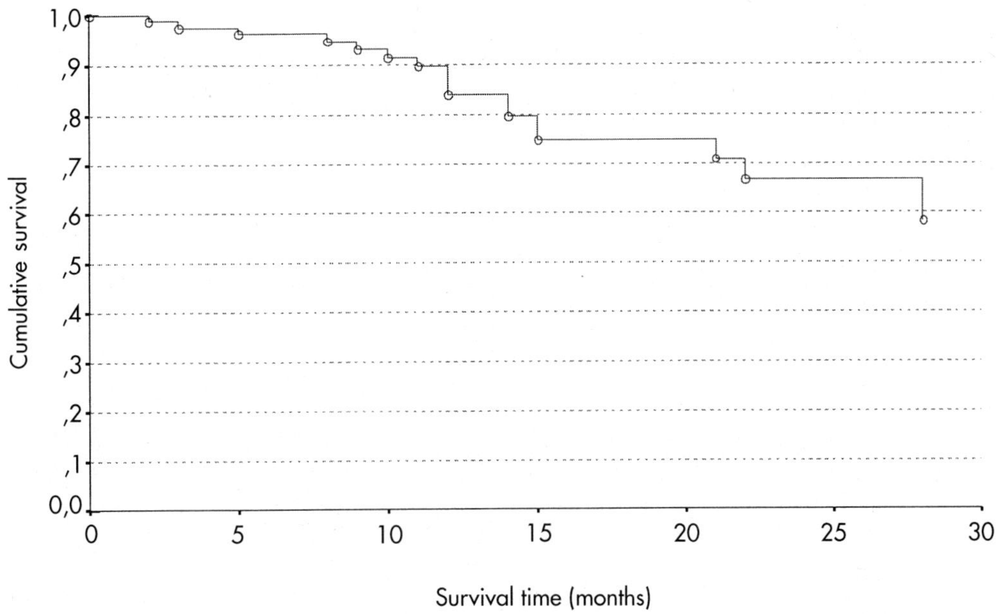

Fig. 40-5. Cumulative survival rate of the consecutive patient series.

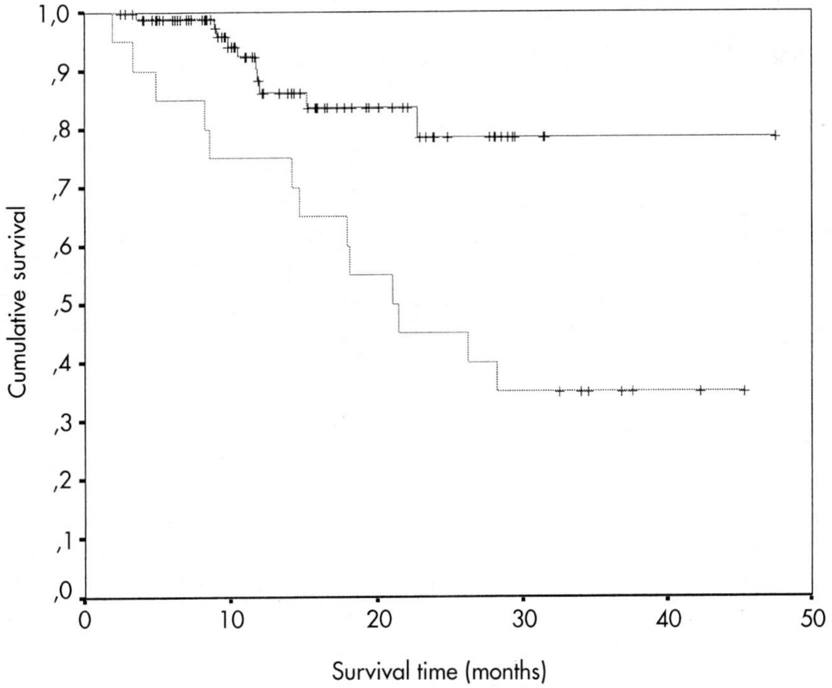

Fig. 40-6. Cumulative survival rates of the consecutive patient series in phase I *(bottom line)* and phase II *(top line)* studies.

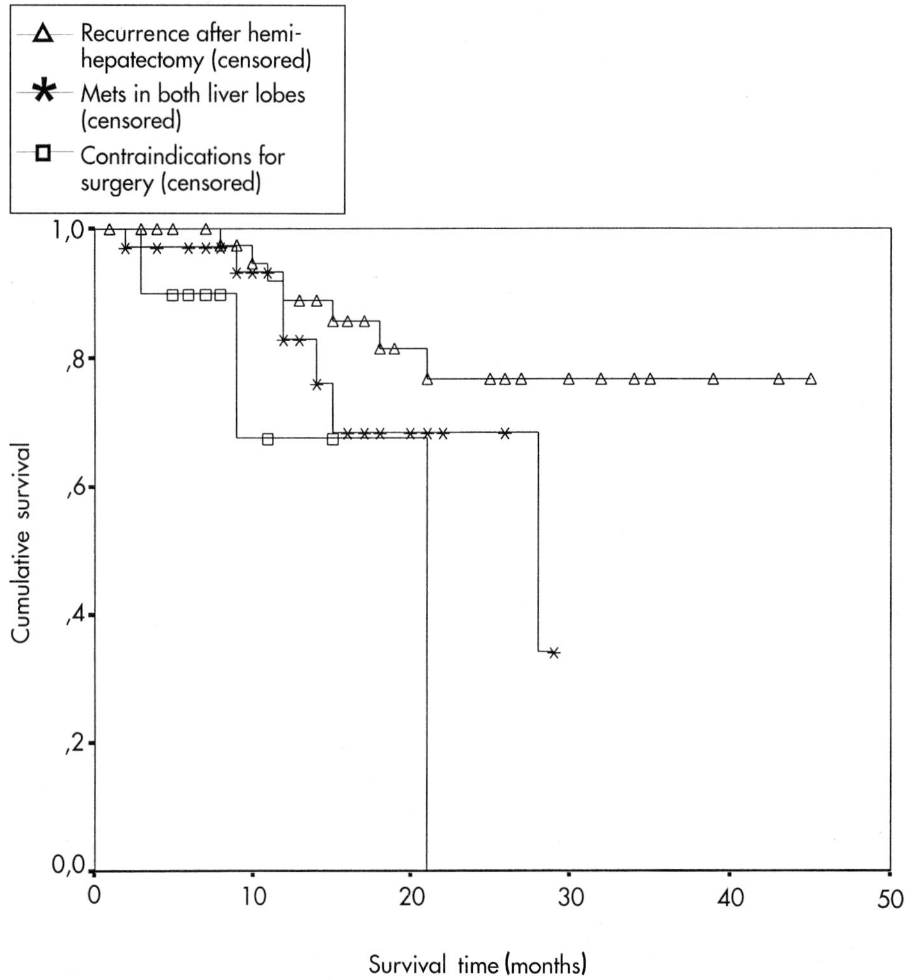

Fig. 40-7. Comparative evaluation of the survival data regarding indications for laser-induced interstitial thermotherapy.

primary disease to diagnosis of metachronous metastases was 16 months. The overall mean survival was 16 months, the overall median survival was 12 months, and the mean survival after diagnosis of the primary tumors was 25 months.

Stangl and others[8] followed up 1099 consecutive patients with colorectal liver metastases, of whom 566 (51.5%) received no treatment; 340 (31%) underwent hepatic resection; 123 (11.2%) received regional chemotherapy; and 70 (6.4%) received systemic therapy. Thirty-four patients died within 30 days as a result of postoperative complications or advanced disease; 48 were excluded because they developed a second primary cancer. After hepatic resection, 60% of all patients survived 2 years, and 32% survived 5 years (median survival, 30 months). In patients who underwent regional or systemic chemotherapy, median survival was 12.7 or 11.1 months, respectively. In patients who did not undergo treatment, 31.3% were alive at 1 year, 7.9% at 2 years, 2.6% at 3 years, and 0.9% at 4 years.

Failures after resection outnumbered cures; disease most frequently recurred in the liver parenchyma. Sugihara, and others[10] reported recurrence in 64 of 109 patients (59%) whose metastases resulting from colorectal cancer were completely resected. Recurrence developed most commonly in the liver (34 of 64 patients) and the lung (20 of 64 patients). The peritoneum was affected in 12 patients. Findings in a more recent study[11] confirmed these results; hepatic recurrence was most often not near the surgical margin. In this series, the mean interval between resection and detection of recurrence was 17 months. This finding confirms the suspicion that many patients who undergo resection have metastases too small to be detected with cross-sectional imaging techniques.

Surgery is the only known cure for hepatic metastases resulting from colorectal carcinoma, but the morbidity associated with hepatic resection is high (15% to 43%).[7,12] Even after apparently successful surgery with complete removal of metastases, disease frequently recurs. Over the past 5 to 10 years, therefore, interest has focused on several minimally invasive interstitial techniques under investigation.

Laser photocoagulation involves heating up a tumor with low-power laser light (Nd:YAG) delivered through optical fibers.

Pilot studies[13-15] using different approaches and techniques have shown that this method is very promising for treatment of liver tumors.

This large study shows that MR-guided LITT can offer several potential management benefits: (1), MRI provides unparalleled accuracy in topographic assessment. (2), The temperature sensitivity of special MR sequences can be used to monitor the temperature elevation in the tumor and surrounding healthy tissues, thus increasing the safety of the procedure. On-line MRI during LITT therefore allows monitoring of treatment effects (e.g., necrosis) and early detection of local complications (e.g., hemorrhage). (3), Recovery times, hospital stays, and the risk of infection and other complications can be reduced compared with conventional surgery. Successful implementation of such minimally invasive procedures would significantly reduce costs compared with surgical procedures. A further, indirect advantage is the psychologic effect caused by avoiding the cosmetic deformities associated with major surgery.

The study yielded an overall cumulative survival rate of 0.86 after 12 months and 0.63 after 28 months. As such, survival data obtained from patients who underwent MR-guided LITT are comparable with data obtained from the literature regarding patients who underwent hepatic resection; these data are better than the data obtained from patients who received chemotherapy or no management. Because 61 patients (52%) already had hepatic resection, and 47 (37.6%) were not candidates for surgery because of metastases in both liver lobes, these results establish a need for further investigation into the use of LITT as a first-line tool for therapy of hepatic metastases.

Thus, this experience with MR-guided LITT in the management of liver metastases shows survival and local tumor control rates comparable with those of hepatic resection; further advantages associated with minimally invasive LITT make it a very promising method for the management of liver metastases.

SUMMARY

In patients with surgically non-treatable hepatic metastases, treatment with MR-guided LITT provides effective local tumor control, but its clinical benefits on survival have not been verified. This study evaluated the effect of local tumor destruction with LITT on clinical outcome.

All patients tolerated the procedure well under local anesthesia. No severe complications or side effects were observed. During follow-up, 23 of 125 patients died of myocardial infarction ($n = 1$), apoplexia ($n = 1$), and tumor progression in the liver ($n = 13$) or in other locations ($n = 8$). The overall cumulative survival rate was 0.86 after 12 months and 0.63 after 28 months. The mean survival time, calculated with the Kaplan-Meier method, was 35 months. In patients with liver metastases, local tumor destruction using minimally invasive percutaneous LITT under local anesthesia results in improved clinical outcomes and survival rates versus chemotherapy alone. Survival data obtained after minimally invasive LITT are comparable with surgical data obtained from the literature.

REFERENCES

1. Weiss L, and others: Haematogenous metastatic patterns in colonic carcinoma: an analysis of 1541 necropsies, *J Pathol* 150:195, 1986.
2. Goslin R, and others: Factors influencing survival in patients with hepatic metastases from adenocarcinoma of the colon or rectum, *Dis Colon Rectum* 25:749, 1982.
3. Jaffe BM, and others: Factors influencing survival in patients with untreated hepatic metastases, *Surg Gynecol Obstet* 127:1, 1968.
4. Steele G Jr, Ravikumar TS: Resection of hepatic metastases from colorectal cancer: biologic perspective, *Ann Surg* 210:127, 1989.
5. Petrelli N, and others: The modulation of fluorouracil with leucovorin in metastatic colorectal carcinoma: a prospective randomized phase III trial. Gastrointestinal Tumor Study Group [published erratum appears in *J Clin Oncol* 8:185, 1990] *J Clin Oncol* 7:1419, 1989.
6. Butler J, Attiyeh FF, Daly JM: Hepatic resection for metastases of the colon and rectum, *Surg Gynecol Obstet* 162:109, 1986.
7. Hughes KS, and others: Resection of the liver for colorectal carcinoma metastases: a multi-institutional study of long-term survivors, *Dis Colon Rectum* 31:1, 1988.
8. Stangl R, and others: Factors influencing the natural history of colorectal liver metastases, *Lancet* 343:1405, 1994.
9. Palmer M, Petrelli NJ, Herrera L: No treatment option for liver metastases from colorectal adenocarcinoma, *Dis Colon Rectum* 32:698, 1989.
10. Sugihara K, and others: Pattern of recurrence after hepatic resection for colorectal metastases, *Br J Surg* 80:1032, 1993.
11. Harned RK, Chezmar JL, Nelson RC: Recurrent tumor after resection of hepatic metastases from colorectal carcinoma: location and time of discovery as determined by CT, *Am J Roentgenol* 163:93, 1994.
12. Scheele J, and others: Indicators of prognosis after hepatic resection for colorectal secondaries, *Surgery* 110:13, 1991.
13. Amin Z, and others: Hepatic metastases: interstitial laser photocoagulation with real-time US monitoring and dynamic CT evaluation of treatment, *Radiology* 187:339, 1993.
14. Vogl TJ, and others: Malignant liver tumors treated with MR imaging-guided laser-induced thermotherapy: technique and prospective results, *Radiology* 196:257, 1995.
15. Vogl TJ, and others: Recurrent nasopharyngeal tumors: preliminary clinical results with interventional MR imaging–controlled laser-induced thermotherapy, *Radiology* 196:725, 1995.

Chapter 41

MR–GUIDED CHOLECYSTOSTOMY: FEASIBILITY STUDIES

Jörg F. Debatin, Susanne C. Göhde

Bile-filled structures can be displayed on heavily T2-weighted magnetic resonance (MR) sequences without the use of contrast agents. Use of very long repetition times (TRs) and echo times (TEs) results in a selective display of the biliary system, referred to as MR cholangiography.[1,2] The MRI scans are acquired in any desirable plane.

With the availability of open-configuration MR systems, percutaneous biliary interventions under MRI-based guidance and control have become possible.[3,4] Fundamental to safe and expeditious percutaneous access of the biliary tree is the visualization of puncture and manipulative instruments relative to the biliary system. This visualization can be accomplished with electrically active techniques[5] (see Chapter 16).

NEEDLE TRACKING

The MR device tracking technique[5] uses a small radiofrequency (RF) coil, built into the tip of an invasive device, for spatial localization. The coil receives signal only from its immediate vicinity. After nonselective RF excitation, gradient-recalled echoes (GREs) are generated along three orthogonal axes to frequency encode the three-dimensional (3D) position of the coil. Digitized MR signals are sent to a "master" workstation, which computes the coil's position, updating it 20 times per sec for real-time tracking.[6,7] The workstation also receives images via a video link from the MR scanner. The coil position is displayed as a graphic overlay on any previously acquired road map MRI scan. In addition, the master workstation applies coordinate transformations of the coil's position from its initial reference plane to the reference plane of a second display connected to a second "slave" workstation. The slave workstation receives the transformed coordinates from the master workstation and presents a second video display with a graphic overlay representing the position of the coil on a second road map image. The composite images, displaying the instantaneous position of the coil in any two planes, are simultaneously projected onto a screen visible to the operator inside the scan room and are videotaped for archiving purposes. The position of the interventional device can thus be followed simultaneously in real-time on any two images. Moreover, images in one or both planes can be continuously updated, corresponding to the position of the RF coil built into the interventional device. Hence, tracking modes consist of (1) continuous tracking of the device tip on a road map image or (2) intermittent tracking and image acquisition, whereby new images are obtained corresponding to the coil position. The system is entirely flexible with respect to the assignment of tracking modes to displays.

EXPERIMENTAL DESIGN

The 14-gauge prototype MR tracking needle was manufactured by BIP (Munich, Germany). Both stylette and cannula are made of polyethyleneketone (PEEK), a polymer composite. Biocompatibility and durability of PEEK have been documented in conjunction with its use as an orthopedic implant material.[8-10] For reliable cutting, the cutting stylette tip is made of ceramic. A simple untuned copper loop RF coil with an outer diameter of 1.2 mm is incorporated into the stylette immediately distal to the cutting tip. The RF coil is attached to a coaxial cable, which is interfaced to the workstation via a plug at the needle base. The RF coil and the coaxial cable are contained in the biocompatible needle material.

The animal experiments were performed in a superconducting, cryogen-free, 0.5-T, open-configuration interventional MR scanner (Signa SP, GE Medical Systems, Milwaukee, Wis). The tracking software was implemented on two Sparc workstations (Sun Microsystems, Mountain View, Calif). Cholecystostomies were conducted on three fully anesthesized female pigs (40 to 45 kg body weight). The animal experiments had been approved by the appropriate governmental regulatory committees.

The gallbladder and the biliary system were displayed in all three orthogonal planes using a heavily T2-weighted fast spin-echo (FSE) sequence (Fig. 41-1, *A* to *C*). Maximum pixel intensity projections of the biliary system were constructed. The gallbladder was targeted using two approaches: along the axis of the magnet and in a perpendicular plane. For planning

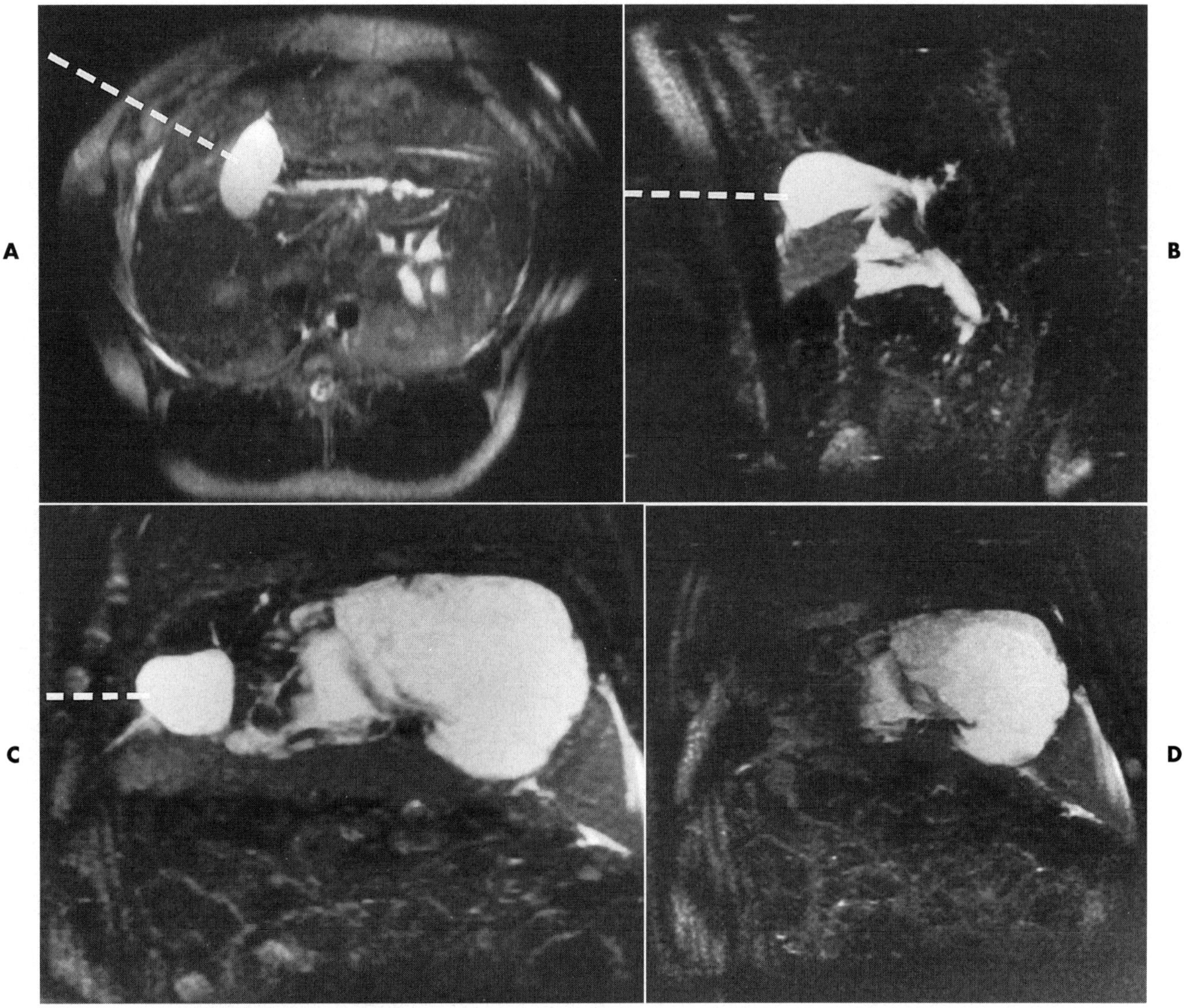

Fig. 41-1. A, Axial; **B,** sagittal; and **C,** coronal maximum intensity projection (MIP) images of the T2-weighted sequence depict the gallbladder of a pig. On the coronal image, the fluid-filled stomach is also displayed as a bright structure. On all three orthogonal images, the position of the needle tip is being projected in real-time *(dotted line)* as it is advanced into the gallbladder. On **D,** the coronal MIP image acquired after bile aspiration, the gallbladder is no longer seen.

purposes, the expected course of the needle was drawn onto the road map images, which were displayed on liquid crystal display monitors in front of the interventionalist, positioned in the opening of the interventional magnet itself.

Based on these "cholangio" road maps, the coaxial MR tracking needle was inserted percutaneously into the gallbladder under continuous MR guidance. Using the MR tracking sequence (TR, 30 msec; TE, 8 msec; flip angle, 60°), the position of the coil was sampled using a Hadamard encoding strategy[11] every 120 msec or 8 times per sec. The position of the needle tip was thus displayed simultaneously on the two cholangio road maps in real-time (less than 10 msec delay from data acquisition).[7] Thus, the biplanar positional information of the needle tip, relative to the biliary tree, became available to the interventionalist as the needle was advanced into the gallbladder (see Fig. 41-1). In addition, updated GRE images were acquired through the tip of the needle every 10 sec in the axial plane. These images document the position of the needle based on the signal void caused by the needle instrument (Fig. 41-2).

Once the needle was positioned inside the gallbladder, the bile was aspirated and the MR cholangiogram was repeated (see Fig. 41-1, *D*).

RESULTS

Based on the heavily T2-weighted MR cholangio road maps, the gallbladder was easily identified. The actual procedure time for the cholecystostomy was less than 5 min. Biplanar MR tracking was robust and remained totally unaffected by the surrounding tissues throughout the interventions (see Figs. 41-1 and 41-2). In all three animals, cholecystostomies were successfully performed under MR guidance and control. The puncture needle was safely guided in real-time using the MR tracking algorithm, displaying the position of the needle simultaneously on two orthogonal cholangio road maps.

A

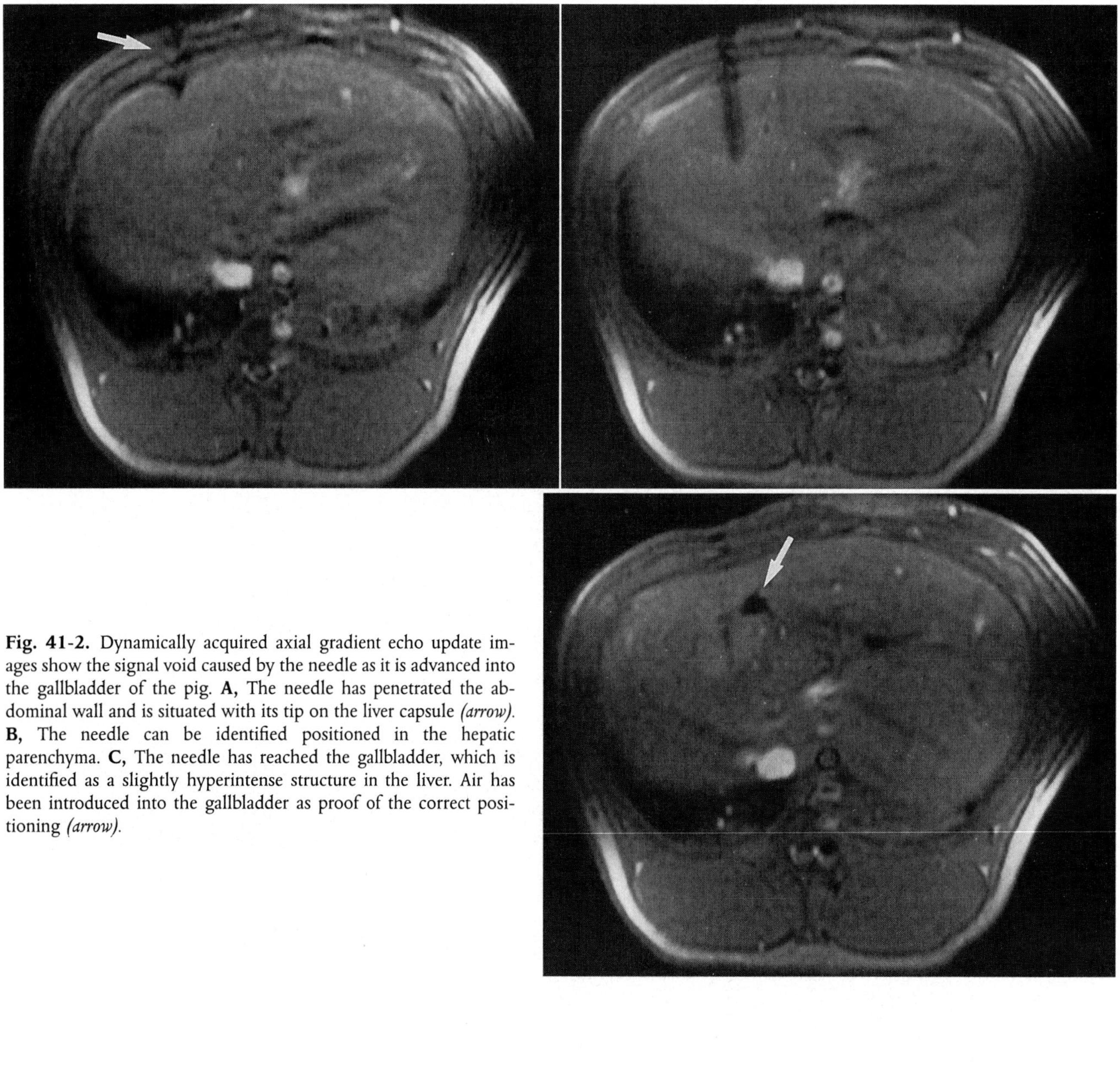

B

C

Fig. 41-2. Dynamically acquired axial gradient echo update images show the signal void caused by the needle as it is advanced into the gallbladder of the pig. **A,** The needle has penetrated the abdominal wall and is situated with its tip on the liver capsule *(arrow)*. **B,** The needle can be identified positioned in the hepatic parenchyma. **C,** The needle has reached the gallbladder, which is identified as a slightly hyperintense structure in the liver. Air has been introduced into the gallbladder as proof of the correct positioning *(arrow)*.

After aspiration of bile from the gallbladder through the cannula of the coaxial MR tracking needle system, MR cholangiograms confirmed a marked reduction in the size of the gallbladder (see Fig. 41-1, *D*).

DISCUSSION

The cholecystostomy procedures performed in animal experiments should be considered the first step with regard to using MR guidance for biliary interventions. The outlined biplanar target-directed active tracking approach appears sufficiently versatile to also permit access to dilated biliary ducts for percutaneous biliary drainage procedures. By visualizing the needle tip in relation to the biliary tree at all times, the drainage cannula can be guided to a most optimal access. Procedure times can be reduced; exposure to ionizing radiation is altogether eliminated. Insertion of coil-tipped MR tracking guidewires and catheters[12] into the biliary tree might enable the performance of more complex biliary interventions.

The present device tracking technique is based on the separation of imaging data acquisition and the collection of the positional data of the device's tip. The device is not identified in the image; instead, its position is determined independent of the morphologic imaging process. The images, based on which the intervention is guided and monitored, can thus be acquired using the highest quality standards, including maximal lesion conspicuity. Images with different inherent contrast properties may be acquired in the same region: one image set will display the dilated biliary system, whereas a second set can be optimized to depict the obstructing tumor in relation to the surrounding vasculature.

In the case that images need to be updated, the positional information of the coil can be used to guide the imaging plane, so new images are acquired corresponding to the coil position. With the biplanar tracking option, updated images can even be acquired in two different planes, displaying the real-time position of the needle tip. The operator can choose whether to track the device on two previously acquired images or to have the scanner provide updated images on one or both displays corresponding to the position of the RF coil.

The results of these preliminary experiments show the feasibility of applying this active device tracking technique to biliary interventions. Fundamental to the functioning of this system is the use of PEEK for the construction of the MR biopsy needle. Two properties of the material make it suitable for this purpose: (1) It is rather inert in an MR environment. No torque is placed on the needle when moved in the magnetic field. The associated susceptibility artifact is sufficiently limited to not dephase the tracking signal originating from the spins inside and outside the coil. Furthermore, susceptibility artifacts and gradient nonlinearities are prevented from affecting the tracked locations by the use of a four excitation–Hadamard encoding scheme.[11] (2) PEEK provides the needle with sufficient stability to penetrate even firm tissues. To enhance the cutting ability, the cutting tip of the stylette is made of ceramic.

The biplanar tracking concept will need to be proven in a clinical environment. The presented data suggest, however, a significant potential for the delivery of diagnostic and therapeutic devices to the biliary system.

REFERENCES

1. Kaufman L, and others: Accessible magnetic resonance imaging, *Magn Reson Q* 5:283, 1989.
2. Schuster DM, Pedrosa MC, Robbins AH: Magnetic resonance cholangiography, *Abdom Imaging* 20:353, 1995.
3. Jolesz FA, Blumenfeld SM: Interventional use of magnetic resonance imaging, *Magn Reson Q* 10:85, 1994.
4. Schenk JF, and others: Superconducting open configuration MR imaging system for image-guided therapy, *Radiology* 195:805, 1995.
5. Dumoulin CL, Souza SP, Darrow RD: Real-time position monitoring of invasive devices using magnetic resonance, *Magn Reson Med* 29:411, 1993.
6. Leung DA, and others: Intravascular MR tracking catheter: preliminary experimental evaluation, *Am J Roentgenol* 164:1265, 1995.
7. Leung DA, and others: Real-time biplanar tracking for interventional MR-imaging procedures, *Radiology* 197:485, 1995.
8. Jokisch KA, and others: Biological response to chopped-carbon-fiber-reinforced PEEK, *J Biomed Mater Res* 26:133, 1992.
9. Maharaj G, and others: Characterization of wear in composite material orthopedic implants: part I. The composite trunnion/ceramic interface, *Biomed Mater Eng* 4:193, 1994.
10. Albert K, and others: Characterization of wear in composite material orthopedic implants. Part II. The implant/bone interface, *Biomed Mater Eng* 4:199, 1994.
11. Dumoulin CL, and others: Simultaneous acquisition of phase contrast angiograms and stationary tissue images with Hadamard encoding of flow-induced phase shifts, *J Magn Reson Imaging* 1:399, 1991.
12. Wildermuth S, and others: MR-guided intravascular procedures: initial demonstration in a pig model, *Radiology* 202:578, 1997.

Chapter 42

MR–GUIDED THERAPY OF THE PROSTATE

Andreas Heuck, Ullrich G. Müller-Lisse, Peter Schneede

Benign prostatic hyperplasia (BPH) occurs in most men older than 60 years and is frequently the cause of severe bladder outflow obstruction.[1] Prostate cancer is the most common human cancer and is found at autopsy in 30% of men aged 50 years and in approximately 80% aged 90 years. Prostate cancer is predominantly latent; however, the annual incidence of the disease has increased considerably during the past decade, with approximately 240,000 cases diagnosed in the United States in 1995.[2]

BPH and prostate cancer are the most common causes for surgical procedures of the prostate. In the United States, approximately 500,000 patients with BPH undergo transurethral resection of the prostate (TURP) each year, and the number of surgical procedures for prostate cancer is estimated to be more than 8000.[3] More recently, thermal modalities have been developed as alternatives for the treatment of BPH and prostate cancer.

This chapter discusses the role of magnetic resonance imaging (MRI) for planning and monitoring of established surgical procedures, especially thermal therapy.

ESTABLISHED MODALITIES FOR TREATMENT OF PROSTATIC DISEASE

Benign prostatic hyperplasia

BPH originates in the transitional zone of the prostate and is the most frequent cause of infravesical obstruction. The most widely established therapy for symptomatic BPH is TURP.[3] Although TURP is highly effective, several side effects and limitations have been described: incorporation of irrigation fluids during the procedure may lead to considerable strain of the cardiovascular system, especially in elderly patients. Furthermore, blood loss requiring blood transfusion occurs in approximately 4% of cases. After TURP, retrograde ejaculation is found in 50% to 68% of patients, erectile dysfunction in up to 15%, urethral stricture in approximately 3%, and incontinence in approximately 2%.[4] In patients with large prostate glands or with frequently recurring hyperplasia, suprapubic prostatectomy may be performed as an alternative to TURP. This open surgical procedure is associated with longer hospitalization and slightly higher mortality than TURP, whereas long-term morbidity is higher after TURP.[3,5]

Prostate cancer

Adenocarcinoma of the prostate is the most common malignancy in men and the second most common cause of death from cancer in men after bronchogenic carcinoma. As stated, according to various autopsy studies, prostate cancer is found in more than 30% of men older than age 50 years. In approximately 70% of cases, prostate cancer appears in the peripheral zone of the gland, whereas approximately 30% of the tumors occur in the central gland. Depending on the tumor stage, operability, and other factors, patients with prostate cancer usually undergo radical prostatectomy, external beam radiotherapy, anti-androgenic therapy, or any combination of these modalities. Radical prostatectomy is the traditional surgical therapy, and improvements in surgical technique allow the neurovascular bundles to be spared in patients with cancer localized to the prostate gland. The neurovascular bundles are critical to the maintenance of erectile function, and sparing of these structures considerably decreases impotency rates after radical prostatectomy. Patients with cancer extending beyond the prostate gland are frequently considered not to benefit from radical prostatectomy and are most often treated primarily with radiation or hormonal therapy. In patients presenting with prostate cancer and infravesical obstruction, TURP may precede radiotherapy or anti-androgenic drugs.

THERMAL AND CRYOSURGICAL MODALITIES IN THE TREATMENT OF PROSTATIC DISEASE

The increasing number of elderly patients who cannot tolerate established surgical treatment and of patients who will not undergo these procedures and their potential risks has led to the development of alternative minimally invasive treatment modalities. These alternative modalities have been designed to decrease complications and side effects associated with the classical surgical procedures. The new treatments include thermal modalities with various energy applications (e.g., medical lasers, microwaves, high-intensity focused ultrasound [US]) and cryosurgical treatment. The common goal of thermal or cryosurgical procedures is to produce focal necrosis and consecutive ablation of targeted tissues (e.g., adenomatous hyperplasia in patients with BPH, tumor in patients with prostate cancer).

Thermal modalities

Laser therapy of the prostate

In most thermal ablation therapies of the prostate, medical lasers are used as energy sources. The term *laser* is an acronym for "light amplification by stimulated emission of radiation" (see Chapter 23). The optical waveguides used in laser ablation of the prostate are fibers of high-purity fused silica glass with minimal optical absorption and scattering. Less than 1% of laser energy is lost during the series of reflections from one sidewall to the opposite sidewall, along the length of the fiber core of a typical optical fiber for medical applications. The active end of the fiber core, the laser applicator, is covered by a layer of lower refractive index glass or plastic termed *cladding* that diffuses the array of laser light beams as it enters the tissue.[6] Depending on the design and properties of the laser applicator, different laser instruments with different properties and modes of tissue interaction result. Sidefire laser applicators are the instruments most frequently used for laser ablation of the prostate.

Energy release from laser applicators into tissues causes a local temperature increase, which results, depending on the temperatures reached, in tissue protein denaturation and coagulation, vaporization, and carbonization.

Endoscopic laser ablation

Endoscopic laser ablation of the prostate is performed by using a transurethral approach and applying sidefire laser applicators in the prostatic urethra in a noncontact mode; laser energy is absorbed by prostatic tissue after passing through urine or water in the urethra. When absorbed, the electromagnetic energy of laser light waves is transformed into thermal energy, which heats the periurethral prostatic tissue and consecutively leads to coagulation necrosis. Endoscopic laser ablation of the prostate has been primarily used for the treatment of BPH, although preliminary experience in the ablation of prostate cancer has been reported.[7-9]

The original refractive right-angle laser delivery system used for endoscopic laser ablation of the prostate was transurethral ultrasonically guided laser prostatectomy (TULIP, IntraSonix, Burlington, Mass). In this device, the laser beam is diverted 90° by a sapphire prism. Reflective sidefire applicators use a gold-plated stainless steel reflector to deflect the laser beam laterally, which results in a higher energy absorption than in refractive systems. Usually, the beam diverges to light a larger surface area (e.g., Urolase, Bard, Marietta, Ga, which has a horizontal beam divergence of 25° and a sagittal divergence of 60°).

In the clinical treatment of BPH, TULIP substantially reduced blood loss, incorporation of irrigation fluids, and the rate of retrograde ejaculation compared with TURP, whereas peak urine flow increases, residual urine volume, and prostate symptom scores decreased considerably.[9] A disadvantage of TULIP is the delayed relief of infravesical obstruction caused by relatively slow removal of coagulated tissue debris and postoperative symptomatic irritation of the bladder.

Another ablation technique using sidefire laser applicators is the visual laser-assisted prostatectomy (VLAP), which uses an approach very similar to TULIP. The main difference lies in the laser device used and in that primary guidance of laser application is performed visually not by US. Randomized trials comparing VLAP and TURP in the treatment of BPH have shown that the functional outcome (urine peak flow, residual urine) of both modalities after 3 to 6 months is similar, whereas prostate symptom scores may be better with TURP.[5] Although sidefire VLAP and TURP use different physical approaches, they are similar in that tissue around the original prostatic urethra, including the transitional epithelium, is removed under endoscopic visual control creating a funnel-like crater primarily depleted of urothelium, which is secondarily reconstituted by urothelial lining.

Interstitial laser ablation

Interstitial laser ablation, also referred to as *laser-induced interstitial thermotherapy* (LITT), of the prostate uses a different approach. Using a transurethral or transperineal approach, the laser applicator is positioned in the prostate in an interstitial location with immediate tissue contact. Laser light is evenly diffused by the applicator and is absorbed in the adjacent tissue, where interstitial tissue temperature increases. After the temperature surpasses 60° C, coagulation necrosis of a roughly ovoid to cylindrical shape occurs. LITT of the prostate has been primarily used as a minimally invasive therapy for BPH,[10-12] whereas its use in the treatment of prostate cancer has not been extensively studied.

The most commonly used laser system for LITT of the prostate is the Dornier fibertom (Dornier Medical Systems, Germering, Germany), operating with a neodymium: yttrium-aluminum-garnet (Nd:YAG) laser generator at a wavelength of 1064 nm.[11,12] As an alternative, the Indigo diode laser system (Indigo IDL 830E, Indigo Medical GmbH, Münster, Germany), operating at a wavelength of 830 nm, may be used for LITT of the prostate; an advantage of this system is the thermoluminescence thermometer at the tip of the applicator, allowing for continuous temperature measurements during LITT.

Another contact laser system consists of a round contact probe having a diameter of 7 mm that is threaded onto a 600 μm optical fiber (Contact Laser System, Surgical Laser Technologies, Oaks, Calif). The surface of this probe has a black coating, which absorbs about 30% of the laser energy, thereby causing intense heating of the probe. Thus, contact between the probe and tissue produces surface vaporization and coagulation necrosis in the subsurface of the tissue. Contact laser systems use a conventional fiberoptic waveguide surrounded by a plastic cooling channel.[6]

Microwave thermotherapy of the prostate

Thermotherapy of the prostate may also be performed by using microwaves as the source of thermal energy. In transurethral microwave therapy (TUMT), a cooled microwave antenna is inserted into the prostatic urethra. Application of microwaves induces coagulation necrosis in the tissues around the urethra where temperatures exceed 45° C. With cooling of the antenna, the urothelial lining and a 3- to 5-mm thick tissue layer around the urethra is preserved from the coagulation process.

In studies comparing TUMT with TURP and sham treatment, clinical effectiveness of TUMT was assessed for at least 6 months after management. Although TUMT improved prostate symptom scores, it did not significantly improve objective functional data, such as urine peak flow and residual urine volume.[13] Thus, as a safe and minimally invasive procedure, TUMT may be considered as a treatment option for patients with mild to moderate symptoms of BPH and can be performed on an outpatient basis.

Focused ultrasound therapy of the prostate

Focused US beams elevate tissue temperature because of energy absorption of the US wave, resulting in different degrees of thermal damage to the tissue under exposure (see Chapter 25). If the tissue temperature increases to greater than 60° C, coagulation of proteins results in tissue necrosis. High-intensity focused US is well-suited for noninvasive local coagulation of deep tissue target volumes under MRI guidance.[14-16] In clinical studies, high-intensity focused US of the prostate showed promising early clinical results in the treatment of BPH including improved peak urine flow and residual urine volume.[17,18]

Cryosurgery

Cryosurgery of the prostate was used in the 1960s for the treatment of prostate cancer (see Chapter 22). Although the reported survival rates were similar to those achieved with conventional therapies,[19] serious complications (e.g., fistula formation, urethral sloughing) were frequent. Therefore, cryosurgery of the prostate was largely abandoned.

With more recent improvements of the technique, including a percutaneous transperineal approach, transrectal US guidance, and urethral warming during the procedure, the morbidity rate of cryosurgical ablation of prostate cancer has been considerably reduced.[20,21] Despite these improvements, complications associated with the procedure, (e.g., impotence, urine retention, tissue sloughing, urinary tract infection) still occur. Impotence rates after cryosurgery of the prostate are as high as 67% to 92%.[20-23]

CURRENT APPLICATIONS OF MAGNETIC RESONANCE IMAGING IN THE PLANNING, MONITORING, AND FOLLOW-UP OF PROSTATIC DISEASE TREATMENT

Magnetic resonance imaging technique and anatomy

Initially, MRI of the prostate was used with conventional body coils,[24-26] a technique that required a large field of view (FOV) to receive sufficient signal from the tissues under investigation. In addition to the prostate, the entire pelvis was usually covered, allowing for simultaneous evaluation of structures adjacent to the prostate (e.g., bladder, rectum, seminal vesicles, lymph nodes). However, the spatial resolution of the prostate itself was limited.

With the use of endorectal surface coils for prostatic imaging, the spatial in-plane resolution could be increased to 0.3 mm with FOVs of 10 to 12 cm.[27,28] The disadvantage of these coils lies in their limited active volume, which allows imaging of only structures close to the rectum with sufficiently high signal-to-noise ratio (SNR). However, evaluation of structures more distant from the coil (e.g., the anterior part of the prostate, the pelvic lymph nodes), is limited or impossible.

External phased-array body coils[29] provide substantially increased SNR compared with conventional body coils,[30] allowing for high-resolution, small FOV imaging of the prostate and adjacent structures without the limitations of endorectal surface coils.

The best MRI of the prostate is provided by the use of an endorectal surface coil combined with a phased-array body coil.[31] This combination allows optimal imaging of the entire prostate gland with simultaneous evaluation of adjacent organs, lymph nodes, and osseous structures.[31,32]

The prostate gland has a chestnut shape, with the base forming the superior end and the apex forming the inferior end. In the healthy gland, the peripheral zone constitutes approximately 70% of the prostatic volume, the central zone 25%, and the periurethral transitional zone approximately 5%. MRI of the prostate is predominantly based on heavily T2-weighted images in the axial, coronal, and sagittal planes. T2-weighted images allow for differentiation of the zonal anatomy of the prostate, including the central, transitional, and peripheral zones; the anterior fibromuscular band; and the prostatic capsule (Fig. 42-1). On T1-weighted images, the internal structure of the prostate usually cannot be differentiated, whereas the gland is clearly delineated from periprostatic fibro-adipose tissue and periprostatic venous plexus. Gadolinium-enhanced T1-weighted images frequently show a rather homogeneous distribution of contrast material throughout the gland on delayed scans.

Role of magnetic resonance imaging for established treatment modalities

Benign prostatic hyperplasia

MRI is very sensitive in detecting morphologic changes of the prostate associated with BPH. MRI findings of BPH consist of heterogeneous signal intensity and enlargement of the periurethral transitional and central zone on T2-weighted images[33] (Fig. 42-2). Depending on the distribution and size of glandular elements and the composition of the surrounding stroma, MRI features vary.[34] The glandular type of BPH shows predominantly high signal intensity, whereas the stromal hyperplasia has an intermediate to low signal intensity. The changes may be distributed symmetrically or asymmetrically throughout the central gland. A pseudocapsule, separating the central gland from the peripheral zone, is displayed with low signal intensity. On T1-weighted images, BPH shows intermediate signal intensity and is not clearly differentiated from the remainder of the prostate.

In patients with classical symptoms of BPH, a digital rectal examination not suspicious for prostate cancer, healthy prostate-specific antigen levels, and typical findings of BPH in transrectal US (TRUS), no further imaging is required before a classic TURP procedure is performed. MRI may be helpful as a problem-solving modality to rule out or detect carcinoma in cases of BPH and to clarify equivocal findings for prostate cancer in one or more of the other examinations.

Despite its sensitivity in diagnosing BPH, MRI has no role in the guidance of the established therapeutic modalities

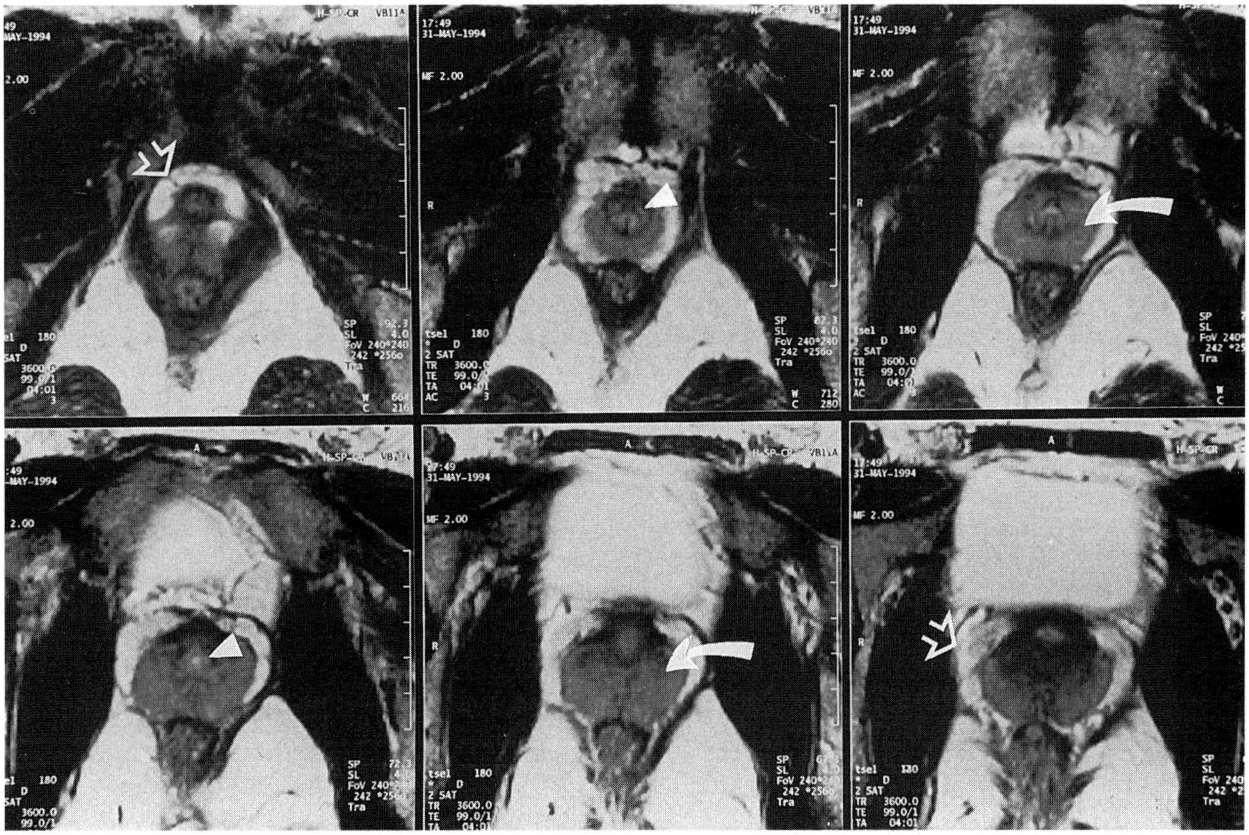

Fig. 42-1. Magnetic resonance imaging anatomy of the healthy prostate of a 30-year-old man (T2-weighted fast spin-echo images). The apex of the gland is seen on the upper left image, and the base on the lower right image. The peripheral zone is displayed with very high signal intensity *(open white arrows)*, the central zone with intermediate signal intensity *(white curved arrows)*, and the periurethral transitional zone with a heterogeneous signal intensity *(arrow heads)*.

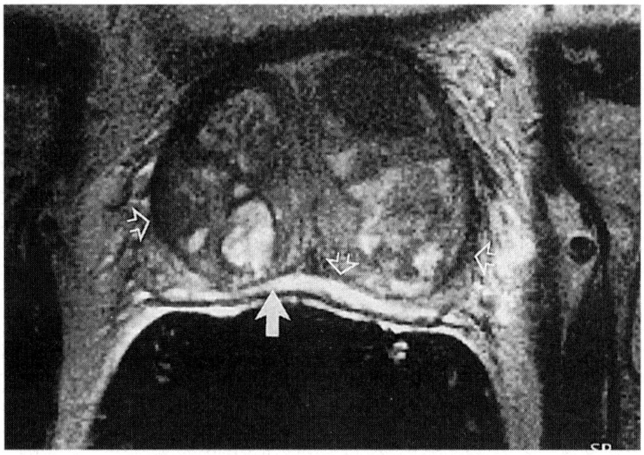

Fig. 42-2. Axial T2-weighted fast spin-echo image of benign prostatic hyperplasia. Considerable enlargement of the periurethral transitional and central zones is seen with hyperplastic glandular elements (high signal intensity) and elements of stromal hyperplasia (low signal intensity). A pseudocapsule *(open arrows)* has developed, separating the central zone from the small peripheral zone (high signal intensity, *arrow*).

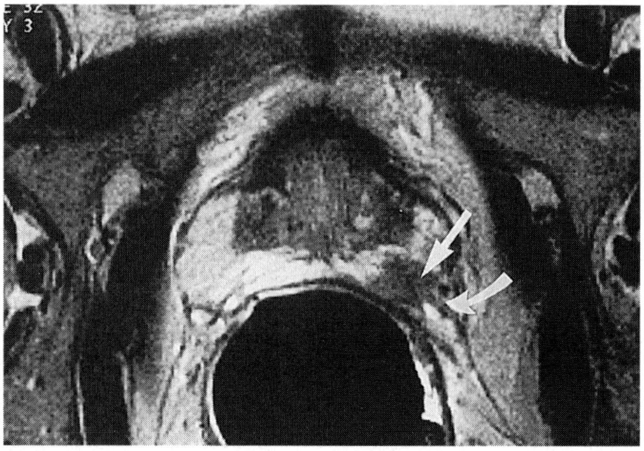

Fig. 42-3. Axial T2-weighted fast spin-echo image of prostate cancer. The tumor is located in the peripheral zone of the left prostatic lobe *(arrow),* displays low signal intensity, and is infiltrating the prostatic capsule and the left neurovascular bundle *(curved arrow).*

mentioned above. In TURP, the resection is carried out under direct visual guidance through the endoscope. MRI has been used, however, in an analysis of morphologic changes in hyperplastic prostate tissues after TURP. Tazaki and others[35] reported the reduction of hyperplastic tissue in the transitional zone of the prostate, re-epithelialization of the prostatic urethra, and narrowing of the TURP-induced urethral channel within 8 to 12 weeks after the procedure. In addition, a decrease of the prostate size over 8 to 12 months and shrinking of the prostate capsule were observed. These imaging findings were paralleled by a 78% to 81% improvement in peak urine flow.

Prostate cancer

Although not very sensitive compared with pathohistologic data, findings on MRI are considered to be the most sensitive for diagnostic imaging of prostate cancer.[25,26,28] More importantly, MRI is the most accurate pretherapeutic technique to determine the extension of prostate cancer, particularly tumor growth beyond the confines of the gland (Fig. 42-3). Because in many institutions transcapsular tumor extension or infiltration of the seminal vesicles is considered a contraindication for radical surgical therapy, MRI can play an important role in pretherapeutic decision-making, particularly in cases with unclear findings on TRUS. Radical prostatectomy performed under direct visual guidance does not require interactive image guidance. Beyond diagnostic applications, MRI has been used for planning treatment with external beam radiotherapy.[36]

Role of magnetic resonance imaging for guidance, monitoring, and follow-up of thermal treatment of the prostate

Endoscopic laser ablation

On-line monitoring of endoscopic laser ablation therapy of the hyperplastic prostate has been reported in only one study.[37] The Urolase (Bard, Marietta, Ga) sidefire laser device used in the study of deSouza and others[37] does not lend itself to permanent on-line monitoring during laser application because (1) it contains a gold-plated stainless steel reflector interfering with the static and dynamic magnetic fields needed for MRI and (2) the technique requires that the operator observe the process of noncontact tissue coagulation permanently through the endoscope.[37] Because of these restrictions, the deep tissue effects of laser irradiation were intermittently monitored with MRI after treatment of one quadrant of hyperplastic prostate tissue in the periurethral, transitional, and central zones, when the Urolase (Bard, Marietta, Ga) device was removed from the patient. T2-weighted images obtained at intermissions showed decreased signal intensity in areas of the prostate treated with VLAP.[37] On T2-weighted images after therapy, a poorly defined region of low signal intensity was found in the tissues around the urethra (Fig. 42-4). After 1 week, this low signal intensity region became less obvious and was replaced by a well-demarcated ring of low signal intensity after a 3-month interval.

Different results for the MR evaluation of endoscopic laser ablation were reported by Tazaki and others.[35,38] In a follow-up study of patients treated with VLAP, necrosis was visualized early by contrast-enhanced T1-weighted images and reached 7- to 10-mm deep into the periurethral prostatic tissues. The necrotic tissue was found to be sloughed off within 8 to 12 weeks, leaving a smoothly outlined cavity with secondary re-epithelialization.

A follow-up study with endorectal MRI before and after VLAP in eight patients with prostate cancer was performed by Huch Böni and others.[39] In this study, MRI findings after VLAP were correlated with macroscopic and histologic findings. Both MRI 3 to 8 days and histology 4 to 9 days after VLAP (Sidefocus applicator and MediLas 4100 generator, Dornier, Keenesaw,

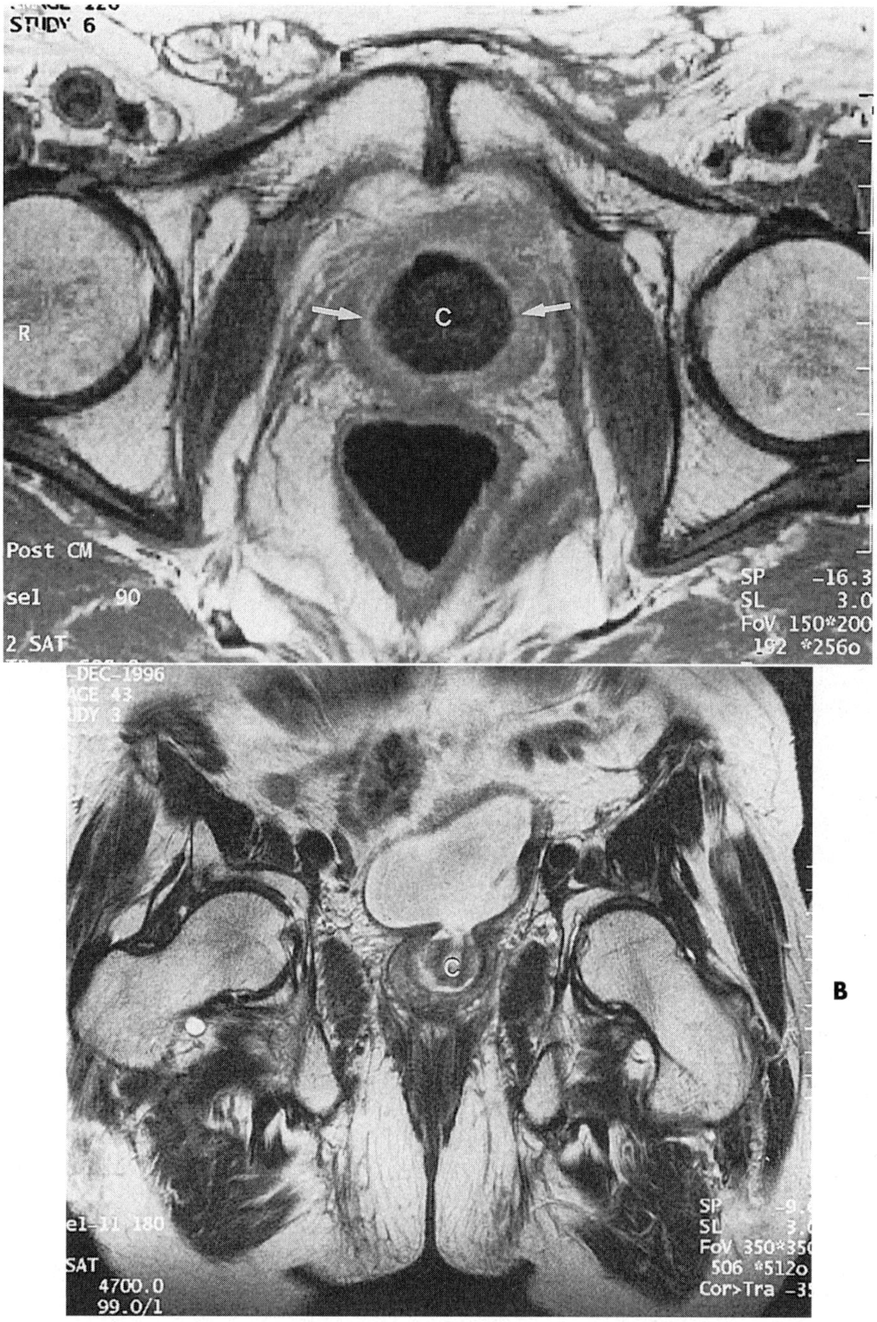

A

B

Fig. 42-4. Appearance of the prostate after endoscopic laser ablation with a sidefire laser device. **A,** Axial T1-weighted contrast-enhanced spin-echo image shows laser-induced coagulation necrosis *(c)* as a nonenhancing low signal intensity lesion in the central part of the prostate. The border of reactive viable tissue is displayed as a moderately enhancing rim *(arrows).* **B,** Coronal T2-weighted fast spin-echo image shows low signal intensity coagulated tissue *(c)* in the central part of the prostate, surrounded by high signal intensity urine. The smoothly outlined funnel displays a low signal intensity border of reactive tissue. (**A** from Müller-Lisse GU, Heuch AF: *Interstitial laser therapy of prostate lesions.* In Debatin J, Adam G, editors: *Interventional magnetic resonance imaging,* Berlin, 1998, Springer-Verlag.)

Ga) revealed periurethral necrosis with considerable interindividual differences (Fig. 42-5). Correlation between the volumes of altered tissue measured on MRI and in macroscopic specimens, respectively, was high ($r = 0.96$). Laser ablation–induced changes were best depicted on gadolinium-enhanced T1-weighted images, whereas plain T1-weighted images and T2-weighted fast spin-echo images were insufficient regarding clear delineation of laser-induced changes from adenomatous tissue.

Interstitial laser ablation

MRI has been used for guidance, on-line monitoring, and posttreatment follow-up of LITT procedures of the prostate in patients with BPH.

A

B

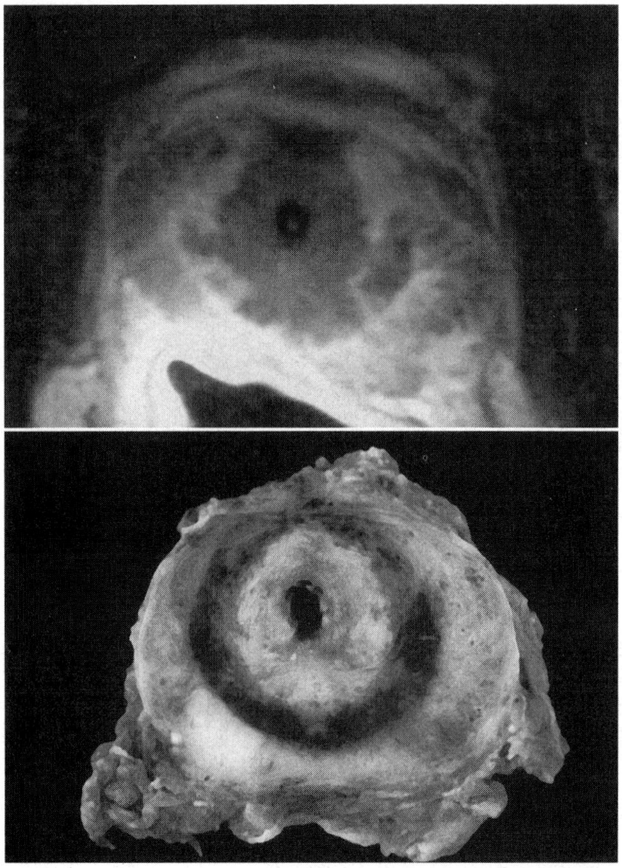

Fig. 42-5. Magnetic resonance imaging findings in a patient with prostate cancer after sidefire laser ablation. **A,** Endorectal axial, T1-weighted, gadolinium-enhanced spin-echo image was obtained 3 days after ablation. The central necrotic periurethral zone is hypointense, whereas the marginal zone shows inhomogeneous contrast enhancement. **B,** Resected prostate 4 days after laser ablation. Macroscopic specimen confirms periurethral necrosis with a hemorrhagic marginal zone. See Color Plate 18. (From Huch Böni RA, and others: Laser ablation-induced changes in the prostate: findings at endorectal MR imaging with histologic correlation, *Radiology* 202:232, 1997. Used with permission.)

Müller-Lisse and others[40] first reported the MR guidance and on-line monitoring of LITT procedures in two patients.[40] In a subsequent study, the same authors described 20 MR-guided LITT procedures of the prostate.[41] Although in these studies the LITT applicator was primarily applied under transurethral endoscopic guidance, its definitive position in the prostate was controlled on T1- or T2-weighted images obtained before laser energy deposition (Fig. 42-6). In four cases, the position of the LITT applicator was insufficient on MRI, and the optical fiber had to be repositioned. During laser energy deposition, an area of decreased signal intensity as compared with healthy prostatic tissue could be observed in the tissue adjacent to the laser applicator on T1-weighted fast low-angle shot (FLASH) images (Fig. 42-7). This low signal intensity area increased centrifugally in size with increasing duration of laser energy application; it completely disappeared after the laser was switched off.

Quantitative evaluation of signal intensity changes in T1-weighted FLASH images showed a high correlation (r = 0.92) with prostate temperature changes. The latter was determined by simultaneous *in vivo* temperature measurements in the human prostate.[41]

Previous *ex vivo* studies investigating the dependence of signal intensity changes in T1-weighted FLASH sequences and interstitial tissue temperature in bovine prostatic tissue had shown a high linear correlation (r = 0.89 to 0.98) of the two parameters between 35° C and 65° C.[40]

In vivo on-line monitoring of prostatic LITT procedures predicted the diameters of laser-induced coagulation necrosis with temperature-sensitive T1-weighted FLASH sequences.[41] Under the assumption that tissue coagulation occurs when tissue temperature reaches 60° C, prostatic interstitial coagulation necroses were correctly predicted in areas where MR signal intensity decreased to a level that correlated with a temperature of 60° C (<87% of average baseline signal intensity).

After successful LITT, intraprostatic coagulation necroses can be delineated by MRI. On T2-weighted images, coagulated prostatic tissue is characterized by an area of low signal intensity, which is surrounded by a high signal intensity rim of reactive edematous and inflammatory tissue (see Fig. 42-6).[42,43] In addition to the typical findings of coagulation necrosis, intraprostatic edema with swelling of the prostate and areas of high signal intensity periprostatic edema were found 24 to 48 hours after LITT on T2-weighted images. Using T1-weighted contrast-enhanced sequences, laser-induced coagulation necroses can be better delineated from the strongly enhancing reactive rim by their lack of contrast enhancement.[42] MR follow-up studies of the prostate, including volumetric assessment over 6 to 12 months after LITT, showed that coagulation necroses shrink to approximately 10% of their original size with an average prostate volume reduction of approximately 20% (total prostatic volume and central zone volume) and a relief of bladder outflow obstruction.

Assessment of prostatic volumes based on MRI is accurate, with intraobserver and interobserver reproducibilities of approximately 5%[43] and a correlation with prostate specimen volumes determined at pathology of approximately 93%.[44] Therefore, and because necrotic areas in the prostate can be outlined on contrast-enhanced images immediately after LITT, a long-term volumetric outcome of the procedure can be predicted at the time of therapy.

Microwave thermotherapy of the prostate

Although TUMT is being investigated in several centers as an alternative to TURP in the treatment of BPH, only one study reports on the MRI findings after TUMT. Tazaki, and others[35] found no remarkable tissue reduction in the transitional zone of the prostate shortly after treatment, but areas of hemorrhagic necrosis beneath the epithelium of the prostatic urethra. In follow-up studies over 8 to 12 weeks, hemorrhagic necrosis was replaced by scar tissue with consecutive widening of the pro-

A

B

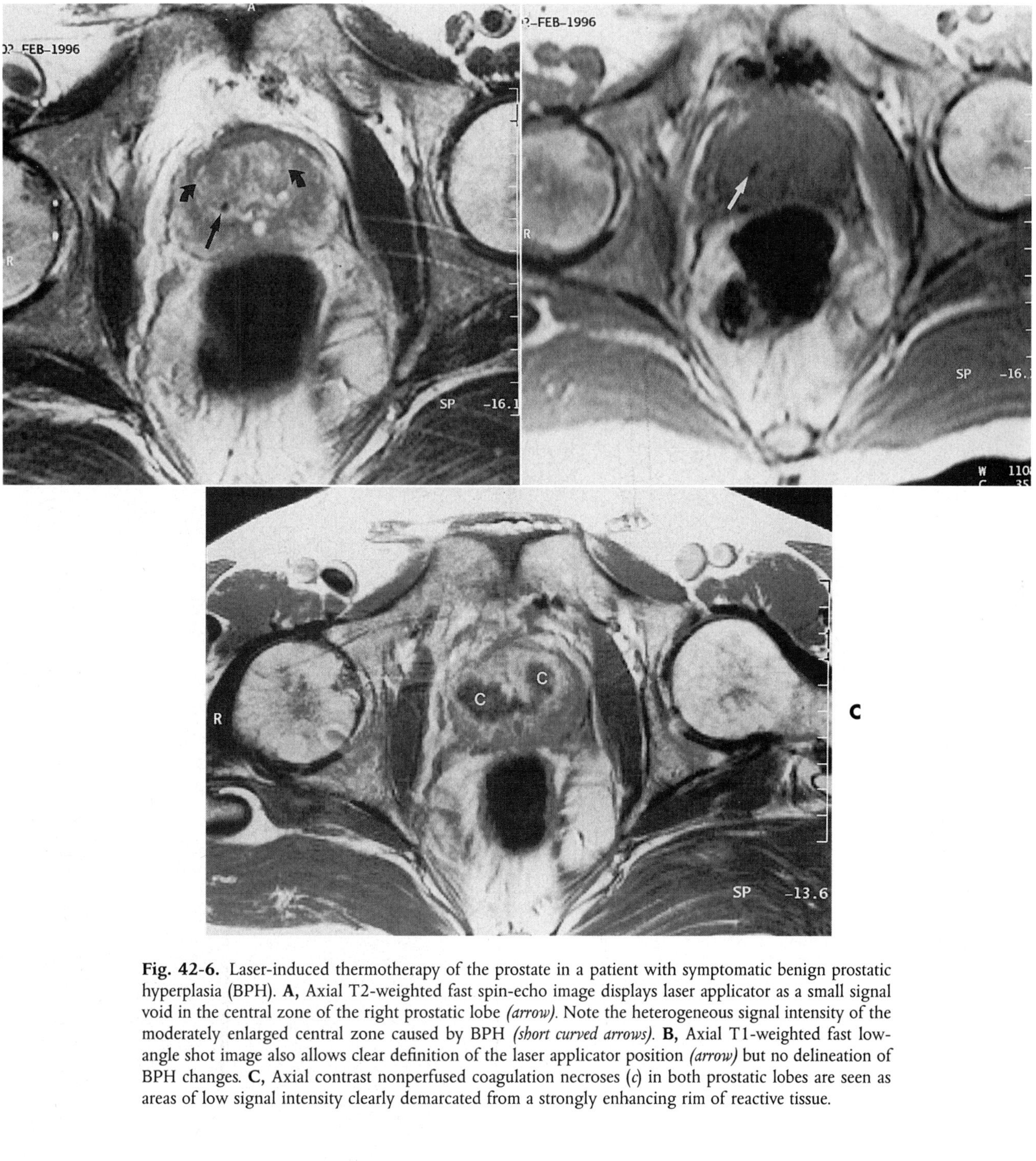

C

Fig. 42-6. Laser-induced thermotherapy of the prostate in a patient with symptomatic benign prostatic hyperplasia (BPH). **A,** Axial T2-weighted fast spin-echo image displays laser applicator as a small signal void in the central zone of the right prostatic lobe *(arrow)*. Note the heterogeneous signal intensity of the moderately enlarged central zone caused by BPH *(short curved arrows)*. **B,** Axial T1-weighted fast low-angle shot image also allows clear definition of the laser applicator position *(arrow)* but no delineation of BPH changes. **C,** Axial contrast nonperfused coagulation necroses (*c*) in both prostatic lobes are seen as areas of low signal intensity clearly demarcated from a strongly enhancing rim of reactive tissue.

static urethra. The urethral lining displayed an intense contrast uptake after intravenous administration of gadolinium in the early and late phases after treatment, suggesting viable urethral epithelium.

Focused ultrasound therapy of the prostate

Focused US has been investigated as an alternative treatment modality for prostatic disease. Preliminary studies on focused US of the prostate have shown some promising early results;[15,17,18] however, despite that MRI is considered very promising for guiding the US beam and for monitoring tissue effects,[16] no study has reported on MRI guidance of prostatic focused US therapy in a clinical setting.

Cryosurgery

MRI and MR spectroscopy have been used to assess the effects and complications of prostatic cryosurgery.[23,45] MRI often shows enlargement of the prostate and loss of zonal anatomy with heterogeneous signal intensity immediately after cryosurgery (Fig. 42-8). Approximately 2 weeks after cryoablation, the prostate volume decreases by 30% to 50% and the zonal anatomy remains indistinct.[23] Necrotic areas can be detected in

A

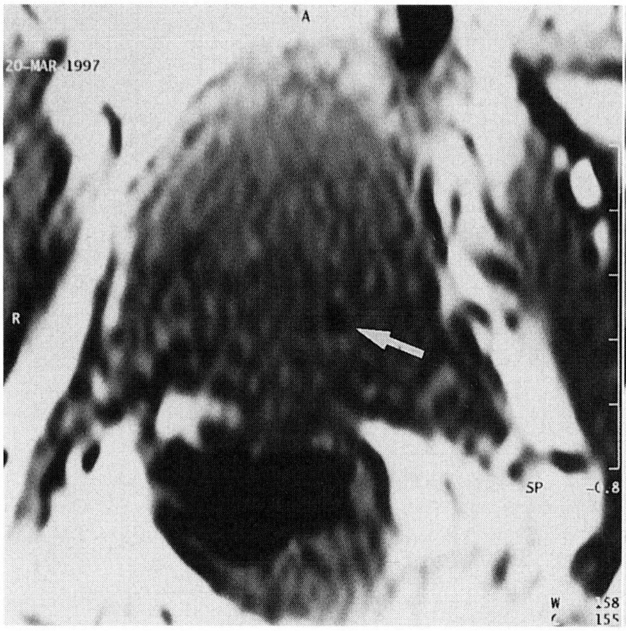

B

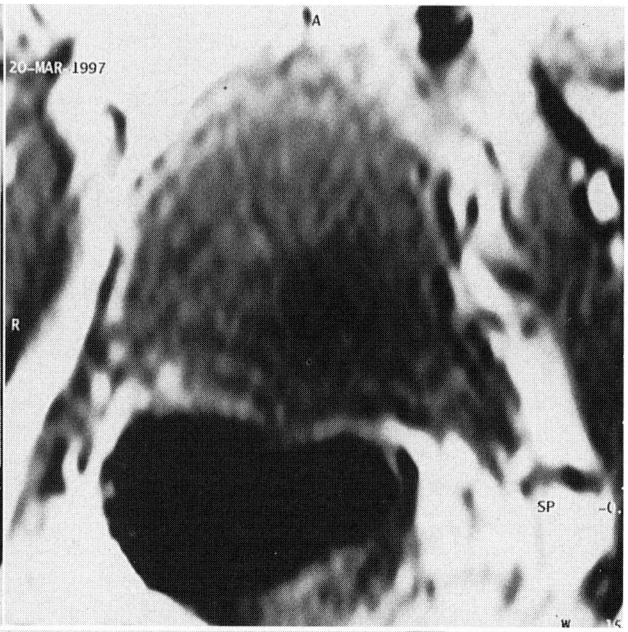

C

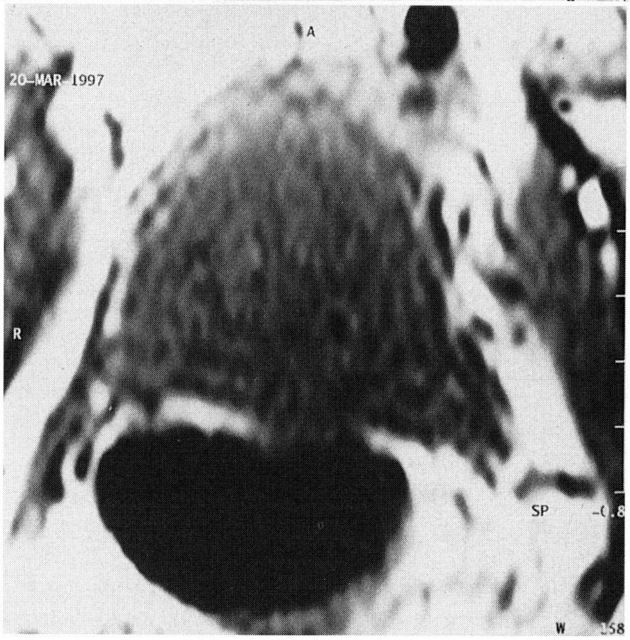

Fig. 42-7. On-line monitoring of prostatic laser-induced interstitial thermotherapy (LITT) with serial T1-weighted fast low-angle shot sequences. **A,** Before laser energy deposition, the signal void of the LITT applicator can be depicted in prostatic tissue *(arrow)*. **B,** After 80 sec of laser treatment a low signal intensity area has developed around the applicator, indicating increased temperature in prostatic tissue. **C,** Approximately 5 min after laser treatment, the low signal intensity around the applicator has partially disappeared. (From Müller-Lisse GU, Heuch AF: *Interstitial laser therapy of prostate lesions.* In Debatin J, Adam G, editors: *Interventional magnetic resonance imaging,* Berlin, 1998, Springer-Verlag.)

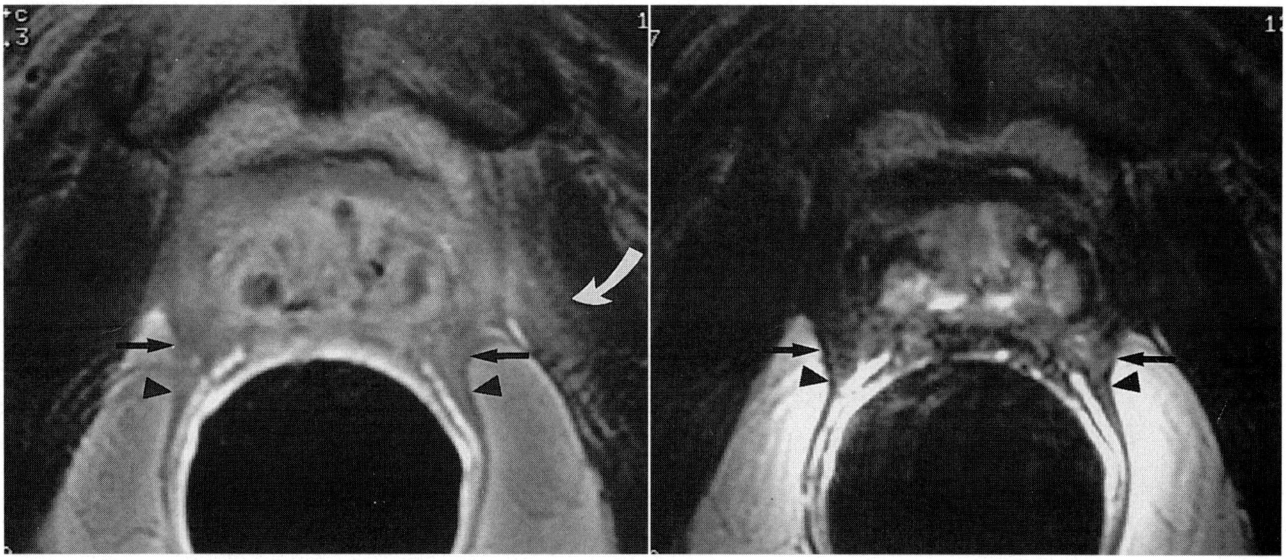

Fig. 42-8. Magnetic resonance imaging (MRI) findings in a patient with prostate cancer after cryosurgery. **A,** Axial postcontrast T1-weighted and **B,** T2-weighted MRI scans show marked heterogeneity throughout the prostate gland after cryosurgery. Multiple low signal intensity areas on the postcontrast T1-weighted image represent necrotic foci. Fibrous tissue can be seen to have enveloped the neurovascular bundles *(straight arrows).* Enhancement of the left internal obturator muscle (*curved arrow* in **A**) is shown. (From Kalbhen CL, and others: Prostate carcinoma: MR imaging findings after cryosurgery, *Radiology* 198:807, 1996. Used with permission.)

approximately 50% of patients and may involve the urethra and the transitional and peripheral zones. In the late follow-up, T2-weighted images frequently display a thick capsule involving the prostate and neurovascular bundles. Appearance of this capsule is correlated with the impotency rate. In the periprostatic tissues, postcryotherapy findings include edematous changes in the levator ani muscles and obturator internus muscles on T2-weighted images and high signal intensity foci in the symphysis pubis, which are thought to represent osteonecrosis. Thus far, on-line MR monitoring during cryotherapy of the human prostate has not been reported in the literature.

REFERENCES

1. Garraway WM, Collins GN, Lee RJ: High prevalence of benign prostatic hypertrophy in community, *Lancet* 338:469, 1991.
2. Wingo PA, Tong T, Bolden S: Cancer statistics, *CA Cancer J Clin* 45:8, 1995.
3. Hinman F: *Atlas of urologic surgery,* Philadelphia, 1989, WB Saunders.
4. Hartung R: Die BPH—ein altes Krankheitsbild—neu betrachtet, *Urologe (A)* 34:77, 1995.
5. Conrad S, and others: Transurethrale Lasertherapie der benignen Prostatahyperplasie (transurethral laser therapy for benign prostatic hyperplasia), *Urologe (A)* 34:25, 1995.
6. Milam DF, Smith JA: Laser prostatectomy devices and their tissue effects, *J Endourol* 9:85, 1995.
7. Sander S, Beisland HO, Fossberg E: Neodymium YAG laser in the treatment of prostatic cancer, *Urol Res* 10:85, 1982.
8. Sander S, Beisland HO: Laser in the treatment of localized prostatic carcinoma, *J Urol* 132:280, 1984.
9. Schulze H, and others: TULIP: experience in over 80 cases, *Urologe (A)* 34:84, 1995.
10. Hofstetter A: Interstitielle Thermokoagulation (ITK) von Prostatatumoren, *Lasermedizin* 7:179, 1991.
11. Muschter R, and others: Die interstitielle laserkoagulation der benignen Prostatahyperplasie, *Urologe (A)* 32:273, 1993.
12. Muschter R, and others: Interstitial laser-induced coagulation of the prostate in the treatment of benign hyperplasia, *Urologe (A)* 34:90, 1995.
13. Höfner K, and others: Thermotherapy in benign prostatic hyperplasia, *Urologe (A)* 34:16, 1995.
14. Hynynen K, and others: MRI-guided noninvasive ultrasound surgery, *Med Phys* 20:107, 1993.
15. Foster RS, and others: High-intensity focused ultrasound in the treatment of prostatic disease, *Eur Urol* 23:29, 1993.
16. Hynynen K: *MR-guided focused ultrasound surgery.* In Debatin J, Adam G, editors: *Interventional magnetic resonance imaging,* Berlin, 1998, Springer-Verlag.
17. Madersbacher S, and others: Effect of high-intensity focused ultrasound on human prostate cancer in vivo, *Cancer Res* 55:3346, 1995.
18. Madersbacher S, and others: Minimal invasive Therapie der benignen Prostatahyperplasie mit fokussiertem Ultraschall, *Urologe (A)* 34:98, 1995.
19. Bonney WW, and others: Cryosurgery in prostate cancer: survival, *Urology* 19:37, 1982.
20. Onik GM, and others: Transrectal ultrasound-guided percutaneous radical cryosurgical ablation of the prostate, *Cancer* 72:1291, 1993.
21. Miller RJ, Cohen JK, Merlotti LA: Percutaneous transpenneal cryosurgical ablation of the prostate for the primary treatment of clinical stage C adenocarcinoma of the prostate, *Urology* 44:170, 1994.
22. Chodak GW: Cryosurgery of the prostate revisited, *Cancer* 72:1145, 1993.
23. Kalbhen CL, and others: Prostate carcinoma: MR imaging findings after cryosurgery, *Radiology* 198:807, 1996.
24. Hricak H, and others: MR imaging of the prostate gland: normal anatomy, *Am J Roentgenol* 148:51, 1987.
25. Schiebler ML, and others: Prostatic carcinoma and benign prostatic hyperplasia: correlation of high-resolution MR and histopathologic findings, *Radiology* 172:131, 1989.
26. Kahn T, and others: Prostatic carcinoma and benign prostatic hyperplasia: MR imaging with histopathologic correlation, *Radiology* 173:847, 1989.

27. Schnall MD, and others: Prostate: MR imaging with an endorectal surface coil, *Radiology* 172:570, 1989.
28. Chelsky MJ, and others: Use of endorectal surface coil magnetic resonance imaging for local staging of prostate carcinoma, *J Urol* 150:391, 1992.
29. Hayes CE, Hattes N, Roemer PB: Volume imaging with phased arrays, *Magn Reson Med* 18:108, 1991.
30. Gauger J, and others: Breathhold imaging of the upper abdomen using a CP-array coil: comparison with standard study coil imaging, *MAGMA* 4:93, 1996.
31. Hricak H, and others: Adenoma of the prostate: MR imaging with pelvic phased-array coil versus integrated endorectal-pelvic phased-array coil, *Radiology* 193:703, 1994.
32. Schnall MD, Connick T, Hayes CE: Imaging of the pelvis with an endorectal-external multicoil array, *J Magn Reson Imaging* 2:229, 1992.
33. Allen KS, and others: Age-related changes of the prostate: evaluation by MR imaging, *Am J Roentgenol* 152:77, 1989.
34. Ishida J, and others: Benign prostatic hyperplasia: value of MR imaging for determining histologic type, *Radiology* 190:329, 1994.
35. Tazaki H, and others: Magnetic resonance imaging following microwave thermotherapy, laser ablation and transurethral resection in patients with BPH, *Urologe (A)* 34:105, 1995.
36. Potter R, and others: *Impact of magnetic resonance imaging assisted simulation on target, treatment, and irradiation volume in treatment planning of prostate cancer.* In Breit A, editor: *Tumor response monitoring and treatment planning,* Berlin, Springer-Verlag.
37. deSouza NM, and others: Endoscopic laser ablation of the prostate: MR appearances during and after treatment and their relation to clinical outcome, *Am J Roentgenol* 164:1429, 1995.
38. Tazaki H, Nakashima J, Nakagawa K: MRI evaluation of cavitation induced by laser prostatectomy, *J Endourol* 9:171, 1995.
39. Huch Böni RA, and others: Laser ablation-induced changes in the prostate: findings at endorectal MR imaging with histologic correlation, *Radiology* 202:232, 1997.
40. Mueller-Lisse GU, and others: MRT: Monitoring vor, während und nach der interstitiellen laserinduzierten Thermotherapie der benignen Prostatahyperplasie. Erste klinische Erfahrungen, *Radiologe (A)* 36:722, 1996.
41. Mueller-Lisse GU, and others: Predictability of the size of laser-induced lesions in T1-weighted MR images obtained during interstitial laser-induced thermotherapy of benign prostatic hyperplasia, *J Magn Reson Imaging* 8:31, 1998.
42. Heuck A, and others: Magnetic resonance imaging in interstitial laser coagulation of benign prostatic hyperplasia: first experience, *Lasermedizin* 11:27, 1995.
43. Mueller-Lisse GU, and others: Postoperative MRI in patients undergoing interstitial laser coagulation thermotherapy of benign prostatic hyperplasia, *J Comput Assist Tomogr* 20:273, 1996.
44. Rahmouni A, and others: Accuracy of in-vivo assessment of prostatic volume by MRI and transrectal ultrasonography, *J Comput Assist Tomogr* 16:935, 1992.
45. Kurhanewicz J, and others: Three-dimensional H-1 MR spectroscopic imaging of the in situ human prostate with high (0.24-0.7-cm^3) spatial resolution, *Radiology* 198:795, 1996.

Chapter 43

MR–GUIDED BONE BIOPSIES

Jörg-Michael Neuerburg

Primary tumors of the bone are relatively uncommon compared with secondary or metastatic neoplasms. Histologic characteristics generally provide the most valuable information concerning the nature of the lesion, but they should be correlated with all other clinical, laboratory, and imaging findings. Diagnosis of bone lesions is most accurate when made in close consultation by the referring physician, the radiologist, and the pathologist. As a less invasive alternative to open surgery or surgical biopsy procedures, pathohistological diagnosis can often be made percutaneously.

In recent years, positioning of biopsy needles in bone lesions has been greatly facilitated by advancements in imaging techniques, such as multi-angle fluoroscopy, computed tomography (CT), a combination of an integrated x-ray fluoroscopy c-arm and CT, and more recently, magnetic resonance imaging (MRI). Percutaneous biopsy under x-ray fluoroscopic guidance is restricted to lesions that can be clearly visualized by fluoroscopy without the need for delineation of significant vulnerable structures in the chosen biopsy path. Fluoroscopy is readily available and enables permanent control of the path of the biopsy needle. The use of biplane fluoroscopy or a c-arm fluoroscopic unit allows control of the needle position in two perpendicular planes without changing the position of the patient. CT guidance is favorable in small bone lesions not clearly depicted by fluoroscopy, in bone lesions with an additional suspected soft-tissue mass, and especially in lesions located in high-risk areas. CT can provide intermittent, reliable three-dimensional (3D) control of the biopsy needle path and allows discrimination of associated soft-tissue masses and vital anatomic vascular and neural structures. An additional integrated mobile fluoroscopic c-arm between the gantry of the CT unit and the examination table allows alternative use of these two imaging modalities for guidance of percutaneous biopsies, which combines the advantages of both methods.[1]

Technical innovations have expanded the use of MRI to various new applications.[2,3] With increasing interest, MRI is used to guide and monitor various interventional procedures. Lack of irradiation, ability to obtain multiplanar and 3D imaging, and high soft-tissue contrast are advantages of MRI guidance over other imaging modalities. However, drawbacks of MRI guidance are evident: requirements for MRI-compatible patient monitoring (e.g., magnetic field and radiofrequency [RF] shielding), limited access to the site of intervention, difficulties in locating instrumentation-based passive image artifacts in the lesion, and inferior spatial resolution compared with CT. The use of MRI to control percutaneous bone biopsies is under investigation. MRI may be complementary to CT and advantageous in lesions not visible with other imaging modalities.

INDICATIONS

Indications for percutaneous bone biopsies include cytologic or histologic evaluation of primary and secondary bone lesions with an unknown etiology and demonstration of the infectious agent in suspected osteomyelitis.[1,4-8] In most instances, MRI may be used as an alternative guidance modality to CT. Thus, the indications for both modalities are similar. MRI guidance may be favorable to visualize lesions not visible with other imaging tools and to avoid x-ray exposure in young patients. MR guidance is appropriate for lesions located in low-risk areas. However, for lesions in high-risk areas, CT guidance is the first choice.[9,10]

Skeletal core biopsies and aspiration biopsies are complementary:[11,12] In small musculoskeletal soft-tissue masses and in small osteolytic bone lesions, fine-needle aspiration techniques may be favorable. In large soft-tissue masses and large osteolytic bone lesions, histologic samples may be obtained with side-slit needles.[5] For osteosclerotic bone tumors, osteosclerotic tumor-like lesions, and bone tumors covered with an intact bony shell, trephine needles are more appropriate. Machine-assisted drilling may become necessary in highly osteosclerotic lesions.[1,5]

MATERIALS AND METHODS

Magnetic resonance scanner

Different MR scanners are suitable for MRI-guided biopsies: open 0.5-T superconducting magnets constructed in a double doughnut configuration with access to the patient between two vertical magnets; partially open horseshoe (0.2-T) and temple-like (0.064-T) low-field magnets; and modified conventional superconducting high-field (1.5-T) MR scanners with or without an integrated x-ray fluoroscopy c-arm (Fig. 43-1).[2]

With an open MRI system, the biopsy procedure can be performed under continual MRI control. However, because of the magnet design, access to the site of intervention may be limited.

If percutaneous bone biopsies are obtained under MRI guidance using a modified conventional superconducting high-field MR scanner, the procedure is similar to the CT-guided technique: i.e., the biopsy should be performed outside the gantry. By moving the examination table, alternative intermittent use of MRI and fluoroscopy is possible to control the path of the biopsy device.

If general anesthesia or neuroleptanalgesia is required, MR-compatible patient monitoring facilities in the MR suite are mandatory.

Magnetic resonance accessories

According to the composition of the bone lesion, biopsy tools are required to sample osteolytic bone lesions and adjacent soft-tissue masses. Bone trephine needles can penetrate lesions covered by intact cortical bone and osteosclerotic lesions. Biopsy procedures under MRI guidance require low-artifact interventional instruments, which can be visualized by MRI and which do not experience torque in the magnetic field. Visualization of instrumentation-based passive image artifacts depends on the susceptibility and configuration of the instrument, pulse-sequence parameters, the field strength B_O, and the orientation of the instrument to B_O.

Various MR-compatible biopsy needles are available for cytologic or histologic sampling of soft-tissue masses or osteolytic bone lesions (Box 43-1). These tools are made of nonferromagnetic components, such as titanium, tantalum, and tungsten alloys with aluminum or vanadium. Configuration, handling, and cutting properties of MR-compatible biopsy needles are similar to those for needles used for fluoroscopic or CT-guided procedures. Side-slit biopsy needles allow multiple sampling, with the outer cannula kept in place while the inner cannula

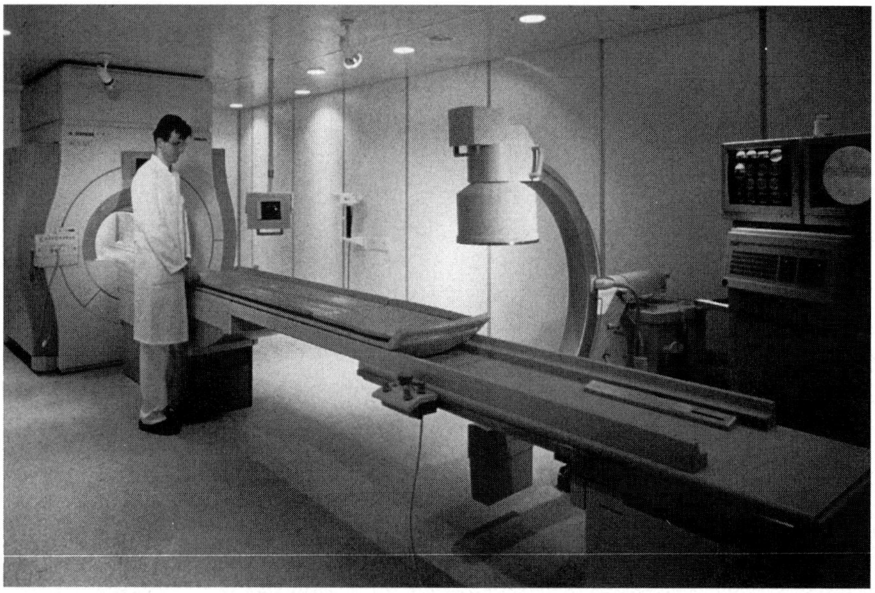

Fig. 43-1. A superconductive 1.5-T magnetic resonance imaging (MRI) system is combined with a conventional c-arm fluoroscopy unit in one room. The two systems are connected via a floating table top. For MR guidance, sequences were started from a panel at the front of the magnet. Images are displayed on a liquid crystal display screen positioned on the magnet.

with the specimen is taken out and replaced. In general, other types of needles are completely withdrawn with the specimen.

Penetration of intact cortical bone or osteosclerotic bone lesions (e.g., osteoid osteomas, osteoplastic metastasis) using cutting needles or sharpened cannulas may be time consuming or even impossible and can cause considerable discomfort to the patient. Although various drill systems are suitable for CT- or fluoroscopic-guided puncture of dense bone lesions, MR-compatible drill systems are not commercially available for this purpose. Thus, a new hand-driven or optionally motor-driven MR- (and CT-) compatible percutaneous bone biopsy system has been developed[10] and is under clinical evaluation (Fig. 43-2). This coaxial bone biopsy system has been developed in cooperation with COOK Europe (William Cook Europe, Bjaeverskov, Denmark). It consists of a 12-gauge guiding cannula with a trocar, a 14-gauge drill with a 16-gauge trocar, a plastic handle with a Luer-Lock for manual use, and a pneumatic turbine with a Luer-Lock and a foot panel for motor-assisted drilling (10 to 250 rotations per min at 6 bar compressed air). If the material obtained by means of the 14-gauge drill is inadequate, an 8-gauge guiding cannula with a 10-gauge trocar and a 10-gauge drill with a 12-gauge trocar can be alternatively used to obtain a larger sample volume.

Guiding cannulas and drills are available in two lengths. While maintaining the outer guiding cannula in place, the coaxial biopsy system allows multiple sampling with one penetration.

Box 43-1. Instruments suitable for magnetic resonance imaging–guided biopsy of osteolytic bone lesions and associated soft-tissue masses

MReye spinal needle (22 gauge, 19.5, or 18 gauge) and MReye Chiba biopsy needle (22 gauge, 19.5, or 18 gauge) (William Cook Europe, Bjaeverskov, Denmark)
MRT biopsy needle (14 gauge or 18 gauge) (Daum Medical, Schwerin, Germany)
Lufkin biopsy needle (22 gauge; 18 or 20 gauge) (E-Z-EM, Westbury, NY; distributed by Guerbet, Sulzbach, Germany)
Soma-Cut MR tool (14 or 18 gauge) (Somatex, Berlin, Germany)

PUNCTURE TECHNIQUE

Anesthesia

In most instances, percutaneous bone biopsies may be performed under local anesthesia. Local anesthesia has the advantage that the patient can inform the physician of radiating pain caused by nerve impingement by the biopsy needle and decreased cardiopulmonary side effects. However, general anesthesia is required for young children, for restless or incooperative patients, and for patients with lesions such as osteoid osteomas,[13] in which drilling of the lesion may be extremely painful.

Localization of the puncture path

For selection of an appropriate percutaneous approach to the bone lesion, several aspects should be analyzed: (1) The possibility of cancer exists in almost every bone lesion. Thus, the percutaneous approach should be planned to avoid unnecessary contamination of tissue planes with tumor cells, which would complicate subsequent surgical resection. In the extremities, biopsies should be obtained when minimal dissection is needed

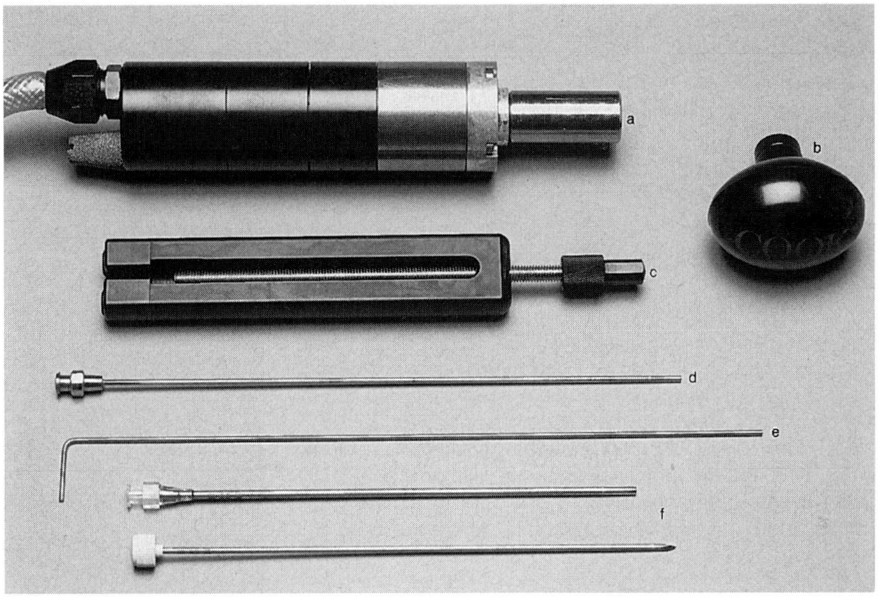

Fig. 43-2. Magnetic resonance–compatible percutaneous coaxial bone biopsy system: *a,* a pneumatic turbine for machine-powered drilling; *b,* a plastic handle for manual drive; *c,* a specimen pusher; *d,* a 14-G drill; *e,* a 16-G obturator; and *f,* a 12-G guiding cannula with trocar.

to reach the tumor. (2) A representative part of the bone lesion should be selected by a careful review of the available imaging modalities (e.g., edema, necrosis, inflammation, vascularity). (3) Areas covered by thin cortical bone, areas with cortical destruction, and soft-tissue components of bone lesions are easier to biopsy than osteosclerotic areas.

Puncture

Using an open MR scanner, the puncture site on the skin can be determined directly under imaging control. The elected entry site on the skin can be easily recognized by manual compression with the finger tip. If a conventional closed MR scanner is used, the entry site can be marked with a grid on the skin. Two grids can be used: For T1-weighted sequences, 9-F plastic tubes are filled with an aqueous gadopentetate solution (Fig. 43-3). For T2-weighted sequences, 9-F plastic tubes are filled with water.

The puncture depth and angle are measured using the standard software of the MR scanner. The chosen entry site is marked on the skin with a permanent pen. Sterile conditions are created. Liberal application of local anaesthetics is recommended because penetration of the periosteum may be very painful. A small skin incision facilitates insertion of the biopsy device into the soft tissues. With a coaxial biopsy system, the guiding cannula is advanced to the periosteum. In lesions that are not covered by intact or by osteosclerotic bone, the biopsy needle can be forced directly into the lesion using moderate axial pressure. In cases in which the coaxial bone biopsy drill system is used, the guiding cannula is pressed against the periosteum. The trocar is exchanged for the drill. The plastic handle is connected to the drill and rotated clockwise using slight axial pressure until representative areas of the lesion are reached.

The path of the needle may be controlled by intermittent MR scans[14] in the open MR system or in the closed magnet by moving the patient (see Fig. 43-1). Use of an MR system with an integrated mobile c-arm allows the procedure to be performed alternatively under fluoroscopic guidance. Although the procedure has been planned under MR guidance, fluoroscopy can be used to show the position of the drill. While drilling through thick cortical or osteosclerotic bone, the drill might become occluded and the specimen hard-packed in the hollow drill. In this situation, the drill should be removed and cleaned or exchanged, which improves the drilling properties and avoids hard-packing of the specimen and alterations in the

A
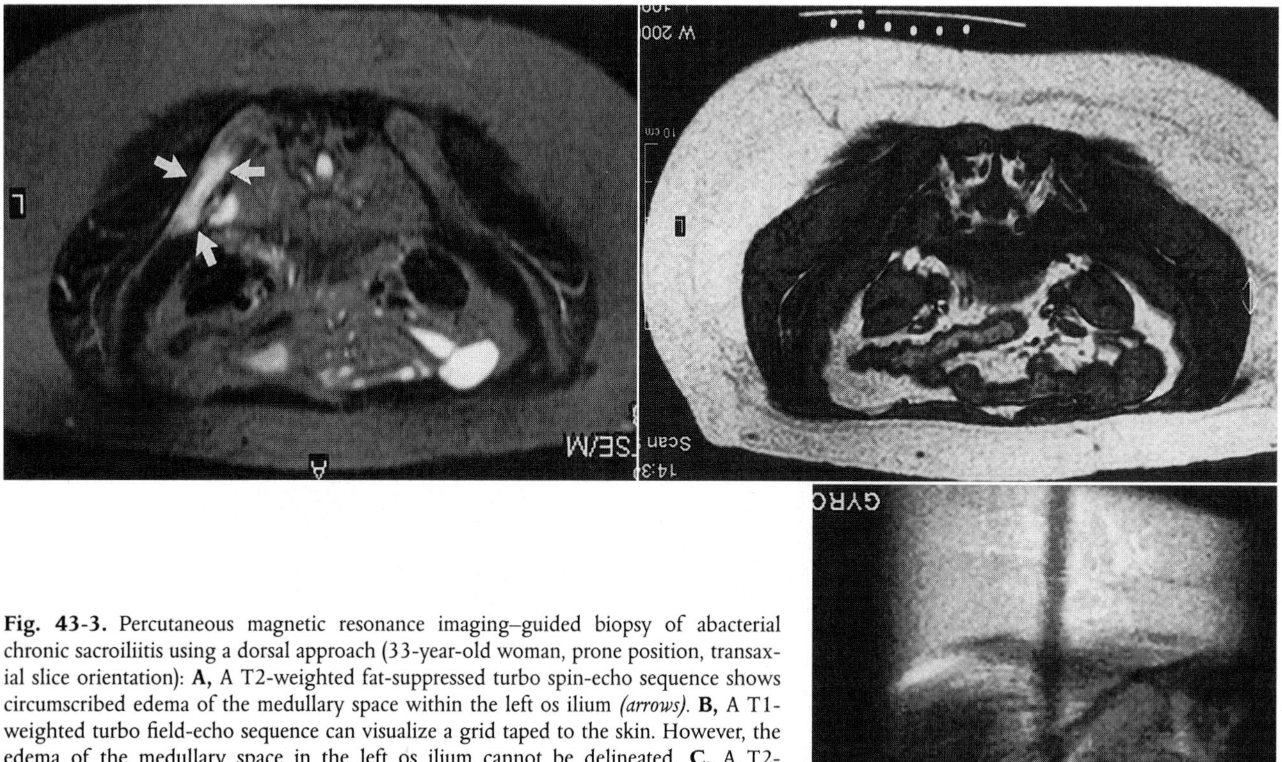
B

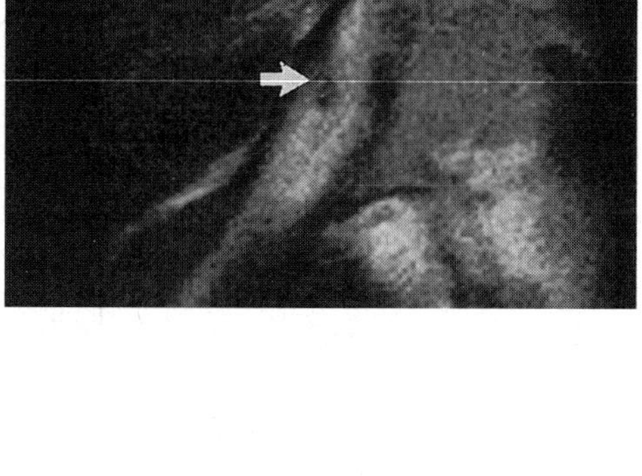
C

Fig. 43-3. Percutaneous magnetic resonance imaging–guided biopsy of abacterial chronic sacroiliitis using a dorsal approach (33-year-old woman, prone position, transaxial slice orientation): **A,** A T2-weighted fat-suppressed turbo spin-echo sequence shows circumscribed edema of the medullary space within the left os ilium *(arrows)*. **B,** A T1-weighted turbo field-echo sequence can visualize a grid taped to the skin. However, the edema of the medullary space in the left os ilium cannot be delineated. **C,** A T2-weighted local look sequence shows the tip of the low-signal 14-G drill in the bone marrow edema *(arrow)*. (From Neuerburg JM, and others: MRI-guided biopsy of bone in a hybrid system, *J Magn Reson Imaging* 8:85, 1998.)

specimen's architecture. During this exchange, the guiding cannula should be firmly pressed against the periosteum to allow a second passage of the drill into the same hole. In addition, a pneumatic turbine with a Luer-Lock is used for infinitely variable motor-assisted drilling connected to 6-bar compressed air (anesthesia equipment). Rotations may vary from 10 to 250 per minute using a foot panel. The specimen obtained with the drill should be ejected by inserting the obturator into the Luer-Lock opening and passing it out the drilling end. However, the specimen may become firmly fixed within the hollow drill. A specimen pusher is used for removal (see Fig. 43-2).

RESULTS AND COMPLICATIONS

Experiences with MRI-guided bone biopsies are limited. In 1996, the author tried to perform all percutaneous diagnostic bone biopsies in his modified interventional MR scanner. Twenty-five patients underwent MRI-guided diagnostic percutaneous bone biopsies for evaluation of bone lesions of unknown etiology or for identification of the infectious agent in cases of suspected osteomyelitis in which surgery was not considered to be the therapy of choice (Table 43-1). One patient was admitted for MRI-guided percutaneous core decompression of an avascular necrosis of the femoral head. Patient age ranged from 9 to 77 years (mean, 49 years); there were 7 males and 18 females. Informed consent was obtained in all patients. The location of the lesions is listed in Table 43-2. The longitudinal extent of the musculoskeletal lesions ranged from 10 to 300 mm.

All but two biopsy procedures were completed in the MR unit, and two patients underwent the procedure using CT guidance (Table 43-3): The first patient had lumbar vertebral osteomyelitis. The preferred approach was directly lateral to the vertebral body through the paravertebral muscles. However, because of the large size of the patient, the drill was not long enough to reach the vertebral body. Thus, a direct approach through the adjacent pedicle was used. The drill and the local anatomy could be more accurately done with CT in this case. The second patient was a child referred for an MR-guided bone biopsy. Because the procedure in this young child required general anesthesia and MR-compatible equipment was not available to monitor general anesthesia, this procedure was performed in the CT suite, where the instruments to control general anesthesia were available.

Table 43-1. Indications for magnetic resonance imaging–guided percutaneous biopsy of bone in 25 patients

Indication	Patients (*n*)
Bone lesion of unknown etiology	20
Demonstration of the infectious agent in suspected osteomyelitis	4
Core decompression (avascular necrosis of the femoral head)	1

Department of Diagnostic Radiology, University of Technology Aachen, January to December 1996; n = 25.

Table 43-2. Location of skeletal lesions detected by magnetic resonance imaging–guided percutaneous biopsy of bone in 25 patients

Location of lesion	Patients (*n*)
Pelvis	10
Femur	9
Tibia	2
Lumbar spine	1
Humerus	1
Sternum	1
Foot	1

Department of Diagnostic Radiology, University of Technology Aachen, January to December 1996; n = 25.

Table 43-3. Results of magnetic resonance imaging–guided percutaneous biopsy of bone in 25 patients

Result	Patients (*n*)
Adequate biopsy	19
Metastasis	3
Aneurysmatic bone cyst	3
Sterile osteomyelitis	3*
Postoperative hemorrhage	2
Chondromyxoidsarcoma	1
Ewing's sarcoma	1
Osteomyelofibrosis	1
Salmonellosis	1
Avascular necrosis	1
Transient osteopenia	1
Stress fracture	1†
Capsule chondroma	1
Inaccurate biopsy	3
Biopsy diagnosis = osteomyelitis; surgical diagnosis = osteosarcoma with secondary inflammation; sampling error	1
Biopsy diagnosis = bone infarction; surgical diagnosis = eosinophilic granuloma; hard-packing distortion	1
Biopsy diagnosis = malignant fibrous histiocytoma; surgical diagnosis = osteosarcoma; hard-packing distortion	1
Inadequate biopsy	3
Biopsy = inadequate sample; surgical diagnosis = solitary bone cyst	
First biopsy = inadequate sample; second biopsy = hemangiopericytoma	
Biopsy = inadequate sample; imaging diagnosis and follow up = fibrous dysplasia	

Department of Diagnostic Radiology, University of Technology Aachen, January to December 1996; *n* = 25.

*One biopsy of a lumbar vertebra was planed with magnetic resonance imaging and completed under computed tomography guidance.

†One biopsy of a tibia in a child was performed under computed tomography guidance under general anesthesia.

MR-guided musculoskeletal biopsy with a side-slit biopsy needle required an average of 45 minutes. The average examination time for biopsies performed with the coaxial prototype drill system was 65 minutes. Four biopsies, obtained with the coaxial prototype drill system, could be completed with manual force only. In 11 cases, the drill was first powered by hand, and the procedure was later completed with the pneumatic turbine for machine-assisted drilling. The reported complication rate of percutaneous bone biopsy is low.[1] Also in the author's series, significant procedural complications did not occur. Rare but typical complications of percutaneous bone biopsy include sequelae caused by nerve or vessel injury, infections, or breakage of the needle or drill.

Nineteen of the twenty-five samples were sufficient, and the histopathologic diagnosis was consistent with the clinical course or other laboratory and imaging findings. However, in three patients the sample revealed inadequate material, and in three patients the sample revealed adequate material but an inaccurate result caused by an improper sample location and two incorrect pathologic interpretations of hard-packed specimens.

Use of the coaxial drill system in lesions covered with thick cortical or osteosclerotic bone has one peculiar problem: In several cases, dense bone formed a hard plug in the hollow drill bit. Thus, the specimen got compressed in the hollow drill, and its histopathologic architecture was altered. This hard-packing was the reason for an inaccurate biopsy result in two cases and occluded the drill in six cases. The occluded drills had to be removed and cleaned with the obturator or exchanged for a new device. When the occluded drill had to be withdrawn, the guiding cannula was pressed against the periosteum. Thus, the second pass of the cleaned or the new drill could be made via the same access.

Also, the puncture techniques using a side-slit biopsy needle permitted multiple samples to be obtained by simply maintaining the outer cannula in place while exchanging the inner cannula, including the specimen.

CONCLUSIONS

Percutaneous biopsy of bone lesions of unknown origin seems to be safe and accurate for diagnosis unless there is a primary indication for surgery. The role of MRI for percutaneous guidance of bone biopsies is under evaluation for various imaging modalities. The accuracy rate of MRI-guided percutaneous biopsy of bone lesions in this limited series of patients is comparable with that reported for the CT-guided technique.[1] For lesions in low-risk areas, MRI may be used as an alternative guidance modality to CT. However, for lesions in high-risk areas, CT guidance is the imaging modality of choice.

REFERENCES

1. Laredo JD, and others: Current status of musculoskeletal interventional radiology, *Radiol Clin North Am* 32:377, 1994.
2. Adam G, and others: Interventional magnetic resonance: initial clinical experience with a 1.5-tesla magnetic resonance system combined with c-arm fluoroscopy, *Invest Radiol* 32:191, 1997.
3. Jolesz FA, Blumenfeld SM: Interventional use of magnetic resonance imaging, *Magn Reson Q* 10:85, 1994.
4. Berning W, Freyschmidt J, Ostertag H: Percutaneous bone biopsy, techniques and indications, *Eur Radiol* 6:875, 1996.
5. Logan PM, and others: Image-guided percutaneous biopsy of musculoskeletal tumors: an algorithm for selection of specific biopsy techniques, *Am J Roentgenol* 166:137, 1996.
6. White LM, and others: Study of osteomyelitis: utility of combined histologic and microbiologic evaluation of percutaneous biopsy samples, *Radiology* 197:840, 1995.
7. Fraser-Hill MA, Renfrew DL, Hilsenrath PE: Percutaneous needle biopsy of musculoskeletal lesions: 2. Cost-effectiveness, *Am J Roentgenol* 158:813, 1992.
8. Ruhs SA, El-Khoury GY, Chrischilles EA: A cost minimization approach to the diagnosis of skeletal neoplasms, *Skeletal Radiol* 25:449, 1996.
9. Reuther G: CT-kontrollierte Biopsien des Achsenskeletts: Zugangswege und Ergebnisse, *Fortschr Röntgenstr* 160:78, 1994.
10. Neuerburg J, and others: Neues MR-kompatibles Knochenbiopsiesystem, *Fortschr Röntgenstr* 165:316, 1996.
11. Schweitzer ME, and others: Percutaneous skeletal aspiration and core biopsy: complementary techniques, *Am J Roentgenol* 166:415, 1996.
12. Tikkakoski T, and others: Combined CT-guided biopsy and cytology in diagnosis of bony lesions, *Acta Radiol* 33:225, 1992.
13. Adam G, and others: Perkutane CT-gesteuerte Behandlung von Osteoidosteomen: kombiniertes Vorgehen mit einem Hohlbohrer und nachfolgender Äthanolinjektion, *Fortschr Röntgenstr* 162:232, 1995.
14. Buecker A, and others: MRI-guided biopsy using a T2-weighted single-shot zoom-imaging sequence (Local Look technique). *J Magn Reson Imaging* (in press).

Chapter 44

VASCULAR INTERVENTIONAL MRI

Gustav K. von Schulthess, Jörg F. Debatin, Paul R. Hilfiker

Vascular interventions is not an obvious choice for magnetic resonance imaging (MRI). X-ray equipment coupled with digital capabilities and contrast media injection provides excellent road maps for vascular interventions, as shown by percutaneous transluminal angioplasties[1] and coronary angioplasties. Therefore, few groups have actively researched the possibility of using MRI as a guiding imaging system for vascular interventions.[2] However, vascular interventional MR has several attractive features:

1. MR has intrinsic flow sensitivity, thus allowing morphologic and functional information[3] to be obtained (e.g., dilatation of a stenosed vessel).
2. MR is not "blind" to the soft tissues surrounding the managed vascular region.
3. MR angiograms are intrinsically three-dimensional (3D).
4. MR can provide very high resolution intravascular imaging if local coils are used. Although such local coil imaging is unacceptable for imaging purposes only, if an intervention is planned, preinterventional imaging with invasive local coils may be very beneficial.
5. Instrument localization techniques can be devised such that the MR computer system "knows" where the instruments are within the sensitive MR volume.
6. The interventionalist is not exposed to ionizing radiation, which is the major hazard in medical interventional procedures.

These benefits make MRI an attractive guidance system for vascular interventions; therefore, it is important that the possibilities inherent in this approach are evaluated.

IMAGING HARDWARE

Any interventional system requires that adequate images be provided so that visualization of the instrument is fast and that images used to guide the instrument contain the necessary information for the interventionalist to successfully carry out the intervention.[4] This provision requires an imaging system that does not unduly restrict patient access. Because standard MR systems usually are cylindrical magnets with a bore length of 170 cm or longer, they are not very useful in this respect. Construction of open MR systems has resulted in the widespread insight that openness and magnetic field strength are intimately linked, such that generation of a high field is difficult in configurations other than cylindrical superconducting horizontal bore systems. At field strengths of 0.6 T or less, more open configurations are possible; several systems are described in Chapters 2 through 4. Typically, open configuration systems have limitations in the achievable main magnetic field strength, the maximum gradient field strength, and gradient slew rates.

The key to vascular interventions is high-resolution, fast vascular angiographic imaging.[5] This type of imaging has been standard with contrast-enhanced x-ray fluoroscopy, whereas MR angiography has had, until recently, severe limitations in providing such information. However, very rapid development in contrast media-enhanced MR angiography has resulted in excellent 3D angiograms with isotropic spatial resolutions in the 1 mm range, which is a prerequisite for MR to be used as a guidance imaging system for vascular interventions.[6] These angiograms can be obtained in a breathhold (i.e., 15 to 20 sec) and thus can serve as road maps similar to those routinely used in x-ray–guided interventions; however the MR angiograms are 3D.[7,8] Acquisition of such fast angiograms requires the most modern gradient systems with very high gradient field strengths (>20 mT/m) and slew rates (>75 mT/m/msec) in conjunction with high main magnetic fields of at least 1 T. Such systems were previously built only in cylindrical superconducting configuration. Vascular interventions usually access the vascular system through the groin, but the site of intervention can be far from the puncture site (frequently 30 to 40 cm). That is, vascular intervention does not require immediate access to the site of intervention as is necessary when biopsies or even surgical interventions are performed.[9,10] Thus, the absolute requirement of high-field and gradient strengths and slew rates combined with the relatively less stringent requirement of limited access make it conceivable that cylindrical bore configuration systems with short bore lengths will soon be built, such that their configuration is not a substantial impediment to carry out vascular interventions. Several manufacturers are marketing cylindrical superconducting systems that have bore lengths of 160 to 170 cm with fast to very fast gradient systems. Such systems may eventually be used for carotid interventions, which typically occur more than 50 cm away from the groin (Fig. 44-1). With a field of view (FOV) of 40 cm, the distance from the magnet entry to the edge of the FOV is 60 to 65 cm in such magnet systems, thus suggesting that an interventionalist could easily manipulate a catheter at the magnet entry and visualize the intervention at the corresponding site (see Fig. 44-1). Because distances between a groin access site and the site of intervention are typically a few centimeters to 60 cm, short-bore cylindrical magnets may eventually be useful for vascular interventions, provided that the gradient system is of high performance. Nevertheless, reducing the length of the cylindrical magnet to 130 to 140 cm will yield even better patient access (see Chapter 5).

INSTRUMENT VISUALIZATION

Visualizing instruments in the MR environment is very different from visualizing instruments in x-ray fluoroscopy. There are two general approaches to instrument visualization in interventional MR. One approach, often termed *passive visualization,* visualizes the instrument by direct effects of the instrument material on the MRI scan.[11] This approach is standard for visualizing instruments in x-ray–guided interventions. However, although in x-ray fluoroscopy high Z material will provide adequate x-ray absorption to make the instrument easily visible, metallic tools in the MR environment will either not show or show susceptibility effects to a variable degree.[12] Plastic tools (e.g., flexible catheters) are not readily visualized by MRI. Various technologies have been explored for instrument visualization in the MR environment. Four possible approaches exist. First, optical guidance systems coupled with virtual reality features can be used to guide interventions, but such systems work only when straight instruments are used; hence, optical guidance is useless for localizing flexible catheter systems.[13]

Second, instruments can be visualized with some metallic implants (e.g. metallic ringlets) or doped with gadolinium.[12] This approach has been tested for the visualization of catheters, but the results are not sufficiently convincing to use the systems clinically. The major problem with this kind of passive visualization is that it is caused by susceptibility artifacts appearing on the images at the site of the instrument.[14] These effects are

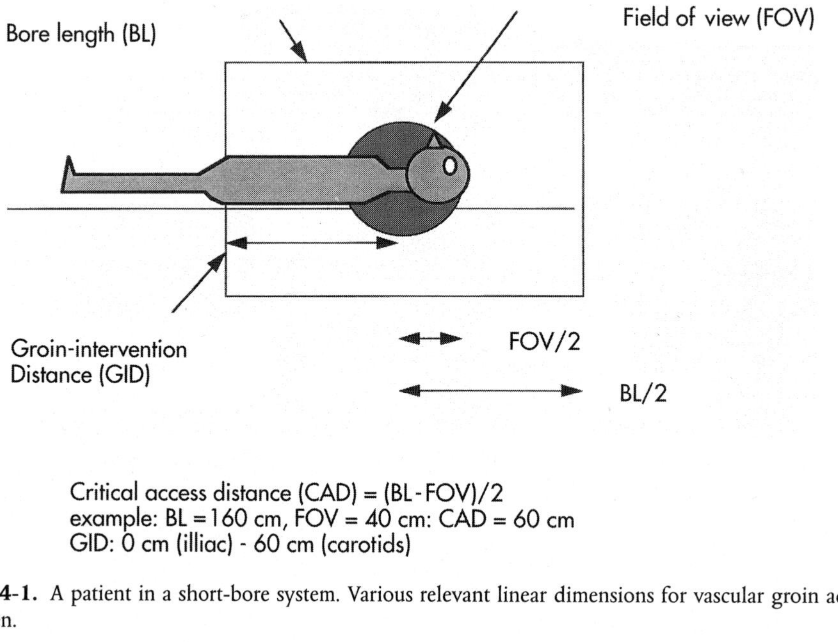

Fig. 44-1. A patient in a short-bore system. Various relevant linear dimensions for vascular groin access are seen.

strongly MR pulse sequence–dependent. When gradient echo pulse sequences are used, the instruments to be visualized can cause uncontrollable artifacts, which also depend on instrument orientation. Because control of interventions uses mainly fast imaging, gradient echo sequences are predominantly used when guiding instruments. Hence, major questions remain whether passive visualization of instruments using susceptibility artifacts will ever be viable.[15] Alternatively, instruments can be impregnated with contrast agents acting on T1 relaxation. The problem with such instruments is that they appear as bright structures. Because the angiograms are also based on T1 contrast agents, the contrast between instruments and the vessels is unfavorable. Other passive approaches have been proposed, such as running an electric current through a non coaxial wire at the tip of an instrument,[16] which produces variable susceptibility artifacts; the results of this approach have not been convincing.

Other promising approaches for instrument visualization are based on active position detection of instruments. These methods are termed *active visualization.*[4,17] Active detection requires that MR signals be obtained from the instruments and that the instruments be outfitted with an MRI device.[2] The most explored approach is called *MR tracking* (see Chapter 16). In this detection approach, a tiny local MR receiver coil is incorporated into the tip of the instrument to be visualized. For better signal-to-noise ratio (SNR), several turns in a solenoidal coil are used, and the coil detects just protons adjacent to the instrument tip. Thus, the MRI scan recorded from such a coil is in essence a point in 3D space. Image reconstruction and identification of instrument position using this set-up are very quick and require no more than 4 alpha pulses in a gradient echo sequence. The tip of an instrument can thus be localized in 20 to 30 msec on any standard MRI scanner.[5] Combination of a 3D MR angiogram as a road map and such a tip-tracking instrument localization technique provides an interventional guidance system in which a flexible catheter can be guided in real-time through the vasculature (Fig. 44-2). For the path of the instrument to be recorded, previous instrument positions should not be erased when a position update is recorded. The methodology has been extensively tested in phantoms and animal experiments; the larger (>2 mm) arterial vessels in animals can be catheterized readily.[1] In an early experiment, a phantom

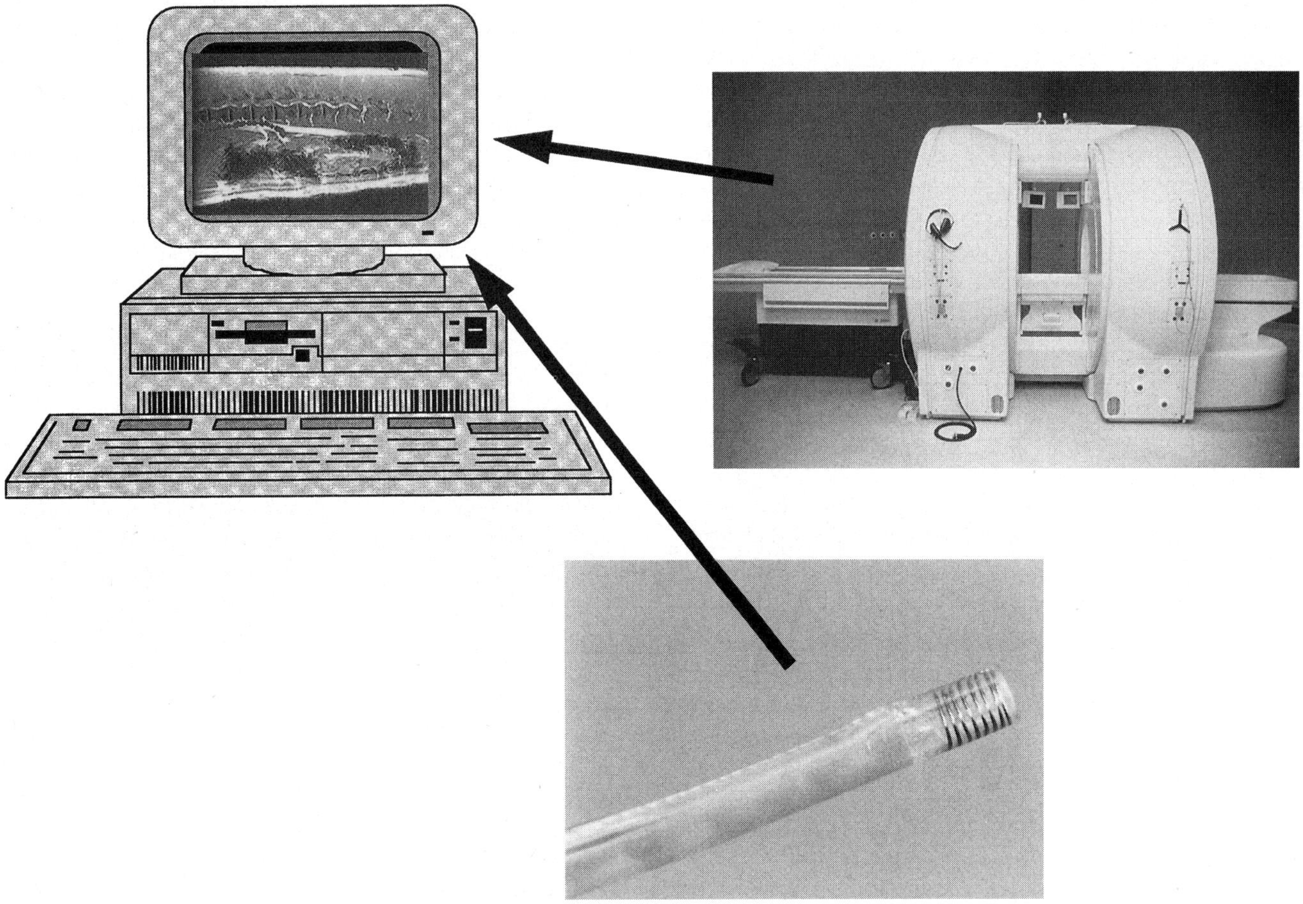

Fig. 44-2. Set-up used for instrument tracking combining a magnetic resonance road map with a tip localization point whose position can be updated in real-time. The tip of the catheter has been placed in the superior mesenteric artery. See Color Plate 19. (From Debatin JF, Adam G, editors: *Interventional magnetic resonance imaging,* Heidelberg, 1998, Springer-Verlag.)

constructed from an *ex vivo* human aorta was prepared and an x-ray opaque catheter with a receiver coil at the tip was constructed. The catheter was placed at various positions in the phantom, and x-rays and MRI scans were obtained. The agreement of the recorded positions was excellent.[18] Using a 1.5-T standard MR system with ultrafast gradients and the open "double-doughnut" configuration 0.5-T system, multiple experiments using pigs were performed, during which guiding of the catheter under MR guidance was tested.[2] Although the catheters used were still relatively big (5 F), the experiments clearly showed that guidance of a flexible catheter into the various vessels of the entire aorta is relatively easy.[18] Furthermore, information can be displayed in a 3D road map in any desired imaging plane.[19] As the system is further developed and its clinical usefulness shown, it is conceivable that stereoscopic goggles will display the field of intervention in which an instrument is guided in 3D fashion. Numerous instruments are equipped with microcoils at the tips.[13] The catheter company Schneider Worldwide (Bülach, Switzerland) and other manufacturers have produced catheters sized 5 F and 7 F, balloon catheters sized 4 to 8 mm, and a prototype plastic guidewire with a diameter of 0.7 mm (Fig. 44-3). The method can, in principle, also be applied in humans.

The other active visualization approach is termed *profiling*. In this approach, the entire distal end of a guidewire is visualized.[11] Extensive electrical engineering design studies determined that the best approach for this way of actively visualizing instruments is to arrange the coils in a braided fashion along the distal 5 or 10 cm (Fig. 44-4). The sensitive volume of such a system is very close to the coils, from the tip to the point where they are soldered to the coaxial cable. Thus, the signal recorded in an image from such a coil corresponds to the few distal centimeters of the instrument. Using the coil to transmit and to receive signal produces better images than when the coil is only used as a receiver (Fig. 44-5). Again, superimposing the image of the instrument tip onto a road map will produce the necessary environment for guidance. In contrast to the tip-tracking approach discussed above, profiling produces a line rather than a point within the sensitive 3D volume of the MRI scanner. As a result, acquisition and reconstruction of the image do not require 4 alpha pulses but rather a more extensive imaging algorithm. At present, four high-resolution position updates can be obtained in 1 sec, which is probably adequate. However, with improved acquisition strategies, this time can be reduced such that 10 updates per second may be obtained.

Active methods have two potential problems: (1) A coaxial cable has to run along the instrument, (i.e., the catheter connecting the local coil to the MRI scanner).[2] If pulse sequences with a high specific absorbtion rate are used, particularly in high field systems, considerable local heating next to the long wire can be induced.[11] This problem is a safety concern that should be investigated thoroughly before the system can be routinely applied in humans. Because the SAR is approximately 10 times smaller at 0.5 T than at 1.5 T, safety concerns with the local coil tracking method are less important. (2) In some environments with few mobile protons, the signal recorded from the coil at the tip of the instrument is not strong enough. Incorporation of a gadolinium-doped fluid pellet in the tip within the coil is the appropriate remedy.[16,18] Even when guidewires are produced, a microscopic lumen at the tip where the coils are located will permit protons from the fluid environment to percolate in the sensitive coil lumen, thus allowing adequate signal in intravascular use.

IMAGING STRATEGIES

Imaging pulse sequences for vascular interventions essentially use gradient echo pulse sequences and, potentially, echo-planar derivatives of such sequences.[20,21] As stated, the first step for intervention is to obtain a 3D MR angiogram road map, onto which the instrument position can be projected.[22,23] The best technique at this time is probably contrast-enhanced MR angiography, which can produce high-quality MR angiograms of any body region except for the coronary vasculature.[8] This technique is a venous injection–based technique and uses a substantial amount of contrast media (0.15 to 0.2 mmol/kg body weight) of small–molecular weight gadolinum chelates.[24] This feature prevents frequent repetitive use of contrast media injection. However, during a real procedure, it is conceivable that the contrast media is injected through the catheter into the vasculature of immediate interest, requiring only reduced amounts of contrast media. Alternatively, intravascular contrast agents can be used. With their prolonged half lives, the vasculature can be imaged repetitively without additional contrast injections, which is a great advantage. The drawback using this type of contrast agent is that arteries and veins are shown simultaneously. Experience is insufficient to offer guidance as to whether multiple injections of contrast media into the region of interest or one injection of intravascular contrast media is better suited to provide adequate road maps. Probably, the combination of 3D data acquisition with intravascular contrast media provides adequate road maps, which can be acquired repetitively so that using them during a vascular interventional MR procedure may be the chosen approach.

Time-of-flight (TOF) and phase-contrast (PC) MR angiography for vascular interventional MR procedures were the principal angiographic techniques on which investigation was based.[16] Inconsistency in the quality of such sequences was a major issue, which should be resolved for vascular interventional MR to become clinically useful; contrast media–enhanced MR angiography resolves this problem. Thus, TOF MR angiography probably will play an inferior role in vascular interventional MR. However, because of its ability to quantify flow and quickly give directional flow information, the PC method may remain an important tool in two respects: PC sequences will provide direct information on the quantitative success of a vascular intervention (e.g., balloon dilatation), and PC MR angiography may provide the relevant flow data to computationally extract arterial from venous vascular structures when contrast media–enhanced angiograms are acquired as repetitive road maps.[2,25] It is conceivable that, in an initial step, a PC an-

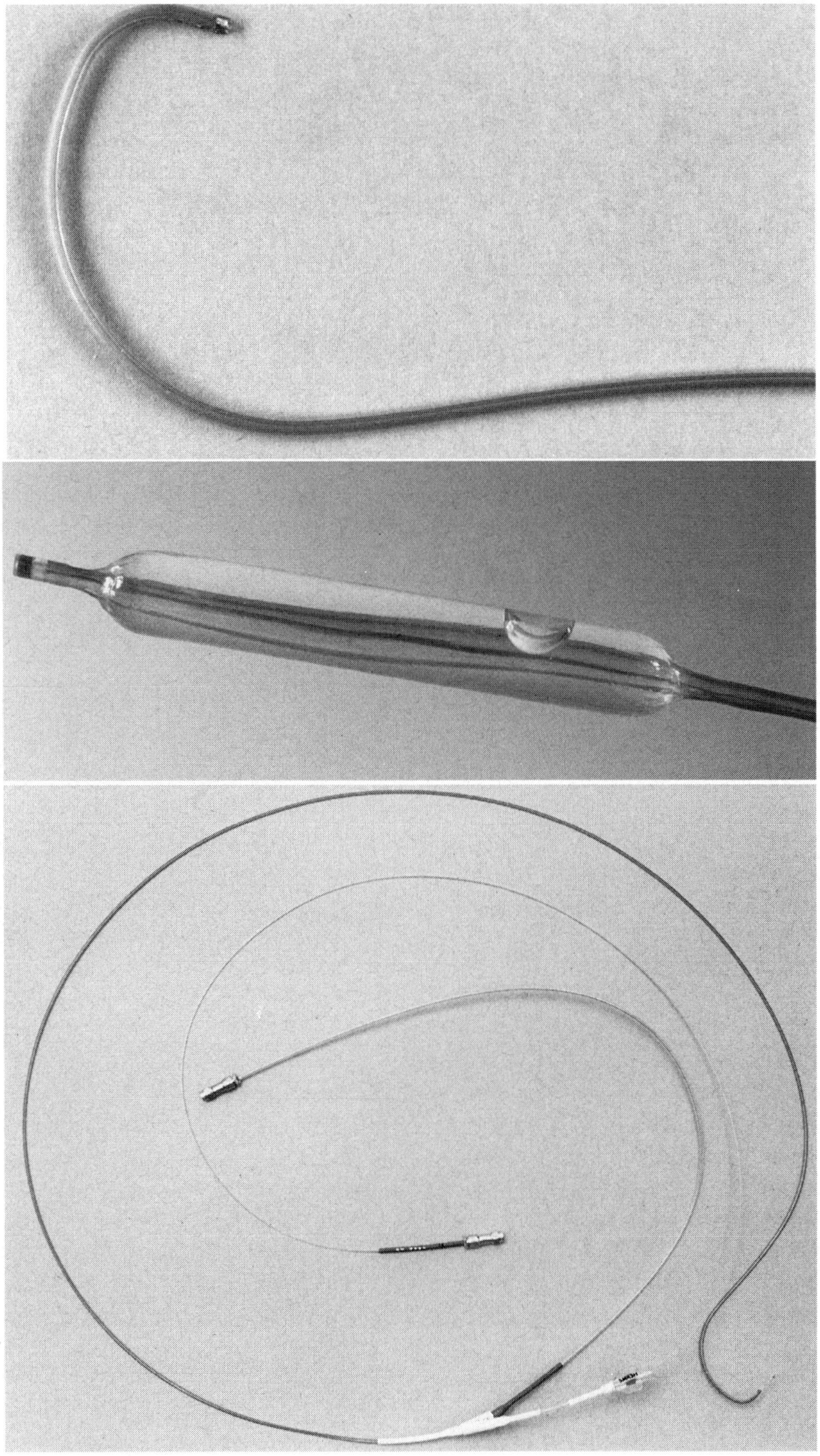

A

B

C

Fig. 44-3. Several prototype interventional systems, equipped with a magnetic resonance (MR) receiver coil. The coil is connected to a coaxial cable running through the instruments. The distal ends of **A,** a standard 5-F catheter; **B,** a balloon catheter; and **C,** a guidewire in a standard 5-F cobra catheter are seen. A plug at the end of the catheter and guidewire connects the tracking coil to the MR system. (From Debatin JF, Adam G, editors: *Interventional magnetic resonance imaging,* Heidelberg, 1998, Springer-Verlag.)

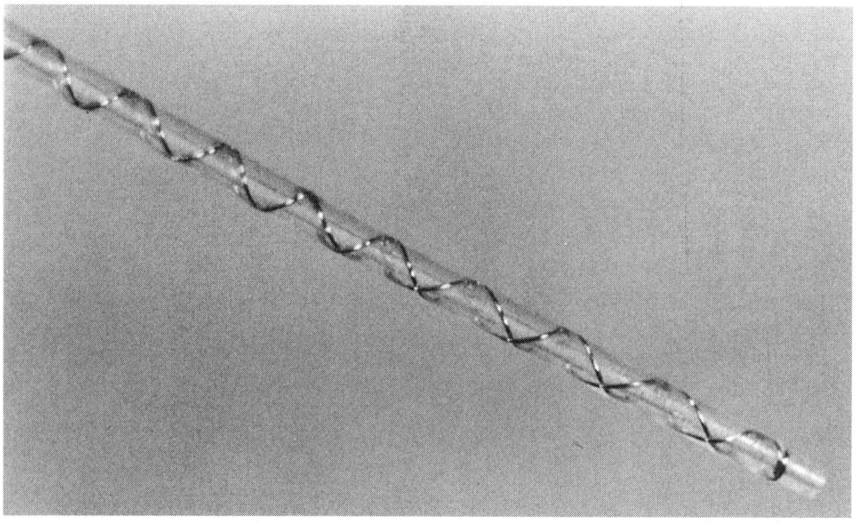

Fig. 44-4. The distal end of a prototype guidewire has wound around the distal few centimeters of a receiver coil. The outer diameter is 0.75 mm (0.035-in guidewire). (From Debatin JF, Adam G, editors: *Interventional magnetic resonance imaging,* Heidelberg, 1998, Springer-Verlag.)

A

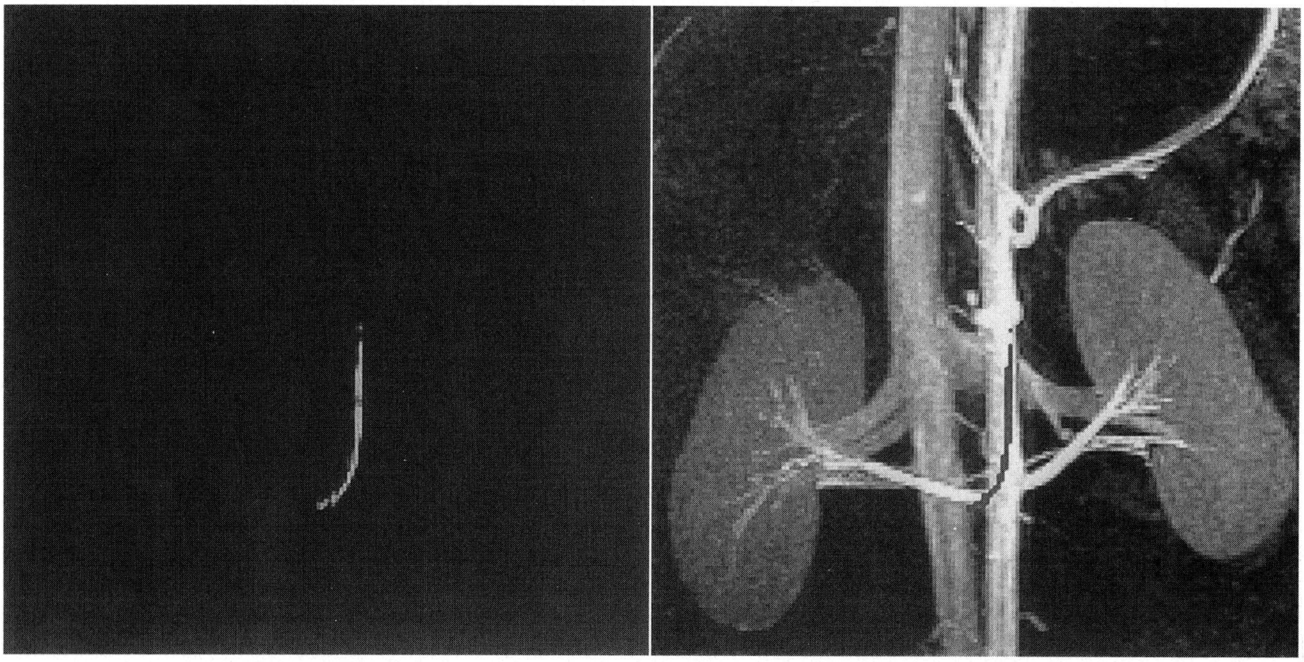

B

Fig. 44-5. Image from a profiling coil shows the distal end of a prototype guidewire **A,** without being superposed on a road map and **B,** after being superposed on a road map, where the track of the instrument is color-coded. See Color Plate 20.

giogram and a contrast media–enhanced MR angiogram are acquired and the vascular structures irrelevant for the interventional procedure are artificially suppressed. Repetitive contrast media–enhanced MR angiograms provide additional road mapping as intervention proceeds. For instrument guidance in the vascular tree, it is unlikely that pulse sequences other than gradient echo–based sequences will play a major role. However, other pulse sequences may be relevant when vascular imaging of the site of intervention before or during the procedure is necessary. An advantage of using MR as the interventional guidance imaging system is its ability to obtain cross-sectional high-contrast images of the structures surrounding the site of vascular intervention. Various imaging questions will be asked by the interventionalist. A relevant issue is the composition of plaques when the endoluminal treatment of an atherosclerotic lesion is planned. For this purpose, multiple pulse sequences are necessary. The literature on plaque imaging is increasing rapidly, and the relevant pulse sequences are spin-echo sequences

A

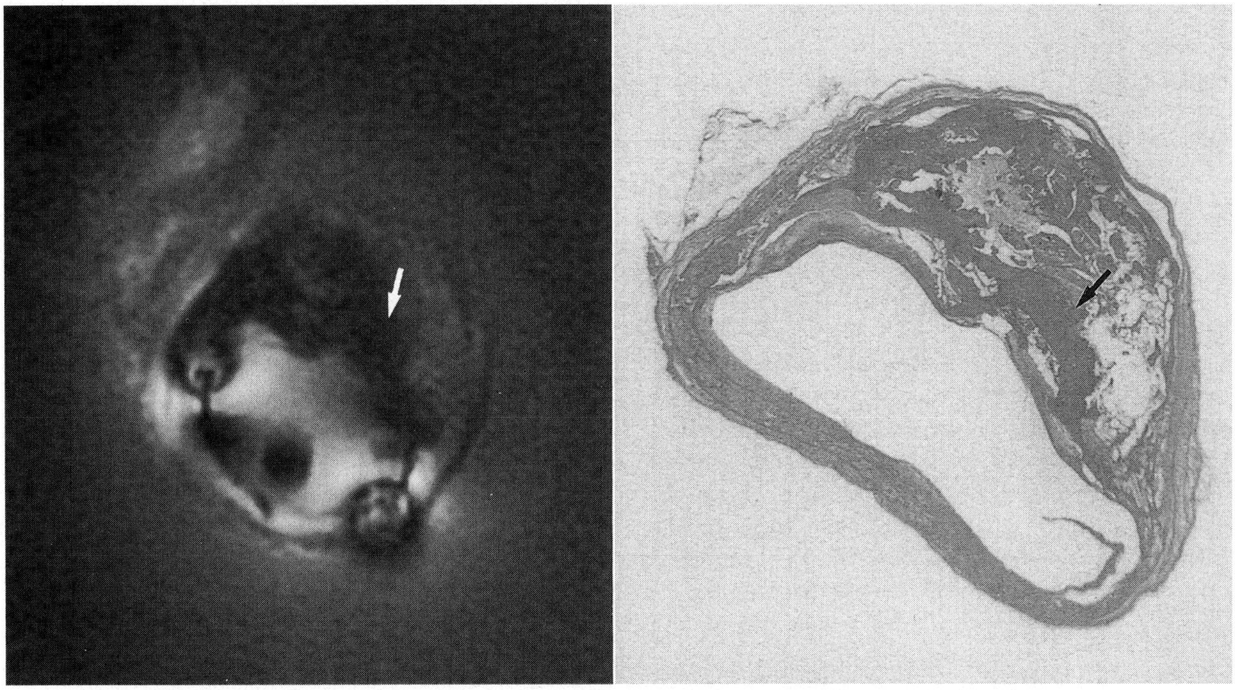

B

Fig. 44-6. *Ex vivo* plaque shows calcifications *(arrow)* on **A,** a T2-weighted image correlating to calcifications in the **B,** histologic section. See Color Plate 21. (From Zimmerman GG, and others: Intravascular MR imaging of atherosclerotic plaque: *ex vivo* analysis of human femoral arteries with histologic correlation, *Radiology* 204:771, 1997.)

(T1-weighted, T2-weighted, and proton-density images).[26,27] Figure 44-6 shows a plaque from an *ex vivo* sample obtained by local coil, high-resolution MRI. It is possible to differentiate with high certainty the presence of calcifications, lipids, and fibrous tissue, including collagen. Aneurysms and their composition are readily analyzed on MRI, and a mural thrombus can be differentiated from an intramural hematoma.[28,29]

Similar to x-ray fluoroscopy–guided interventions, MR interventions using flexible instruments may become relevant in the vascular system and in other lumina (e.g., renal collecting system, pancreaticobiliary tree). Recent applications of MR using very heavily T2-weighted fast MR pulse sequences have shown excellent images of these structures, which clearly could serve as road maps for MR-guided interventions in these hollow structures.[30] Once the structure has been accessed, it still is too early to determine whether contrast media–enhanced MR angiography techniques will be relevant during intervention.

ENDOLUMINAL IMAGING

Early researchers explored the possibility of endovascular MRI by inserting local coils into the vascular system in the region of interest. This same approach may be used in other luminal structures.[31] Because MRI is an intrinsically noninvasive technique using, at most, the injection of some intravenous contrast agent, arterial puncture for the placement of such endoluminal coils is unacceptable for imaging purposes only. As a result, the literature on this subject is scant.[32] However, the relevance of such an imaging approach increases drastically when an endoluminal intervention is planned because invasive access should be gained for other purposes. Studies have therefore begun to extensively explore systems for endoluminal imaging.[33] For the access route to be minimized, the endoluminal imaging device should be expandable or should provide adequate images from a thin linear structure.[34] The latter, although simplest to implement, may be the least effective because the range over which a local coil provides good imaging characteristics is related to its linear dimensions. In the case of a loop fitting through a 5-F catheter, the two transaxial linear dimensions are less than 1 mm; hence, adequate image quality beyond the device is unlikely. Thus, designs for intravascular MRI coils based on expandable structures, mainly balloon-mounted coils and coils made of Nitinol, have been explored.[27] The advantage of such devices is that they assume the axial dimensions of the imaged vessel, which is typically several millimeters; therefore, the axial imaging FOV is also several millimeters, which clearly allows imaging of the relevant structures of the vessel walls. The favored design is a balloon-mounted copper single-loop coil, which provides adequate images with inherent artifacts that can be relatively easily controlled. Other coil designs have been explored experimentally and theoretically and have not yielded comparable imaging results. Such a device has been able to obtain high-resolution images, with in-plane resolutions of less than 0.1 mm and axial resolutions of 3 mm, which are adequate for plaque characterization in any part of the body. The advantage of a balloon-mounted coil is its ability to suppress flow-related artifacts; during imaging, the inflated balloon prevents flow, although a system could be devised that, through a central lumen, would allow for some distal perfusion in the vessel occluded during imaging. Flow artifacts during intravascular imaging are caused by two effects. If the device is not securely fastened against the vessel wall, it may meander in the vessel because of streaming blood; therefore, motion artifacts may become prominent. Such artifacts will be present to a lesser degree when the device is fastened against the wall, as with an expandable Nitinol loop, but flow next to the loop is prominent. Figure 44-7 shows a balloon-mounted endovascular single-loop prototype coil. Extensive experience using such devices was gained on rabbits fed atherogenetic diets. High-resolution vascular imaging without the use of endoluminal coils is only possible in vessels very close to the surface; even in vessels such as the common carotid or the superficial femoral arteries, images using surface rather then endoluminal coils will not provide adequate information. One of the problems to be explored *in vivo* is vascular obstruction, which is highly relevant in the carotids and essentially irrelevant in the arteries feeding the lower limbs. No substantial technical problems would prevent the use of such systems.

IN VIVO RESULTS AND POTENTIAL APPLICATIONS

Vascular or, more generally, endoluminal interventional MR may have many applications, which range from all procedures used to treat arteriosclerotic disease to therapies such as transluminal portosystemic shunt placements[2,35] and from tumor embolization to the repair of congenital heart lesions and ablation of cardiac arrythmogenic foci. With implementation and expansion of MR technology, which has an extremely rich 50 year history, many other procedures may soon become routine.

At this point, the following can be inferred: With the exception of the coronary arteries and the small intracranial vessels, the spatial resolution of contrast media–enhanced MR angiography is high enough that such angiograms can serve as adequate road maps for instrument guidance for interventions in such vessels. Thus, embolization procedures of larger vessels (Fig. 44-8) are feasible.[2] Percutaneous transluminal angioplasty can be performed, and the first human *in vivo* results of such procedures under MR guidance in a 0.5-T magnet are under study (Pfammatter, Personal communication). MR-guided per-

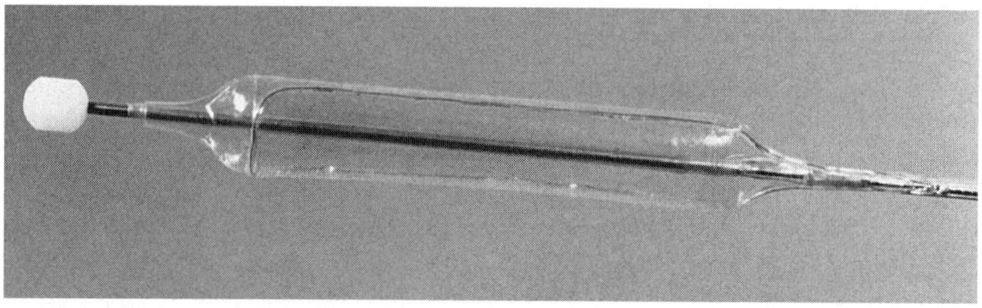

Fig. 44-7. A balloon-mounted endovascular single-loop prototype coil (6-mm diameter). (From Zimmerman GG, Erhart P, Schneider J: Intravascular MR imaging of atherosclerotic plaque: ex vivo analysis of human femoral arteries with histologic correlation, *Radiology* 204:770, 1997.)

A

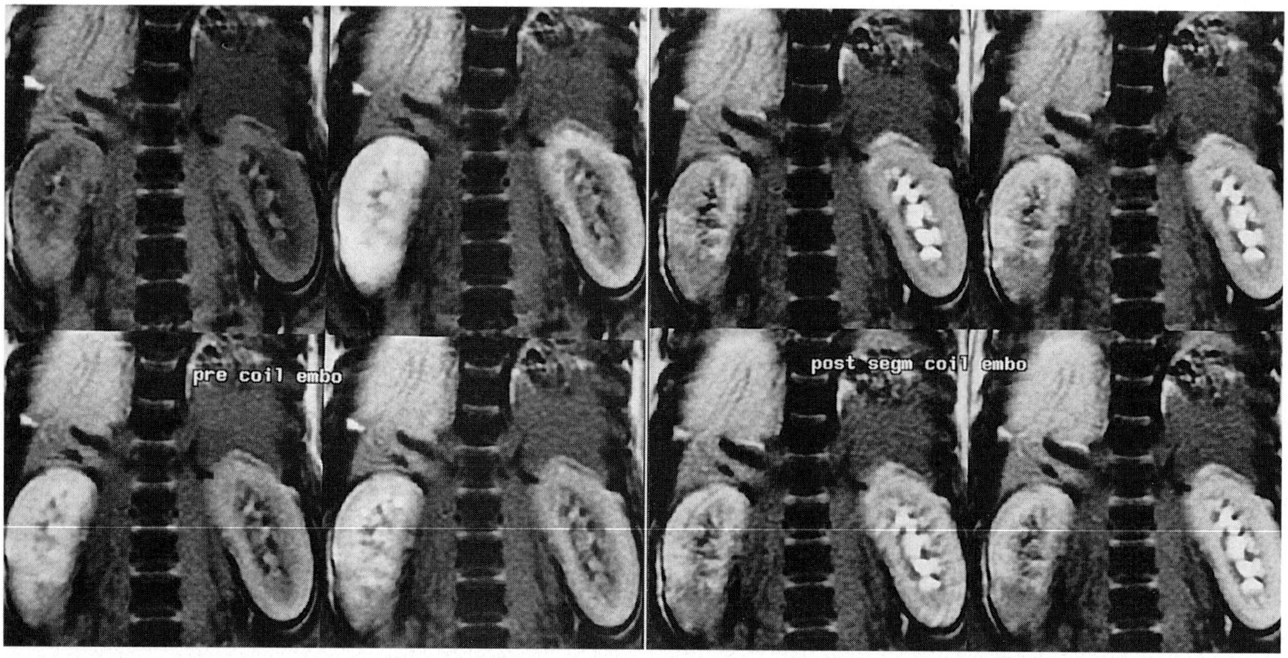

B

Fig. 44-8. Magnetic resonance image of the kidneys **A**, and **B**, after embolization of the right renal artery in a swine.

cutaneous transluminal angioplasty procedures could become standard in vessels such as the common or internal carotids, the iliac and femoral vessels, and some abdominal vessels. Although catheter technology exists in prototypes, the short-bore MR systems are not widely available. How the additional imaging capabilities, compared with x-ray guidance, are going to be helpful is a matter of conjecture. Instant flow mapping, local analysis of plaque structure, and postdilatation effects will be possible, but it is unclear how they could affect the outcome. Because stents are made of metal, imaging artifacts may be relevant after stenting. Plastic stents are being developed, so this problem may soon be solved. Other more complex procedures could also greatly benefit from MR guidance, such as transluminal portosystemic shunt placement, which has been performed experimentally in swine, and minimally invasive cardiac procedures, such as radiofrequency ablation of unwanted electric atrial foci.

CONCLUSIONS

Vascular interventional MRI is a very interesting field of research. Potential applications and benefits of using MR as a guiding system abound, but technology development is needed. No fundamental physical hurdles make the application of MR in this setting impossible. The next decade will show whether MRI can replace x-ray fluoroscopy.

REFERENCES

1. Wildermuth S, and others: MR guided percutaneous angioplasty: assessment of tracking safety, catheter handling and functionality, *Cardiovasc Intervent Radiol* 1998 (in press).
2. Wildermuth S, and others: MR imaging-guided intravascular procedures: initial demonstration in a pig model, *Radiology* 202:578, 1997.
3. Edelmann MR: MR angiography: present and future, *Am J Roentgenol* 161:1, 1977.
4. Dumoulin CL, Souza SP, Darrow RD: Real-time position monitoring of invasive devices using magnetic resonance, *Magn Reson Med* 29:411, 1993.
5. Dumoulin CL, and others: Simultaneous acquisition of phase-contrast angiograms and stationary-tissue images with Hadamard encoding of flow-induced phase shifts, *J Magn Reson Imaging* 1:399, 1991.
6. Lewin JS, Laub G, Hausmann R: Three-dimensional time-of-flight MR angiography: applications in the abdomen and thorax, *Radiology* 179:261, 1991.
7. Holland GA, and others: Breath-hold ultrafast three-dimensional gadolinium-enhanced MR angiography of the aorta and the renal and other visceral abdominal arteries, *Am J Roentgenol* 166:971, 1996.
8. Snidow JJ, and others: Three-dimensional gadolinium-enhanced MR angiography for aortoiliac inflow assessment plus renal artery screening in a single breath hold, *Radiology* 198:725, 1996.
9. Lufkin RB: Interventional MR imaging, *Radiology* 197:16, 1995 (editorial; comment).
10. Hagspiel KD, Kandarpa K, Jolesz FA: Interventional MR imaging, *J Vasc Interv Radiol* 8:745, 1997.
11. Ladd ME, and others: Guidewire antennas for MR fluoroscopy, *Magn Reson Med* 37:891, 1997.
12. Schenck JF, and others: Superconducting open-configuration MR imaging system for image-guided therapy, *Radiology* 195:805, 1995.
13. Steiner P, and others: Active biplanar MR tracking for biopsies in humans, *Am J Roentgenol* 169:735, 1997.
14. Frahm C, and others: Visualization of magnetic resonance-compatible needles at 1.5 and 0.2 Tesla, *Cardiovasc Intervent Radiol* 19:335, 1996.
15. Ladd ME, and others: Biopsy needle susceptibility artifacts, *Magn Reson Med* 36:646, 1996.
16. McKinnon GC, and others: Towards active guidewire visualization in interventional magnetic resonance imaging, *MAGMA* 4:13, 1996.
17. Ackermann JL, and others: *Rapid 3 D tracking of small RF coils: book of abstracts,* Berkeley, Calif, 1986, Society of Magnetic Resonance in Medicine.
18. Leung DA, and others: Intravascular MR tracking catheter: preliminary experimental evaluation, *Am J Roentgenol* 164:1265, 1995.
19. Leung DA, and others: Real-time biplanar needle tracking for interventional MR imaging procedures, *Radiology* 197:485, 1995.
20. Prince MR, and others: Dynamic gadolinium-enhanced three-dimensional abdominal MR arteriography, *J Magn Reson Imaging* 3:877, 1993.
21. Debatin JF, and others: Advances in vascular echoplanar imaging, *Cardiovasc Intervent Radiol* 18:277, 1995.
22. Leung DA, Debatin JF: Three-dimensional contrast-enhanced magnetic resonance angiography of the thoracic vasculature, *Eur Radiol* 7:981, 1997.
23. Hany TF, and others: Evaluation of the aortoiliac and renal arteries: comparison of breath-hold, contrast-enhanced, three-dimensional MR angiography with conventional catheter angiography, *Radiology* 204:357, 1997.
24. Hany TF, and others: Optimization of contrast timing for breath-hold three-dimensional MR angiography, *J Magn Reson Imaging* 7:551, 1997.
25. Pelc NJ, and others: Encoding strategies for three-direction phase-contrast MR imaging of flow, *J Magn Reson Imaging* 1:405, 1991.
26. Martin AJ, Plewes DB, Henkelman RM: MR imaging of blood vessels with an intravascular coil, *J Magn Reson Imaging* 2:421, 1992.
27. Zimmermann GG, and others: Intravascular MR-imaging: first in vivo experience with an arteriosclerotic animal model, *Fortschr Geb Rontgenstr Nuklearmed Erganzungsbd* 162:180, 1997.
28. Murray JG, and others: Intramural hematoma of the thoracic aorta: MR image findings and their prognostic implications, *Radiology* 204:349, 1997.
29. Bluemke DA: Definitive diagnosis of intramural hematoma of the thoracic aorta with MR imaging, *Radiology* 204:319, 1997 (editorial; comment).
30. Gohde SC, and others: MR-guided cholecystostomy: assessment of biplanar, real-time needle tracking in three pigs, *Cardiovasc Intervent Radiol* 20:295, 1997.
31. Martin AJ, Gotlieb AI, Henkelman RM: High-resolution MR imaging of human arteries, *J Magn Reson Imaging* 5:93, 1995.
32. Hurst GC, and others: Intravascular (catheter) NMR receiver probe: preliminary design analysis and application to canine iliofemoral imaging, *Magn Reson Med* 24:343, 1992.
33. Zimmermann GG, and others: Intravascular MR imaging of atheriosclerotic plaque: 'ex vivo' analysis of human femoral arteries with histologic correlation, *Radiology* 204:769, 1997.
34. Martin AJ, Henkelman RM: Intravascular MR imaging in a porcine animal model, *Magn Reson Med* 32:224, 1994.
35. Skeens J, Semba C, Dake M: Transjugular intrahepatic portosystemic shunts, *Annu Rev Med* 46:95, 1995.

INDEX

Note: An *f* following page numbers indicates figures; *t* indicates table.

K

L

M

Q

R

S